Medical Management of Type 1 Diabetes

Medical Management of Type 1 Diabetes

Editor: Eric Gregory

AMERICAN
MEDICAL PUBLISHERS
www.americanmedicalpublishers.com

AMERICAN
MEDICAL PUBLISHERS
www.americanmedicalpublishers.com

Cataloging-in-Publication Data

Medical management of type 1 diabetes / edited by Eric Gregory.
p. cm.
Includes bibliographical references and index.
ISBN 979-8-88740-251-2
1. Diabetes. 2. Diabetes--Treatment. 3. Diabetes--Treatment--Methodology.
4. Diabetes--Complications. 5. Diabetes--Diagnosis. 6. Disease management.
I. Gregory, Eric.
RC660 .M43 2023
616.462--dc23

American Medical Publishers,
41 Flatbush Avenue,
1st Floor, New York,
NY 11217, USA

ISBN 979-8-88740-251-2 (Hardback)

Contents

Preface

Type 1 diabetes is a chronic health condition characterized by the destruction of beta cells in the pancreas. In this condition, the pancreas produces little or no insulin, a hormone that enables sugar to enter cells to produce energy. The major symptoms of type 1 diabetes are dry mouth, upset stomach and vomiting, frequent urination, unexplained weight loss, fatigue, blurry vision, and frequent infections of skin, urinary tract, vagina, etc. Glycated hemoglobin (A1C) test, random blood sugar test, and fasting blood sugar tests are major diagnostic tests used for type 1 diabetes. Its treatment is aimed at keeping blood sugar level under control and includes insulin administration, frequent blood sugar monitoring, eating healthy foods, exercising regularly and maintaining a healthy weight. This book is compiled in such a manner, that it will provide in-depth knowledge about the medical management of type 1 diabetes. Its extensive content provides the readers with a thorough understanding of this medical condition. This book will prove immensely beneficial to professionals and students involved in the study and management of diabetes at various levels.

The information shared in this book is based on empirical researches made by veterans in this field of study. The elaborative information provided in this book will help the readers further their scope of knowledge leading to advancements in this field.

Finally, I would like to thank my fellow researchers who gave constructive feedback and my family members who supported me at every step of my research.

Editor

1

IL-10 Deficiency Accelerates Type 1 Diabetes Development *via* Modulation of Innate and Adaptive Immune Cells and Gut Microbiota in *BDC2.5* NOD Mice

Juan Huang[1,2], Qiyuan Tan[2,3], Ningwen Tai[2†], James Alexander Pearson[2,4†], Yangyang Li[2,5], Chen Chao[1], Lucy Zhang[2], Jian Peng[2], Yanpeng Xing[2,6], Luyao Zhang[2,6], Youjia Hu[2], Zhiguang Zhou[1], F. Susan Wong[4] and Li Wen[2]*

[1] National Clinical Research Center for Metabolic Diseases, Key Laboratory of Diabetes Immunology (Central South University), Ministry of Education, and Department of Metabolism and Endocrinology, The Second Xiangya Hospital, Central South University, Changsha, China, [2] Section of Endocrinology, Department of Internal Medicine, School of Medicine, Yale University, New Haven, CT, United States, [3] Department of Endocrinology and Metabolism, Shanghai Jiaotong University Affiliated Sixth People's Hospital, Shanghai, China, [4] Division of Infection and Immunity, School of Medicine, Cardiff University, Cardiff, United Kingdom, [5] Department of Endocrinology, The Second Hospital of Jilin University, Changchun, China, [6] Department of Gastrointestinal Surgery, The First Hospital of Jilin University, Changchun, China

***Correspondence:**
Li Wen
li.wen@yale.edu

[†]These authors have contributed equally to this work

Type 1 diabetes is an autoimmune disease caused by T cell-mediated destruction of insulin-producing β cells. *BDC2.5* T cells in *BDC2.5* CD4$^+$ T cell receptor transgenic Non-Obese Diabetic (NOD) mice (*BDC2.5*$^+$ NOD mice) can abruptly invade the pancreatic islets resulting in severe insulitis that progresses rapidly but rarely leads to spontaneous diabetes. This prevention of diabetes is mediated by T regulatory (Treg) cells in these mice. In this study, we investigated the role of interleukin 10 (IL-10) in the inhibition of diabetes in *BDC2.5*$^+$ NOD mice by generating *Il-10*-deficient *BDC2.5*$^+$ NOD mice (*BDC2.5*$^+$*Il-10*$^{-/-}$ NOD mice). Our results showed that *BDC2.5*$^+$*Il-10*$^{-/-}$ NOD mice displayed robust and accelerated diabetes development. *Il-10* deficiency in *BDC2.5*$^+$ NOD mice promoted the generation of neutrophils in the bone marrow and increased the proportions of neutrophils in the periphery (blood, spleen, and islets), accompanied by altered intestinal immunity and gut microbiota composition. *In vitro* studies showed that the gut microbiota from *BDC2.5*$^+$*Il-10*$^{-/-}$ NOD mice can expand neutrophil populations. Moreover, *in vivo* studies demonstrated that the depletion of endogenous gut microbiota by antibiotic treatment decreased the proportion of neutrophils. Although *Il-10* deficiency in *BDC2.5*$^+$ NOD mice had no obvious effects on the proportion and function of Treg cells, it affected the immune response and activation of CD4$^+$ T cells. Moreover, the pathogenicity of CD4$^+$ T cells was much increased, and this significantly accelerated the development of diabetes when these CD4+ T cells were transferred into immune-deficient NOD mice. Our study provides novel insights into the role of IL-10 in the modulation of neutrophils and CD4+ T cells in *BDC2.5*+ NOD mice, and suggests important crosstalk between gut microbiota and neutrophils in type 1 diabetes development.

Keywords: type 1 diabetes, interleukin-10, neutrophils, gut microbiota, CD4+ T cells

INTRODUCTION

Type 1 diabetes (T1D) is an autoimmune disease that results from the destruction of insulin-producing β cells. T cells are the predominant component of the infiltrates in these pancreatic islet lesions (1, 2). Reports from bone marrow transplantation studies in identical twins in humans (3) and adoptive transfer of T cells from diabetic Non-Obese Diabetic (NOD) mouse donors to non-diabetic NOD mouse recipients (4) demonstrated that type 1 diabetes is an immune cell-mediated disease. T cell receptor (TCR) transgenic NOD mice provide critical tools for investigation of the important roles that T cells play in the immunopathogenesis of T1D development.

The *BDC2.5* TCR transgenic NOD (*BDC2.5*+ NOD) mouse was generated from a diabetogenic CD4+ T cell clone, designated as *BDC2.5*, from a new-onset diabetic NOD mouse (5). In these mice, ~90% CD4+ T cells express the transgenic TCR (6). Interestingly, despite the potent ability of the parental *BDC2.5* T clone in inducing type 1 diabetes development, *BDC2.5*+ NOD mice showed severe insulitis as young as 2-3 weeks of age but rarely developed diabetes (7, 8). However, *BDC2.5*+ CD4+ T cells from the *BDC2.5*+ NOD mouse could rapidly transfer diabetes into severe combined immune-deficient NOD (NOD.*scid*) recipients after activation *in vitro* (9). Moreover, if *BDC2.5*+ NOD mice are on an immunodeficient background, such as a recombination-activating gene (*Rag*) deficiency (10) or NOD.*scid* (9), the mice develop rapid diabetes at a very early age, suggesting intrinsic immune regulatory factors suppress the development of diabetes in *BDC2.5*+ NOD mice in immuno-sufficient hosts. Studies have shown that Foxp3+CD4+ regulatory T (Treg) cells play a protective role by regulating autoimmune responses in *BDC2.5*+ NOD mice (11–13). Our previous studies found that B cell depletion in *BDC2.5*+ NOD mice induced transient aggressive behavior in diabetogenic *BDC2.5*+ CD4+ T cells with reduction in Treg cell number and Treg cell suppressive functions (14). However, after B cell reconstitution, *BDC2.5*+ CD4+ T cells were less aggressively pathogenic due to the increased number of Treg cells and enhanced suppressive function of Tregs cells to CD4+CD25- T effector cells, as well as increasing IL-10 producing Bregs (14).

Although the destruction of insulin-producing pancreatic beta cells seen in type 1 diabetes is primarily characterized by autoreactive T cells, recent studies suggest that neutrophils also play an essential role in the development of type 1 diabetes. Diana et al. found that neutrophils infiltrate the islets of NOD mice at an early age, which was required for the initiation of the diabetogenic T cell response (15). The authors also showed that neutrophils interacted with B-1a cells and plasmacytoid dendritic cells in the development of type 1 diabetes (15). Their further study showed that macrophages and β-cells in the pancreas were responsible for neutrophil recruitment to the pancreas (16). In patients with type 1 diabetes, the level of circulating neutrophil elastase released from activated neutrophils was positively associated with the numbers and titers of the autoantibodies against β-cell-specific antigens, suggesting that neutrophil activation leading to the elevated proteases might be involved in the process of β-cell autoimmunity (17). Moreover, the changes in circulating neutrophil numbers were found to be associated with β-cell specific autoimmunity and the HLA-DR3-DQ2/DR4-DQ8 high risk genotype (18–22). Studies have shown that gut microbiota also regulated neutrophil aging and homeostasis (23, 24) and increasing evidence suggests that gut microbiota play an important role in modulating type 1 diabetes development in NOD mice (25–29) and in patients with type 1 diabetes (30, 31). It is known that IL-10 is an important immuno-regulatory cytokine in homeostasis of gut mucosal immunity (32–34) and IL-10 also mediates immune supression by Treg cells (35–37). However, it is not clear how IL-10 mediates the immune regulation seen in *BDC2.5*+ NOD mice and if gut microbiota also modulate islet β cell autoimmunity through regulation of neutrophil homeostasis in *BDC2.5*+ NOD mice. To fill those knowledge gaps, we generated *BDC2.5*+ NOD mice with *Il-10* deficiency (*BDC2.5*+*Il-10*-/- NOD mice) and investigated the action of IL-10 in modulating diabetogenic CD4+ T cells, neutrophils and the gut microbiota in type 1 diabetes development.

METHODS AND MATERIALS

Mice

Mice used in this study were housed in specific pathogen-free (SPF) facilities with a 12-hour-dark/light cycle at Yale University. NOD mice, *BDC2.5*+ NOD mice, *Il-10*-/- NOD mice and NOD.*scid* mice were originally obtained from the Jackson Laboratory and maintained at Yale University. *BDC2.5*+*Il-10*+/+ NOD mice and *BDC2.5*+*Il-10*-/- NOD mice were generated by

Abbreviations: FITC, fluorescein isothiocyanate; G-CSF, granulocyte colony-stimulating factor; IL-10, interleukin 10; MyD88, myeloid differentiation factor 88; NOD, non-obese diabetic; OTU, operational taxonomic unit; PBS, Phosphate Buffered Saline; PCoA, Principal Coordinate Analysis; PLN, pancreatic lymph node; Rag, recombination-activating gene; Scid, severe combined immune deficiency; SPF, specific pathogen-free; TLR4, Toll-like receptor 4.

breeding *BDC2.5*$^+$ NOD mice with *Il-10*$^{-/-}$ NOD mice, followed by intercrossing the *BDC2.5*$^+$*Il-10*$^{+/-}$ NOD mice. The use of animals in this study was approved by the Institutional Animal Care and Use Committee of Yale University (approval number 2016-07911). Except for the experiments to observe diabetes incidence and adoptive transfer experiments using splenocytes from diabetic mice, all the other experiments were performed using 4-5 week-old non-diabetic mice. The detail of the number of animals used and the number of replicates are included in the figure legends for each experiment and also see **Table S1**.

Natural History of Diabetes Development

BDC2.5$^+$*Il-10*$^{+/+}$ NOD mice and *BDC2.5*$^+$*Il-10*$^{-/-}$ NOD mice (both sexes) were observed for spontaneous diabetes development by screening for glycosuria (Bayer Diastix) weekly and diabetes onset was confirmed by blood glucose ≥ 250 mg/dl (13.9 mmol/l).

Islet and Islet-Infiltrating Immune Cell Isolation

Pancreata removed from 4-week-old *BDC2.5*$^+$*Il-10*$^{+/+}$ NOD mice and *BDC2.5*$^+$*Il-10*$^{-/-}$ NOD mice were agitated in a 37°C shaking water bath after addition of 1.5 mg/ml collagenase (Sigma) and 62.5 units/ml DNase-I (Sigma). Collagenase activity was stopped by adding complete RPMI-1640 media after digestion. Islets were hand-picked under a light microscope, and subsequently incubated in a 37°C water bath for 6 minutes in the presence of 500 µl Cell Dissociation Buffer (Gibco), for immune cell isolation. After washing, isolated immune cells were filtered and re-suspended in complete RPMI-1640 media before staining.

Intraperitoneal Glucose Tolerance Test (IPGTT)

BDC2.5$^+$*Il-10*$^{+/+}$ NOD mice and *BDC2.5*$^+$*Il-10*$^{-/-}$ NOD mice were fasted overnight prior to intraperitoneal injection with 20% glucose (2 g/kg). Blood glucose was measured before glucose injection and at different time points after glucose injection.

Cell Purification

CD4$^+$ T cells, antigen-presenting cells, Treg cells and neutrophils were each purified from the splenocytes of 4-week-old *BDC2.5*$^+$*Il-10*$^{+/+}$ NOD mice, *BDC2.5*$^+$*Il-10*$^{-/-}$ NOD mice, or wild type NOD mice. Splenic CD4$^+$ T cells were purified by depletion, of CD8$^+$ T cells (clone T1B105), MHC class II$^+$ cells (clone 10.2.16), and B cells (anti-mouse IgM and IgG), incubating the cells with monoclonal antibody (mAb) hybridoma supernatants, followed by magnetic bead separation. For splenic antigen-presenting cell (APC) isolation, anti-Thyl (Y19) mAb hybridoma supernatant and complement was used to remove Thyl$^+$ T cells. The supernatants of different mAb hybridomas were kindly provided by the late Charles Janeway (Yale University). Magnetic beads conjugated with goat anti-mouse IgG, goat anti-mouse IgM, or goat anti-rat IgG were purchased from QIAGEN. Treg cells were isolated using MojoSort™ Mouse CD4$^+$ T cell Isolation Kit (BioLegend), followed by CD25 positive isolation using a PE-anti-mouse CD25 antibody (Clone, PC61, BioLegend) and MojoSort™ Mouse anti-PE Nanobeads (BioLegend). The remaining CD4$^+$CD25$^-$ T cells were used as effector CD4$^+$ T cells. Neutrophils were isolated according to the manufacturer's instructions using MojoSort™ Mouse Neutrophil Isolation kit (BioLegend).

In Vitro Culture

Splenic CD4$^+$ T cells (1 × 10^5/well) purified from 4-week-old *BDC2.5*$^+$*Il-10*$^{+/+}$ NOD mice and *BDC2.5*$^+$*Il-10*$^{-/-}$ NOD mice were stimulated with different concentrations of mimotope peptide in the presence of mitomycin-c-treated APCs for 3 days at 37°C. CD4$^+$CD25$^+$ Tregs (5 × 10^4/well) purified from 4-week-old *BDC2.5*$^+$*Il-10*$^{+/+}$ NOD mice and *BDC2.5*$^+$*Il-10*$^{-/-}$ NOD were co-cultured with effector CD4$^+$ T cells (CD4$^+$CD25$^-$ T cells, 1 × 10^5/well) from either *BDC2.5*$^+$*Il-10*$^{+/+}$ NOD mice or *BDC2.5*$^+$*Il-10*$^{-/-}$ NOD mice, in the presence of 5 ng/ml mimotope peptide (amino acid sequence RTRPLWVRME) and mitomycin-c-treated APCs (5 × 10^4/well), which were purified from wild-type NOD mice. Cells were incubated for 3 days at 37°C. Purified splenic neutrophils (5 × 10^4/well) from *BDC2.5*$^+$*Il-10*$^{+/+}$ NOD mice and *BDC2.5*$^+$*Il-10*$^{-/-}$ NOD mice were co-cultured with purified splenic CD4$^+$ T cells (1 × 10^5/well) isolated from either *BDC2.5*$^+$*Il-10*$^{+/+}$ NOD mice or *BDC2.5*$^+$*Il-10*$^{-/-}$ NOD mice in the presence of mitomycin-treated APCs (5 × 10^4/well) from wild type NOD mice and mimotope peptide (5 ng/ml). Cell proliferation was determined by ^{3}H-thymidine incorporation over 16 hours, with supernatants collected prior to ^{3}H-thymidine addition.

Adoptive Transfer Experiments

Total splenocytes (10 × 10^6) from diabetic *BDC2.5*$^+$*Il-10*$^{+/+}$ NOD mice and *BDC2.5*$^+$*Il-10*$^{-/-}$ NOD mice were injected (*i.v.*) into irradiated 4-week-old wild-type NOD mice. Total splenocytes (10 × 10^6), or purified splenic CD4$^+$ T cells (7 × 10^6) from non-diabetic *BDC2.5*$^+$*Il-10*$^{+/+}$ NOD mice and *BDC2.5*$^+$*Il-10*$^{-/-}$ NOD mice were transferred (*i.v.*) into 4-week-old NOD.*scid* mice. Recipients were monitored for glycosuria (Bayer Diastix) weekly and diabetes was confirmed by blood glucose ≥ 250 mg/dl (13.9 mmol/l).

Extraction of Gut Bacterial DNA

Fecal pellets collected from 4-week-old *BDC2.5*$^+$*Il-10*$^{+/+}$ NOD mice and *BDC2.5*$^+$*Il-10*$^{-/-}$ NOD mice were resuspended in 300 µl Tris-EDTA buffer (10 mM Tris and 1 mM EDTA, pH8) containing 7.5 µl 0.5% SDS and 3 µl Proteinase K (200 µg/ml). The samples were then incubated at 37°C for 1 h and homogenized in solution, containing one volume of phenol/chloroform/isoamyl alcohol (25:24:1), 200 µl 20% SDS and 0.3 g zirconium silica beads, with a mini-bead-beater (BioSpec) for 2 minutes. Phenol/chloroform/isoamyl alcohol was then added to the samples prior to centrifugation (4°C, 12000 g, 15 mins), with the upper aqueous layer, containing DNA, transferred to a new tube. Bacterial DNA was subsequently precipitated with isopropanol, washed with 70% ethanol, air-dried, and resuspended in 100 µl of sterile water.

16S rRNA Sequencing and Data Analysis

The V4 region of the bacterial 16S rRNA gene was amplified from each DNA sample by PCR using barcoded broadly-conserved primer pairs (5'-GTGCCAGCMGCCGCGGTAA-3') and (5'-GGACTACHVGGGTWTCTAAT-3'). The PCR products were purified using gel extraction kits (QIAGEN) with DNA concentration quantified on a Nanodrop spectrophotometer. Equimolar amounts of each sample were pooled for pyrosequencing using the Ion Torrent Personal Genome Machine (PGM) sequencing system (Life Technologies). The sequencing results were analyzed with the Quantitative Insights Into Microbial Ecology (QIIME) software package (version 1.8) and UPARSE pipeline (version 7.0). β-diversity was analyzed to compare differences between microbial communities, and the data are shown as a Principal Coordinate Analysis (PCoA). Taxonomy assignment was performed at various levels using representative sequences of each operational taxonomic unit (OTU).

Pre- and Neo-Natal Antibiotic Treatment *In Vivo*

For depletion of endogenous commensal microbiota, *BDC2.5$^+$Il-10$^{+/-}$* NOD breeders were treated with an antibiotic cocktail containing 0.5 g/l vancomycin, 1 g/l ampicillin, 1 g/l metronidazole, and 1 g/l neomycin added in drinking water, from one week before delivery to 4 weeks after birth.

Cytokine ELISA

Murine IL-17A, IL-10 and IFN-γ from the serum and gut flush from different sections of the intestine were measured using the Mouse ELISA kits (BioLegend), following the manufacturer's instructions. Serum samples were diluted 1:100 in PBS before measurement. Gut flush was obtained by infusing 10 ml PBS to the gut lumen, after termination of the mice, and removal of the intestine. The collected fluid used for ELISA, after removing the solid material by centrifugation (12,000 g, 5 min, RT).

Gut Permeability Assay

Four-week-old *BDC2.5$^+$Il-10$^{+/+}$* NOD mice and *BDC2.5$^+$Il-10$^{-/-}$* NOD mice were fasted overnight for 13 hours. Food was resupplied to the mice two hours post-gavage with 0.6 mg/g FITC-dextran (MW 3,000-5,000, Sigma). Blood samples were collected from the mice two hours after food restoration and were centrifuged (2300 g, 5 min, RT) for serum separation. Serum samples were diluted 1:1 in PBS with the FITC-dextran concentration determined using a fluorescence spectrophotometer (Perkin Elmer). Standard curves were generated using known concentrations of FITC-dextran, diluted in serum from untreated NOD mice. The concentrations in serum from FITC-dextran gavaged *BDC2.5$^+$Il-10$^{+/+}$* NOD mice and *BDC2.5$^+$Il-10$^{-/-}$* NOD mice were determined using linear regression.

In Vitro Bacterial Stimulation

Fresh stool samples, collected from 4-week-old *BDC2.5$^+$Il-10$^{+/+}$* NOD mice and *BDC2.5$^+$Il-10$^{-/-}$* NOD mice, were resuspended at 1 g/mL in sterile PBS, and homogenized by vortexing vigorously for 30 secs. The samples were then centrifuged (300 g, 1 min, RT) to remove large debris and subsequently further centrifuged at 12,000 g for 5 minutes to pellet the bacteria. Bacteria from *BDC2.5$^+$Il-10$^{+/+}$* NOD mice and *BDC2.5$^+$Il-10$^{-/-}$* NOD mice were re-suspended in sterile PBS, heat-inactivated at 95°C for 30 min, and co-cultured overnight (10^8 CFU) with 2 million total splenocytes or purified splenic neutrophils from *BDC2.5$^+$Il-10$^{+/+}$* and *BDC2.5$^+$Il-10$^{-/-}$* NOD mice. Stimulated splenocytes or neutrophils were further analyzed by flow cytometry and real-time qPCR.

Real Time Quantitative PCR (qPCR)

RNA from purified neutrophils (un-stimulated or stimulated with gut microbiota) or small intestinal tissue was extracted using Trizol reagent and an RNeasy mini plus kit (QIAGEN). After quantification, RNA was used for cDNA synthesis using the iScript cDNA synthesis kit (Invitrogen). Samples were analyzed on an iCycler qPCR machine (Bio-rad). Gene expression level was determined using the $2^{-\Delta\Delta Ct}$ method and normalized with the housekeeping gene, *Gapdh*. Primers sequences are listed in **Table 1**. Each sample was assayed in duplicate and the experiments were repeated at least twice.

Flow Cytometry

0.5 - 1 × 10^6 single-cell suspensions from different lymphoid tissues were incubated with Fc block at room temperature for 20 min, before cell surface staining. For intracellular cytokine staining, cells were incubated at 37°C for 4 h in the presence of 10 ng/ml phorbol myristate acetate (PMA, Sigma), 500 ng/ml of ionomycin (Sigma) and 1 µl of Golgi plug™ (BD Bioscience), followed by cell surface staining, washing, fixation and permeabilization and intracellular cytokine staining. For intranuclear staining, cells were fixed and permeabilized using the Transcription Factor Staining Buffer Set (Tonbo Biosciences).

TABLE 1 | Primer information.

Genes	Primers	Sequence
Tnf-α	Forward	CAAATGGCCTCCCTCTCAT
	Reverse	TGGGCTACAGGCTTGTCACT
Il-1β	Forward	TGGAGAACACCACTTGTTGCTCCA
	Reverse	AAACAGATGAAGTGCTCCTTCGAGG
Inos	Forward	AGATTGGAGTTCGAGACTTCTG
	Reverse	TGGCTAGTGCTTCAGACTTC
Nos2	Forward	CCAAGCCCTCACCTACTTCC
	Reverse	CTCTGAGGGCTGACACAAGG
Arg1	Forward	CTCCAAGCCAAAGTCCTTAGAG
	Reverse	AGGAGCTGTCATTAGGGACATC
Caspase9	Forward	TCCTGGTACATCGAGACCTTG
	Reverse	AAGTCCCTTTCGCAGAAACAG
Zonulin1	Forward	CACCGGAGTGATGGTTTTCT
	Reverse	CCACCTCTGTCCAGCTCTTC
Reg3β	Forward	CTGCCTTAGACCGTGCTTTC
	Reverse	CCCTTGTCCATGATGCTCTT
Reg3γ	Forward	TTCCTGTCCTCCATGATCAAAA
	Reverse	CATCCACCTCTGTTGGGTTCA
Defcr6	Forward	CAGGCTGTGTCTGTCTCTTTTG
	Reverse	TAAATGACCCTTTCTGCAGGTC
Gapdh	Forward	GGGGTCGTTGATGGCAACA
	Reverse	TGTAGACCATGTAGTTGAGGTCA

After incubation, the cells were stained with an anti-Foxp3 antibody (clone: FJK-16s, eBioscience) and T-bet (clone:4B10, BioLegend). Cells were stained with mAbs to the following surface markers: CD45 (clone: 30-F11), TCR-β (clone: H57-597), CD4 (clone: GK1.5), CD8 (clone: 53-6.7), CD11b (clone: M1/70), CD62L (clone: MEL-14), ICOS (clone: 15F9), CD69 (clone: H1.2F3), CD25 (clone: 3C7), CD19 (clone: 6D5), all from BioLegend, and Ly6G (clone: 1A8) from BD Biosciences. mAbs to intracellular cytokines include TNF-α (clone: MP6-XT22), IFN-γ (clone: XMG1.2) and IL-17A (clone: TC11-18H10.1) were purchased from Biolegend. Samples were analyzed on a BD LSRII flow cytometer and subsequently analyzed by FlowJo 8.8.6 software (Tree star). Immune cells were gated based on their FSC-A/SSC-A properties. Single cells and subsequent live cells were gated on their FSC-A/FSC-H properties and live/dead staining, respectively.

Statistics

Diabetes incidence was compared using a log-rank test for survival. Insulitis scores were analyzed using a *Chi*-square test. Statistical analysis of microbial β-diversity was conducted using an analysis of similarities (ANOSIM). Differences between microbial species were determined following analysis using multiple *t*-tests with Bonferroni correction. Data from experiments *in vitro* were assessed for normality and subsequently analyzed using a two-tailed Student's *t* test (if data were normally distributed), a two-tailed Mann-Whitney test (if data were not normally distributed), or a two-way ANOVA. $P < 0.05$ was considered statistically significant.

RESULTS

In the Absence of IL-10, BDC2.5$^+$ NOD Mice Develop Accelerated Diabetes at a Very Young Age

To assess the role of IL-10 in diabetes protection observed in *BDC2.5*$^+$ NOD mice, we first monitored the natural history of type 1 diabetes development in *BDC2.5*$^+$*Il-10*$^{+/+}$ NOD mice and *BDC2.5*$^+$*Il-10*$^{-/-}$ NOD mice. Interestingly, both female and male *BDC2.5*$^+$*Il-10*$^{-/-}$ NOD mice developed accelerated diabetes at a very young age (**Figures 1A, B**). In line with islet β cell destruction, *BDC2.5*$^+$*Il-10*$^{-/-}$ NOD mice displayed impaired glucose tolerance compared with *BDC2.5*$^+$*Il-10*$^{+/+}$ NOD mice (**Figure 1C**). We found no significant difference in severity of insulitis between *BDC2.5*$^+$*Il-10*$^{+/+}$ and *BDC2.5*$^+$*Il-10*$^{-/-}$ NOD

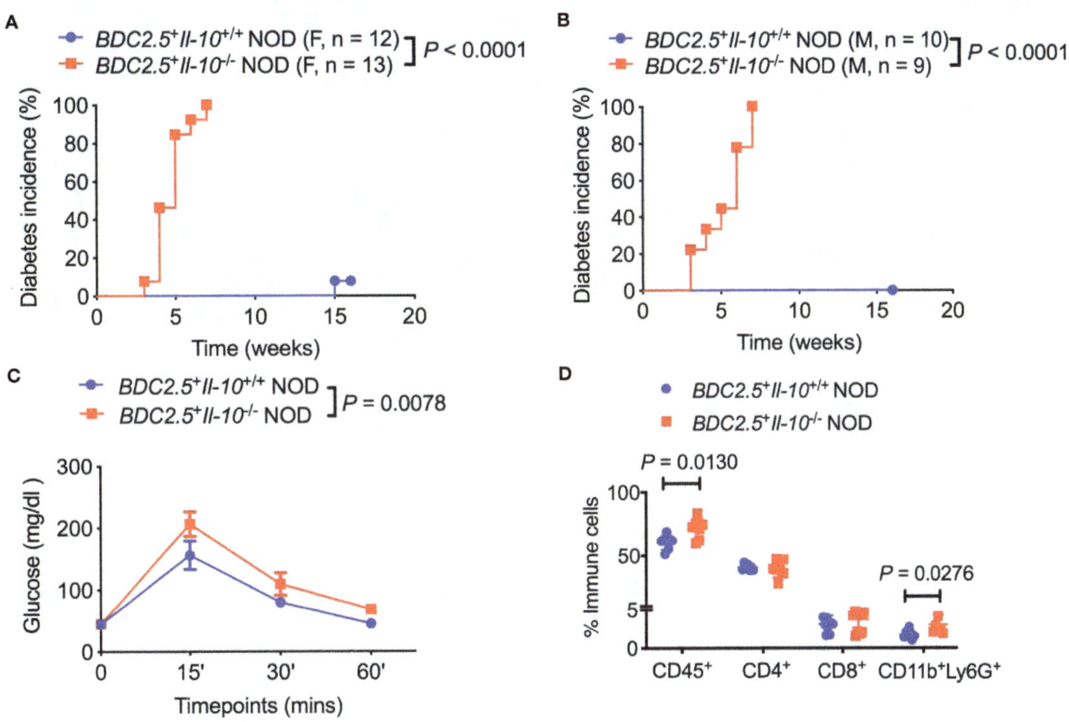

FIGURE 1 | *Il-10* deficiency in *BDC2.5*$^+$ NOD mice induced rapid development of type 1 diabetes. **(A, B)** Natural history of type 1 diabetes development in *BDC2.5*$^+$*Il-10*$^{+/+}$ NOD mice and *BDC2.5*$^+$*Il-10*$^{-/-}$ NOD littermates from females [**(A)**, n = 12-13/group] and males [**(B)**, n = 9-10/group]. **(C)** Intraperitoneal glucose tolerance test (IPGTT) in *BDC2.5*$^+$*Il-10*$^{+/+}$ NOD mice and *BDC2.5*$^+$*Il-10*$^{-/-}$ NOD mice (n = 5/group). **(D)** Infiltrated immune cells in the islets of mice (*n* = 7-11/group). In flow cytometric analysis, CD45$^+$ immune cells were gated from live cells. CD4$^+$ T cells, CD8$^+$ T cells, CD11b$^+$Ly6G$^+$ neutrophils were gated from CD45$^+$ immune cells. Data in **(A, B, D)** were pooled from two or more independent experiments. The experiment in **(C)** was performed twice, and consistent results were obtained. Data were analyzed using a log-rank test for survival **(A, B)**, a two-way ANOVA **(C)**, or a two-tailed Student's *t*-test [**(D)**, Data are presented as mean ± SD]. $P < 0.05$ was considered statistically significant.

mice (**Figures S1A, B**); however, *BDC2.5*$^{+}$*Il-10*$^{-/-}$ NOD mice had more CD45^{+} immune cells, especially CD11b^{+}Ly6G^{+} neutrophils, infiltrating the islets than *BDC2.5*$^{+}$*Il-10*$^{+/+}$ NOD mice, but no significant differences in the proportion of CD4^{+} T cells, CD8^{+} T cells, B cells, macrophages, and dendritic cells (**Figure 1D** and data not shown). Our data showed that in the absence of IL-10, *BDC2.5*$^{+}$ NOD mice develop accelerated diabetes at a very young age.

IL-10 Deficiency Promotes the Expansion of Bone Marrow and Peripheral Neutrophils in BDC2.5^{+} NOD Mice

We observed an increased frequency of neutrophils infiltrating the islets of *BDC2.5*$^{+}$*Il-10*$^{-/-}$ NOD mice (**Figure 1D**). To investigate the crosstalk between IL-10 and neutrophils, we assessed the neutrophil population in both the bone marrow and peripheral tissues of *BDC2.5*$^{+}$*Il-10*$^{+/+}$ and *BDC2.5*$^{+}$*Il-10*$^{-/-}$ NOD mice. Consistent with the results from the islets, we also found a higher percentage of neutrophils in the spleen, bone marrow and blood of *BDC2.5*$^{+}$*Il-10*$^{-/-}$ NOD mice, compared to *BDC2.5*$^{+}$*Il-10*$^{+/+}$ NOD mice (**Figures 2A–E and S2A, B**). Moreover, there was a higher proportion of IFN-γ-producing splenic neutrophils in *BDC2.5*$^{+}$*Il-10*$^{-/-}$ NOD mice compared with *BDC2.5*$^{+}$*Il-10*$^{+/+}$ NOD mice (**Figures 2F, G**). The expression levels of cytokines in the neutrophils from the blood and islets in *BDC2.5*$^{+}$*Il-10*$^{+/+}$ NOD mice were the same as those in *BDC2.5*$^{+}$*Il-10*$^{-/-}$ NOD mice (**Figures S3A–G**). Additionally, we found that neutrophils from the islets of the *BDC2.5*$^{+}$*Il-10*$^{+/+}$ NOD mice had lower levels of CD62L (**Figure 2H**). We then purified neutrophils and found no significant differences in the gene expression of *Inos*, *Nos2*, *Arg1*, and *Caspase9* in the spleen (**Figures S4A–D**); however, we found increased *Nos2* and *Il-1β* in purified neutrophils from the bone marrow of *BDC2.5*$^{+}$*Il-10*$^{-/-}$ NOD mice (**Figures 2I, J**), but no significant differences in the expressions of *Inos*, *Arg1*, *Caspase 9*, and *Mmp9* (**Figures S4E–H**). Next, we assessed the phagocytotic ability of neutrophils

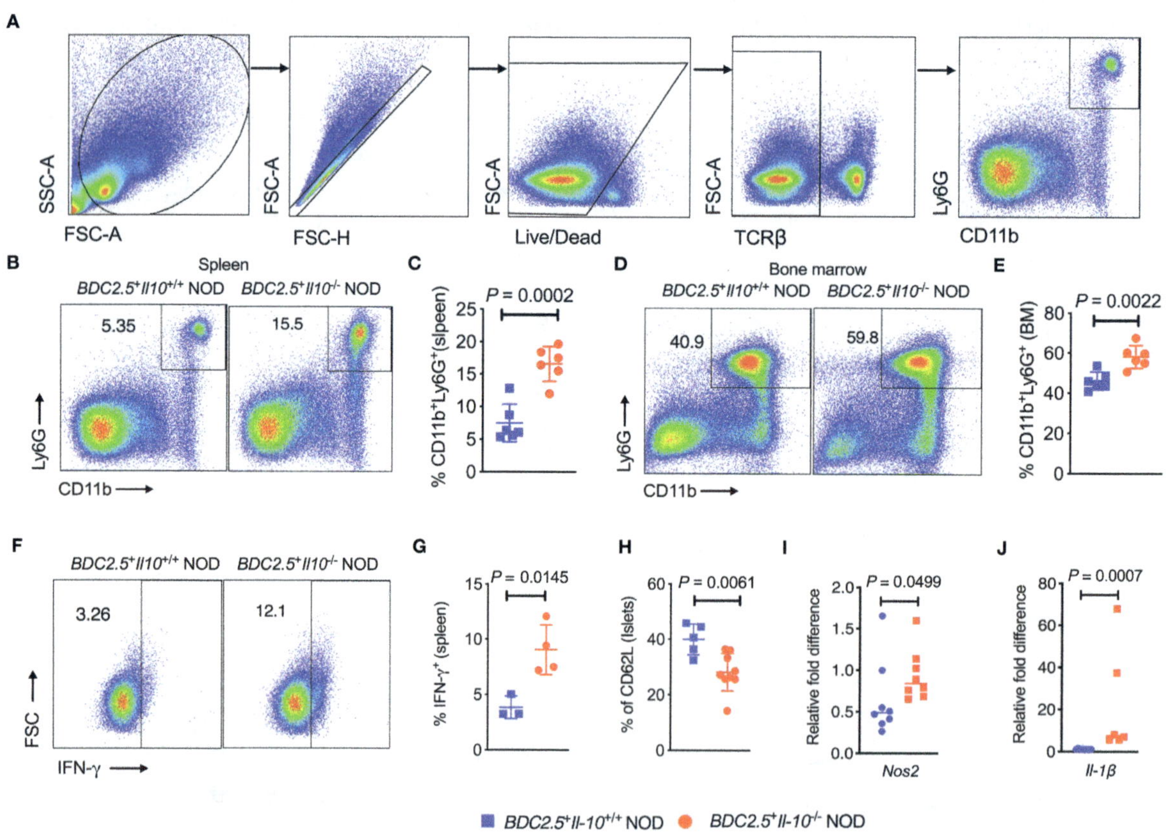

FIGURE 2 | Altered neutrophil homeostasis in *BDC2.5*$^{+}$*Il-10*$^{-/-}$ NOD mice compared with *BDC2.5*$^{+}$*Il-10*$^{+/+}$ NOD mice. **(A)** Gating strategies of CD11b^{+}Ly6G^{+} neutrophils from the spleen. **(B, C)** Proportion of CD11b^{+}Ly6G^{+} neutrophils in the spleen (n = 6/group). Representative flow cytometric profiles **(B)**, and summary of CD11b^{+}Ly6G^{+} neutrophils gated from TCR-β^{-} cells **(C)**. **(D, E)** Proportion of CD11b^{+}Ly6G^{+} neutrophils in the bone marrow (n = 6/group). Representative flow cytometric profiles **(D)**, and summary of CD11b^{+}Ly6G^{+} neutrophils gated from TCRβ^{-} cells **(E)**. **(F, G)** IFN-γ expression in splenic CD11b^{+}Ly6G^{+} neutrophils (n = 3-4/group). Representative flow cytometric profiles **(F)**, and summary of IFN-γ expression **(G)**. **(H)** CD62L expression in pancreatic CD11b^{+}Ly6G^{+} neutrophils (n = 5-9/group). **(I, J)** Gene expression of *Nos2* **(I)** *and Il-1β* **(J)** in splenic neutrophils from *BDC2.5*$^{+}$*Il-10*$^{+/+}$ NOD mice and *BDC2.5*$^{+}$*Il-10*$^{-/-}$ NOD mice (n = 6-8/group). Data in **(C, E, H–J)** were combined from two or more independent experiments. The experiment in **(G)** was performed twice and consistent results were obtained. Data in **(C, E, G, H)** are shown as mean ± SD and were analyzed using a two-tailed Student's t-test. Data in **(I, J)** are presented as median and were analyzed using a two-tailed Mann-Whitney test. $P < 0.05$ was considered statistically significant.

and found that neutrophils from *BDC2.5*$^{+}$*Il-10*$^{-/-}$ NOD mice were not different from those from *BDC2.5*$^{+}$*Il-10*$^{+/+}$ NOD mice (**Figures S5A, B**). Taken together, our data suggested that *Il-10* deficiency altered neutrophil homeostasis in *BDC2.5*$^{+}$ NOD mice.

In the Absence of IL-10, CD4^{+} T Cells Are More Activated and Pathogenic in BDC2.5^{+} NOD Mice

Next, we assessed the phenotype and function of different T cell populations in *BDC2.5*$^{+}$*Il-10*$^{-/-}$ NOD mice. Interestingly, unlike the composition of the immune cells seen in the islet infiltrate (**Figure 1D**), *BDC2.5*$^{+}$*Il-10*$^{-/-}$ NOD mice had a higher proportion of splenic CD4^{+} T cells when compared with *BDC2.5*$^{+}$*Il-10*$^{+/+}$ NOD mice (**Figure 3A**), while no significant difference was found in the percentage of CD8^{+} T cells (**Figure 3A**). The proportions of both CD4^{+} and CD8^{+} T cells were increased in the pancreatic lymph node (PLN) of *BDC2.5*$^{+}$*Il-10*$^{-/-}$ NOD mice (**Figure 3B**). We found that splenic CD4^{+} T cells from *BDC2.5*$^{+}$*Il-10*$^{-/-}$ mice expressed a higher proportion of ICOS, T-bet and CD69 (**Figure 3C**) while splenic CD8^{+} T cells expressed higher level of T-bet only (**Figure 3D**). Moreover, splenic CD4^{+} T cells from *BDC2.5*$^{+}$*Il-10*$^{-/-}$ mice showed increased expressions of inflammatory cytokines including IFN-γ and IL-17A in the spleen (**Figure 3E**) and more TNF-α in CD4^{+} T cells from PLN (**Figure 3F**). Additionally, splenic CD8^{+} T cells in *BDC2.5*$^{+}$*Il-10*$^{-/-}$ NOD mice expressed more TNF-α (**Figure 3G**). Interestingly, splenic CD4^{+} T cells from *BDC2.5*$^{+}$*Il-10*$^{-/-}$ NOD mice showed stronger proliferative responses to their antigenic peptide

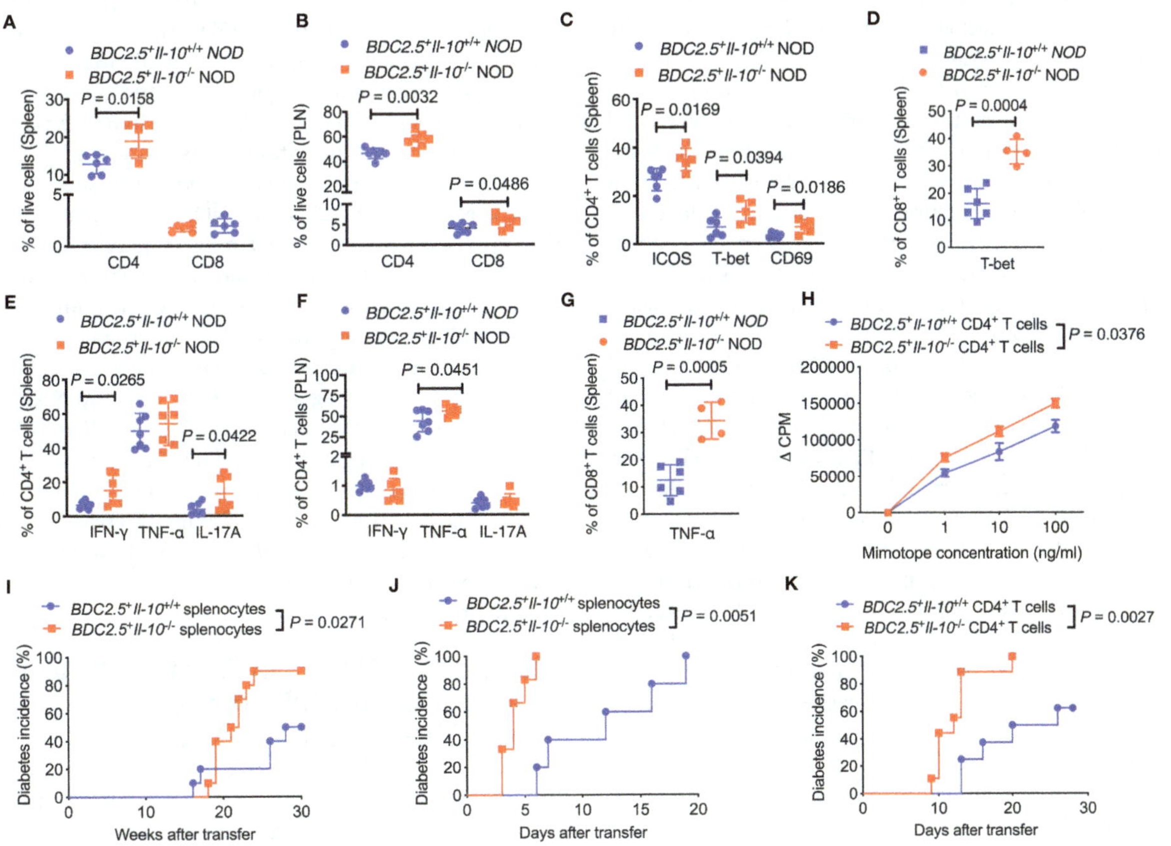

FIGURE 3 | *BDC2.5*$^{+}$*Il-10*$^{-/-}$ NOD mice have more activated and pathogenic CD4^{+} T cells. **(A)** The percentage of CD4^{+} T cells and CD8^{+} T cells in the spleen of *BDC2.5*$^{+}$*Il-10*$^{+/+}$ NOD mice and *BDC2.5*$^{+}$*Il-10*$^{-/-}$ NOD mice (n = 6/group). **(B)** The percentage of CD4^{+} T cells and CD8^{+} T cells in the pancreatic lymph node (PLN) of *BDC2.5*$^{+}$*Il-10*$^{+/+}$ NOD mice and *BDC2.5*$^{+}$*Il-10*$^{-/-}$ NOD mice (n = 7/group). **(C)** The proportion of ICOS^{+}, T-bet^{+} and CD69^{+} splenic CD4^{+} T cells in *BDC2.5*$^{+}$*Il-10*$^{+/+}$ NOD mice and *BDC2.5*$^{+}$*Il-10*$^{-/-}$ NOD mice (n = 5-6/group). **(D)** The proportion of T-bet^{+} splenic CD8^{+} T cells in *BDC2.5*$^{+}$*Il-10*$^{+/+}$ NOD mice and *BDC2.5*$^{+}$*Il-10*$^{-/-}$ NOD mice (n = 4-6/group). **(E)** The proportion of IFN-γ^{+}, TNF-α^{+}, and IL-17A^{+} splenic CD4^{+} T cells in *BDC2.5*$^{+}$*Il-10*$^{+/+}$ NOD mice and *BDC2.5*$^{+}$*Il-10*$^{-/-}$ NOD mice (n = 7/group). **(F)** The proportion of IFN-γ^{+}, TNF-α^{+}, and IL-17A^{+} CD4^{+} T cells in the PLN from *BDC2.5*$^{+}$*Il-10*$^{+/+}$ NOD mice and *BDC2.5*$^{+}$*Il-10*$^{-/-}$ NOD mice (n = 7/group). **(G)** The proportion of TNF-α^{+} splenic CD8^{+} T cells in *BDC2.5*$^{+}$*Il-10*$^{+/+}$ NOD mice and *BDC2.5*$^{+}$*Il-10*$^{-/-}$ NOD mice (n = 4-6/group). **(H)** Proliferation of purified splenic CD4^{+} T cells from *BDC2.5*$^{+}$*Il-10*$^{+/+}$ NOD mice and *BDC2.5*$^{+}$*Il-10*$^{-/-}$ NOD mice in the presence of different concentrations of mimotope. **(I)** Adoptive transfer of diabetic splenocytes from *BDC2.5*$^{+}$*Il-10*$^{+/+}$ NOD mice and *BDC2.5*$^{+}$*Il-10*$^{-/-}$ NOD mice into irradiated wild-type NOD mice (n = 10/group). **(J)** Adoptive transfer of non-diabetic splenocytes from *BDC2.5*$^{+}$*Il-10*$^{+/+}$ NOD mice and *BDC2.5*$^{+}$*Il-10*$^{-/-}$ NOD mice into NOD-*scid* mice (n = 7-9/group). **(K)** Adoptive transfer of purified splenic CD4^{+} into NOD-*scid* mice (n = 8-9/group). Data in **(A–C, E, F, I–K)** were combined from two or more independent experiments. The experiments in **(D, G, H)** were performed two or more times, with similar results obtained. Data in **(A–G)** are shown as mean ± SD. Data were analyzed using a two-tailed Student's *t*-test **(A–G)**, a two-way ANOVA **(H)**, or log-rank test for survival **(I–K)**. $P < 0.05$ was considered statistically significant.

(mimotope) compared to CD4$^+$ T cells from *BDC2.5$^+$Il-10$^{+/+}$* splenocytes (**Figure 3H**). No significant differences were found in the proportion of CD8$^+$ T cells expressing IFN-γ, TNF-α, or IL-17A in the PLN between *BDC2.5$^+$Il-10$^{+/+}$* and *BDC2.5$^+$Il-10$^{-/-}$* NOD mice (**Figures S6A–C**). To determine the effect of IL-10 on diabetogenicity of the T cells from *BDC2.5$^+$Il-10$^{-/-}$* NOD mice *in vivo*, we adoptively transferred total splenocytes from diabetic *BDC2.5$^+$Il-10$^{-/-}$* or *BDC2.5$^+$Il-10$^{+/+}$* NOD mice into 4-week-old irradiated wild-type female NOD mice. Supporting the *in vitro* data, splenocytes from diabetic *BDC2.5$^+$Il-10$^{-/-}$* NOD mice showed more potent diabetogenicity by inducing a higher incidence of diabetes in the recipients, compared with the splenocytes from *BDC2.5$^+$Il-10$^{+/+}$* NOD mice (**Figure 3I**). Moreover, when we transferred total splenocytes from non-diabetic *BDC2.5$^+$Il-10$^{-/-}$* or *BDC2.5$^+$Il-10$^{+/+}$* NOD mice into NOD.*scid* mice, splenocytes from *BDC2.5$^+$Il-10$^{-/-}$* mice induced rapid diabetes in the NOD.*scid* recipients as early as 3-days after transfer (**Figure 3J**). We further confirmed the enhanced diabetogenicity by BDC2.5 CD4$^+$ T cells by adoptive transfer with purified splenic CD4$^+$ T cells from non-diabetic *BDC2.5$^+$Il-10$^{-/-}$* or *BDC2.5$^+$Il-10$^{+/+}$* NOD mice into NOD.*scid* recipients. Similar to the adoptive transfer with total splenocytes, CD4$^+$ T cells from *BDC2.5$^+$Il-10$^{-/-}$* NOD mice induced rapid onset of diabetes compared to their counterparts from *BDC2.5$^+$Il-10$^{+/+}$* NOD mice (**Figure 3K**). To determine the effects of neutrophils on CD4$^+$ T cells, we performed criss-cross co-culture in which purified splenic neutrophils from *BDC2.5$^+$Il-10$^{+/+}$ or BDC2.5$^+$Il-10$^{-/-}$* NOD mice were cultured with purified splenic CD4$^+$ T cells from *BDC2.5$^+$Il-10$^{-/-}$* or *BDC2.5$^+$Il-10$^{+/+}$* NOD mice. Interestingly, neutrophils from both *BDC2.5$^+$Il-10$^{+/+}$* and *BDC2.5$^+$Il-10$^{-/-}$* NOD mice effectively inhibited the proliferation of CD4$^+$ T cells from *BDC2.5$^+$Il-10$^{+/+}$* and *BDC2.5$^+$Il-10$^{-/-}$* NOD mice when stimulated by antigenic peptide (**Figures S7A, B**). However, there was no significant difference in the inhibitory effect of neutrophils from *BDC2.5$^+$Il-10$^{+/+}$* and *BDC2.5$^+$Il-10$^{-/-}$* NOD mice (**Figures S7A, B**). When we transferred purified splenic CD4$^+$ T cells alone or purified splenic neutrophils together with CD4$^+$ T cells from *BDC2.5$^+$Il-10$^{-/-}$* NOD mice into *Rag$^{-/-}$* NOD mice, no significant difference in the diabetes incidence was found, indicating that the altered neutrophils in *BDC2.5$^+$Il-10$^{-/-}$* NOD mice may contribute to the disease development, but not by direct effects on CD4$^+$ T cells (**Figure S7C**). We examined the Treg cells in *BDC2.5$^+$Il-10$^{-/-}$* NOD mice. Surprisingly, there were no significant differences in both the proportion and the suppressive function of Treg cells between *BDC2.5$^+$Il-10$^{+/+}$* and *BDC2.5$^+$Il-10$^{-/-}$* NOD mice (**Figures S8A–C**). Taken together, our data showed that in the absence of *Il-10*, CD4$^+$ T cells in *BDC2.5$^+$* NOD mice were more activated and highly pathogenic. However, Tregs did not appear to be directly affected by the absence of *Il-10*.

IL-10 Deficiency Alters the Composition of Gut Bacteria and Intestinal Immunity in BDC2.5$^+$ NOD Mice

To study whether *Il-10* deficiency also alters the gut bacteria of TCR transgenic *BDC2.5$^+$* NOD hosts, we investigated the gut bacterial composition of *BDC2.5$^+$Il-10$^{+/+}$* and *BDC2.5$^+$Il-10$^{-/-}$* NOD mice. *Il-10*-deficient *BDC2.5$^+$* NOD mice had an altered composition of gut bacteria, indicated by β-diversity of the gut microbiota shown in the Principal Coordinate Analysis (PCOA; **Figure 4A**), compared to *Il-10*-sufficient *BDC2.5$^+$* NOD mice. Further analysis also revealed differences at the phylum, class, and species levels. At the phylum level, *BDC2.5$^+$Il-10$^{-/-}$* NOD mice had increased levels of *Proteobacteria* compared with *BDC2.5$^+$Il-10$^{+/+}$* NOD mice (**Figures 4B, C**), with increased abundance of *Epsilonproteobacteria* and *Gammaproteobacteria* (**Figure 4D**). Moreover, the relative abundance of *Escherichia* from *Proteobacteria* was significantly different between the two groups (**Figure 4E**). We also assessed gut permeability *in vivo* to determine whether the altered gut bacteria affected the gut barrier in *Il-10*-deficient *BDC2.5$^+$* NOD mice. Indeed, *BDC2.5$^+$Il-10$^{-/-}$* NOD mice exhibited increased gut permeability compared to *BDC2.5$^+$Il-10$^{+/+}$* NOD mice as demonstrated by the increased concentration of serum FITC-dextran (**Figure 5A**). We found decreased expression of the intestinal tight junction protein *Zonulin1* in *BDC2.5$^+$Il-10$^{-/-}$* NOD mice (**Figure 5B**), but not *Claudin2* or *Occludin* (data not shown). Moreover, when we assessed the inflammatory cytokines in the gut lumen, we found an increased level of IL-17A (**Figure 5C**) in *BDC2.5$^+$Il-10$^{-/-}$* NOD mice. Additionally, the intestinal expression of *Myd88*, which plays an essential role in the activation of innate immunity, was also increased in *BDC2.5$^+$Il-10$^{-/-}$* NOD mice when compared with that in *BDC2.5$^+$Il-10$^{+/+}$* NOD mice (**Figure 5D**). Interestingly, *BDC2.5$^+$Il-10$^{-/-}$* NOD mice showed increased expression of intestinal antimicrobial peptide genes, including *Crp*, *Defcr6*, *Reg3γ*, and *Reg3β* (**Figures 5E–H**), which could be induced to defend against the altered bacteria in the gut. Additionally, we found that the percentages of TCR-γδ$^+$ cells and NKP46$^+$ (one of the ILC markers) cells decreased in *BDC2.5$^+$Il-10$^{-/-}$* NOD mice, but no significant differences in CD11c$^+$ cells, IFN-γ$^+$CD4$^+$ (Th1) cells, IL-17$^+$CD4$^+$ (Th17) cells, and CD117$^+$ (one of the ILC markers) cells between the two groups (**Figures S9A–F**). Taken together, *Il-10* deficiency in *BDC2.5$^+$* NOD mice not only altered the gut bacterial composition, but also changed the intestinal immune responses of the host.

Altered Gut Bacteria Contribute to the Altered Neutrophil Homeostasis in *BDC2.5$^+$Il-10$^{-/-}$*s NOD Mice

To determine whether the altered gut bacteria in *BDC2.5$^+$Il-10$^{-/-}$* NOD mice contribute to the increased frequency of neutrophils, we first depleted the endogenous commensal bacteria of *BDC2.5$^+$Il-10$^{+/-}$* NOD breeders by treating the mice with a cocktail of antibiotics (0.5 g/L vancomycin, 1 g/L ampicillin, 1 g/L metronidazole, and 1 g/L neomycin) in drinking water and investigated the changes in neutrophils. Our results revealed that the antibiotic treatment significantly decreased the proportions of neutrophils in the islet, bone marrow, spleen and peripheral blood (**Figures 6A–H**). We also had the wildtype mice (*BDC2.5$^+$Il-10$^{+/+}$*) as controls, treated with or without antibiotic, and found that neutrophils were only decreased in the spleen in *BDC2.5$^+$Il-10$^{+/+}$* NOD mice (**Figure S10**). To further confirm the role of gut microbiota from *BDC2.5$^+$Il-10$^{-/-}$* NOD mice in modulating neutrophil homeostasis, we co-cultured *BDC2.5$^+$Il-10$^{-/-}$* NOD

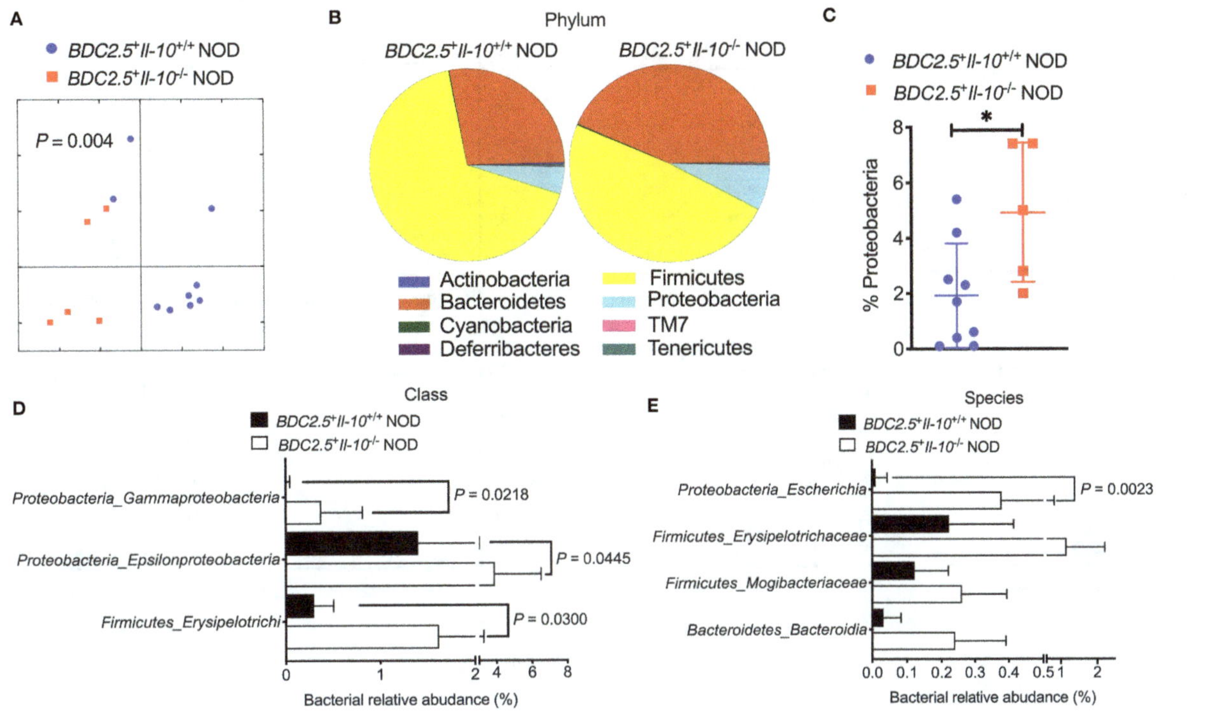

FIGURE 4 | Gut bacterial composition of *BDC2.5*$^{+}$*Il-10*$^{-/-}$ NOD mice showed distinct differences compared with *BDC2.5*$^{+}$*Il-10*$^{-/-}$ NOD mice. Gut bacteria in fecal pellets were analyzed by 16S rRNA sequencing (n = 5-9/group). **(A)** β-diversity of the gut bacteria indicated by unweighted PCoA. **(B, C)** Gut bacterial composition at the phylum level including representative composition **(B)** and summarized percentage of *Proteobacteria* as an example **(C)**. **(D)** Gut bacterial composition at the class level. **(E)** Gut bacterial composition at the species level. Statistical analysis was performed by an analysis of similarities (ANOSIM) **(A)**, a two-tailed Student's t-test **(C)**, or multiple t-tests with Bonferroni correction **(D, E)**. $P < 0.05$ was considered statistically significant. $^{*}P = 0.0261$.

splenocytes *in vitro* with heat-inactivated gut bacteria from either *BDC2.5*$^{+}$*Il-10*$^{+/+}$ or *BDC2.5*$^{+}$*Il-10*$^{-/-}$ NOD mice. Interestingly, we found that gut microbiota from *BDC2.5*$^{+}$*Il-10*$^{-/-}$ NOD further expanded the neutrophil population significantly (**Figures 6I, J**). Next, we purified splenic neutrophils from *BDC2.5*$^{+}$*Il-10*$^{-/-}$ NOD mice and stimulated them with heat-inactivated gut bacteria from either *BDC2.5*$^{+}$*Il-10*$^{+/+}$ or *BDC2.5*$^{+}$*Il-10*$^{-/-}$ NOD mice, followed by assessment of gene expression. Our qPCR results showed that *BDC2.5*$^{+}$*Il-10*$^{-/-}$ NOD gut microbiota promoted *Ifn-γ* gene expression (**Figure 6K**), which was consistent with the intracellular cytokine staining results seen in *BDC2.5*$^{+}$*Il-10*$^{-/-}$ NOD mice (**Figures 2F, G**). Similar to the results using fresh *ex-vivo* splenic neutrophils (**Figures S4A, B**), there were no significant differences in the gene expressions of *Inos* and *Nos2* in the neutrophils after *in vitro* stimulation (**Figures 6L, M**). Taken together, our data suggested that altered gut bacteria from *BDC2.5*$^{+}$*Il-10*$^{-/-}$ NOD mice modulated neutrophil homeostasis, which play a role in the development of type 1 diabetes.

DISCUSSION

In this study, we developed a markedly accelerated model of type 1 diabetes by introducing an *Il-10* deficiency to *BDC2.5*$^{+}$ NOD mice, whereas *Il-10* sufficient *BDC2.5*$^{+}$ NOD mice develop a very low incidence and delayed spontaneous diabetes. Although no significant difference was found in the severity of insulitis between *BDC2.5*$^{+}$*Il-10*$^{+/+}$ NOD mice and *BDC2.5*$^{+}$*Il*-10$^{-/-}$ NOD mice, *BDC2.5*$^{+}$*Il-10*$^{-/-}$ NOD mice had more immune cells, especially neutrophils, infiltrating into the islets. In this mouse model, *BDC2.5*$^{+}$ NOD CD4^{+} T cells are more activated and pathogenic than CD4^{+} T cells from *Il-10* sufficient *BDC2.5*$^{+}$ NOD mice. Furthermore, *BDC2.5*$^{+}$*Il-10*$^{-/-}$ NOD mice displayed increased proportions of neutrophils in the bone marrow, peripheral blood and spleen, which was closely associated with altered gut microbiota. We postulate that the altered microbiota may be central in increasing the neutrophils, which also play a role in increasing pathogenic CD4^{+} T cells.

IL-10 is a multifunctional cytokine that plays crucial roles in limiting the immune response and regulating the growth and/or differentiation a variety of immune cells (38, 39). The reports of the role of IL-10 in the development of type 1 diabetes are conflicting. It has been documented that early exposure to IL-10 accelerates the disease development (40), while IL-10 exposure during the later prediabetic phase inhibits disease (41). Additionally, the effects of IL-10 on autoimmune diabetes of NOD mice are associated with the location of IL-10 expression. Pancreatic expression of IL-10 can up-regulate the expression of intercellular adhesion molecule 1 (ICAM-1) on vascular endothelium (42) and promotes diabetes development (43),

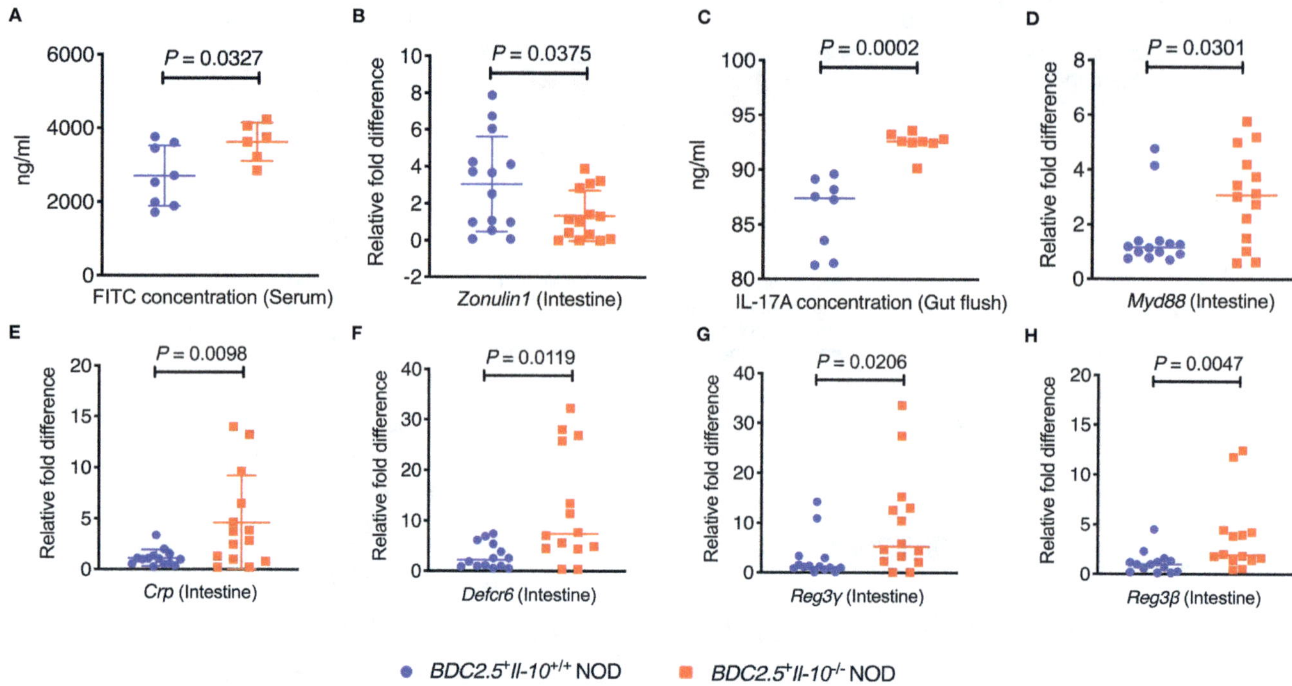

FIGURE 5 | *BDC2.5*$^{+}$*Il-10*$^{-/-}$ NOD mice showed altered intestinal responses compared with *BDC2.5*$^{+}$*Il-10*$^{+/+}$ NOD mice. **(A)** Gut permeability assessed following FITC-dextran uptake into the blood from the gut (n = 6-8/group). **(B)** Gene expression of *Zonulin1* (n = 14/group). **(C)** IL-17A concentration in the gut flush of the large intestine (n = 8/group). **(D)** Gene expression of *Myd88* (n = 14/group). **(E–H)** Gene expression of intestinal antimicrobial peptide genes, including *Crp* **(E)**, *Defcr6* **(F)**, *Reg3γ* **(G)**, and *Reg3β* **(H)** (n = 14/group). Data in **(A–H)** were combined from two or more independent experiments are presented as mean ± SD **(A, B, E)** or Median **(C, D, F–H)**. Statistical analysis was performed by a two-tailed Student's t-test **(A, B, E)** or a two-tailed Mann-Whitney test **(C, D, F–H)**. $P < 0.05$ was considered statistically significant.

but systemic IL-10 is dispensable for autoimmune diabetes (44). IL-10 has the ability to drive the generation and differentiation of Treg cells that can inhibit the antigen-specific immune responses (45, 46). Moreover, IL-10 also affects the function of Treg cells (35). In NOD mice, overexpression of IL-10 can dramatically induce Treg cells and therefore ameliorates the development of type 1 diabetes (47). However, we found that *Il-10* deficiency in *BDC2.5*$^{+}$ NOD mice did not affect the frequency and function of Treg cells. Consistent with previous findings that IL-10 strongly inhibited the cytokine production (48) and the proliferation of CD4^{+} T cells (49), we found that *Il-10* deficiency significantly affected the cytokine expression in CD4^{+} T cells and enhanced the immune response of *BDC2.5*$^{+}$ CD4^{+} T cells to specific antigen stimulation. Moreover, *Il-10* deficiency modulated the activation of *BDC2.5*$^{+}$ NOD CD4^{+} T cells, with increased expression of T-bet, CD69, IFN-γ, TNF-α and IL-17A. Most importantly, *Il-10* deficiency changed the function of CD4^{+} T cells as *BDC2.5*$^{+}$*Il-10*$^{-/-}$ CD4^{+} T cells were more pathogenic and induced rapid diabetes onset in NOD.*scid* mice compared with those CD4^{+} T cells from *BDC2.5*$^{+}$*Il-10*$^{+/+}$ NOD mice. Therefore, *Il-10* deficiency in *BDC2.5*$^{+}$ NOD mice significantly affects the activation, proliferation, and function of CD4^{+} T cells, and thus contributes to the development of type 1 diabetes.

Although T cells have been well documented to play predominant roles in type 1 diabetes development, there is increasing evidence from both animal models and human beings that neutrophils from the innate immune system also contribute the initiation and progression of type 1 diabetes (15, 17, 21, 22). In addition to any effects on CD4^{+} T cells, *Il-10* deficiency had a significant impact on homeostasis of neutrophils in different tissues and expanded neutrophils in the bone marrow, peripheral blood, spleen, and islets in *BDC2.5*$^{+}$ NOD mice. Interestingly, we found that the change in the frequency of neutrophils was mediated by the altered gut microbiota in *BDC2.5*$^{+}$*Il-10*$^{-/-}$ NOD mice, as this expansion was ameliorated by the depletion of the endogenous commensal microbiota *via* antibiotic treatment. Our work furthers the current understanding from other studies where gut microbiota was shown to regulate the host immunity by influencing neutrophil production and activation (50). Khosravi et al. also demonstrated that germ-free (GF) animals displayed reduced proportions of neutrophils in bone marrow and spleen (51). Microbially-derived components can regulate neutrophil homeostasis as the neutrophil reduction was rescued by treatment with microbe-associated molecular patterns from heat-killed *E coli* or autoclaved cecal content (51). Gut microbiota have been documented to regulate granulocytosis and neutrophil homeostasis by influencing the intestinal IL-17-producing cells and the release of granulocyte colony-stimulating factor (G-CSF) in a Toll-like receptor 4 (TLR4)/myeloid differentiation factor 88 (MyD88)-dependent manner (23). Additionally, Zhang and colleagues found that gut

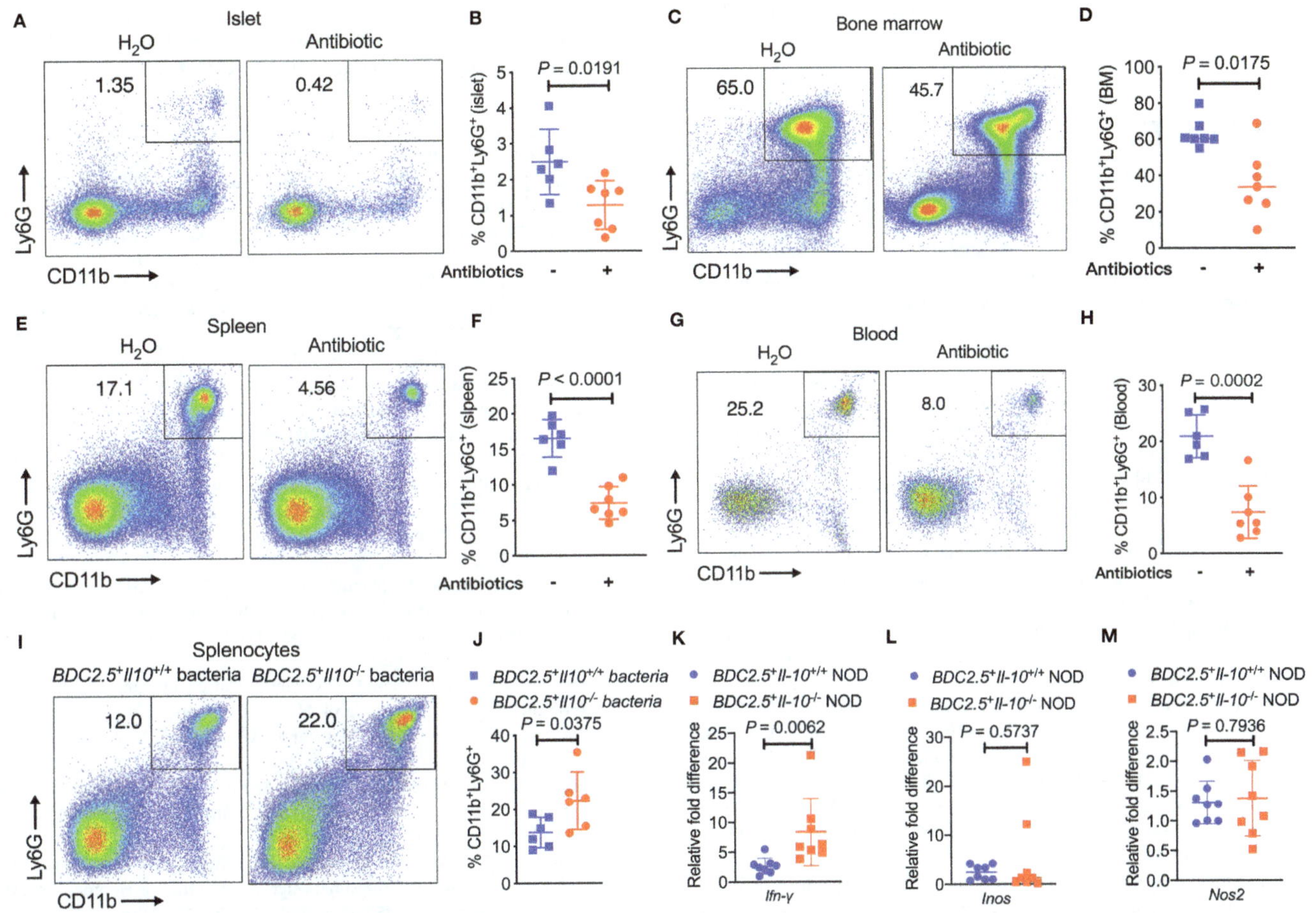

FIGURE 6 | $BDC2.5^{+}Il\text{-}10^{-/-}$ NOD gut bacteria modulate neutrophil homeostasis. **(A–H)** $BDC2.5^{+}Il\text{-}10^{-/-}$ NOD mice showed altered percentages of neutrophils after antibiotic treatment (n = 6-7/group). Representative flow cytometric profiles, and summary of $CD11b^{+}Ly6G^{+}$ neutrophils in the islets gated from $CD45^{+}$ immune cells **(A, B)**, in the bone marrow gated from $TCR\beta^{-}$ cells **(C, D)**, in the spleen gated from $TCR\beta^{-}$ cells **(E, F)**, and in the blood gated from live cells **(G, H)**. **(I, J)** Proportion of $CD11b^{+}Ly6G^{+}$ neutrophils in the splenocytes stimulated with heat-inactivated gut bacteria from either $BDC2.5^{+}Il\text{-}10^{+/+}$ NOD mice or $BDC2.5^{+}Il\text{-}10^{-/-}$ NOD mice (n = 6/group). Representative flow cytometric profiles **(I)**, and summary of $CD11b^{+}Ly6G^{+}$ neutrophils gated from $TCR\text{-}\beta^{-}$ cells **(J)**. **(K–M)** Gene expression of *Ifn-γ* **(K)**, *Inos* **(L)**, and *Nos2* **(M)** from purified splenic neutrophils after stimulation with heat-inactivated gut bacteria from either $BDC2.5^{+}Il\text{-}10^{+/+}$ NOD mice or $BDC2.5^{+}Il\text{-}10^{-/-}$ NOD mice (n = 8/group). Data in **(B, D, F, H, J–M)** were combined from two or more independent experiments. Data in **(B, F, H, J, K, M)** are presented as mean ± SD and statistical analysis was performed by a two-tailed Student's *t*-test. Data in **(D, L)** are presented as Median and were analyzed using a two-tailed Mann-Whitney test. $P < 0.05$ was considered statistically significant.

microbiota modulate the neutrophil ageing and the depletion of the microbiota can significantly reduce the number of circulating aged neutrophils (24). Our studies suggest that gut microbiota might affect type 1 diabetes development through modulating neutrophil hemostasis, especially by increasing neutrophil infiltration in the islets. Further investigation is needed to elucidate how gut microbiota modulate neutrophils and their role in the development of type 1 diabetes. To better understand the role of IL-10 in regulation of gut microbiota and gut microbiota-associated neutrophil hemostasis, the ideal approach would be to generate germ free *Il-10* deficient mice. This would be our future direction.

Taken together, by depleting *Il-10* in *BDC2.5*$^{+}$ NOD mice, we generated a markedly accelerated model of type 1 diabetes. Our studies showed that *Il-10* deficiency in *BDC2.5*$^{+}$ NOD mice significantly altered the immune response and function of $CD4^{+}$ T cells. Importantly, we showed that the effect of IL-10 on the homeostasis of neutrophils was mediated by the altered gut microbiota. Thus, our study suggests that gut microbiota might contribute to the development of type 1 diabetes by regulation of neutrophil homeostasis. These findings may provide novel insights into the role of IL-10 in the modulation of both innate immune cells and adaptive immune cells and the development of autoimmunity, such as type 1 diabetes.

AUTHOR CONTRIBUTIONS

LW conceived the project. JH, QT, NT, JAP, YL, CC, LZ, JP, YX, LYZ, and YH researched the data. ZZ contributed to the discussion. JH wrote the manuscript. LW, FW, and JAP revised the manuscript. All authors contributed to the article and approved the submitted version.

ACKNOWLEDGMENTS

The authors thank the technicians, especially Juan Carlos Roman, for taking care the animals used in the study.

REFERENCES

1. Miyazaki A, Hanafusa T, Yamada K, Miyagawa J, Fujino-Kurihara H, Nakajima H, et al. Predominance of T Lymphocytes in Pancreatic Islets and Spleen of Pre-Diabetic Non-Obese Diabetic (NOD) Mice: A Longitudinal Study. *Clin Exp Immunol* (1985) 60(3):622–30.
2. Hanafusa T, Miyazaki A, Miyagawa J, Tamura S, Inada M, Yamada K, et al. Examination of Islets in the Pancreas Biopsy Specimens From Newly Diagnosed Type 1 (Insulin-Dependent) Diabetic Patients. *Diabetologia* (1990) 33(2):105–11. doi: 10.1007/BF00401048
3. Lampeter EF, Homberg M, Quabeck K, Schaefer UW, Wernet P, Bertrams J, et al. Transfer of Insulin-Dependent Diabetes Between HLA-Identical Siblings by Bone Marrow Transplantation. *Lancet* (1993) 341(8855):1243–4. doi: 10.1016/0140-6736(93)91148-F
4. Wicker LS, Miller BJ, Mullen Y. Transfer of Autoimmune Diabetes Mellitus With Splenocytes From Nonobese Diabetic (NOD) Mice. *Diabetes* (1986) 35 (8):855–60. doi: 10.2337/diabetes.35.8.855
5. Haskins K, Portas M, Bradley B, Wegmann D, Lafferty K. T-Lymphocyte Clone Specific for Pancreatic Islet Antigen. *Diabetes* (1988) 37(10):1444–8. doi: 10.2337/diab.37.10.1444
6. Katz JD, Wang B, Haskins K, Benoist C, Mathis D. Following a Diabetogenic T Cell From Genesis Through Pathogenesis. *Cell* (1993) 74(6):1089–100. doi: 10.1016/0092-8674(93)90730-E
7. Hoglund P, Mintern J, Waltzinger C, Heath W, Benoist C, Mathis D. Initiation of Autoimmune Diabetes by Developmentally Regulated Presentation of Islet Cell Antigens in the Pancreatic Lymph Nodes. *J Exp Med* (1999) 189(2):331–9. doi: 10.1084/jem.189.2.331
8. Gonzalez A, Katz JD, Mattei MG, Kikutani H, Benoist C, Mathis D. Genetic Control of Diabetes Progression. *Immunity* (1997) 7(6):873–83. doi: 10.1016/S1074-7613(00)80405-7
9. Kurrer MO, Pakala SV, Hanson HL, Katz JD. Beta Cell Apoptosis in T Cell-Mediated Autoimmune Diabetes. *Proc Natl Acad Sci USA* (1997) 94(1):213–8. doi: 10.1073/pnas.94.1.213
10. Gonzalez A, Andre-Schmutz I, Carnaud C, Mathis D, Benoist C. Damage Control, Rather Than Unresponsiveness, Effected by Protective DX5+ T Cells in Autoimmune Diabetes. *Nat Immunol* (2001) 2(12):1117–25. doi: 10.1038/ni738
11. Tang Q, Henriksen KJ, Bi M, Finger EB, Szot G, Ye J, et al. In Vitro-Expanded Antigen-Specific Regulatory T Cells Suppress Autoimmune Diabetes. *J Exp Med* (2004) 199(11):1455–65. doi: 10.1084/jem.20040139
12. Tarbell KV, Yamazaki S, Olson K, Toy P, Steinman RM. CD25+ CD4+ T Cells, Expanded With Dendritic Cells Presenting a Single Autoantigenic Peptide, Suppress Autoimmune Diabetes. *J Exp Med* (2004) 199(11):1467–77. doi: 10.1084/jem.20040180
13. Feuerer M, Shen Y, Littman DR, Benoist C, Mathis D. How Punctual Ablation of Regulatory T Cells Unleashes an Autoimmune Lesion Within the Pancreatic Islets. *Immunity* (2009) 31(4):654–64. doi: 10.1016/j.immuni.2009.08.023
14. Xiang Y, Peng J, Tai N, Hu C, Zhou Z, Wong FS, et al. The Dual Effects of B Cell Depletion on Antigen-Specific T Cells in BDC2.5NOD Mice. *J Immunol* (2012) 188(10):4747–58. doi: 10.4049/jimmunol.1103055
15. Diana J, Simoni Y, Furio L, Beaudoin L, Agerberth B, Barrat F, et al. Crosstalk Between Neutrophils, B-1a Cells and Plasmacytoid Dendritic Cells Initiates Autoimmune Diabetes. *Nat Med* (2013) 19(1):65–73. doi: 10.1038/nm.3042
16. Diana J, Lehuen A. Macrophages and Beta-Cells Are Responsible for CXCR2-Mediated Neutrophil Infiltration of the Pancreas During Autoimmune Diabetes. *EMBO Mol Med* (2014) 6(8):1090–104. doi: 10.15252/emmm.201404144
17. Wang Y, Xiao Y, Zhong L, Ye D, Zhang J, Tu Y, et al. Increased Neutrophil Elastase and Proteinase 3 and Augmented NETosis Are Closely Associated With Beta-Cell Autoimmunity in Patients With Type 1 Diabetes. *Diabetes* (2014) 63(12):4239–48. doi: 10.2337/db14-0480
18. Valle A, Giamporcaro GM, Scavini M, Stabilini A, Grogan P, Bianconi E, et al. Reduction of Circulating Neutrophils Precedes and Accompanies Type 1 Diabetes. *Diabetes* (2013) 62(6):2072–7. doi: 10.2337/db12-1345
19. Harsunen MH, Puff R, D'Orlando O, Giannopoulou E, Lachmann L, Beyerlein A, et al. Reduced Blood Leukocyte and Neutrophil Numbers in the Pathogenesis of Type 1 Diabetes. *Horm Metab Res* (2013) 45(6):467–70. doi: 10.1055/s-0032-1331226
20. Huang J, Xiao Y, Zheng P, Zhou W, Wang Y, Huang G, et al. Distinct Neutrophil Counts and Functions in Newly Diagnosed Type 1 Diabetes, Latent Autoimmune Diabetes in Adults, and Type 2 Diabetes. *Diabetes Metab Res Rev* (2019) 35(1):e3064. doi: 10.1002/dmrr.3064
21. Salami F, Lee HS, Freyhult E, Elding Larsson H, Lernmark A, Torn C, et al. Reduction in White Blood Cell, Neutrophil, and Red Blood Cell Counts Related to Sex, HLA, and Islet Autoantibodies in Swedish TEDDY Children at Increased Risk for Type 1 Diabetes. *Diabetes* (2018) 67(11):2329–36. doi: 10.2337/db18-0355
22. Vecchio F, Lo Buono N, Stabilini A, Nigi L, Dufort MJ, Geyer S, et al. Abnormal Neutrophil Signature in the Blood and Pancreas of Presymptomatic and Symptomatic Type 1 Diabetes. *JCI Insight* (2018) 3(18): e122146. doi: 10.1172/jci.insight.122146
23. Deshmukh HS, Liu Y, Menkiti OR, Mei J, Dai N, O'Leary CE, et al. The Microbiota Regulates Neutrophil Homeostasis and Host Resistance to Escherichia Coli K1 Sepsis in Neonatal Mice. *Nat Med* (2014) 20(5):524–30. doi: 10.1038/nm.3542
24. Zhang D, Chen G, Manwani D, Mortha A, Xu C, Faith JJ, et al. Neutrophil Ageing Is Regulated by the Microbiome. *Nature* (2015) 525(7570):528–32. doi: 10.1038/nature15367
25. Wen L, Ley RE, Volchkov PY, Stranges PB, Avanesyan L, Stonebraker AC, et al. Innate Immunity and Intestinal Microbiota in the Development of Type 1 Diabetes. *Nature* (2008) 455(7216):1109–13. doi: 10.1038/nature07336
26. Hu Y, Peng J, Li F, Wong FS, Wen L. Evaluation of Different Mucosal Microbiota Leads to Gut Microbiota-Based Prediction of Type 1 Diabetes in NOD Mice. *Sci Rep* (2018) 8(1):15451. doi: 10.1038/s41598-018-33571-z
27. Tai N, Peng J, Liu F, Gulden E, Hu Y, Zhang X, et al. Microbial Antigen Mimics Activate Diabetogenic CD8 T Cells in NOD Mice. *J Exp Med* (2016) 213(10):2129–46. doi: 10.1084/jem.20160526
28. Livanos AE, Greiner TU, Vangay P, Pathmasiri W, Stewart D, McRitchie S, et al. Antibiotic-Mediated Gut Microbiome Perturbation Accelerates Development of Type 1 Diabetes in Mice. *Nat Microbiol* (2016) 1 (11):16140. doi: 10.1038/nmicrobiol.2016.140
29. Mullaney JA, Stephens JE, Costello ME, Fong C, Geeling BE, Gavin PG, et al. Type 1 Diabetes Susceptibility Alleles Are Associated With Distinct Alterations in the Gut Microbiota. *Microbiome* (2018) 6(1):35. doi: 10.1186/s40168-018-0438-z
30. Kostic AD, Gevers D, Siljander H, Vatanen T, Hyotylainen T, Hamalainen AM, et al. The Dynamics of the Human Infant Gut Microbiome in Development and in Progression Toward Type 1 Diabetes. *Cell Host Microbe* (2015) 17(2):260–73. doi: 10.1016/j.chom.2015.01.001
31. Vatanen T, Franzosa EA, Schwager R, Tripathi S, Arthur TD, Vehik K, et al. The Human Gut Microbiome in Early-Onset Type 1 Diabetes From the TEDDY Study. *Nature* (2018) 562(7728):589–94. doi: 10.1038/s41586-018-0620-2
32. Herfarth HH, Mohanty SP, Rath HC, Tonkonogy S, Sartor RB. Interleukin 10 Suppresses Experimental Chronic, Granulomatous Inflammation Induced by Bacterial Cell Wall Polymers. *Gut* (1996) 39(6):836–45. doi: 10.1136/gut.39.6.836
33. Steidler L, Hans W, Schotte L, Neirynck S, Obermeier F, Falk W, et al. Treatment of Murine Colitis by Lactococcus Lactis Secreting Interleukin-10. *Science* (2000) 289(5483):1352–5. doi: 10.1126/science.289.5483.1352

34. Wu C, Sartor RB, Huang K, Tonkonogy SL. Transient Activation of Mucosal Effector Immune Responses by Resident Intestinal Bacteria in Normal Hosts Is Regulated by Interleukin-10 Signalling. *Immunology* (2016) 148(3):304–14. doi: 10.1111/imm.12612
35. Asseman C, Mauze S, Leach MW, Coffman RL, Powrie F. An Essential Role for Interleukin 10 in the Function of Regulatory T Cells That Inhibit Intestinal Inflammation. *J Exp Med* (1999) 190(7):995–1004. doi: 10.1084/jem.190.7.995
36. Kingsley CI, Karim M, Bushell AR, Wood KJ. CD25+CD4+ Regulatory T Cells Prevent Graft Rejection: CTLA-4- and IL-10-Dependent Immunoregulation of Alloresponses. *J Immunol* (2002) 168(3):1080–6. doi: 10.4049/jimmunol.168.3.1080
37. Chaudhry A, Samstein RM, Treuting P, Liang Y, Pils MC, Heinrich JM, et al. Interleukin-10 Signaling in Regulatory T Cells Is Required for Suppression of Th17 Cell-Mediated Inflammation. *Immunity* (2011) 34(4):566–78. doi: 10.1016/j.immuni.2011.03.018
38. Saraiva M, O'Garra A. The Regulation of IL-10 Production by Immune Cells. *Nat Rev Immunol* (2010) 10(3):170–81. doi: 10.1038/nri2711
39. Moore KW, de Waal Malefyt R, Coffman RL, O'Garra A. Interleukin-10 and the Interleukin-10 Receptor. *Annu Rev Immunol* (2001) 19:683–765. doi: 10.1146/annurev.immunol.19.1.683
40. Balasa B, Davies JD, Lee J, Good A, Yeung BT, Sarvetnick N. IL-10 Impacts Autoimmune Diabetes via a CD8+ T Cell Pathway Circumventing the Requirement for CD4+ T and B Lymphocytes. *J Immunol* (1998) 161 (8):4420–7.
41. Pennline KJ, Roque-Gaffney E, Monahan M. Recombinant Human IL-10 Prevents the Onset of Diabetes in the Nonobese Diabetic Mouse. *Clin Immunol Immunopathol* (1994) 71(2):169–75. doi: 10.1006/clin.1994.1068
42. Wogensen L, Huang X, Sarvetnick N. Leukocyte Extravasation Into the Pancreatic Tissue in Transgenic Mice Expressing Interleukin 10 in the Islets of Langerhans. *J Exp Med* (1993) 178(1):175–85. doi: 10.1084/jem.178.1.175
43. Balasa B, Van Gunst K, Jung N, Balakrishna D, Santamaria P, Hanafusa T, et al. Islet-Specific Expression of IL-10 Promotes Diabetes in Nonobese Diabetic Mice Independent of Fas, Perforin, TNF Receptor-1, and TNF Receptor-2 Molecules. *J Immunol* (2000) 165(5):2841–9. doi: 10.4049/jimmunol.165.5.2841
44. Balasa B, Van Gunst K, Jung N, Katz JD, Sarvetnick N. IL-10 Deficiency Does Not Inhibit Insulitis and Accelerates Cyclophosphamide-Induced Diabetes in the Nonobese Diabetic Mouse. *Cell Immunol* (2000) 202(2):97–102. doi: 10.1006/cimm.2000.1658
45. Groux H, O'Garra A, Bigler M, Rouleau M, Antonenko S, de Vries JE. Roncarolo MG. A CD4+ T-Cell Subset Inhibits Antigen-Specific T-Cell Responses and Prevents Colitis. *Nature* (1997) 389(6652):737–42. doi: 10.1038/39614
46. Levings MK, Sangregorio R, Galbiati F, Squadrone S, de Waal Malefyt R, Roncarolo MG. IFN-Alpha and IL-10 Induce the Differentiation of Human Type 1 T Regulatory Cells. *J Immunol* (2001) 166(9):5530–9. doi: 10.4049/jimmunol.166.9.5530
47. Goudy KS, Burkhardt BR, Wasserfall C, Song S, Campbell-Thompson ML, Brusko T, et al. Systemic Overexpression of IL-10 Induces CD4+CD25+ Cell Populations In Vivo and Ameliorates Type 1 Diabetes in Nonobese Diabetic Mice in a Dose-Dependent Fashion. *J Immunol* (2003) 171(5):2270–8. doi: 10.4049/jimmunol.171.5.2270
48. Fiorentino DF, Zlotnik A, Vieira P, Mosmann TR, Howard M, Moore KW, et al. IL-10 Acts on the Antigen-Presenting Cell to Inhibit Cytokine Production by Th1 Cells. *J Immunol* (1991) 146(10):3444–51.
49. de Waal Malefyt R, Haanen J, Spits H, Roncarolo MG, te Velde A, Figdor C, et al. Interleukin 10 (IL-10) and Viral IL-10 Strongly Reduce Antigen-Specific Human T Cell Proliferation by Diminishing the Antigen-Presenting Capacity of Monocytes via Downregulation of Class II Major Histocompatibility Complex Expression. *J Exp Med* (1991) 174(4):915–24. doi: 10.1084/jem.174.4.915
50. Zhang D, Frenette PS. Cross Talk Between Neutrophils and the Microbiota. *Blood* (2019) 133(20):2168–77. doi: 10.1182/blood-2018-11-844555
51. Khosravi A, Yanez A, Price JG, Chow A, Merad M, Goodridge HS, et al. Gut Microbiota Promote Hematopoiesis to Control Bacterial Infection. *Cell Host Microbe* (2014) 15(3):374–81. doi: 10.1016/j.chom.2014.02.006

2

Insights from Single Cell RNA Sequencing Into the Immunology of Type 1 Diabetes-Cell Phenotypes and Antigen Specificity

Stephanie J. Hanna[1*]*, Danijela Tatovic*[1]*, Terri C. Thayer*[1,2] *and Colin M. Dayan*[1,3]

Diabetes Research Group, Division of Infection and Immunity, School of Medicine, Cardiff University, Cardiff, United Kingdom, Department of Biological and Chemical Sciences, School of Natural and Social Sciences, Roberts Wesleyan College, Rochester, NY, United States, [3] *Wellcome Centre for Human Genetics, University of Oxford, Oxford, United Kingdom*

Correspondence:
Stephanie J. Hanna
HannaSJ@cf.ac.uk

In the past few years, huge advances have been made in techniques to analyse cells at an individual level using RNA sequencing, and many of these have precipitated exciting discoveries in the immunology of type 1 diabetes (T1D). This review will cover the first papers to use scRNAseq to characterise human lymphocyte phenotypes in T1D in the peripheral blood, pancreatic lymph nodes and islets. These have revealed specific genes such as IL-32 that are differentially expressed in islet –specific T cells in T1D. scRNAseq has also revealed wider gene expression patterns that are involved in T1D and can predict its development even predating autoantibody production. Single cell sequencing of TCRs has revealed V genes and CDR3 motifs that are commonly used to target islet autoantigens, although truly public TCRs remain elusive. Little is known about BCR repertoires in T1D, but scRNAseq approaches have revealed that insulin binding BCRs commonly use specific J genes, share motifs between donors and frequently demonstrate poly-reactivity. This review will also summarise new developments in scRNAseq technology, the insights they have given into other diseases and how they could be leveraged to advance research in the type 1 diabetes field to identify novel biomarkers and targets for immunotherapy.

Keywords: type 1 diabetes, scRNAseq, immunology, lymphocytes, TCR - T cell receptor, BCR - B cell receptor

INTRODUCTION

It is widely accepted that in T1D "there remains a paucity of robust and accepted biomarkers that can effectively inform on the activity of T cells during the natural history of the disease or in response to treatment" (1). Furthermore, the phenotype and roles of autoreactive B cells in T1D have received less attention than T cells (2–4). Whilst flow and mass cytometry approaches have

Abbreviations: AAB+, Autoantibody positive; DE cell, dual expressor cell reported to express both a TCR and a BCR'; DEG, differentially expressed genes; GEX, gene expression; scRNAseq, single cell RNA sequencing.

enabled many insights into cell phenotypes and antigen specificity in type 1 diabetes [reviewed (5)], they allow detection of a relatively small number of markers, limiting the potential to discover truly novel biomarkers. In turn this limits the ability to monitor the natural history of diabetes development and patient responses to immunotherapy. In addition, although a number of immunomodulatory agents are in clinical trials for type 1 diabetes, these are generally non-specific in their actions (for example targeting CD3 or CD20) (6), and there remains a need to identify and target pathways that are perturbed specifically in islet-antigen specific lymphocytes.

Traditional RNA sequencing involves taking all cells of interest, and combining their RNA in a single sample before sequencing. In contrast, single cell RNA sequencing isolates individual cells, either through sorting into wells, or using droplet based technology (7). Transcripts from each cell are barcoded (a unique molecular identifier is also added to each transcript to circumvent any amplification bias), before being combined for sequencing. This allows quantification of the expression of every gene in every individual cell, so that cell phenotypes and heterogeneity can be fully elucidated. Of particular interest to immunologists are scRNAseq methods that allow sequencing across the V(D)J region of TCRs and BCRs. This allows capture of the paired TCRα and β chains (or paired heavy and light chains of BCRs) which is key to determining antigen specificity (8, 9) and being able to reconstitute the receptor in a cell line or to express it as a secreted antibody. A single cell sequencing approach also avoids much of the bias of bulk RNAseq of receptors (10).

There are a variety of methods used for scRNAseq [reviewed (7)] although the 10x Genomics platform has come to dominate the field, due to the relatively large number of cells that can be sampled and options of combining, for example, protein expression and V(D)J sequencing with standard gene expression (GEX) data (11, 12). In parallel, there has been an explosion in techniques to deal with the vast quantity of data generated, perform quality control and extract meaningful findings (13).

However, scRNAseq also comes with a number of caveats. Firstly it is technically challenging and poor sample preparation can lead to doublet formation in a similar manner to that seen in flow cytometry, but in addition scRNAseq samples are susceptible to contamination with RNA from dying cells and the downstream clustering algorithms can also produce seemingly novel cell populations which are in fact artefacts (14). Secondly, the high cost can make it somewhat inaccessible and limit sample numbers and sizes. Lastly, it requires stringent statistical analysis to avoid type 1 errors, preferably backed up by follow up experiments to verify findings (13).

Nevertheless, scRNAseq offers an exciting opportunity to identify novel biomarkers that could be indicative of diabetes progression in at risk individuals, and allow real-time monitoring of clinical trials through tracking expression of specific immuno-receptor sequences and cell phenotypes. Furthermore, it has the potential to discover novel targets for immunotherapy of type 1 diabetes, through the identification of genes that are differentially expressed in islet-antigen specific lymphocytes.

USING scRNAseq TO IDENTIFY BIOMARKERS FOR PROGRESSION TO TYPE 1 DIABETES AND PHENOTYPES IN T1D

scRNAseq's potential is demonstrated in a paper by Kallionpää et al. They revealed that high IL-32 expression in PBMCs was strongly associated with seroconversion and progression to T1D, contributed mainly by activated, highly differentiated, T cells and NK cells. Interestingly insulin (INS), glucagon (GCG), and REG1A were found to be upregulated in T1D and AAB+ individuals in the bulk RNAseq of PBMC but not in scRNAseq (15). These genes are normally associated with the pancreas, but expressed at the mRNA level in whole blood and lymph nodes at much lower levels (www.genecards.org). For insulin in particular this wider expression is thought to be involved in peripheral maintenance of tolerance (16).

We can also glean insight into the immunology of T1D from scRNAseq studies of the pancreas, as in T1D these will include infiltrating immune cells. For example, the Vahedi group performed scRNAseq of human pancreatic islet cells and found particular enrichment of antigen-presenting cells and macrophages in T1D (17). In a strong replication of Kallionpää et al.'s findings, an analysis of differentially expressed genes (DEG) in immune cells between healthy and type 1 diabetes pancreas samples identified REG1B, REG1A, INS and REG3A and IL-32 as highly differentially expressed (17). As with INS, GCG and REG1A, REG1B and REG3A are highly expressed in the pancreas but at lower levels in the blood and lymph nodes. Furthermore REG genes are reported to be upregulated in the pancreas not only in people that have T1D, but also those who are autoantibody positive (18). They are upregulated in inflammatory conditions and are thought to be important in the survival of beta cells in T1D (18). An alternative explanation for the association of these RNA transcripts with immune cells is that RNA transcripts from dying beta cells are contaminating other cell types during the scRNAseq process (19). A similar scRNAseq analysis of the NOD mouse pancreas has also been conducted (20) and scRNAseq has been used to characterise hESCs differentiating into beta cells (21). Studies using scRNAseq to investigate the human pancreas and T1D are summarised in **Table 1**.

Closely related to scRNAseq is scATACseq, whereby the DNA from individual cell nuclei is analysed to identify open or accessible chromatin regions and hence predict which genes are being expressed in each cell. Recently, Chiou et al. combined scATACseq with bulk ATACseq and scRNAseq approaches to link cis-regulatory elements (CREs e.g. gene promoters and enhancers) in peripheral blood cells and pancreatic cells with GWAS of diabetes risk (23). As would be expected this identified

TABLE 1 | human scRNAseq gene expression studies relevant to type 1 diabetes.

Paper	Tissues	Antigen receptors	T1D status	Citation	Notes
Fasolino et al.	Pancreas	no	Healthy donors, AAB+, T1D	(17)	
Kallionpää et al.	PBMC	no	Healthy donors, AAB+	(15)	Children <3 2/4 AAB+ rapidly developed T1D
Xin et al.	Pancreas	no	Healthy donors, T1D	(22)	All islet cells sequenced, but analysis of beta cells only
Chiou et al.	PBMC pancreas	no	Healthy donors, T1D	(23)	scATACseq of PBMCs and pancreas of healthy donors. Reanalysis of healthy donor and T1D islet scRNAseq (22)
Cerosaletti et al.	PBMC	TCRs	Healthy donors, T1D	(24)	Islet-reactive T cells
Fuchs YF et al.	PBMC	TCRs	Healthy donors, T1D	(25)	Only one T1D sample
Culina S et al.	PBMC	TCRs	Healthy donors, T1D	(26)	Sorted ZnT8 186-194 MMr+CD8+ T cells.
Heninger et al.	PBMC	TCRs	Healthy donors, children who later progressed to T1D	(27)	GAD65- and proinsulin-responsive CD4+ T cells, limited genes sequenced in scRNAseq
Ahmed R, et al.	PBMC	TCRs, BCRs	T1D	(28)	Single donor
Hao Y et al.	Pancreas	no	Healthy children-older adults (29) Unspecified (30) Unspecified (31) Healthy controls and T2D (32) Healthy controls and T2D (33) Unspecified (34) Healthy controls (35)	(12)	Combines multiple previous scRNAseq datasets to make a reference dataset and app, Azimuth

many CREs used in T cells and beta cells that had genetic variants associated with T1D susceptibility. For example CREs that controlled CTLA4 and CCR7 expression in T cells had variants associated with T1D. Importantly, this paper also identified CREs used in pancreatic cells that had polymorphisms associated with T1D risk, particularly those used in acinar and ductal cells. They were further able to map the T1D risk allele of rs7795896 to a CRE used in ductal cells. The risk variant was associated with decreased CFTR expression in ductal cells. Mutations in CFTR itself cause cystic fibrosis, frequently associated with pancreatic exocrine and endocrine abnormalities, but this is this first demonstration of a role for it, and may other genes expressed in the exocrine pancreas, in T1D pathogenesis. This paper also produced a reference map of single-cell chromatin accessibility from T1D-relevant cells from healthy donors (i.e. lymphoid, myeloid and pancreatic endocrine and non-endocrine cells). Interestingly scRNAseq of the human pancreas also identified multiple changes in gene expression in ductal cells in T1D (17). In particular expression of MHC Class II pathway and interferon alpha and beta pathway genes were increased. Other developments in the field of epigenetics of T1D and the interplay with environmental triggers [reviewed (36–38)] have also started to yield evidence of pathogenic roles for molecules such as BACH2, IL23A, IL6R and IL6ST in T cell function in T1D (39). It will be of great interest to see how our understanding of epigenetics in T1D develops at the single cell level.

scRNAseq OF TCRS

Methods to Identify Antigen Specific T Cells

As discussed above, there are many advantages of single cell sequencing TCRs over bulk TCR repertoire sequencing. Before the advent of large scale scRNAseq, many people in the type 1 diabetes field appreciated the importance of sequencing immunoreceptors on a single cell basis and linking this to antigen specificity and affinity (40–42). As of 2017 there were 1655 clonotypes of known specificity for T1D autoantigens (41), a number which has increased substantially with the advent of higher throughput scRNAseq.

These have been identified through a numbers of methods. HLA class I or class II multimers may be used to select antigen specific T cells. This has the advantage of being able to select cells from the peripheral blood but is limited by HLA restriction and to known epitopes or mimotopes (43). In addition non-specific binding may yield false-positive TCRs. Alternatively peripheral blood T cells can be stimulated *in vitro* with islet peptide pools and selected on the basis of upregulation of activation markers, allowing wider specificities and HLA compatibilities, but with the risk of bystander activation again resulting in false negatives. A third approach is to sample T cells directly from the pLN or pancreas, where islet-specific T cells will be massively enriched. These cells can then either be stimulated *in vitro* with peptide pools the TCRs re-expressed *ex vivo* to determine specificity. Alternatively, TCR sequences can be compared to those in the literature known to be islet antigen specific.

Diabetes Autoantigen- Specific Paired TCRs in the Peripheral Blood

Eugster and colleagues performed an heroic effort to sequence paired TCRs from 1650 T cells that either bound a GAD tetramer or responded to GAD *in vitro*, by sorting single cells from the peripheral blood and performing plate based scRNAseq (44). GAD specific TCRs were highly heterogenous both within and between donors, with no shared TCRs between donors, although individual TCRα or TCRβ chains were often shared. Moreover, there was limited overlap between the TCRs identified by tetramer binding and T cell activation methods, indicating that epitope recognition and MHC usage by GAD specific TCRs was likely to be broad (44).

Cerosaletti et al. performed scRNAseq of islet-reactive TCRs from the peripheral blood (identified by *ex vivo* response to stimulation with islet-peptide pools). They found that T cells from T1D had higher numbers of identical CDR3, which had arisen by clonal expansion (i.e. T cells with identical TCRα and TCRβ chains, that have arisen by division of a parent cell), rather than convergent recombination (24). By re-expressing the TCRs in cell lines it was found that many of these TCRs in people with T1D were IGRP specific (24). It was further shown that donors with T1D had large clonal expansions of IGRP-reactive T cells in the peripheral blood and frequently used a specific shared TCRα chain, which was paired with different beta chains in each donor (45). Preferential usage of TRAJ53 and TRAV29 and TCRα chains bearing the motif SGGSNYKLTF were identified in single cell TCR sequencing of people with T1D. When a bulk sequencing approach was taken, a particular TCRα chain bearing this motif was highly enriched in the memory CD8+ T cells of autoantibody positive people and those with T1D compared to controls. Clones bearing the motif were also shown to directly kill IGRP- peptide bearing cells (45). T cell clones bearing both IGRP (24, 45) and hybrid insulin peptide-responsive TCRs are persistent over time (46). However, others have examined TCR repertoires in children progressing to diabetes and shared TCRs were not seen either between children or within the same child over time, indicating high diversity in the peripheral blood at this age (27).

Diabetes Autoantigen- Specific Paired TCRs in the Pancreas and Pancreatic Lymph Nodes

Early work examined T cells from the pancreatic lymph nodes (pLN) of people with T1D and found high clonal expansions (47). Additionally there were many T cells that shared a TCRβ but had divergent TCRα. Many clonally expanded CD4+ T cells recognised insulin A1-15 in the context of DR4 (47). Pathiraja et al. grew out CD4+T cells from the pancreatic islets of a donor with T1D using anti CD3 and cytokine stimulation. Over 25% of these clones had TCRs that responded to proinsulin peptides restricted by HLA-DQ8 or the HLA-DQ8 transdimer and 30% of clones used TRBV5–1*01 (48). Whilst it is difficult to make direct comparisons to frequencies of islet-reactive T cells in the peripheral blood (26), it is clear that in the peripheral blood frequencies are much lower [around 0.01-0.05% of T cells in people with T1D (3, 44, 49)]. Most T cells isolated from the pancreas had unique clonotypes, whilst the majority of *in vivo* clonally expanded T cells were specific for proinsulin (48). It has also been found that ZnT8- reactive T cells were present at similar frequencies in the blood of healthy controls and people with T1D, but were enriched in the pancreas of the latter (26). Single cell sequencing of TCRs found a public ZnT8 specific CDR3B in the peripheral blood, and enriched in the pancreas of people with T1D, although the full TCRβ had divergent sequences due to different gene usages. ZnT8 reactive T cells also showed a bias towards TRBV19 and TRAV12-2 usage (26).

Seay et al. also found sharing of CDR3s between donors in the pancreas, with a TCRβ with homology to a known GAD reactive TCR found in 7/18 T1D donors (50). Furthermore a shared CDR3β chain was found in all people with T1D in the conventional T cell compartment, whilst in healthy controls it was predominantly in the Treg compartment (50). Interestingly TCR sequencing of GAD-responsive CD4+IL-13+ T cells from patients who had received injected GAD Alum found that they often used a highly public TCRβ (TCRα sequencing was not available) (51).

Direct capture of pancreatic T cells by the Nakayama group enabled single cell TCR sequencing and confirmed infiltration of proinsulin specific cells into the pancreas in T1D. Of the hundreds of TCRs sequenced, most were present only on a single cell, indicating a diversity of response even years after diagnosis. Clonal expansions were more likely in CD8+ T cells and these clones were found in multiple islets from the same donor, indicating *in vivo* migration. Furthermore, across three donors it was noted that whilst there were no identical TCRs, there were identical TCRα sequences and TCR subunits (52). When the TCRs were re-expressed, the B9-23 reactive TCRs isolated from the pancreas induced much higher IL-2 secretion compared to control B9-23 TCRs isolated from peripheral blood (52) which may indicate the former have a higher affinity for B9-23. Moreover, only the pancreas-derived TCRs were capable of a response to whole proinsulin presented by APCs (52).

Recently the Nakayama group has reconstructed individual TCRs from the pancreas of people with T1D. TCRs were selected for re-expression on the basis of clonal expansion or V gene usage previously associated with proinsulin C19-A3 specificity, and were found to recognise epitopes across preproinsulin and presented by a variety of MHC class II (53). Many TCRs recognised peptides in the region of B9-23, but others, (many from clonally expanded cells) recognised peptide right across from the signal peptide to the A chain. Furthermore, these TCRs recognised peptides in the context of diverse MHCII, although a preference was shown for DQ (53). Even with these constraints of the selection criteria in this study, this single cell approach showed a diversity of peptide and MHCII specificity that would have been missed using tetramers.

New Avenues for scRNAseq of TCRs

Taken together, the evidence suggests that T cells with TCRs with higher affinity for diabetes autoantigens are more likely to be found in the pancreas than in the peripheral circulation. This represents a major challenge in T1D research as in other autoimmune diseases it is relatively straightforward to obtain samples from the site of autoimmune attack (54). For example in psoriatic arthritis, extraction of viable T cells directly from the affected joints enabled sequencing of paired TCR receptors and scRNAseq profiling of cells phenotypes (55). Even in the pancreas, clonal expansion is modest and whilst CDR3 sequences specific for many diabetes autoantigens are shared between donors, there is not yet evidence of truly public TCRs with identical TCRα and β chains. However, more widespread use of the VDJdb repository (56), IEDB (57) and the JDRF/nPOD CloneSearch might allow enriched motifs to become apparent across different experiments, although this would still be limited by HLA restriction. To further complicate the picture, scRNAseq has demonstrated that islet antigen –reactive T cells (24) and HIP reactive T cells in particular (58) sometimes express two TCRα chains, which are known to contribute to autoimmunity (59, 60).

Phenotypes of Antigen-Specific T Cells: Combining TCR Sequencing With Gene Expression

Combining TCR sequencing (or selection based on autoantigen reactivity), with scRNAseq has the potential to give further insights into T cell function. This has not always been straightforward to demonstrate, for example analysis of IGRP- specific T cells from the peripheral blood did not show a distinctive gene expression (GEX) pattern in response to stimulation (25). Similarly scRNAseq of ZnT8 reactive cells from the peripheral blood of people with T1D showed similar GEX profiles to healthy controls, indicating that these peripheral T cells may not be playing a driving role in T1D, although T1D patients had higher expression of aryl hydrocarbon receptor (AHR) and aurora kinase A (AURKA) and lower expression of RORA (26).

The approach was more successful for Heninger et al, who demonstrated that proinflammatory responses to diabetes autoantigens were dominant in children who progressed to autoantibody positivity, whilst regulatory T cell responses were seen in those who didn't (27). An algorithm based on gene expression in response to autoantigens enabled identification of which children would later progress to autoantibody positivity. As this group developed autoantibodies the GEX profiles of their CD4+ T cells changed towards increased expression of Th1 genes (27). These findings suggest that biomarkers of T1D susceptibility may allow identification of at risk children prior to seroconversion (61).

In addition, Cerosaletti et al. used islet peptide pools to stimulate T cells from the peripheral blood *in vitro* and characterised those that activated by scRNAseq. They did not observe a significant level of differentially expressed genes between healthy controls to those from people with T1D. However, when they focussed on cells from people with T1D that were highly clonally expanded (termed T1D-E cells), they found that these cells did have a unique transcriptional profile compared to islet reactive T cells from healthy controls or those from people with T1D that were not clonally expanded. T1D-E cells preferentially expressed genes associated with T cell activation and leukocyte differentiation (24). These experiments demonstrate how focussing on antigen specificity can enhance findings from scRNAseq.

scRNAseq OF BCRS

Early Work to Determine Antibody Sequences

Early interest in autoantibodies in T1D, before the advent of scRNAseq, focussed on isolating GAD-specific B cells from people with T1D (62) and sequencing the BCRs from clones, which provided evidence that GAD autoantibodies have frequently undergone somatic maturation and are therefore from antigen-experienced B cells (63, 64). Similarly IA-2 specific antibodies sequenced from B cells from people with T1D also show evidence of somatic mutation (65–67). Anti-insulin antibodies have been sequenced from people with T1D, but may have arisen in response to injected insulin rather than endogenous insulin (68, 69) [reviewed (70)]. BCR sequencing combined with phenotyping of B cells has given great insight into B cell response in other autoimmune diseases (71) and in response to vaccinations (72) and in B cell lymphoma (73). Yet without the equivalent of a tetramer approach to identifying autoreactive B cells, phenotyping and characterisation of the BCR has lagged behind T cell research in T1D.

Identifying Islet-Reactive BCRs in the Periphery, Pancreatic Lymph Nodes and Pancreas

Smith et al. developed an approach to isolate insulin reactive B cells from the peripheral blood of people with T1D, by flow cytometric sorting B cells that bound insulin conjugated to fluorescent tags. The authors were then able to sequence BCRs from individual cells. They demonstrated that insulin binding BCRs preferentially used JH6 gene segments which have previously been associated with autoreactivity and were biased towards use of positively charged amino acids in the CDR3 region (74). When re-expressed as antibodies, BCRs from anergic naive IgD^+, IgM^- B cells demonstrated binding at levels thought to induce anergic B cell responses, whilst those from naïve B cells bound weakly and would likely be ignorant of insulin under physiological conditions (74).

scRNAseq has been used to characterise a novel lymphocyte population that express both TCRs and BCRs (28). It is suggested that these "dual expressors" (DE) are increased in frequency in type 1 diabetes and that in people with type 1 diabetes there is a public BCR which can stimulate insulin-reactive CD4+ T cells. However, this work remains controversial as others have been unable to replicate the enrichment of DE in T1D nor the specific public BCR sequence (75). This highlights the importance of good quality control at every step of scRNAseq experiments.

Isolation of CD19+IgG+ B cells from pancreatic lymph nodes from autoantibody positive donors and single cell sequencing of their BCRs demonstrated that no clonally expanded B cells were identified in the pLN. Antibodies were reconstructed from BCR sequencing, although very few of these were found to be specific for IA2 (none were specific for GAD and insulin was not tested) (76). Seay et al. also sorted and single cell sequenced the BCRs from pancreatic LNs. They found an enrichment of insulin binding motifs in pLN from people with T1D compared to controls (50). They also observed sequence overlap with autoreactive BCRs cloned from precursor (early immature) B cells from healthy donors previously published by Wardemann et al. (77). Wardemann et al. observed that not only are many BCRs from healthy donor precursor B cells insulin reactive, they are often also polyreactive to other autoantigens for example dsDNA, ssDNA or nuclear proteins (77). This polyreactivity has also been noted for both IgM and IgG insulin antibodies (68).

Similarly Smith et al. demonstrated that all of their high affinity insulin binding BCRs were also reactive to LPS and chromatin (74). Polyreactive antibodies have been postulated to play a key role in the healthy immune system but are also implicated in a variety of autoimmune diseases (78, 79). It therefore appears that autoreactive B cells in T1D may span a wide range of phenotypes and the antibodies produced may often be polyreactive, however the limited number of studies make it difficult to draw firm conclusions.

FUTURE PERSPECTIVES ON scRNAseq IN TYPE 1 DIABETES

New Single Cell Methods and Analysis Tools

scRNAseq is beginning to give fascinating insights into type 1 diabetes and new approaches may yield further discoveries. The first of these is spatial transcriptomics (80). In this technique, indexed oligos capture RNA from either fresh-frozen or formalin-fixed, paraffin-embedded tissue sections. This allows determination of gene expression on a level that is fast approaching single cell resolution. It has already been used to give insights into cell interactions in other diseases such as rheumatoid arthritis, where infiltrating leukocytes interact with target cells (81, 82). Spatial transcriptomics therefore has great potential to unravel lymphocyte interactions with beta cells in the pancreas and to give insight into different patterns of immune cell infiltration (2). In both type 1 (23) and type 2 diabetes (83) scATACseq has recently been used to link GWAS to epigenetic regulation of gene expression. New methodologies enabling combination of ATACseq, and CITEseq with scRNAseq in the same experiment will also contribute to the field (84). New analysis tools such as CellPhoneDB give the ability to map interactions between subsets of cells, based on DEG in scRNAseq datasets, which would allow identification of novel interactions between immune cells and beta cells in the pancreas (85, 86). This may become increasingly important as we begin to understand the role of beta cell stress and signalling in type 1 diabetes (6) as well as the involvement of other pancreatic cells in diabetes development (23). CellPhoneDB has been used to identify crosstalk between T cells and epithelial cells in ulcerative colitis (87) whilst in rheumatoid arthritis scRNAseq has revealed interaction pathways between B cells, fibroblasts and monocytes (88). Additionally, recent work from the Satija lab has brought together previously published scRNAseq datasets of pancreatic cells, including immune cells from healthy pancreatic samples (12), which will facilitate this type of analysis. This would be further enhanced were there a unified repository for T1D scRNAseq datasets, similar to those for COVID-19 (89).

Technological and Analytical Approaches to Enhance Immunoreceptor Sequencing

We have seen how combining GEX with V(D)J sequencing has increased insights into T1D. The recent development of DNA barcoded multimers will allow now the determination of T cell antigen specificity in scRNAseq experiments (90, 91), whilst conjugation of whole proteins or large folded protein fragments to DNA barcodes will facilitate identification of antigen specific B cells (92).

Computational approaches to determine the likely interaction of an immunoreceptor with target antigen also have the potential to revolutionise the search for antigen specific TCRs and BCRs. Approaches such as tcrdist (93), GLIPH (94) and immune receptor network generation for BCRs (95) enable BCR and TCR sequences to be mapped and visualised, and those that differ by only one or two amino acids are assumed to target the same antigens. NetTCR (96) and TCRex (97) use neural networks and machine learning algorithms to cluster TCRs predicited to bind the same epitope. Recent advances such as ICON and TCRAI leverage scRNAseq technology along with oligo labelled dextramers. They utilise the paired TCRα and TCRβ transcripts to build libraries of antigen specific receptors, with a neural network to predict antigen specificity of TCRs. However, many of these approaches have been validated using viral or tumour antigens with well-defined epitopes. As we have seen in the sections above, whilst there definitely are peptide sequences from diabetes autoantigens that are widely recognised, the immune response also targets diverse sequences in different individuals. Furthermore, auto-antigenic TCRs tend to bind pMHC with lower affinity than TCRs targeting pathogens (98, 99) as high affinity self-reactive TCRs are generally deleted in the thymus. It is not clear how this lower affinity and lack of public TCRs may impact upon the usefulness of computational approaches for T1D.

Biomarkers in Clinical Trials

In 2019, it was demonstrated that teplizumab could delay progression to T1D in high risk individuals (100). Further work confirmed a correlation between fold change in C-peptide and change in frequency of CD8+KLRG1+TIGIT+ T cells (101). scRNAseq of T cells from the clinical trials of teplizumab and other immunotherapies in T1D could offer an amazing opportunity to identify all biomarkers predictive of successful treatment. For example, scRNAseq studies have shown a variety of phenotypic markers induced *in vitro* with anti-CD3 antibodies in human PBMC, including a variety of interleukin receptors and markers of regulation and exhaustion including FOXP3, CTLA4, TNFRSF18, LAG3 and PDCD1 (102). In contrast, anti-CD3/CD28 stimulation of PBMC analysed with scRNAseq and CITEseq, showed phenotypes strongly associated with activation (although memory subsets also upregulated senescence) (103).

In the future, a deeper understanding of TCRs and BCRs has the potential to better quantify the risk of progression in autoantibody positive people. Monitoring the abundance and phenotypes of lymphocytes bearing specific CDR3 sequences or using specific V genes may also prove useful in monitoring immunotherapies, particularly antigen specific immunotherapies, where phenotypic changes in whole lymphocyte populations may not be so obvious (1, 104–106). In addition, BCRs also have the potential to be used in CAR-Treg cell immunotherapy as has been demonstrated in the NOD mouse (107).

A Computational Approach to Move Beyond scRNAseq

scRNAseq has demonstrated its great potential to identify novel biomarkers both in T1D and other autoimmune diseases. However, it is both technically challenging and expensive. Therefore it is crucial that researchers should be able to translate findings from scRNAseq into more accessible diagnostic and monitoring tests, for example using standardised flow cytometry or qPCR panels as is starting to happen in cancer research (108, 109). Similarly in IBD, a machine learning approach allowed identification of a CD8+ T cell signature that could predict prognosis. These biomarkers were then developed into a commercially available whole blood qPCR test to facilitate personalised therapy (110).

In T1D, recent advances in computational analysis are beginning to allow discrimination of changes in cell subsets from bulk RNAseq. Mehdi et al. identified a peripheral blood transcriptomic signature that predicted autoantibody development (111). Of the DEG identified, many were associated with the ubiquitin-proteasome pathway, DC and T cell function and were potentially targets of drugs approved for other conditions (111). Xhonneux et al. (112), demonstrated from transcriptomics of whole blood that they could undertake "digital cytometry", by mapping groups of genes back to cell types. Children who developed autoantibodies against insulin first, had a signature of increased NK cells and CD4+ memory T cells. In contrast, those who first developed autoantibodies to GAD had a reduced percentage of CD4+ memory T cells and NK cells, but increased activated NK cells. Harmonizome (113) was used to identify a G protein–coupled receptor, GPR171, predicted to control the immune signature found in IAA+ children (112). Adding gene expression information to predictive models, increased their accuracy in predicting later T1D development in children under 18 months (112).

DISCUSSION

The first papers to analyse lymphocytes from type 1 diabetes using scRNAseq have provided fascinating insights into phenotypes involved in driving the disease and identified new potential targets for immunotherapy, such as IL-32 (15, 17). scRNAseq of TCRs involved in T1D has revealed that autoantigen specific TCRs have a wide range of targets and that whilst single chains or CDR3s are often shared between donors, it is rare to see TCRs with both chains identical in multiple donors; hence public TCRs remain elusive. In the peripheral blood, diabetes autoantigen reactive cells do not always have distinct phenotypes in healthy donors compared to those with T1D (25, 26), and enrichment of islet reactive cells is much more pronounced in the pancreas and pancreatic lymph nodes. Combining TCR sequencing with T cell phenotyping has led to a deeper understanding of islet antigen-specific cells in the peripheral blood (24, 27). A key challenge, for which scRNAseq is ideally suited, will be to develop methods to identify which T cells in the periphery are truly involved in beta cell destruction, and which are simply able to bind islet antigen multimers but are not capable of either trafficking to the islets or contributing to beta cell killing. Looking to the future, it is clear that combining antigen specificity with scRNA phenotyping and new computational approaches, such as those that can give insight into interactions between islet cells and infiltrating lymphocytes, have the potential to revolutionise the field.

Relatively few papers have tackled single cell sequencing (or indeed bulk sequencing) of BCRs repertoires in T1D, but those available suggest that these BCRs have unique properties and are often polyreactive (50, 74, 77). New approaches to identify islet-antigen specific B cells with scRNAseq (92) will therefore have much to contribute to our knowledge of how islet autoantibodies develop and are involved in disease progression.

scRNAseq is ideally suited to identifying subtle phenotypic differences between cohorts and has demonstrated promise in identifying differentially expressed genes in people that will later progress to autoantibody positivity and T1D (27). Developing this approach will be key to identifying at-risk individuals and matching them to a novel immunotherapy that is appropriate for their stage and phenotype of disease (100, 101, 114, 115). Furthermore, new analytical approaches will enable scRNAseq findings to be translated into new immunotherapies and biomarkers to monitor effectiveness of those already in clinical trials.

AUTHOR CONTRIBUTIONS

SH wrote the first draft of the manuscript. All authors contributed to the article and approved the submitted version.

REFERENCES

1. Ahmed S, Cerosaletti K, James E, Long SA, Mannering S, Speake C, et al. Standardizing T-Cell Biomarkers in Type 1 Diabetes: Challenges and Recent Advances. *Diabetes* (2019) 68:1366–79. doi: 10.2337/db19-0119
2. Leete P, Oram RA, McDonald TJ, Shields BM, Ziller CTIGI study team, et al. Studies of Insulin and Proinsulin in Pancreas and Serum Support the Existence of Aetiopathological Endotypes of Type 1 Diabetes Associated With Age at Diagnosis. *Diabetologia* (2020) 63:1258–67. doi: 10.1007/s00125-020-05115-6
3. Hanna SJ, Powell WE, Long AE, Robinson EJS, Davies J, Megson C, et al. Slow Progressors to Type 1 Diabetes Lose Islet Autoantibodies Over Time, Have Few Islet Antigen-Specific CD8+ T Cells and Exhibit a Distinct CD95hi B Cell Phenotype. *Diabetologia* (2020) 63:1174–85. doi: 10.1007/s00125-020-05114-7
4. Powell WE, Hanna SJ, Hocter CN, Robinson E, Davies J, Dunseath GJ, et al. Loss of CXCR3 Expression on Memory B Cells in Individuals With Long-Standing Type 1 Diabetes. *Diabetologia* (2018) 61:1794–803. doi: 10.1007/s00125-018-4651-x
5. Rahman AH, Homann D. Mass Cytometry and Type 1 Diabetes Research in the Age of Single-Cell Data Science. *Curr Opin Endocrinol Diabetes Obes* (2020) 27:231–9. doi: 10.1097/MED.0000000000000549
6. von Scholten BJ, Kreiner FF, Gough SCL, von Herrath M. Current and Future Therapies for Type 1 Diabetes. *Diabetologia* (2021) 64:1037–48. doi: 10.1007/s00125-021-05398-3
7. Ding J, Adiconis X, Simmons SK, Kowalczyk MS, Hession CC, Marjanovic ND, et al. Systematic Comparison of Single-Cell and Single-Nucleus RNA-Sequencing Methods. *Nat Biotechnol* (2020) 38:737–46. doi: 10.1038/s41587-020-0465-8
8. Efremova M, Vento-Tormo R, Park J-E, Teichmann SA, James KR. Immunology in the Era of Single-Cell Technologies. *Annu Rev Immunol* (2020) 38:727–57. doi: 10.1146/annurev-immunol-090419-020340

9. Carter JA, Preall JB, Grigaityte K, Goldfless SJ, Jeffery E, Briggs AW, et al. Single T Cell Sequencing Demonstrates the Functional Role of αβ TCR Pairing in Cell Lineage and Antigen Specificity. *Front Immunol* (2019) 10:1516. doi: 10.3389/fimmu.2019.01516
10. Barennes P, Quiniou V, Shugay M, Egorov ES, Davydov AN, Chudakov DM, et al. Benchmarking of T Cell Receptor Repertoire Profiling Methods Reveals Large Systematic Biases. *Nat Biotechnol* (2021) 39:236–45. doi: 10.1038/s41587-020-0656-3
11. See P, Lum J, Chen J. Ginhoux F. A Single-Cell Sequencing Guide for Immunologists. *Front Immunol* (2018) 9:2425. doi: 10.3389/fimmu.2018.02425
12. Hao Y, Hao S, Andersen-Nissen E, Mauck WM, Zheng S, Butler A, et al. Integrated Analysis of Multimodal Single-Cell Data. *Cell* (2021) 184:3573–87.e29. doi: 10.1016/j.cell.2021.04.048
13. Andrews TS, Kiselev VY, McCarthy D, Hemberg M. Tutorial: Guidelines for the Computational Analysis of Single-Cell RNA Sequencing Data. *Nat Protoc* (2021) 16:1–9. doi: 10.1038/s41596-020-00409-w
14. Sun B, Bugarin-Estrada E, Overend LE, Walker CE, Tucci FA, Bashford-Rogers RJM. Double-Jeopardy: scRNA-Seq Doublet/Multiplet Detection Using Multi-Omic Profiling. *Cell Rep Methods* (2021) 1:100008. doi: 10.1016/j.crmeth.2021.100008
15. Kallionpää H, Somani J, Tuomela S, Ullah U, de Albuquerque R, Lönnberg T, et al. Early Detection of Peripheral Blood Cell Signature in Children Developing β-Cell Autoimmunity at a Young Age. *Diabetes* (2019) 68:2024–34. doi: 10.2337/db19-0287
16. Thayer TC, Pearson JA, De Leenheer E, Hanna SJ, Boldison J, Davies J, et al. Peripheral Proinsulin Expression Controls Low-Avidity Proinsulin-Reactive CD8 T Cells in Type 1 Diabetes. *Diabetes* (2016) 65:3429–39. doi: 10.2337/db15-1649
17. Fasolino M, Schwartz GW, Golson ML, Wang YJ, Morgan A, Liu C, et al. Multiomics Single-Cell Analysis of Human Pancreatic Islets Reveals Novel Cellular States in Health and Type 1 Diabetes. *Genomics* (2021). doi: 10.1101/2021.01.28.428598
18. Nyalwidhe JO, Grzesik WJ, Burch TC, Semeraro ML, Waseem T, Gerling IC, et al. Comparative Quantitative Proteomic Analysis of Disease Stratified Laser Captured Microdissected Human Islets Identifies Proteins and Pathways Potentially Related to Type 1 Diabetes. *PloS One* (2017) 12: e0183908. doi: 10.1371/journal.pone.0183908
19. AlRashidi FT, Gillespie KM. Biomarkers in Islet Cell Transplantation for Type 1 Diabetes. *Curr Diabetes Rep* (2018) 18:94. doi: 10.1007/s11892-018-1059-4
20. Zakharov PN, Hu H, Wan X, Unanue ER. Single-Cell RNA Sequencing of Murine Islets Shows High Cellular Complexity at All Stages of Autoimmune Diabetes. *J Exp Med* (2020) 217:e20192362. doi: 10.1084/jem.20192362
21. Sharon N, Vanderhooft J, Straubhaar J, Mueller J, Chawla R, Zhou Q, et al. Wnt Signaling Separates the Progenitor and Endocrine Compartments During Pancreas Development. *Cell Rep* (2019) 27:2281–91.e5. doi: 10.1016/j.celrep.2019.04.083
22. Xin Y, Dominguez Gutierrez G, Okamoto H, Kim J, Lee A-H, Adler C, et al. Pseudotime Ordering of Single Human β-Cells Reveals States of Insulin Production and Unfolded Protein Response. *Diabetes* (2018) 67:1783–94. doi: 10.2337/db18-0365
23. Chiou J, Geusz RJ, Okino M-L, Han JY, Miller M, Melton R, et al. Interpreting Type 1 Diabetes Risk With Genetics and Single-Cell Epigenomics. *Nature* (2021) 594:398–402. doi: 10.1038/s41586-021-03552-w
24. Cerosaletti K, Barahmand-pour-Whitman F, Yang J, DeBerg HA, Dufort MJ, Murray SA, et al. Single-Cell RNA Sequencing Reveals Expanded Clones of Islet Antigen-Reactive CD4 $^+$ T Cells in Peripheral Blood of Subjects With Type 1 Diabetes. *JI* (2017) 199:323–35. doi: 10.4049/jimmunol.1700172
25. Fuchs YF, Sharma V, Eugster A, Kraus G, Morgenstern R, Dahl A, et al. Gene Expression-Based Identification of Antigen-Responsive CD8+ T Cells on a Single-Cell Level. *Front Immunol* (2019) 10:2568. doi: 10.3389/fimmu.2019.02568
26. Culina S, Lalanne AI, Afonso G, Cerosaletti K, Pinto S, Sebastiani G, et al. Islet-Reactive CD8 $^+$ T Cell Frequencies in the Pancreas, But Not in Blood, Distinguish Type 1 Diabetic Patients From Healthy Donors. *Sci Immunol* (2018) 3:eaao4013. doi: 10.1126/sciimmunol.aao4013
27. Heninger A-K, Eugster A, Kuehn D, Buettner F, Kuhn M, Lindner A, et al. A Divergent Population of Autoantigen-Responsive CD4 $^+$ T Cells in Infants Prior to β Cell Autoimmunity. *Sci Transl Med* (2017) 9:eaaf8848. doi: 10.1126/scitranslmed.aaf8848
28. Ahmed R, Omidian Z, Giwa A, Cornwell B, Majety N, Bell DR, et al. A Public BCR Present in a Unique Dual-Receptor-Expressing Lymphocyte From Type 1 Diabetes Patients Encodes a Potent T Cell Autoantigen. *Cell* (2019) 177:1583–99.e16. doi: 10.1016/j.cell.2019.05.007
29. Enge M, Arda HE, Mignardi M, Beausang J, Bottino R, Kim SK, et al. Single-Cell Analysis of Human Pancreas Reveals Transcriptional Signatures of Aging and Somatic Mutation Patterns. *Cell* (2017) 171:321–30.e14. doi: 10.1016/j.cell.2017.09.004
30. Grün D, Muraro MJ, Boisset J-C, Wiebrands K, Lyubimova A, Dharmadhikari G, et al. De Novo Prediction of Stem Cell Identity Using Single-Cell Transcriptome Data. *Cell Stem Cell* (2016) 19:266–77. doi: 10.1016/j.stem.2016.05.010
31. Muraro MJ, Dharmadhikari G, Grün D, Groen N, Dielen T, Jansen E, et al. A Single-Cell Transcriptome Atlas of the Human Pancreas. *Cell Syst* (2016) 3:385–94.e3. doi: 10.1016/j.cels.2016.09.002
32. Segerstolpe Å, Palasantza A, Eliasson P, Andersson E-M, Andréasson A-C, Sun X, et al. Single-Cell Transcriptome Profiling of Human Pancreatic Islets in Health and Type 2 Diabetes. *Cell Metab* (2016) 24:593–607. doi: 10.1016/j.cmet.2016.08.020
33. Lawlor N, George J, Bolisetty M, Kursawe R, Sun L, Sivakamasundari V, et al. Single-Cell Transcriptomes Identify Human Islet Cell Signatures and Reveal Cell-Type–Specific Expression Changes in Type 2 Diabetes. *Genome Res* (2017) 27:208–22. doi: 10.1101/gr.212720.116
34. Baron M, Veres A, Wolock SL, Faust AL, Gaujoux R, Vetere A, et al. A Single-Cell Transcriptomic Map of the Human and Mouse Pancreas Reveals Inter- and Intra-Cell Population Structure. *Cell Syst* (2016) 3:346–60.e4. doi: 10.1016/j.cels.2016.08.011
35. Xin Y, Adler C, Kim J, Ding Y, Ni M, Wei Y, et al. Single-Cell RNA Sequencing and Analysis of Human Pancreatic Islets. *JoVE* (2019) 149. doi: 10.3791/59866
36. Zhang J, Chen L-M, Zou Y, Zhang S, Xiong F, Wang C-Y. Implication of Epigenetic Factors in the Pathogenesis of Type 1 Diabetes. *Chin Med J* (2021) 134:1031–42. doi: 10.1097/CM9.0000000000001450
37. Esposito S, Toni G, Tascini G, Santi E, Berioli MG, Principi N. Environmental Factors Associated With Type 1 Diabetes. *Front Endocrinol* (2019) 10:592. doi: 10.3389/fendo.2019.00592
38. Xie Z, Chang C, Huang G, Zhou Z. The Role of Epigenetics in Type 1 Diabetes. In: Chang C, Lu Q, editors. *Epigenetics in Allergy and Autoimmunity Advances in Experimental Medicine and Biology*. Singapore: Springer Singapore (2020). p. 223–57. doi: 10.1007/978-981-15-3449-2_9
39. Robertson CC, Inshaw JRJ, Onengut-Gumuscu S, Chen W-M, Santa Cruz DF, Yang H, et al. Fine-Mapping, Trans-Ancestral and Genomic Analyses Identify Causal Variants, Cells, Genes and Drug Targets for Type 1 Diabetes. *Nat Genet* (2021) 53:962–71. doi: 10.1038/s41588-021-00880-5
40. Clark M, Kroger CJ, Ke Q, Tisch RM. The Role of T Cell Receptor Signaling in the Development of Type 1 Diabetes. *Front Immunol* (2021) 11:615371. doi: 10.3389/fimmu.2020.615371
41. Jacobsen LM, Posgai A, Seay HR, Haller MJ. Brusko TM. T Cell Receptor Profiling in Type 1 Diabetes. *Curr Diabetes Rep* (2017) 17:118. doi: 10.1007/s11892-017-0946-4
42. Wang Y, Sosinowski T, Novikov A, Crawford F, White J, Jin N, et al. How C-Terminal Additions to Insulin B-Chain Fragments Create Superagonists for T Cells in Mouse and Human Type 1 Diabetes. *Sci Immunol* (2019) 4: eaav7517. doi: 10.1126/sciimmunol.aav7517
43. James EA, Mallone R, Kent SC. DiLorenzo TP. T-Cell Epitopes and Neo-Epitopes in Type 1 Diabetes: A Comprehensive Update and Reappraisal. *Diabetes* (2020) 69:1311–35. doi: 10.2337/dbi19-0022
44. Eugster A, Lindner A, Catani M, Heninger A-K, Dahl A, Klemroth S, et al. High Diversity in the TCR Repertoire of GAD65 Autoantigen-Specific Human CD4 $^+$ T Cells. *JI* (2015) 194:2531–8. doi: 10.4049/jimmunol.1403031
45. Fuchs YF, Eugster A, Dietz S, Sebelefsky C, Kühn D, Wilhelm C, et al. CD8+ T Cells Specific for the Islet Autoantigen IGRP Are Restricted in Their T Cell

Receptor Chain Usage. *Sci Rep* (2017) 7:44661. doi: 10.1038/srep44661

46. Baker RL, Rihanek M, Hohenstein AC, Nakayama M, Michels A, Gottlieb PA, et al. Hybrid Insulin Peptides Are Autoantigens in Type 1 Diabetes. *Diabetes* (2019) 68:1830–40. doi: 10.2337/db19-0128
47. Kent SC, Chen Y, Bregoli L, Clemmings SM, Kenyon NS, Ricordi C, et al. Expanded T Cells From Pancreatic Lymph Nodes of Type 1 Diabetic Subjects Recognize an Insulin Epitope. *Nature* (2005) 435:224–8. doi: 10.1038/nature03625
48. Pathiraja V, Kuehlich JP, Campbell PD, Krishnamurthy B, Loudovaris T, Coates PTH, et al. Proinsulin-Specific, HLA-DQ8, and HLA-DQ8-Transdimer–Restricted CD4 $^+$ T Cells Infiltrate Islets in Type 1 Diabetes. *Diabetes* (2015) 64:172–82. doi: 10.2337/db14-0858
49. Skowera A, Ladell K, McLaren JE, Dolton G, Matthews KK, Gostick E, et al. β-Cell–Specific CD8 T Cell Phenotype in Type 1 Diabetes Reflects Chronic Autoantigen Exposure. *Diabetes* (2015) 64:916–25. doi: 10.2337/db14-0332
50. Seay HR, Yusko E, Rothweiler SJ, Zhang L, Posgai AL, Campbell-Thompson M, et al. Tissue Distribution and Clonal Diversity of the T and B Cell Repertoire in Type 1 Diabetes. *JCI Insight* (2016) 1:e88242. doi: 10.1172/jci.insight.88242
51. Arif S, Gomez-Tourino I, Kamra Y, Pujol-Autonell I, Hanton E, Tree T, et al. GAD-Alum Immunotherapy in Type 1 Diabetes Expands Bifunctional Th1/Th2 Autoreactive CD4 T Cells. *Diabetologia* (2020) 63:1186–98. doi: 10.1007/s00125-020-05130-7
52. Michels AW, Landry LG, McDaniel KA, Yu L, Campbell-Thompson M, Kwok WW, et al. Islet-Derived CD4 T Cells Targeting Proinsulin in Human Autoimmune Diabetes. *Diabetes* (2017) 66:722–34. doi: 10.2337/db16-1025
53. Landry LG, Anderson AM, Russ HA, Yu L, Kent SC, Atkinson MA, et al. Proinsulin-Reactive CD4 T Cells in the Islets of Type 1 Diabetes Organ Donors. *Front Endocrinol* (2021) 12:622647. doi: 10.3389/fendo.2021.622647
54. Zhao M, Jiang J, Zhao M, Chang C, Wu H, Lu Q. The Application of Single-Cell RNA Sequencing in Studies of Autoimmune Diseases: A Comprehensive Review. *Clinic Rev Allerg Immunol* (2021) 60:68–86. doi: 10.1007/s12016-020-08813-6
55. Penkava F, Velasco-Herrera MDC, Young MD, Yager N, Nwosu LN, Pratt AG, et al. Single-Cell Sequencing Reveals Clonal Expansions of Pro-Inflammatory Synovial CD8 T Cells Expressing Tissue-Homing Receptors in Psoriatic Arthritis. *Nat Commun* (2020) 11:4767. doi: 10.1038/s41467-020-18513-6
56. Bagaev DV, Vroomans RMA, Samir J, Stervbo U, Rius C, Dolton G, et al. VDJdb in 2019: Database Extension, New Analysis Infrastructure and a T-Cell Receptor Motif Compendium. *Nucleic Acids Res* (2020) 48:D1057–62. doi: 10.1093/nar/gkz874
57. Vita R, Mahajan S, Overton JA, Dhanda SK, Martini S, Cantrell JR, et al. The Immune Epitope Database (IEDB): 2018 Update. *Nucleic Acids Res* (2019) 47:D339–43. doi: 10.1093/nar/gky1006
58. Wiles TA, Hohenstein A, Landry LG, Dang M, Powell R, Guyer P, et al. Characterization of Human CD4 T Cells Specific for a C-Peptide/C-Peptide Hybrid Insulin Peptide. *Front Immunol* (2021) 12:668680. doi: 10.3389/fimmu.2021.668680
59. Ji Q, Perchellet A, Goverman JM. Viral Infection Triggers Central Nervous System Autoimmunity *via* Activation of CD8+ T Cells Expressing Dual TCRs. *Nat Immunol* (2010) 11:628–34. doi: 10.1038/ni.1888
60. Schuldt NJ, Auger JL, Spanier JA, Martinov T, Breed ER, Fife BT, et al. Cutting Edge: Dual Tcrα Expression Poses an Autoimmune Hazard by Limiting Regulatory T Cell Generation. *JI* (2017) 199:33–8. doi: 10.4049/jimmunol.1700406
61. Schallenberg S, Kretschmer K. New Insight Into Type 1 Diabetes Development: Resolving Early Diabetogenic CD4+ T Cell Responses That Precede Seroconversion. *Ann Transl Med* (2018) 6:58–8. doi: 10.21037/atm.2017.12.14
62. Richter W, Endl J, Eiermann TH, Brandt M, Kientsch-Engel R, Thivolet C, et al. Human Monoclonal Islet Cell Antibodies From a Patient With Insulin-Dependent Diabetes Mellitus Reveal Glutamate Decarboxylase as the Target Antigen. *Proc Natl Acad Sci* (1992) 89:8467–71. doi: 10.1073/pnas.89.18.8467
63. Madec AM, Rousset F, Ho S, Robert F, Thivolet C, Orgiazzi J, et al. Four IgG Anti-Islet Human Monoclonal Antibodies Isolated From a Type 1 Diabetes Patient Recognize Distinct Epitopes of Glutamic Acid Decarboxylase 65 and Are Somatically Mutated. *J Immunol* (1996) 156:3541–9.
64. Jury KM, Loeffler D, Eiermann TH, Ziegler B, Boehm BO, Richter W. Evidence for Somatic Mutation and Affinity Maturation of Diabetes Associated Human Autoantibodies to Glutamate Decarboxylase. *J Autoimmun* (1996) 9:371–7. doi: 10.1006/jaut.1996.0050
65. Kolm-Litty V, Berlo S, Bonifacio E, Bearzatto M, Engel AM, Christie M, et al. Human Monoclonal Antibodies Isolated From Type I Diabetes Patients Define Multiple Epitopes in the Protein Tyrosine Phosphatase-Like IA-2 Antigen. *J Immunol* (2000) 165:4676–84. doi: 10.4049/jimmunol.165.8.4676
66. Ananieva-Jordanova R, Evans M, Nakamatsu T, Premawardhana LDKE, Sanders J, Powell M, et al. Isolation and Characterisation of a Human Monoclonal Autoantibody to the Islet Cell Autoantigen IA-2. *J Autoimmun* (2005) 24:337–45. doi: 10.1016/j.jaut.2005.03.003
67. Weenink SM, Lo J, Stephenson CR, McKinney PA, Ananieva-Jordanova R, Rees Smith B, et al. Autoantibodies and Associated T-Cell Responses to Determinants Within the 831–860 Region of the Autoantigen IA-2 in Type 1 Diabetes. *J Autoimmun* (2009) 33:147–54. doi: 10.1016/j.jaut.2009.04.002
68. Ikematsu H, Ichiyoshi Y, Schettino EW, Nakamura M, Casali P. VH and V Kappa Segment Structure of Anti-Insulin IgG Autoantibodies in Patients With Insulin-Dependent Diabetes Mellitus. Evidence for Somatic Selection. *J Immunol* (1994) 152:1430–41.
69. Ichiyoshi Y, Zhou M, Casali P. A Human Anti-Insulin IgG Autoantibody Apparently Arises Through Clonal Selection From an Insulin-Specific "Germ-Line" Natural Antibody Template. Analysis by V Gene Segment Reassortment and Site-Directed Mutagenesis. *J Immunol* (1995) 154:226–38.
70. Potter KN, Wilkin TJ. The Molecular Specificity of Insulin Autoantibodies. *Diabetes Metab Res Rev* (2000) 16:338–53. doi: 10.1002/1520-7560(2000)9999:9999<::aid-dmrr145>3.0.co;2-l
71. Bashford-Rogers RJM, Bergamaschi L, McKinney EF, Pombal DC, Mescia F, Lee JC, et al. Analysis of the B Cell Receptor Repertoire in Six Immune-Mediated Diseases. *Nature* (2019) 574:122–6. doi: 10.1038/s41586-019-1595-3
72. Horns F, Dekker CL, Quake SR. Memory B Cell Activation, Broad Anti-Influenza Antibodies, and Bystander Activation Revealed by Single-Cell Transcriptomics. *Cell Rep* (2020) 30:905–13.e6. doi: 10.1016/j.celrep.2019.12.063
73. Milpied P, Cervera-Marzal I, Mollichella M-L, Tesson B, Brisou G, Traverse-Glehen A, et al. Human Germinal Center Transcriptional Programs Are De-Synchronized in B Cell Lymphoma. *Nat Immunol* (2018) 19:1013–24. doi: 10.1038/s41590-018-0181-4
74. Smith MJ, Packard TA, O'Neill SK, Henry Dunand CJ, Huang M, Fitzgerald-Miller L, et al. Loss of Anergic B Cells in Prediabetic and New-Onset Type 1 Diabetic Patients. *Diabetes* (2015) 64:1703–12. doi: 10.2337/db13-1798
75. Japp AS, Meng W, Rosenfeld AM, Perry DJ, Thirawatananond P, Bacher RL, et al. TCR+/BCR+ Dual-Expressing Cells and Their Associated Public BCR Clonotype Are Not Enriched in Type 1 Diabetes. *Cell* (2021) 184:827–39.e14. doi: 10.1016/j.cell.2020.11.035
76. Catani M, Walther D, Christie MR, McLaughlin KA, Bonifacio E, Eugster A. Isolation of Human Monoclonal Autoantibodies Derived From Pancreatic Lymph Node and Peripheral Blood B Cells of Islet Autoantibody-Positive Patients. *Diabetologia* (2016) 59:294–8. doi: 10.1007/s00125-015-3792-4
77. Wardemann H. Predominant Autoantibody Production by Early Human B Cell Precursors. *Science* (2003) 301:1374–7. doi: 10.1126/science.1086907
78. Avrameas S, Alexopoulos H, Moutsopoulos HM. Natural Autoantibodies: An Undersugn Hero of the Immune System and Autoimmune Disorders—A Point of View. *Front Immunol* (2018) 9:1320. doi: 10.3389/fimmu.2018.01320
79. Zhou Z-H, Tzioufas AG, Notkins AL. Properties and Function of Polyreactive Antibodies and Polyreactive Antigen-Binding B Cells. *J Autoimmun* (2007) 29:219–28. doi: 10.1016/j.jaut.2007.07.015
80. Ståhl PL, Salmén F, Vickovic S, Lundmark A, Navarro JF, Magnusson J, et al. Visualization and Analysis of Gene Expression in Tissue Sections by Spatial Transcriptomics. *Science* (2016) 353:78–82. doi: 10.1126/science.aaf2403
81. Carlberg K, Korotkova M, Larsson L, Catrina AI, Ståhl PL, Malmström V. Exploring Inflammatory Signatures in Arthritic Joint Biopsies With Spatial Transcriptomics. *Sci Rep* (2019) 9:18975. doi: 10.1038/s41598-019-55441-y

82. Vickovic S, Schapiro D, Carlberg K, Lötstedt B, Larsson L, Korotkova M, et al. Three-Dimensional Spatial Transcriptomics Uncovers Cell Type Dynamics in the Rheumatoid Arthritis Synovium. *Genomics* (2020). doi: 10.1101/2020.12.10.420463
83. Rai V, Quang DX, Erdos MR, Cusanovich DA, Daza RM, Narisu N, et al. Single-Cell ATAC-Seq in Human Pancreatic Islets and Deep Learning Upscaling of Rare Cells Reveals Cell-Specific Type 2 Diabetes Regulatory Signatures. *Mol Metab* (2020) 32:109–21. doi: 10.1016/j.molmet.2019.12.006
84. Mimitou EP, Lareau CA, Chen KY, Zorzetto-Fernandes AL, Hao Y, Takeshima Y, et al. Scalable, Multimodal Profiling of Chromatin Accessibility, Gene Expression and Protein Levels in Single Cells. *Nat Biotechnol* (2021). doi: 10.1038/s41587-021-00927-2
85. Efremova M, Vento-Tormo M, Teichmann SA, Vento-Tormo R. CellPhoneDB: Inferring Cell–Cell Communication From Combined Expression of Multi-Subunit Ligand–Receptor Complexes. *Nat Protoc* (2020) 15:1484–506. doi: 10.1038/s41596-020-0292-x
86. Hao S, Yan K-K, Ding L, Qian C, Chi H, Yu J. Network Approaches for Dissecting the Immune System. *iScience* (2020) 23:101354. doi: 10.1016/j.isci.2020.101354
87. Corridoni D, Antanaviciute A, Gupta T, Fawkner-Corbett D, Aulicino A, Jagielowicz M, et al. Single-Cell Atlas of Colonic CD8+ T Cells in Ulcerative Colitis. *Nat Med* (2020) 26:1480–90. doi: 10.1038/s41591-020-1003-4
88. Palla G, Ferrero E. Latent Factor Modeling of scRNA-Seq Data Uncovers Dysregulated Pathways in Autoimmune Disease Patients. *iScience* (2020) 23:101451. doi: 10.1016/j.isci.2020.101451
89. Chan Zuckerberg Initiative Single-Cell COVID-19 Consortia, Ballestar E, Farber DL, Glover S, Horwitz B, Meyer K, et al. Single Cell Profiling of COVID-19 Patients: An International Data Resource From Multiple Tissues. *MedRxiv* (2020). doi: 10.1101/2020.11.20.20227355
90. Bentzen AK, Marquard AM, Lyngaa R, Saini SK, Ramskov S, Donia M, et al. Large-Scale Detection of Antigen-Specific T Cells Using Peptide-MHC-I Multimers Labeled With DNA Barcodes. *Nat Biotechnol* (2016) 34:1037–45. doi: 10.1038/nbt.3662
91. Minervina AA, Pogorelyy MV, Kirk AM, Allen EK, Allison KJ, Lin C-Y, et al. Convergent Epitope-Specific T Cell Responses After SARS-CoV-2 Infection and Vaccination. *MedRxiv* (2021). doi: 10.1101/2021.07.12.21260227
92. Setliff I, Shiakolas AR, Pilewski KA, Murji AA, Mapengo RE, Janowska K, et al. High-Throughput Mapping of B Cell Receptor Sequences to Antigen Specificity. *Cell* (2019) 179:1636–46.e15. doi: 10.1016/j.cell.2019.11.003
93. Dash P, Fiore-Gartland AJ, Hertz T, Wang GC, Sharma S, Souquette A, et al. Quantifiable Predictive Features Define Epitope-Specific T Cell Receptor Repertoires. *Nature* (2017) 547:89–93. doi: 10.1038/nature22383
94. Glanville J, Huang H, Nau A, Hatton O, Wagar LE, Rubelt F, et al. Identifying Specificity Groups in the T Cell Receptor Repertoire. *Nature* (2017) 547:94–8. doi: 10.1038/nature22976
95. Bashford-Rogers RJM, Palser AL, Huntly BJ, Rance R, Vassiliou GS, Follows GA, et al. Network Properties Derived From Deep Sequencing of Human B-Cell Receptor Repertoires Delineate B-Cell Populations. *Genome Res* (2013) 23:1874–84. doi: 10.1101/gr.154815.113
96. Montemurro A, Schuster V, Povlsen HR, Bentzen AK, Jurtz V, Chronister WD, et al. NetTCR-2.0 Enables Accurate Prediction of TCR-Peptide Binding by Using Paired TCRα and β Sequence Data. *Commun Biol* (2021) 4:1060. doi: 10.1038/s42003-021-02610-3
97. Gielis S, Moris P, Bittremieux W, De Neuter N, Ogunjimi B, Laukens K, et al. Detection of Enriched T Cell Epitope Specificity in Full T Cell Receptor Sequence Repertoires. *Front Immunol* (2019) 10:2820. doi: 10.3389/fimmu.2019.02820
98. Bridgeman JS, Sewell AK, Miles JJ, Price DA, Cole DK. Structural and Biophysical Determinants of αβ T-Cell Antigen Recognition: T-Cell Antigen Recognition. *Immunology* (2012) 135:9–18. doi: 10.1111/j.1365-2567.2011.03515.x
99. Cole DK, Bulek AM, Dolton G, Schauenberg AJ, Szomolay B, Rittase W, et al. Hotspot Autoimmune T Cell Receptor Binding Underlies Pathogen and Insulin Peptide Cross-Reactivity. *J Clin Invest* (2016) 126:2191–204. doi: 10.1172/JCI85679
100. Herold KC, Bundy BN, Long SA, Bluestone JA, DiMeglio LA, Dufort MJ, et al. An Anti-CD3 Antibody, Teplizumab, in Relatives at Risk for Type 1 Diabetes. *N Engl J Med* (2019) 381:603–13. doi: 10.1056/NEJMoa1902226
101. Sims EK, Bundy BN, Stier K, Serti E, Lim N, Long SA, et al. Teplizumab Improves and Stabilizes Beta Cell Function in Antibody-Positive High-Risk Individuals. *Sci Transl Med* (2021) 13:eabc8980. doi: 10.1126/scitranslmed.abc8980
102. Sousa IG, Simi KCR, do Almo MM, Bezerra MAG, Doose G, Raiol T, et al. Gene Expression Profile of Human T Cells Following a Single Stimulation of Peripheral Blood Mononuclear Cells With Anti-CD3 Antibodies. *BMC Genomics* (2019) 20:593. doi: 10.1186/s12864-019-5967-8
103. Lawlor N, Nehar-Belaid D, Grassmann JDS, Stoeckius M, Smibert P, Stitzel ML, et al. Single Cell Analysis of Blood Mononuclear Cells Stimulated Through Either LPS or Anti-CD3 and Anti-Cd28. *Front Immunol* (2021) 12:636720. doi: 10.3389/fimmu.2021.636720
104. Alhadj Ali M, Liu Y-F, Arif S, Tatovic D, Shariff H, Gibson VB, et al. Metabolic and Immune Effects of Immunotherapy With Proinsulin Peptide in Human New-Onset Type 1 Diabetes. *Sci Transl Med* (2017) 9:eaaf7779. doi: 10.1126/scitranslmed.aaf7779
105. Casas R, Dietrich F, Barcenilla H, Tavira B, Wahlberg J, Achenbach P, et al. Glutamic Acid Decarboxylase Injection Into Lymph Nodes: Beta Cell Function and Immune Responses in Recent Onset Type 1 Diabetes Patients. *Front Immunol* (2020) 11:564921. doi: 10.3389/fimmu.2020.564921
106. Assfalg R, Knoop J, Hoffman KL, Pfirrmann M, Zapardiel-Gonzalo JM, Hofelich A, et al. Oral Insulin Immunotherapy in Children at Risk for Type 1 Diabetes in a Randomised Controlled Trial. *Diabetologia* (2021) 64:1079–92. doi: 10.1007/s00125-020-05376-1
107. Tenspolde M, Zimmermann K, Weber LC, Hapke M, Lieber M, Dywicki J, et al. Regulatory T Cells Engineered With a Novel Insulin-Specific Chimeric Antigen Receptor as a Candidate Immunotherapy for Type 1 Diabetes. *J Autoimmun* (2019) 103:102289. doi: 10.1016/j.jaut.2019.05.017
108. Zheng l, Li l, Xie j, Jin h, Zhu n. Six Novel Biomarkers for Diagnosis and Prognosis of Esophageal Squamous Cell Carcinoma: Validated by scRNA-Seq and qPCR. *J Cancer* (2021) 12:899–911. doi: 10.7150/jca.50443
109. Liu J, Xu T, Jin Y, Huang B, Zhang Y. Progress and Clinical Application of Single-Cell Transcriptional Sequencing Technology in Cancer Research. *Front Oncol* (2021) 10:593085. doi: 10.3389/fonc.2020.593085
110. Biasci D, Lee JC, Noor NM, Pombal DR, Hou M, Lewis N, et al. A Blood-Based Prognostic Biomarker in IBD. *Gut* (2019) 68:1386–95. doi: 10.1136/gutjnl-2019-318343
111. Mehdi AM, Hamilton-Williams EE, Cristino A, Ziegler A, Bonifacio E, Le Cao K-A, et al. A Peripheral Blood Transcriptomic Signature Predicts Autoantibody Development in Infants at Risk of Type 1 Diabetes. *JCI Insight* (2018) 3:e98212. doi: 10.1172/jci.insight.98212
112. Xhonneux L-P, Knight O, Lernmark Å, Bonifacio E, Hagopian WA, Rewers MJ, et al. Transcriptional Networks in at-Risk Individuals Identify Signatures of Type 1 Diabetes Progression. *Sci Transl Med* (2021) 13:eabd5666. doi: 10.1126/scitranslmed.abd5666
113. Rouillard AD, Gundersen GW, Fernandez NF, Wang Z, Monteiro CD, McDermott MG, et al. The Harmonizome: A Collection of Processed Datasets Gathered to Serve and Mine Knowledge About Genes and Proteins. *Database* (2016) 2016:baw100. doi: 10.1093/database/baw100
114. Jacobsen LM, Bundy BN, Greco MN, Schatz DA, Atkinson MA, Brusko TM, et al. Comparing Beta Cell Preservation Across Clinical Trials in Recent-Onset Type 1 Diabetes. *Diabetes Technol Ther* (2020) 22:948–53. doi: 10.1089/dia.2020.0305
115. Sosenko JM, Skyler JS, Herold KC, Schatz DA, Haller MJ, Pugliese A, et al. Slowed Metabolic Decline After 1 Year of Oral Insulin Treatment Among Individuals at High Risk for Type 1 Diabetes in the Diabetes Prevention Trial–Type 1 (DPT-1) and TrialNet Oral Insulin Prevention Trials. *Diabetes* (2020) 69:1827–32. doi: 10.2337/db20-0166

3

Patient and Healthcare Professionals Perspectives on the Delivery of Exercise Education for Patients with Type 1 Diabetes

Ian Litchfield[1*], *Rob C. Andrews*[2,3], *Parth Narendran*[4,5] *and Sheila Greenfield*[1]
On behalf of the EXTOD Education Programme Development team

[1] *Institute of Applied Health Research, University of Birmingham, Birmingham, United Kingdom,* [2] *Medical School, University of Exeter, Exeter, United Kingdom,* [3] *Taunton and Somerset NHS Foundation Trust, Musgrove Park Hospital, Taunton, United Kingdom,* [4] *Institute of Immunology and Immunotherapy, University of Birmingham, Birmingham, United Kingdom,* [5] *University Hospitals Birmingham NHS Foundation Trust, Queen Elizabeth Hospital, Birmingham, United Kingdom*

Correspondence:
Ian Litchfield
i.litchfield@bham.ac.uk

Objective: One way of improving the prognosis for the growing numbers of people with type 1 diabetes (T1D) is to increase their frequency of exercise. One known barrier to this is the lack of cohesive support and information from care providers. To better understand the issues around existing support for patients wishing to exercise and inform the design of an education package specifically to facilitate safe exercise we interviewed care providers and patients about the existing provision of support.

Research Design and Methods: The study was based within two large UK teaching hospitals where four focus groups were undertaken two consisting of patients diagnosed with T1D who undertook regular exercise, and two with health care providers (HCPs) that were part of the diabetes care team. In all 14 patients and 11 staff were involved. These were complemented by two 1:1 interviews with staff unable to attend group discussions.

Results: We found the successful provision of education and advice was influenced by factors relating to the individual patient and their service provider. Patient factors included the type of activity and complexity of the exercise regime, the level of engagement with their condition and care and health literacy. Service-related factors included inconsistent training, a lack of capacity and continuity, and limited coherence of information from across their care team.

Conclusions: Any education package developed to support exercise in patients with type 1 diabetes should be offered at a time following diagnosis in accordance with patients' preferences and priorities, contain information on how to manage regular and irregular bouts of exercise. Patients described how they related more closely to the stories of their peers than famous sports stars and one way this can be facilitated is by group delivery. The content and relevance of any supporting materials should be closely considered. Training in the delivery of a novel education package should be made available to staff across the care team to enable them to either deliver the course or increase their confidence in offering salient advice as part of routine care.

Keywords: type 1 diabetes (T1D), exercise, service delivery and organization, structured education program, staff development

INTRODUCTION

The number of individuals affected by Type 1 Diabetes (T1D) continues to increase with some 20 million affected globally (1). In the United States the estimated 3 million with the condition is set to treble by 2050 (2, 3) with a concomitant increase in economic burden that is currently estimated at some $14.4 billion annually (4). One way in which the effects of T1D might be mitigated and the associated costs might be reduced is by meeting the recommendations for patients with T1D to undertake regular moderate-intensity exercise (5–9)[1]. The potential benefits both for patients and service utilization of their maintaining such a regime are numerous (10, 11) including a reduced risk of cardiovascular disease (12, 13), microvascular complications, hypoglycaemia (14) as well as enhanced psychological well-being (15). Existing guidelines recommend that patients with T1D should exercise regularly[1,2] however, with a reported 50% undertaking little or no physical activity either in Europe (14) or the United States (16), the need to increase the amount of sustained exercise and physical activity undertaken by patients with T1D remains[1] (17). To this end research on both sides of the Atlantic (18–21) has identified a number of barriers that might inhibit patients with T1D exercising including a lack of concerted information on exercise management. In the United States, it's recommended that patients seek the advice of physiologists or fitness coaches with experience of managing patients with T1D (22) whereas in the UK its expected support will be provided by dieticians, specialist diabetic nurses, educators and consultants as part of their routine care[1].

The content of any advice is frequently generic focussing on the basics of carbohydrate counting and insulin management. However, the implementation of this advice is influenced by numerous factors such as the duration and intensity of physical activity (23), the presence of co-morbidities (24), the level of patient engagement (25), and environmental parameters such as temperature (26). All of these contribute to variable glycaemic responses that make uniform recommendations challenging (22). In the UK patients attempting to negotiate these multiple influences are often dependent upon multiple care providers, with diverse levels of training and experience (27–29) with a recent survey reporting that two thirds were unfamiliar with the evidence-based guidance[1] leaving them unable to offer basic advice on insulin action (27).

There appears to be a clear need in T1D care both in the UK and elsewhere for a structured educational package specifically addressing safe exercise. Our study "Supporting adults with Type 1 Diabetes to undertake exercise; Developing and piloting an Education programme for exercise in Type 1 Diabetes" (EXTOD) was established to co-design an education package to support the management of exercise by both patients and staff[3]. The initial phase used focus groups to better understand the existing provision of advice and education on exercise that explored both patient and provider perspectives and preferences. The findings presented here describe for the first time the existing influences on how successfully the content of the information provided and the processes by which it is delivered meets the needs of patients. In doing so we offer valuable insight into the requirements of patients with T1D and their care providers as they attempt to maintain or increase levels of exercise. Our findings can inform the actions of all providers supporting patients with exercise and have been integral in the development of the EXTOD educational package.

METHODS

Settings

The study took place in two hospitals in the UK. Taunton and Somerset NHS Foundation trust which is a medium sized hospital in the Southwest that provides care for people living in a mixture of rural and urban environments and the Queen Elizabeth Hospital Birmingham. This is a large teaching hospital in the West Midlands that provides care for people living predominantly in an urbanized Metropolitan environment.

Recruitment

Patients

To participate in the study patients must have a clinical diagnosis of T1D, be aged between 18 and 70, be on a basal bolus insulin regime, and have attended their local approved T1D Education Programme [DAFNE, BERTIE, Living with diabetes, or equivalent[4,5] (30)]. Finally they should be exercising regularly or starting to train for a specific sporting event. All eligible patients were approached directly in diabetes clinics in a consecutive manner in each hospital by healthcare professionals aware of their existing or planned exercise activities. Those that expressed an interest were provided with an information sheet

[1] https://www.nice.org.uk/guidance/ng17 (accessed October 2017)

[2] American Diabetes Association Diabetes Care (2018). 41(Supplement 1):S38–50.

[3] http://www.isrctn.com/ISRCTN61403534?q=&filters=&sort=&offset=5&totalResults=14839&page=1&pageSize=10&searchType=basic-search(accessed November 2017)

[4] https://www.bertieonline.org.uk/ (accessed November 2017)

[5] https://www.nhs.uk/conditions/type-1-diabetes/living-with/ (accessed October 2017)

and offered an appointment with the research nurse who would answer their queries, discuss eligibility, and consent participants.

Staff

Any Health Care Professional (HCP) involved in the care of patients with T1D across the Southwest and West Midlands were contacted via email by the research teams in each hospital to ask if they would be interested in taking part in this study. As with patients those that expressed an interest were provided with an information sheet and offered an appointment to see the research nurse to discuss their involvement, to check their eligibility and to be consented.

Ethics

This study was carried out in accordance with the recommendations of the National Health Service Health Research Authority, through the Coventry and Warwickshire research Ethics Committee. The protocol was approved by the same committee and given the reference code 16/WM/0034. All subjects gave written informed consent in accordance with the Declaration of Helsinki.

Data Collection

We collected data on experiences of existing exercise education provision from staff and patients using focus groups or for those unable to attend the groups by semi-structured telephone interviews. Focus groups were chosen as the primary method of data collection as they offer opportunity for participants to reflect and test ideas rather than formulate ideas on the spot (31). The uninhibited discussion can also serve to remind participants of their past experiences and produce new thoughts about the delivery of education on exercise. In this study, the ability to generate information on collective views is useful to generate consensus to inform the nascent education package (31).

Two focus groups, were convened at each hospital (32). One was comprised of people with T1D and the second multi-disciplinary HCPs involved in T1D patient care. Each group was facilitated by IL a research fellow with extensive experience of qualitative methodologies used in improving health service delivery. A topic guide was used, tailored to either patients (see **Box 1**) or providers (see **Box 2**) and designed to allow themes and issues to arise naturally from the interaction of the group during the course of the meeting (33).

Box 1 | Patient Topic guide

Your own exercise programme

1. Can you tell me about the sort of exercise you regularly take each week?
   Prompts; When, who with, length/intensity/frequency, type of sport
2. Do you do anything special to prepare yourself – before, during or after exercising?
   Prompts: Food, diet, drinks - including alcohol
3. Do you have any problems when you exercise?
   Prompts: Tiredness, muscle fatigue, other
4. Is there anything that makes it easier/more difficult to exercise?
   Prompts: T1D, other medical condition, related non-medical factors

Current provision of information around exercise and managing your condition

5. Who have you spoken with about T1D and exercise?
   Prompts: Consultant, other hospital doctor, GP, nurse, dietician, other
6. When did you discuss this?
   Prompts: At diagnosis, at each consultation, every so often, a specific session
7. What was the content of the discussion?
   Prompts: Condition related - insulin, glucose levels, what to do about hypos Other health related - exercising when feeling unwell (colds etc.) Exercise related - different types of exercise and how much Preparation for exercise – steps to take during and recovering from exercise Diet - different foods, liquid and alcohol intake Environmental factors - the influence of hot/cold weather Personal characteristics – age, any other barriers and facilitators
8. Did you use additional sources of information?
   Prompts: Webinar, peer group, online, correspondence course, booklet

Analysis

Focus groups in the South West were conducted and analyzed first. These began with the patient focus group and were followed by the HCP group. This allowed for a preliminary analysis to inform the topic guide of the second set of focus groups conducted in the West Midlands. Staggering the focus groups and their analysis helped ensure that the key points were recognized and explored. Semi-structured interviews were carried out with participants unable to attend by the researcher using the same topic guide as in the focus groups.

The patient and staff transcripts from the focus groups conducted in the South West were independently coded by IL and SG a medical sociologist. Although IL moderated the focus groups and conducted the interviews the potential for bias was checked by the close involvement of SG who was not involved in data collection. All data were analyzed using thematic analysis (33) and underwent three key phases of coding. The first involved multiple detailed codes relating to the various responses of the participants following the first two focus groups. During the second phase these were grouped into broader over-arching themes which IL discussed with SG who had independently read the same two transcripts. The final phase was again conducted with SG where the over-arching themes and sub-themes were agreed following the final two focus groups and 1:1 interviews. IL and SG then met and agreed emerging themes and sub-themes from across both patient and staff groups. This then became the coding framework for the remaining focus groups at the West Midlands site and the semi-structured interviews. Initially the patient and HCP transcripts were coded separately but when IL and SG discussed the coding it was apparent that the initial overarching themes extended across all the interviews. As a result the data from all transcripts were combined and the results presented together.

Group discussions were digitally audio-recorded with permission, and transcribed verbatim for analysis, Data were managed using N-Vivo software. The intention in this instance was not to reach data saturation but instead to use the content

Box 2 | Staff topic guide

Current provision of information around exercise and T1D

1. What aspects of exercise do you usually discuss with patients?
   Prompts: The impact of different sports, length/intensity/frequency aerobic vs. anaerobic
2. When do you introduce this topic
   Prompts: At diagnosis, at each consultation, every so often, in a separate or targeted session (e.g. DAFNE)
3. Are there any particular types of patients with whom you find it easier/more difficult to talk about exercise with?
   Prompts: Age, ethnicity, gender, preferred exercise
4. What are the barriers if any to your discussing exercise?
   Prompts: Time, lack of knowledge
5. Which healthcare professionals should talk to patients about exercise?
   Prompts: Consultant, other hospital doctor, GP, nurse, dietician, other
6. What sorts of issues do you discuss?
   Prompts: Condition related - insulin, glucose levels, what to do about hypos; Other health related - exercising when feeling unwell (colds etc.) Exercise related - different types of exercise and how much, Preparation for exercise – including steps taken during and recovering Diet - different foods, liquid and alcohol intake Environmental factors - the influence of hot/cold weather

TABLE 1 | Patient participants.

Study ID	Time since diagnosis (years)	Exercise regime (Sessions per week)
SOUTH WEST (SW)		
P1	3.5	Gym x2, Karate x2
P2	20	Dance x4, Perform x1
P3	5	Hockey training x4, Play at the weekend
P4	3	Football x1, Cycle commute and run regularly
P5	50+	Gym x2, Keep fit class x1
P6	5.5	Horse riding x7 (Competes on weekends)
P7	3	Gym x3
P8	4	Cycling x2, Gym x1
WEST MIDLANDS (WM)		
P9	17.5	Gardening, Aikido x3
P10	2	Swim x1, Keep fit x1
P11	56	Gardening, Walking, Infrequent cycling
P12	36	Walking short distances x7
P13	6	Badminton x3
P14	6	Squash x1, Cycling x5

of the various discussions to inform the content and format of a novel education package[3]. However, by the end of the four focus groups and interviews no new themes or sub-themes were emerging.

RESULTS

Patients

Two focus groups were conducted consisting of a total of 14 patients. They were aged from 22 to 71 of which eight were males and six female. The group in the South West (SW) contained four male and four female participants and the time since diagnosis varied from 3 to 50 years. Those that exercised or competed regularly were predominantly found in the SW group, where five of the eight regularly exercised a minimum of four times a week. The discussion here lasted 80 min. In the West Midlands (WM) group there were four male participants and two female with a slightly broader range in the time since diagnosis than the SW group of between two and 60 years. They tended to exercise less in this group with only one participant undertaking exercise more than three times a week. The discussion lasted 86 min. The characteristics of all patient participants are summarized in **Table 1**.

Health Care Professionals

A total of 11 staff were interviewed in the two focus groups; of the five participants in SW three were dieticians and two were specialist diabetes nurses with between 6 and 21 years experience, four of them had taught on DAFNE or equivalent courses. The discussion lasted 69 min. The group from the West Midlands consisted of three specialist nurses, two dieticians and a speciality doctor, their experience ranged from between 4 and 15 years, four had experience of teaching on DAFNE or equivalent courses and the group ran for 75 min. Two semi-structured interviews were conducted both with consultant diabetologists from the South West (HCP6 and HCP7) who were unable to attend the focus groups as originally intended. The interviews lasted between 45 and 55 min. The characteristics of staff participants are summarized in **Table 2**.

Analysis

Themes were combined across patient and staff groups and four emerged which are presented together below. The first concerns the nature of the exercise regime undertaken by each individual relating to both its complexity in terms of the types and combination of exercise and the consistency in the pattern of exercise. The second theme centers on patient engagement, specifically how their ability to manage health is affected by the knowledge, skills and confidence they possess as reflected in their preferences, the use of self-management techniques and level of health literacy. The third theme is related to organizational factors concerning staff training, limits of capacity, consistency of care, and existing education strategies. These themes and sub-themes are summarized in **Table 3** and below we present exemplar quotes for each alongside the key characteristics of the participant that provided them. Additional and extended quotes can be found in **Supplementary Table 1**.

Exercise Regime

The types of exercise individuals enjoyed, the consistency of their exercise regime and the intensity of the activity all impacted

TABLE 2 | Staff participants.

Study ID	Job title	Time in post (years)	Exercise education provided
SOUTH WEST			
HCP1	Diabetes dietician	21	Teach on carbohydrate counting course (plus 4 h a week research)
HCP2	Diabetes dietician	8	Teaches on carbohydrate counting course, specialist interest in sport
HCP3	Diabetes dietician		Pediatrician (previously adult) Teaches on carbohydrate counting course
HCP4	Diabetes specialist nurse	6	Teaches on carbohydrate counting course
HCP5	Diabetes specialist nurse	12	1 day a week "pumps adviser"
HCP 6	Consultant in diabetes endocrinology, acute and general internal medicine	13	Proactive enquiry around exercise during consultation. Advises on range of exercise and activity
HCP 7	Consultant diabetes endocrinologist, and the clinical lead for patient specialities	8	Advises patients on recreational exercise and events such as marathons
WEST MIDLANDS			
HCP8	Speciality Doctor	8	Educates patients on exercise in response to their enquiries
HCP9	Diabetes dietician	2	Deliver the exercise section of the carbohydrate counting course.
HCP10	Specialist dietician	4	Teaches exercise as part of education programmes for both Type 1 and Type 2 diabetes.
HCP11	Diabetes specialist nurse	15	Teaches on carbohydrate counting course
HCP12	Diabetes specialist nurse	15	Teaches on carbohydrate counting course
HCP13	Diabetes specialist nurse	14.5	Teaches on carbohydrate counting course

TABLE 3 | Influences on the successful delivery of exercise education: themes and sub-themes.

Theme	Sub theme 1	Sub theme 2
1.0 Exercise regime	1.1 Type of exercise	Predictable intensity Anaerobic exercise Specialized sport
	1.2 Patterns of exercise	Routine vs. sporadic
	1.3 Intensity	Competitive vs. non-competitive
2.0 Patient engagement	2.1 Patient preference	Priority of exercise
	2.2 Self-management	Monitoring Carbohydrate counting
	2.3 Health Literacy	Understanding advice
3.0 Organizational factors	3.1 Staff training	Limited knowledge of the effects of exercise Deskilling
	3.2 Capacity	Limited access to education packages Limited access to specialist providers Length of consultation
	3.3 Coherence of care	Consistency of message Continuity of care
4.0 Existing education strategies	4.1 Structured education package	Criteria for inclusion
	4.2 Format and content	Patient stories Generic written information

on the ability of staff to advise them how to safely conduct this exercise.

Type of Exercise

Predictable Intensity

The nature of the exercise being undertaken was a key indicator of how confident staff felt in delivering appropriate advice. Staff described feeling most comfortable presenting advice to individuals who took part in relatively consistent bouts of aerobic exercise such as long-distance running or cycling.

> "... the longer distance runners, triathletes, and cyclists I tend to find a bit easier to work with, ... maybe because their activity is a bit more predictable? They tend to have... more structured training, and more obvious responses to their activity."
> - *HCP6 Consultant*

Patients reflected on how difficult it was to accurately predict the varying intensity of an individual bout of exercise and the difficulty this presented in managing their body's response.

> "... with the intensity, because that varies depending on just even how you're feeling on the day... you might not feel like you want to go too far... and therefore you get different readings than what you might have done a week ago doing the same distance, or length in time of exercise, or whatever."
> – *Patient 8*

Anaerobic Exercise

A notable area of uncertainty was instructing patients about anaerobic exercise such as weight-training. One diabetic specialist nurse (DSN) described how it felt counter-intuitive that blood sugar levels should rise after lifting weights and the struggle they had in coming to terms with the concept.

> "I still find it a bit hard around the anaerobic sport, when they're doing weights and things like that, and actually their blood sugars go up, so one guy I mentioned he does that first thing in the morning, so he has no breakfast and three units of insulin and

> goes to the gym, and then his blood sugars are okay. I sort in my head think "Oh!" [laughter] but it does work. But that took a lot on both of us gradually edging that up, but it doesn't seem right does it?"
> - *HCP5 Diabetes Specialist Nurse*

Patients also recognized the different effects on their physiology of aerobic as opposed to anaerobic exercise.

> " ...you know what to do for let's say, I don't know, spin class, you know how you need to fuel yourself for that, then if you want to change what exercise you do, if you want, I don't know... a spin class and a weight class affects me completely differently and I have to fuel differently for that,"
> – *Patient 7*

Specialized Sport

Staff spoke about how their personal experience of a particular sport would inform the advice they provided. Where patients undertook more specialized or unusual forms of exercise they felt less able to offer advice. For example one DSN described how her lack of understanding of the physical demand of extreme triathlons made it harder for her to provide relevant advice.

> "I get quite... we've got a couple that one is training to do the iron man competition, and one is doing a triathlon and I have absolutely no idea where to start, because I don't understand the sports themselves and exactly what they're actually trying to achieve. So not knowing what they're doing it's hard to give advice when you don't know, and I'm certainly not going to go and do a triathlon [laughs]."
> - *HCP13, Diabetes Specialist Nurse*

Patterns of Exercise

Routine vs. Sporadic

Whether the individual's exercise regime was predictable impacted on how readily it might be managed and the level of sophistication of advice and education they required. For example one patient expressed their uncertainty of how to manage change in their exercise routine.

> "...it's any kind change to your routine, if you can stick to your routine you're fine, but I find any kind of change is when I have problems."
> -*Patient 10*

Staff also described the issues they had informing patients who took on a variety of sports in various combinations. For example, one dietician described their apprehension in advising those that played an aerobically intense sport like rugby in the winter then a sport of lengthier duration with bursts of aerobic and anaerobic exercise such as cricket.

> "I think people that have a routine where they do things, the same exercise, are easier to advise, but those people like you were saying who do a different sport, or do cricket in the summer, rugby in the winter, and actually need to do very different things, and there's parts of the year when you're doing both."
> – *HCP5, Diabetes Specialist Nurse*

Intensity

Competitive vs. Non-competitive

Another factor central to the level of confidence of staff in speaking to patients about managing exercise was the standard at which individuals exercised or played sport. In the view of one dietician the sporting ability of a patient would impact on their own confidence to offer appropriate advice.

> "I think my difficulty comes when I've got people who are very sporty, either competitive sport or are training for something specific like for a marathon or something. Then I feel it stops my confidence not theirs, and that might rub off on them, I don't know, because then it becomes quite difficult, because you're managing quite a lot regarding their diabetes, and I suppose that's just experience of what to do with people that are very sporty or training..."
> – *HCP12, Diabetes Specialist Nurse*

One patient described how the impact of aerobically demanding competitive sport is more difficult to manage.

> "I used to event, luckily I don't event anymore, I just do dressage, so it's very controlled, so it's not a huge high impact thing. You work hard but your heart rate never [rapidly increases]... it probably does through adrenaline, but not like a run or if you're cycling hundreds of miles, it's quite controlled."
> – *Patient 6*

Patient Engagement

Patient engagement is defined as an individual's knowledge, skills, ability, and willingness to manage their own health and care[6]. Here we describe three factors related to the level of this engagement amongst our patients and how it shaped the support they requested, received, and assimilated. These factors are, their preference for the content of consultations, the level of competence in their self-management, and related to this, their level of health literacy.

Patient Preference

Priority of Exercise

We found that the content of any advice provided around exercise was frequently led by patient enquiry and related to their preferences and priorities. If regular exercise was a central activity prior to diagnosis then patients would be more likely to ask additional questions and require greater detail in the response. In this example a DSN described how the importance of exercise to the individual would be apparent from the first consultation and shape subsequent conversations.

> "It all depends very much on the patient because you might have somebody who is newly diagnosed who is a regular sportsperson and they're doing a particular activity, and they want to know whether they can keep it going, and they would introduce the fact that they need to have the advice, whereas you might have another person who is fairly newly diagnosed who actually wants to just concentrate on getting to terms with diabetes without looking

[6]https://www.kingsfund.org.uk/projects/gp-inquiry/patient-engagement-involvement (accessed October 2017)

at other things that can affect it. So it's all very much down to the individual."
– *HCP13, Diabetes Specialist Nurse*

Self-Management

Self-management describes the capability of an individual to recognize, treat, and manage their own health whether independently or in partnership with the healthcare system[7]. The basic advice offered to any patients with T1D irrespective of exercise regimen involves a number of self-management techniques, in particular how to monitor and record blood glucose levels, and count the carbohydrates they have consumed. The ability or willingness of patients to consistently fulfill these tasks would vary.

Monitoring

For clinicians to provide salient advice they must have some understanding of an individual's metabolic response to the exercise they undertake and the carbohydrates they consume. One patient who cycled for lengthy periods described how they would monitor their blood glucose sugar as often as every 30 min.

"...you've got to try and work it out like we've said before. But I think they said that every half an hour you've got to re-evaluate the situation, so when you're doing something like four and a half hours, I'm sure with cycling and things, if you do cycling you've got to look at it every half an hour and just take on fuel, it's hard work."
- *Patient 4*

However, some patients outwardly interested in undertaking regular exercise would fail to provide any information on their blood glucose levels. In its absence providers felt unable to offer relevant advice. For example a dietician described an instance where a patient wanted to increase their level of exercise without collecting or presenting the relevant information.

"...and I think the problem is we are generally presented with a person who maybe wants to increase activity or who has got problems, but presents you with no testing and no information, and then you say to them "Well you've got to go away, you've got to do some testing...."
– *HCP5, Diabetes Specialist Nurse*

Carbohydrate Counting

A basic knowledge of carbohydrate counting is necessary to exercise safely with T1D yet patients did not always possess this capability. One dietician described how patients with a keen interest in sport would not be able to complete the basic task of carbohydrate counting.

"Some people who come to you want to specifically talk about their interest in sport and how to manage it. But I find that some of them aren't even carbohydrate counting or have any of the foundations. So where you've set out to think this is all going to be targeted around sport you then begin stripping it back and doing all the foundations of the basic principles or carbohydrate counting and dose adjustment. So I found that it's pointless giving much information until they've even got that foundation, because otherwise that's more important than then tailoring for all the sports advice."
– *HCP2, Diabetes Dietician*

Related to this a patient described how they only learnt to control their body's response to training after an extended period of trial and error.

"Mine is a little bit involved with diet as well. So I tend to reduce the amount of insulin I'm having if I'm training, but if I'm performing at the weekend? I tend to carb load the day before, and then I have less [food] but fully protein based the day off, so that [way] my liver doesn't go into overdrive with my blood sugar spikes. It took me quite a while to work out how to manage that."
– *Patient 2*

Health Literacy

Understanding Advice

The term health literacy describes the ability of a patient to understand and assimilate health-related information[8]. Health literate patients with T1DM were able to independently use the written information contained within the booklets or pamphlets provided as part of their structured education package. For example a patient described how one such booklet provided by their diabetes team remained a useful reference point and allowed them to cope with some of the less common side-effects.

"I know that when I've been quite ill and I've used sick day rules through DAFNE, I'm glad I can grab that leaflet and that booklet and I can read, because it's hard to remember it because you don't often get ketones when you get ill, but if you've got good control you know you're getting ill and you can keep your levels low enough that you don't get ketones."
– *Patient 6*

In terms of communicating to patients one HCP described how they would use the "talking test" to help a patient understand the various levels of intensity of their exercise.

Talk about the talking test, whether they can talk and how red in the face they go, that's what we talk about, to calibrate it.
- *HCP7*

Organizational Factors

Organizational factors are related to the levels of staff training (and the ensuing confidence they have in imparting advice), the limited capacity of the system to cope with large numbers of patients, and the coherence of care provided across the patient's care team.

[7] https://www.england.nhs.uk/ourwork/patient-participation/self-care/ (accessed November 2017)

[8] https://www.hee.nhs.uk/our-work/health-literacy (accessed November 2017)

Staff Training

Limited Knowledge of the Effects of Exercise

Both staff and patients recognized there was a gap in providers' knowledge beyond a certain intensity or duration of exercise. One dietician described how they would impart advice on the basic tenets of carbohydrate counting and the principles of managing exercise but if asked to provide specific information they would instead refer the patient to a consultant.

> "The DAFNE and all our in-house carbohydrate counting covers the basic aspects of sport management but we were finding that we were getting people referred for they're going to climb Mount Kilimanjaro, and they're going to... and because it's slightly out of our depth we were finding that we were then referring a lot of those patients up to [specialist consultant] and there was a gap in terms of the basic level of education to the more elite, and whilst I was trying to bridge the gap and give information I didn't really feel fully qualified to give."
> – *HCP2, Diabetes Dietician*

The apparent reluctance of some HCPs to entertain discussions around exercise was also noted by patients. One felt that dieticians were very supportive of the general management of diabetes but hesitant to discuss exercise.

> "The dieticians in the formalized setting have been brilliant with everything else, so they would say to me "keep a diary, come back, let's see what did you do here?" And "that's the result of this," and "you've got the ratios correct, they're working for me". But the nurses and the dieticians whenever it comes to exercise they step back..."
> – *Patient 13*

Some of the carbohydrate counting courses offered to patients incorporated a practical element with patients measuring blood glucose levels before and after a spell of exercise. The HCPs we spoke to raised concerns around their involvement in any such element, at least without appropriate support. For example one Specialist Diabetic Nurse felt unwilling to take patients for a supervised gym session without being accompanied by a specialist member of staff.

> "...I wouldn't feel comfortable to take a group of people to a gym for multiple reasons. If it was a trainer now that's different... people who knew what they were doing and specialists in that field then fine, but not if it was just nurse and a dietician."
> - *HCP10, Specialist dietician*

Deskilling

The UK's guidance produced by the National Institute for Health and Care Excellence (NICE) recommends that carbohydrate counting courses be delivered by a trained educator (7). One unforeseen consequence of bringing in a specialist educator was that other members of the multidisciplinary team that would otherwise be involved in delivering the programme can become deskilled. One DSN described how the diabetes team were unfamiliar with the format of a new blood glucose diary as they had not been involved in its conception or introduction to patients.

> "I think the other thing is what we find when we have got some individual educators for DAFNE or whatever courses that are in a trust, and then what happens is they go back to their regular care, and that the other specialist consultant, or the registrar or the other DSN isn't geared up enough to deal with their new blood glucose diary they're faced with."
> – *HCP12, Diabetes Specialist Nurse*

Limited Capacity

The number of patients with T1D is growing and staff described how the ability of the service to provide education to all patients was inhibited by limited places on structured education programmes, shortages of relevant staff, and constraints on lengths of consultations.

Limited Access to Education Packages

The NICE guidance recommends that all those diagnosed with T1D should be offered a place on a structured education course between 6 and 12 months after diagnosis[1]. However, a consultant in the South West described how places on the course at their hospital were limited and expressed regret that they could not offer a place to everyone eligible.

> "It's not for every patient unfortunately. It would be lovely to have it for [everyone]... is just the SWIFT course is completely chocka for the next how many months, because it's multidisciplinary teaching, quite intensive, it takes the days out of their normal work..."
> – HCP 7, *Consultant diabetologist*

Limited Access to Specialist Providers

The restricted availability of specialist diabetic nurses was reported by one consultant who described how patients were unable to follow a prescribed care plan that involved reviews by specialist nurses because of a lack of appointments within the relevant time frame.

> "I will pick up the problem probably so, for those that I don't transfer out, I'll pick up what I think should... set out a plan, and I'll ask the nursing team to pick up in a follow up. The problem we have is actually the nursing clinic appointments are full, they do get longer with patients but there's little availability and sometimes I will have seen the patient again before the nurses have seen them. So that's obviously a barrier to getting good information off."
> – HCP7 *Consultant*

Length of Consultation

Both dieticians and consultants described how limits on the time they could spend with individual patients prevented a more detailed dialogue around exercise. The time constraints meant they would prioritize other aspects of T1D management in accordance with patient preference or clinical urgency.

> "Time is a nightmare. I think if I go into activity in detail I reckon you're looking at 45 minutes minimum, if you're trying to unpick... so I have a 20 minute slot and I'll spend 45 minutes with

someone who's doing regular sport and we're trying to unpick things, because by the time you have unpicked other stuff and you've dealt with other questions ... "
- HCP7 *Consultant*

"It's the time element as well; somebody is coming to you with [exercise] just up to a certain level - which may be their weekend football session with their pub team or something - that's okay, and I think that's fine and you can manage that within normal sessions. But if you've got somebody who is becoming a higher level, more competitive, or training for something, and quite big, then it takes a lot of your time up as well and you don't always get *that* amount of time to see the patient.."
- HCP12, Diabetes Specialist Nurse

Coherence of Care

Consistency of Message

Within the multi-disciplinary T1D care team staff possess varying levels of training, experience and interest and these differences appeared to lead to patients receiving inconsistent messages from even quite senior staff. For example, one consultant acknowledged that varied levels of awareness of the impact of exercising with T1D might mean advice differs depending on which consultant a patient speaks to.

"So we've got a number of consultants here, and I think you will... there's a couple of us who are much more interested than the others, and I am not sure you would get entirely consistent advice across the consultant group let alone a broader body."
- HCP7 Consultant

Issues emerged around inconsistent information from clinicians with expertise in other specialities whether based in secondary or primary care settings. One DSN described how colleagues in cardiology had experienced a patient with diabetes having hypoglycaemic episodes and so tried to prevent them from attending future cardio-rehabilitation classes.

"We've had people go to the cardiac rehab and we have phone calls because they've had hypos and they want to stop their exercise sessions at the cardiac rehab, and you're like "Yes but we can manage the hypos, the whole point of the cardiac rehab is after their heart attack or whatever else they've had..." and that is then a barrier but it's other healthcare professionals putting that barrier of a person doing the activity."
- HCP12, Diabetes Specialist Nurse

This variation in knowledge of TID between clinicians was also experienced by patients in primary care. One patient described how a locum general practitioner had failed to grasp the differences between Type 1 and Type 2 Diabetes.

"Like the GP thing - when I first started having conversations about the fact that I increase my exercise way back then, and then I was doing DAFNE, we had a locum GP and he said, "Well just low carb anything," and that was his response, and I went, "I'm Type 1!" he went, "It's the same thing." So I didn't listen to anything he said..."
- Patient 2

Continuity of Care

The benefits of continuity of care have been widely recognized across many healthcare settings (34, 35). The knowledge of the physical and mental characteristics of patients gained over time help to inform clinical decision making. In offering individual advice on exercising with T1D staff acknowledged the benefits of building up a relationship with a patient over time, and the increased understanding of how their body responded to exercise.

"It's just really individual. I think though when you are talking to certain people and you might get it right for their training, and then they have a race, and then their training then pushes their blood sugars up so they've got to do something different that day. So it's very hard to go 'I'll just go and get from the cupboard, because this is what you need...' because it is really individual, so you have to really know that person, how fit they are, what preparation they can and will do, and then try and tailor it that way to keep them safe and perform well."
- HCP2, Diabetes Dietician

A patient described how continuity of care was inhibited by a perceived lack of communication between primary and secondary clinicians.

"I think part of my problem with my GP surgery is they seem to think all of my care is being done by the hospital, the hospital thinks some of it is being done by the GP and I'm left in limbo with do I need to book an appointment with the GP, do I just wait for my letter to say I'm coming into the hospital?"
- Patient 8

Existing Education Strategies

Current guidance recommends that all patients are offered a place on a structured education package that teaches the basic skills of how to self-manage their condition between 6 and 12 months from diagnosis. The criteria used to determine who should be invited to attend and when was queried by patients. As well as taught courses a variety of written information is also made available to patients via their care provider and the design and content of some of these materials was also questioned.

Criteria for Invitation to Existing Packages

Criteria for Inclusion

Current guidelines recommend a period of 6 months before patients attend a course teaching them the basics of carbohydrate counting and insulin management as this would allow for their T1D to stabilize. However, some patients felt they would have benefitted from attending closer to their diagnosis, feeling the information would have been valuable to them earlier, particularly with relevance to their desire to exercise.

"...I personally feel that if I had been able to access DAFNE when I first started I would have handled it in such a different way. The National Health isn't giving individual choice of at what level you want to consume and take control. So a gentleman who had come on the DAFNE he had just been diagnosed, and it was all just too much for him and basically he had to leave. But for me it was just

the most... I wish that I didn't have the complications, if I had DAFNE five years ago I would have been able to handle it and my body would have been a lot better than what it is. So that's one thing that the National Health needs to do, it's one fits all kind of thing."
– *Patient 13*

Another criterion applied to the selection of patients for attendance on the course was the level of an individual's insulin consumption. One patient reported how they were not invited to attend because staff felt their insulin consumption was too low to justify attendance. However, the patient felt that information contained in the course would still have been useful as they had experienced difficulties in maintaining blood sugar levels from the beginning.

"I think you should be put on it quite quickly, even if you're not necessarily going to use the information they've given you. I wasn't on it until... I didn't go on DAFNE until May, and I think that was too late for me, it was just because I wasn't taking enough insulin to warrant going on it, but I don't think they should really use that, because especially - not necessarily for situations at home, because you know that you're cooking and stuff - but when you go out and things like that? It's really, it's difficult enough at home when you're just starting, it's really difficult to get it right, and I found that I was always way off my insulin when I was out, or if I was on holiday or something like that. But I think even if you're not necessarily going to use the information just have it there so that you can access it if you need to would have been helpful."
– *Patient 7*

Format and Content

Patient Stories

One educational tool frequently used as part of the structured education package but also via other platforms was the "patient story," a device that uses real-world examples to provide context for the learning point and so enable patients to more readily assimilate the information[9]. The stories used in T1D frequently involved elite sports stars whose experiences were so different to the patient's experience of living and exercising with T1D that little could be drawn from them[10].

"Look at the way they performed and they had all the back up in the world that you could ever want. Steve Redgrave is a whopper! His wife is a doctor, so she's there checking him out and pumping him full of insulin when he needs it. Danny McGrain and Mabbutt would have had the sports physios and all the doctors that professional footballers had on tap. Now the rest of us had to do it ourselves."
– *Patient 11*

In contrast to the stories of famous athletes several patients spoke of the value of the support they gained from people with T1D involved in similar sports and competing at a comparable level.

"I was lucky when I started, I had one of the guys on our mat, higher grade than me, he had been Type 1 since he was six... and I said to him one day, 'What is happening? I never know if I'm going to be finishing on 3.6 or ten.' He said, 'that's the way it is; don't fret because if you fret it will make it go higher.' So that was actually my most useful bit of information I had, 'don't fret'..."
– *Patient 9*

"I think it would maybe help more to have somebody that does exercise, somebody that is in this, somebody that's on the same page that lives it and knows it would definitely help."
– *Patient 1*

Generic Written Materials

Educational materials for patients with T1D are provided in a number of formats including booklets and posters. The design and content of these elements was questioned by some of our participants. One patient expressed disappointment at the tone of a poster in a shared waiting area and felt it was uninspiring, particularly during the period they were adjusting to their diagnosis.

"I suppose if you think about the psychology right, you've got all of these hospital appointments that you never used to have to do, you go and sit in some God awful waiting room with all these posters of cartoon characters, about having a carrot or something like that, and it's all this "Here's how your plate's divided." It's quite patronizing a lot of it, it's just it's not very enticing is it?"
– *Patient 10*

DISCUSSION

Key Findings

Though exercise avoidance and physical inactivity are common in patients with T1D this is the first time that the impact of the provision of advice and education on exercising safely has been explored simultaneously with patients and providers. Subsequently we have identified a number of interrelated influences on the success of this provision, these were; the nature of an individual's exercise regime including its intensity, type, and frequency; the degree of patient engagement relating to their preference, the self-management techniques employed, and individual health literacy; Organizational factors that affected staff training, and the capacity and coherence of the system; and finally issues around existing education strategies including access to structured education packages and the content and format of written materials.

Strengths and Limitations

We have gained a number of novel insights into issues specific to educating patients with T1D on how to exercise regularly and safely. The sample was relatively small and though the intention of this qualitative work was primarily to inform the content and format of a novel education package and not necessarily to reach data saturation, the staff, and patients that took part reflect a

[9] https://improvement.nhs.uk/documents/2140/patient-stories.pdf(accessed November 2017)
[10] https://www.diabetes.co.uk/celebrities/gary-mabbutt.html(accessed October 2017)

varied range of characteristics and by its completion saturation was reached (33). The inclusion criteria for the study meant all the patients we spoke to engaged in regular exercise and included a range of abilities, sports and exercise regimes. We recognize that patients with less ability or interest in exercise might have expressed different views and may need different support and education to encourage them to start to exercise or to exercise more regularly and safely. Similarly it is understood that staff and patients at non-participating sites may have offered alternative opinions due to differences in ethos and experience present at their facility.

Specific Findings/Existing Literature

Staff Training

Deficits in the training of health care providers (HCPs) to deliver advice on exercise were identified. The reported gaps in the knowledge of diabetes specialists reflect broader existing evidence of the repeated failure to equip clinicians with the basic knowledge, confidence and skills to promote physical activity (36, 37). There have been prior calls to train clinicians to prescribe exercise with the same regularity and level of detail as pharmaceutical options (38) and such targeted training has been shown to increase the frequency of exercise counseling for patients with chronic disease (39) including diabetes (40). In the UK and abroad recent initiatives have emerged specifically to educate care providers and patients about exercising with T1D such as JDRF's Performance in Exercise and Knowledge (PEAK) programme (41). However, it seems important that any such training initiative should be offered across the patient's entire care team. This is because we found that not only did dieticians and SDNs describe their lack of confidence in delivering advice on anything but routine and predictable exercise, but patients and staff described the conflicting advice offered to patients between staff groups, specialities, and care settings. One alternative way of ensuring advice remains consistent is to include exercise specialists as part of the existing multi-disciplinary teams (42, 43). However, staff we spoke to reported feeling deskilled as a result of using specialist educators and though effective in the short-term their presence may actually limit the ability of other providers to offer meaningful advice.

Lack of Capacity/Adherence to Guidelines

Despite current recommendations exercise did not routinely form part of current consultations among our study participants due at least in part to constraints on time and a reliance on patients to prompt any discussion on exercise. There is a lack of precision in the UK guidelines about the provision of support[1] for patients wishing to exercise. This is mirrored in the advice of the American Diabetic Association which though making a number of valuable recommendations for patients with T1D regards exercise and carbohydrate intake only suggests that patients may benefit from working with fitness experts that understand diabetes (44). There is no further stipulation of who should educate patients on the principles of managing exercise, when this should be introduced, who should provide continued and responsive support, and the explicit role of self-management (44).

Self-Management

In any chronic disease utilizing and improving the capacity of patients to self-manage is a key component of effective care leading to improved patient outcomes, adherence, and efficiency of healthcare utilization (45–48) and this includes patients with T1D (49). The need for effective education to enable patients to self-manage was apparent considering we heard how some keen on exercise failed to understand the importance of self-monitoring blood glucose levels (50). One of the current aims of the UK's National Diabetes Treatment and Care Programme is to improve the uptake of structured education packages designed to "facilitate the knowledge skills and ability for diabetes self-management" (51, 52). Currently the nationally reported take-up is <30% (53) perhaps due in part to the limitations in availability described by some providers we spoke to.

Existing Provision

The lack of capacity within the system places more importance on sources of educational material that can be independently accessed. The design and content of educational material for patients deserves careful consideration as it influences their satisfaction, adherence, and health outcomes (54) yet patients' needs are varied and their ability to independently assimilate this information determined by numerous factors including age, socio-economic status, education, and ethnicity (55–58). Some we spoke to described their antipathy toward aspects of existing diabetes educational material, including generic "diabetes" posters that failed to differentiate between T1D and Type II Diabetes. One particular source of frustration amongst patient participants was selecting elite sportspeople to tell their patient story[11]. Used appropriately these stories can be a powerful tool and through their familiarity, become especially vivid (35) yet many existing examples bore little resemblance to patients' everyday experience of living and exercising with T1D. Instead patients spoke of the value of peer-to-peer contact where the benefits of discussing relatable strategies and solutions would be more readily applicable. The benefits of this type of peer-to-peer mentoring in diabetes have been recognized previously and appear an underutilized resource in supporting those wishing to exercise (59).

CONCLUSION

Drawing on both patient and staff perspectives, our findings provide persuasive evidence of the need for a more responsive and directed education programme for patients with T1D that exercise regularly alongside a similar programme for providers to enable them to offer ongoing advice for this level of activity. Currently there is no such educational package available for patients with T1D and the findings we present here will inform the content and delivery of an educational package that can support patients not only in the UK but also internationally. The nascent EXTOD education package will be offered to all patients based on their interests and preferences and not dictated solely by the time since diagnosis. It will contain advice on

[11]http://www.diabetesadvice.co.uk/real-stories/sir-steve-redgraves-winning-ways-with-type-2-diabetes (accessed October 2017)

the management of regular and irregular bouts of aerobic and anaerobic exercise alongside how to prepare for specific events. The patient stories utilized will more closely reflect the everyday experiences of patients with T1D supported by group education that both facilitates peer-to-peer interaction and minimizes costs to the provider. Perhaps most importantly it will incorporate a section that trains staff across the diabetes care team to enable them to contribute to the course directly or more confidently offer applicable advice as part of their routine patient contact.

AUTHOR CONTRIBUTIONS

The overall concept of the project was devised by RA and PN. The data collection was conducted by IL and the analysis performed by IL and SG. IL produced the original draft this was then critically revised by SG, RA, and PN for important intellectual content. A further draft was produced and all authors approved the final submitted manuscript. Each author certifies that this material or similar material has not been and will not be submitted to or published in any other publication. IL is the guarantor who takes full responsibility for the work as a whole, including, access to data, and the decision to submit and publish the manuscript.

EXTOD EDUCATION PROGRAMME DEVELOPMENT TEAM

Yvonne Doherty, June Sorensen, Janette Barnette, Ian Gallen, Dinesh Nagi, Melanie Davies, Lindsey Apps, Janet Gorton, Heather Daley, Catherine Thompson, Manyee Li, Barbara Hudson.

REFERENCES

1. International Diabetes Federation. *Diabetes Atlas.* 6th ed. Brussels: International Diabetes Federation (2013).
2. Menke A, Orchard TJ, Imperatore G, Bullard KM, Mayer-Davis E, Cowie CC. The prevalence of type 1 diabetes in the United States. *Epidemiology* (2013) 24:773–4. doi: 10.1097/EDE.0b013e31829ef01a
3. Imperatore G, Boyle JP, Thompson TJ, Case D, Dabelea D, Hamman RF, et al. Projections of type 1 and type 2 diabetes burden in the U.S. population aged <20 years through 2050: dynamic modeling of incidence, mortality, and population growth. *Diabetes Care* (2012) 35:2515–20. doi: 10.2337/dc12-0669
4. Tao B, Pietropaolo M, Atkinson M, Schatz D, Taylor D. Estimating the cost of type 1 diabetes in the U.S.: a propensity score matching method. *PLoS ONE* (2010) 5:e11501. doi: 10.1371/journal.pone.0011501
5. Hex N, Bartlett C, Wright D, Taylor M, Varley D. Estimating the current and future costs of Type 1 and Type 2 diabetes in the UK, including direct health costs and indirect societal and productivity costs. *Diabet Med.* (2012) 29:855–62. doi: 10.1111/j.1464-5491.2012.03698.x
6. Office of Disease Prevention and Health Promotion. *2008 Physical Activity Guidelines for Americans Summary* (2008). Available online at: https://health.gov/paguidelines/guidelines/summary.aspx (Accessed Oct 2017).
7. Moy CS, Songer TJ, LaPorte RE, Dorman JS, Kriska AM, Orchard TJ, et al. Insulin-dependent diabetes mellitus, physical activity, and death. *Am J Epidemiol.* (1993) 137:74–81.
8. Chimen M, Kennedy A, Nirantharakumar K, Pang TT, Andrews R, Narendran P. What are the health benefits of physical activity in type 1 diabetes mellitus? A literature review. *Diabetologia* (2012) 55:542–51. doi: 10.1007/s00125-011-2403-2
9. American Diabetes Association. Physical activity/exercise and diabetes. *Diabetes Care* (2004) 27 (Suppl. 1):S58–62. doi: 10.2337/diacare.27.2007.S58
10. Tonoli C, Heyman E, Roelands B, Buyse L, Piacentini MF, Berthoin S, et al. Diabetes associated cognitive decline, is there a role for exercise? *J Diabetes Metab.* (2013) S10:006. doi: 10.4172/2155-6156.S10-006
11. Chiang JL, Kirkman S, Laffel LMB, Peters AL. Type 1 diabetes through the life span: a position statement of the American Diabetes Association. *Diabetes Care* (2014) 37:2034–54. doi: 10.2337/dc14-1140
12. Laaksonen DE, Atalay M, Niskanen LK, Mustonen J, Sen CK, Lakka TA, et al. Aerobic exercise and the lipid profile in type 1 diabetic men: a randomized controlled trial. *Med Sci Sports Exerc.* (2000) 32:1541–8. doi: 10.1097/00005768-200009000-00003
13. Lehmann R, Kaplan V, Bingisser R, Bloch KE, Spinas GA. Impact of physical activity on cardiovascular risk factors in IDDM. *Diabetes Care* (1997) 20:1603–11.
14. Bohn B, Herbst A, Pfeifer M, Krakow D, Zimny S, Kopp F, et al. Impact of physical activity on glycemic control and prevalence of cardiovascular risk factors in adults with type 1 diabetes: a cross-sectional multicenter study of 18,028 patients. *Diabetes Care* (2015) 38:1536–43. doi: 10.2337/dc15-0030
15. Steppel JH, Horton ES. Exercise in the management of type 1 diabetes mellitus. *Rev Endocr Metab Disord.* (2003) 4:355–60. doi: 10.1023/A:1027302112655
16. McCarthy MM, Funk M, Grey M. Cardiovascular health in adults with type 1 diabetes. *Prev Med.* (2016) 91:138–43. doi: 10.1016/j.ypmed.2016.08.019
17. Nadeau KJ, Regensteiner JG, Bauer TA, Brown MS, Dorosz JL, Hull A, et al. Insulin resistance in adolescents with type 1 diabetes and its relationship to cardiovascular function. *J Clin Endocrinol Metab.* (2010) 95:513–21. doi: 10.1210/jc.2009-1756
18. Lascar N, Kennedy A, Hancock B, Jenkins D, Andrews RC, Greenfield S, et al. Attitudes and barriers to exercise in adults with type 1 diabetes (T1DM) and how best to address them: a qualitative study. *PLoS ONE* (2014) 9:e108019. doi: 10.1371/journal.pone.0108019
19. Pierre-Louis B, Guddati AK, Syed MKH, Gorospe VE, Manguerra M, Bagchi C, et al. Exercise capacity as an independent risk factor for adverse cardiovascular outcomes among nondiabetic and diabetic patients. *Arch Med Sci.* (2014) 10:25–32. doi: 10.5114/aoms.2014.40731
20. Brazaeu A, Rabasa-Lhoret R, Strychar I, Mircescu H. Barries to physical activity among patients with type 1 diabetes. *Diabetes Care* (2008) 31:2108–09. doi: 10.2337/dc08-0720
21. Jabbour G, Henderson M, Mathieu ME. Barriers to active lifestyles in children with type 1 diabetes. *Can J Diabetes* (2016) 40:170–2. doi: 10.1016/j.jcjd.2015.12.001
22. Colberg SR. Key points from the updated guidelines on exercise and diabetes. *Front Endocrinol.* (2017) 8:33. doi: 10.3389/fendo.2017.00033
23. Reddy M, Rilstone S, Cooper P, Oliver NS. Type 1 diabetes in adults: supporting self management. *BMJ* (2016) 352:i998. doi: 10.1136/bmj.i998
24. Franzese A, Mozzillo E, Nugnes R, Falco M, Fattorusso V. *Type 1 Diabetes Mellitus and Co-morbidities, Type 1 Diabetes.* London: IntechOpen.
25. Due-Christensen M, Zoffmann V, Willaing I, Hopkins D, Forbes A. The process of adaptation following a new diagnosis of type 1 diabetes in adulthood: a meta-synthesis. *Qual Health Res.* (2018) 28:245–58. doi: 10.1177/1049732317745100
26. Kenny GP, Sigal RJ, McGinn R. Body temperature regulation in diabetes. *Temp Multidiscip Biomed J.* (2016) 3:119–45. doi: 10.1080/23328940.2015.1131506
27. Knight CJ, Lowe R, Edwards M, Yardley JE, Bain SC, Bracken RM. Type 1 diabetes and physical activity: an assessment of knowledge and needs in healthcare practitioners. *J Diabetes Nurs.* (2016) 20:271–7.
28. Kennedy A, Narendran P, Andrews RC, Daley A, Greenfield SM, for the EXTOD Group. Attitudes and barriers to exercise in adults with a recent diagnosis of type 1 diabetes: a qualitative study of participants in the Exercise for Type 1 Diabetes (EXTOD) study. *BMJ Open* (2018) 8:e017813. doi: 10.1136/bmjopen-2017-017813

29. Campbell MD, Kime N, McKenna J. Exercise and physical activity in patients with type 1 diabetes. *Lancet Diabetes Endocrinol.* (2017) 5:493–4. doi: 10.1016/S2213-8587(17)30168-7
30. Gill P, Stewart K, Treasure E, Chadwick B. Methods of data collection in qualitative research. *Br Dent J.* (2008) 204:291–5. doi: 10.1038/bdj.2008.192
31. Stewart DW, Shamdasani PM. *Focus Groups. Theory and Practice.* London: Sage (1990).
32. Morgan DL, editor. Future directions in focus group research. In: *Succesful Focus Groups.* London: Sage (1993) 224–244.
33. Cassell C, Symon G. *Essential Guide to Qualitative Methods in Organizational Research.* London: SAGE Publications (2004).
34. Guthrie B, Saultz JW, Freeman GK, Haggerty JL. Continuity of care matters. *BMJ* (2008) 337:a867. doi: 10.1136/bmj.a867
35. Pereira Gray DJ, Sidaway-Lee K, White E, Thorne A, Evans PH. Continuity of care with doctors—a matter of life and death? A systematic review of continuity of care and mortality. *BMJ Open* (2018) 8:e021161. doi: 10.1136/bmjopen-2017-021161
36. Weiler R, Chew S, Coombs N, Hamer M, Stamatakis E. Physical activity education in the undergraduate curricula of all UK medical schools. Are tomorrow's doctors equipped to follow clinical guidelines? *Br J Sports Med.* (2012) 46:1–3. doi: 10.1136/bjsports-2012-091380
37. Thornton JS, Fremoont P, Khan K, Poirier P, Fowles J, Wells GD, et al. Physical activity prescription: a critical opportunity to address a modifiable risk factor for the prevention and management of chronic disease: a position statement by the Canadian Academy of Sport and Exercise Medicine. *Br J Sports Med.* (2016) 50:1109–14. doi: 10.1136/bjsports-2016-096291
38. Nunan D. Doctors should be able to prescribe exercise like a drug. *BMJ* (2016) 353:i2468. doi: 10.1136/bmj.i2468
39. Joyce CL, O'Tuathaigh CM. Increased training of general practitioners in Ireland may increase the frequency of exercise counselling in patients with chronic illness: a cross-sectional study. *Eur J Gen Pract.* (2014) 20:314–9. doi: 10.3109/13814788.2014.900534
40. Shields CA, Fowles JR, Dunbar P, Barron B, McQuaid S, Dillman CJ. Increasing diabetes educators' confidence in physical activity and exercise counselling: the effectiveness of the "physical activity and exercise toolkit" training intervention. *Can J Diabetes* (2013) 37:381–7. doi: 10.1016/j.jcjd.2013.08.265
41. JDRF, TypeOneNation. *T1D Performance in Exercise and Knowledge.* Available online at: www.jdrf.org/peak (Accessed Oct 2017).
42. Cheema BS, Robergs RA, Askew CD. Exercise physiologists emerge as allied healthcare professionals in the era of non-communicable disease pandemics: a report from Australia, 2006–2012. *Sports Med.* (2014) 44:869–77. doi: 10.1007/s40279-014-0173-y
43. Johnson ST, Mundt C, Qiu W, Soprovich A, Wozniak L, Plotnikoff RC, et al. Increase in daily steps after an exercise specialist led lifestyle intervention for adults with type 2 diabetes in primary care: a controlled implementation trial. *J Phys Act Health* (2015) 12:1492–9. doi: 10.1123/jpah.2014-0200
44. Colberg SR, Sigal RJ, Yardley JE, Riddell MC, Dunstan DW, Dempsey PC, et al. Physical activity/exercise and diabetes: a position statement of the American Diabetes Association. *Diabetes Care* (2016) 39:2065–79. doi: 10.2337/dc16-1728
45. Schulman-Green D, Jaser S, Martin F, Alonzo A, Grey M, McCorkle R, et al. Processes of self-management in chronic illness. *J Nurs Scholarship* (2012) 44:136–44. doi: 10.1111/j.1547-5069.2012.01444.x
46. Corbin JM, Strauss A. *Unending Work and Care: Managing Chronic Illness at Home.* San Francisco, CA: Jossey-Bass (1998).
47. Dunbar SB, Clark PC, Quinn C, Gary RA, Kaslow NJ. Family influences on heart failure self-care and outcomes. *J Cardiovasc Nurs.* (2008) 23:258–65. doi: 10.1097/01.JCN.0000305093.20012.b8
48. Grey M, Knafl K, McCorkle R. A framework for the study of self and family management of chronic conditions. *Nurs Outlook* (2006) 54:278–86. doi: 10.1016/j.outlook.2006.06.004
49. Kovatchev BP, Cox DJ, Straume M, Farhy LS. Association of self-monitoring blood glucose profiles with glycosylated haemoglobin in patients with insulin-dependent diabetes. *Methods Enzymol.* (2000) 321:410–7. doi: 10.1016/S0076-6879(00)21205-6
50. Wei N, Zheng H, Nathan DM. Empirically establishing blood glucose targets to achieve HbA1c goals. *Diabetes Care* (2014) 37:1048–51. doi: 10.2337/dc13-2173
51. NHS. *National Diabetes Treatment and Care Programme* (2016). Available online at: https://www.england.nhs.uk/wp-content/uploads/2016/12/diabetes-call-to-bid.pdf (Accessed Oct 2017).
52. Group TNA. *National Diabetes Audit 2012-2013 Report 1: Care Processes and Treatment Targets.* Health and Social Care Information Centre (2014).
53. Gadsby R, Young B. Diabetes care in England and Wales: information from the 2010-2011 National Diabetes Audit. *Diabet Med.* (2013) 30:799–802. doi: 10.1111/dme.1218
54. National Voices. *Improving Information and Understanding: A Summary of the Evidence* (2014). Available online at: https://www.nationalvoices.org.uk/sites/default/files/public/publications/improving_information.pdf (Accessed Oct 2017).
55. Davis TC, Dolan NC, Ferreira MR, Tomori C, Green KW, Sipler AM, et al. The role of inadequate health literacy skills in colorectal cancer screening. *Cancer Investig.* (2001) 19:193–200. doi: 10.1081/CNV-100000154
56. Williams MV, Baker DW, Parker RM, Nurss JR. Relationship of functional health literacy to patients' knowledge of their chronic disease. A study of patients with hypertension and diabetes. *Arch Intern Med.* (1998) 158:166–72.
57. Lukoschek P, Fazzari M, Marantz P. Patient and physician factors predict patients' comprehension of health information. *Patient Educ Counsel.* (2003) 50:201–10. doi: 10.1016/S0738-3991(02)00128-3
58. National Institute for Care and Health Excellence (NICE). *Patient Experience in Adult NHS Services: Improving the Experience of Care for People Using Adult NHS Services.* (2012). Available online at: https://www.nice.org.uk/guidance/cg138 (Accessed Oct 2017).
59. Knox L, Huff J, Graham D, Henry M, Bracho A, Henderson C, et al. What peer mentoring adds to already good patient care: implementing the Carpeta Roja Peer Mentoring Program in a well-resourced health care system. *Ann Fam Med.* (2015) 13(Suppl. 1):S59–65. doi: 10.1370/afm.1804

4

Transient Depletion of Foxp3$^+$ Regulatory T Cells Selectively Promotes Aggressive β Cell Autoimmunity in Genetically Susceptible DEREG Mice

Deepika Watts[1,2,3], *Marthe Janßen*[1,2,3], *Mangesh Jaykar*[1], *Francesco Palmucci*[1,2,3], *Marc Weigelt*[4], *Cathleen Petzold*[1], *Angela Hommel*[4], *Tim Sparwasser*[5], *Ezio Bonifacio*[2,3,4] *and Karsten Kretschmer*[1,2,3]*

[1] Molecular and Cellular Immunology/Immune Regulation, Center for Regenerative Therapies Dresden (CRTD), Center for Molecular and Cellular Bioengineering (CMCB), Technische Universität Dresden, Dresden, Germany, [2] Paul Langerhans Institute Dresden (PLID) of the Helmholtz Zentrum München at the University Hospital and Medical Faculty Carl Gustav Carus of TU Dresden, Dresden, Germany, [3] German Center for Diabetes Research (DZD e.V.), Neuherberg, Germany, [4] Regenerative Therapies for Diabetes, Center for Regenerative Therapies Dresden (CRTD), Center for Molecular and Cellular Bioengineering (CMCB), Technische Universität Dresden, Dresden, Germany, [5] Institute of Infection Immunology, TWINCORE/Centre for Experimental and Clinical Infection Research, Hanover, Germany

Correspondence:
Karsten Kretschmer
karsten.kretschmer@tu-dresden.de

Type 1 diabetes (T1D) represents a hallmark of the fatal multiorgan autoimmune syndrome affecting humans with abrogated Foxp3$^+$ regulatory T (Treg) cell function due to *Foxp3* gene mutations, but whether the loss of Foxp3$^+$ Treg cell activity is indeed sufficient to promote β cell autoimmunity requires further scrutiny. As opposed to human Treg cell deficiency, β cell autoimmunity has not been observed in non-autoimmune-prone mice with constitutive *Foxp3* deficiency or after diphtheria toxin receptor (DTR)-mediated ablation of Foxp3$^+$ Treg cells. In the spontaneous nonobese diabetic (NOD) mouse model of T1D, constitutive Foxp3 deficiency did not result in invasive insulitis and hyperglycemia, and previous studies on Foxp3$^+$ Treg cell ablation focused on Foxp3^{DTR} NOD mice, in which expression of a transgenic BDC2.5 T cell receptor (TCR) restricted the CD4$^+$ TCR repertoire to a single diabetogenic specificity. Here we revisited the effect of acute Foxp3$^+$ Treg cell ablation on β cell autoimmunity in NOD mice in the context of a polyclonal TCR repertoire. For this, we took advantage of the well-established DTR/GFP transgene of DEREG mice, which allows for specific ablation of Foxp3$^+$ Treg cells without promoting catastrophic autoimmune diseases. We show that the transient loss of Foxp3$^+$ Treg cells in prediabetic NOD.DEREG mice is sufficient to precipitate severe insulitis and persistent hyperglycemia within 5 days after DT administration. Importantly, DT-treated NOD.DEREG mice preserved many clinical features of spontaneous diabetes progression in the NOD model, including a prominent role of diabetogenic CD8$^+$ T cells in terminal β cell destruction. Despite the severity of destructive β cell autoimmunity, anti-CD3 mAb therapy of DT-treated mice interfered with the progression to overt diabetes, indicating that the novel NOD.DEREG model can be exploited for preclinical studies on T1D under experimental conditions of synchronized, advanced β cell autoimmunity. Overall, our studies highlight the continuous requirement of Foxp3+ Treg cell activity for the control of genetically pre-installed autoimmune diabetes.

Keywords: type 1 diabetes, immune regulation, Treg cells, Foxp3, cell ablation

INTRODUCTION

Type 1 diabetes (T1D) is a chronic disease under complex environmental, immunological and genetic control, which is manifested by the autoimmune destruction of functional insulin-producing β cells of pancreatic islets caused by islet-infiltrating diabetogenic CD4+ and CD8+ T cells (1, 2). The concept of Foxp3+ regulatory T (Treg) cell-based therapies to interfere with β cell autoimmunity in T1D has been fueled in large part by evidence indicating that diminished Treg cell activity may contribute to disease pathogenesis. In fact, many of the T1D genetic susceptibility loci have been implicated in Foxp3+ Treg cell function, either through indirect (e.g., *IL2*) or direct (e.g., *IL2R, CTLA4, PTPN22, IL10*) mechanisms (2). Likewise, T1D is considered a hallmark (3) of the fatal multiorgan autoimmune syndrome (IPEX; immune dysfunction, polyendocrinopathy, enteropathy, X-linked) affecting humans with abrogated Treg cell function due to genetic *FOXP3* gene mutations (4, 5), demonstrating that a severe Treg cell defect is sufficient to promote destructive β cell autoimmunity independently of other genetic and environmental factors. However, loss-of-function studies in non-autoimmune and diabetes-prone mice have not been able to demonstrate an unequivocal link between Foxp3+ Treg cell deficiency and catastrophic β cell autoimmunity. In mice on a non-autoimmune genetic background, constitutive genetic *Foxp3* deficiency (6, 7) or acute Foxp3+ Treg cell ablation based on Foxp3-driven expression of a human diphtheria toxin receptor (DTR) (8–10) recapitulates many clinical features of the human IPEX syndrome, but the manifestation of β cell autoimmunity has not been reported. Moreover, Foxp3-deficient *scurfy* mice on the diabetes-prone NOD background (NOD.Foxp3^{sf}) develop exocrine pancreatitis and peri-insulitis, but do not develop insulitis and overt diabetes, unless the CD4+ T cell receptor (TCR) repertoire of NOD.Foxp3^{sf} mice is artificially restricted to a single highly diabetogenic specificity by transgenic expression of the BDC2.5 TCR (11). These observations could be interpreted as evidence that Foxp3+ Treg cells are dispensable for the autoimmune β cell protection in the NOD model, but the interpretation of data in the constitutive absence of Treg cells is hampered by potentially confounding effects of immune adaptations and severe systemic autoimmunity, including premature death and alterations in thymic T cell development (12). The administration of mAbs directed against CD25 as 'surrogate' Treg cell marker largely preserves systemic immune homeostasis and has been employed to examine the role of Foxp3+ Treg cells in the control of β cell autoimmunity. However, CD25 is not uniquely expressed on Foxp3+ Treg cells, and anti-CD25 mAb treatment has been proposed to act on Treg cells by functional inactivation, rather than physical depletion (13–15), while sparing Foxp3+ Treg cells with a CD25− phenotype. These limitations in specificity and efficiency of CD25-targeted interference with Foxp3+ Treg cell activity may account for the largely contradictory range of data in the NOD model, including precipitation of overt diabetes (16–19), accelerated diabetes progression in young but not adult mice (20), as well as maintenance of β cell tolerance (21–23), or even delayed onset of diabetes (22).

Foxp3-driven DTR expression has been successfully employed for the specific and temporally controlled ablation of Foxp3+ Treg cells (8–10, 24), while the outcome can considerably differ between independent Foxp3^{DTR} mouse lines, depending on the transgenic strategy of Foxp3-driven DTR/GFP expression. In 'knock-in' mice expressing a DTR/GFP fusion protein from an IRES down-stream of the endogenous *Foxp3* gene (Foxp3$^{IRES\text{-}DTR/GFP}$) on a non-autoimmune genetic background, DT-mediated Treg cell-ablation in young and adult Foxp3$^{IRES\text{-}DTR/GFP}$ mice resulted in an autoimmune disease similar to that observed in Foxp3-deficient mice (8). In the DEREG ('depletion of regulatory T cell') model, in which DTR/GFP is expressed from a transgenic Foxp3 bacterial artificial chromosome (Foxp3$^{BAC\text{-}DTR/GFP}$), administration of DT into newborns resulted in *scurfy*-like symptoms, while adults were found to be protected from autoimmune diseases, despite efficient GFP+ Treg cell depletion (9). In fact, and as opposed to Foxp3$^{IRES\text{-}DTR/GFP}$ mice, the Foxp3$^{BAC\text{-}DTR/GFP}$ transgene of DEREG mice is not physically linked to the endogenous *Foxp3* gene, allowing for the accumulation of DT-resistant Foxp3+GFP− Treg cells (25–28). These unique features prompted us to hypothesize that the DEREG model is particularly suited to study the role of Foxp3+ Treg cells in organ-specific autoimmunity in mice on a genetically susceptible genetic background, while keeping collateral autoimmune damage to a minimum. In previous studies employing a NOD model, in which the spontaneous diabetes development was constrained by transgenic BDC2.5 TCR expression on all CD4+ T cells (29), acute Foxp3+ Treg cell ablation was shown to unleash a highly aggressive form of autoimmune diabetes (30), which fully abrogated the sex bias usually observed in spontaneous diabetes progression of NOD mice (31). Here, we report on the specific effects of acute Foxp3+ Treg cell ablation on the physiologic disease course in autoimmune diabetes-prone DEREG mice in the context of a polyclonal TCR repertoire.

MATERIALS AND METHODS

Mice

NOD/ShiLtJ, NOD.Rag1$^{-/-}$, NOD.BDC2.5 mice (all Jackson Laboratories, Bar Harbor, USA), and DEREG mice (9) on different genetic backgrounds (C57BL/6, BALB/c, or NOD) were housed and bred at the Animal Facility of the CRTD under specific pathogen-free conditions. NOD.DEREG mice were obtained by backcrossing C57BL/6.DEREG mice onto the NOD/ShiLtJ background for ≥13 generations. NOD.DEREG mice were intercrossed with NOD.BDC2.5 mice to obtain NOD.DEREG × BDC2.5 mice. All NOD mouse lines were fed with NIH #31M rodent diet (Altromin, Germany). Blood glucose levels were measured using whole blood from the tail vein and Accu-Chek® Aviva (Roche). If not stated otherwise, blood glucose levels were routinely determined once a week. Mice were considered diabetic at blood glucose levels above 200 mg/dl on at least two consecutive measurements or with blood glucose levels once above 400 mg/dl. All animal experiments were performed as approved by the Landesdirektion Dresden (24-9168.24-1/2014-1, DD 24-5131/338/38 (TVV37/2015).

DT-mediated Foxp3$^+$ Treg Cell Ablation and Adoptive Cell Transfers

Mice were *i.p.* injected with 0.5 μg DT (Merck Millipore - Calbiochem, Darmstadt, Germany) in 200 μl of sterile PBS on two consecutive days, if not stated otherwise. Where indicated, DT-treated NOD.DEREG mice were additionally *i.v.* injected with 5 μg anti-CD3e mAb (145-2C11). For total splenocyte transfers, single-cell suspensions were prepared from pooled spleens of 4-5-week-old (n = 4) and 16-18-week-old (n = 6) NOD.DEREG females, and 5 x 10^6 total cells were *i.v.* injected into NOD.Rag$^{-/-}$ recipient mice, followed by two consecutive injections of DT at day 7 and 8. For CD4$^+$BDC2.5$^+$ T cell transfers, conventional T (Tcon) cells (CD4$^+$CD62L^{hi}Vβ-4$^+$CD25$^-$GFP$^-$) and Foxp3$^+$ Treg cells (CD4$^+$Vβ-4$^+$CD25^{high}GFP$^+$) were FACS-isolated (99.3 – 99.8% purity) from pooled spleen and LN of NOD.DEREG × BDC2.5 mice. FACS-purified DTR$^-$ Treg cells (CD4$^+$Vβ-4$^+$CD25^{high}) from DEREG$^-$ NOD.BDC2.5 mice were included to control for DT toxicity. Diabetogenic Tcon cells (5 × 10^5) were *i.v.* injected into NOD.Rag$^{-/-}$ recipient mice, either alone or co-injected with DTR$^+$ or DTR$^-$ Treg cells (1 × 10^5), followed by DT injection on three consecutive days in week 6 after adoptive transfer.

Immunohistochemistry

Pancreatic cryosections (5μm) were fixed in 4% formalin and stained for C-peptide using polyclonal rabbit anti-C-peptide Ab (Cell Signaling, Germany), followed by Alexa Fluor 488-labeled polyclonal goat anti-rabbit IgG Ab (Invitrogen). Subsequently, detection of CD3 was carried out using rat anti-CD3 mAb (CD3-12) (AbD Serotec), followed by staining with Alexa Fluor 568-labeled polyclonal goat anti-rat secondary Ab (Invitrogen). Nuclei were visualized using 4′-6-Diamidino-2-phenylindole (DAPI). Slides were mounted with Vectashield (Vector Laboratories, Burlingame, CA, USA), using standard protocols. All images were acquired with a Leica SP5 upright Laser Scanning confocal microscope. For evaluation of lymphocyte infiltration (insulitis), at least three sections were collected at 50 μm intervals and 6-12 pictures per pancreas were taken, using the following scale (32): 0, no infiltration; 1, minimal focal infiltration; 2, peri-islet infiltration (<50%); 3, intra-islet infiltration (>50%); 4, extensive infiltration (100%).

Flow Cytometry and Cell Sorting

Pancreatic islets were isolated by collagenase digestion (0.7 mg/ml) (Sigma-Aldrich Chemie GmbH) and discontinuous Ficoll density gradient. Single-cell suspensions of pancreatic islets and lymphoid tissues were prepared using 70 μm cell strainers (Becton Dickinson, San Diego, CA, USA) and Hank's buffer [1 x HBSS, 5% (v/v) FCS, 10mM HEPES; all Invitrogen]. Single cell suspensions from spleen were additionally subjected to red blood cell lysis (erythrocyte lysis buffer EL, Qiagen). Peripheral blood mononuclear cells (PBMCs) were obtained by retro-orbital sinus puncture [PBS supplemented with 10% (v/v) Heparin (Biochrom AG, Berlin, Germany)] and Ficoll (VWR, Darmstadt, Germany) gradient centrifugation. mAbs to CD3 (145-2C11), CD4 (RM4-5, GK1.5), CD8 (53–6.7), CD25 (PC61, 7D4), CD44 (IM7), CD62L (MEL-14), Vβ-4 (KT4), and CD49b (R1-2) were purchased from eBioscience (Frankfurt, Germany) or BD (Heidelberg). The samples were analyzed using a LSRII or sorted on a FACS Aria (all BD). Data were analyzed with the FlowJo software (Tree Star).

Immunophenotyping

For flow cytometry-based immunophenotyping, male and female cohorts of adult, age-matched NOD.DEREG mice were either left untreated or injected with DT on two consecutive days. Pancreatic islets, pancreatic lymph nodes (pLN), and a collection of other lymphoid tissues [subcutaneous LN (scLN), spleen, and thymus] were harvested before (day 0) or at different days after (day 1-7, day 10) administration of the first dose of DT (3-6 mice per timepoint). Single-cell suspensions were subjected to multicolor flow cytometry for the quantification of immune subsets (αβ T cells, NKT cells, and NK cells: mAbs directed against CD3, CD4, CD8, CD25, and CD49b; B cells, granulocytes, macrophages, and dendritic cells: mAbs directed against CD19, Gr1, CD11b, and CD11c).

Gene Expression Analysis

Freshly isolated pancreata were subjected to rapid freezing and grinding in liquid nitrogen, followed by total RNA extraction using Trizol® (Life Technologies), the RNeasy Mini Kit, and DNase I digestion (Qiagen, Hilden, Germany). Total RNA was extracted from pLN using the RNeasy Mini Kit, DNase I digestion. For real-time RT-PCR, cDNA was synthesized using Oligo-d(T) primers and SuperScript II reverse transcriptase (Invitrogen) according to the manufacturer's recommendations. The QuantiFast SYBR Green PCR kit (Qiagen) and a Mastercycler ep realplex thermal cycler (Eppendorf) was used to analyze cDNA in replicates. The following primers were used: β-Actin, 5'-TGG AAT CCT GTG GCA TCC ATG AAA C-3' and 5'- TAA AAC GCA GCT CAG TAA CAG TCC G-3'; GzmA, 5'-TTT CAT CCT GTA ATT GGA CTA A-3' and 5'-GCG ATC TCC ACA CTT CTC-3'; IFN-γ, 5'-GGC TGT TAC TGC CAC GGC ACA-3' and 5'-CAC CAT CCT TTT GCC AGT TCC TCC-3'; GITR, 5'-GAC GGT CAC TGC AGA CTT TG-3' and 5'-GCC ATG ACC AGG

AAG ATG AC-3'; NKG2D, 5'-ACG TTT CAG CCA GTA TTG TGC-3' and 5'-GGA AGC TTG GCT CTG GTT C-3'.

RESULTS

Generation of Autoimmune Diabetes-Prone DEREG Mice

The DEREG mouse line was originally developed on the non-autoimmune prone C57BL/6 background (9). Here, we introduced the $Foxp3^{BAC\text{-}DTR/GFP}$ transgene of DEREG mice into the autoimmune diabetes-susceptible NOD background by extensive backcrossing (see *Materials and Methods*). We preferred this strategy, rather than generating a novel Foxp3-DTR transgenic line directly on the NOD genetic background, because adult DEREG mice on a non-autoimmune prone genetic background have been shown to be resistant to autoimmune diseases or *scurfy*-like symptoms after DT treatment (9, 25, 26). Confirming the validity of our NOD.DEREG model, DT-untreated female mice spontaneously developed overt diabetes, which was accompanied by an early onset of insulitis at ≤ 4 weeks of age and progressive loss of insulin-producing β cells (see below), resulting in the manifestation of hyperglycemia from 12 weeks of age (**Supplementary Figure S1**). In line with previous reports on efficient Treg cell depletion in C57BL/6.DEREG mice (9), administration of two consecutive daily doses of DT into NOD.DEREG mice resulted in an > 98% depletion of $CD4^+GFP^+$ Treg cells in peripheral blood (day 3, **Figure 1A**), while total $CD4^+$ T cell proportions (mean ± SD: day 0: 58.3 ± 5.0, day 3: 53.3 ± 4.3, day 7: 52.6 ± 6.0) did not significantly change over time (Unpaired t-test, n = 8). We observed a similar efficiency of

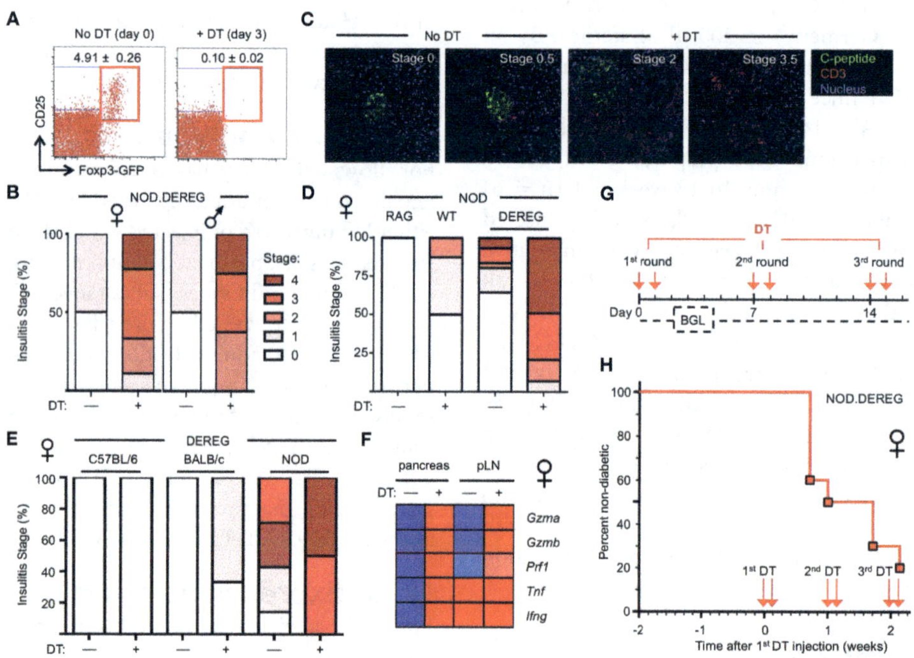

FIGURE 1 | Rapid progression to overt diabetes after acute Treg cell ablation in adult NOD.DEREG females. Mice were either left untreated or injected with DT on two consecutive days, and subjected to further analysis on day 14, unless otherwise stated. **(A)** Efficiency of Treg cell ablation. Representative dot plots of CD4-gated cells from peripheral blood of 16-week-old NOD.DEREG females before (day 0) and after (day 3) injection with DT. Numbers in dots plots indicate mean percentage ± SD of 8 mice (unpaired t-test, p < 0.001) from a single experiment representative of 6 experiments performed (5-9 mice per experiment).
(B–E) Pancreatic pathohistological changes. Histological sections were scored as described in Materials and Methods. **(B)** Insulitis scores of 4-5-week-old female (left, n = 10) and male (right, n = 9) NOD.DEREG mice. As all mice remained normoglycemic by day 7 after the first DT injection, two additional doses of DT were administered (day 7 and 8) prior to histology on day 14. **(C)** Representative histology and **(D)** insulitis score of 8-9-week-old NOD.DEREG females (8-10 mice per group). Untreated NOD.RAG (n = 4) and DT-injected $DEREG^-$ NOD (n = 5) females were included as controls. **(E)** Insulitis scores of 16-week-old DEREG females on different genetic backgrounds (4-7 mice per group). **(F)** Expression of mRNA encoding immune effector molecules with known function in autoimmune β cell destruction. Freshly isolated mRNA from pancreas and pLN (pooled from 4-5 mice per group) of 10-12-week-old NOD.DEREG females was subjected to real-time RT-PCR using β-Actin for normalization. Heat map (row normalized) shows mean values of triplicate samples from a single experiment representative of at least two independent experiments performed. Blue and red represent lowest and highest gene expression values, respectively. Pancreas, Unpaired t-test: p < 0.001: *Gzma, Gzmb, Prf1, Tnf*; p ≤ 0.01: *Ifng*. pLN, Unpaired t-test: p <0.001: *Gzma, Gzmb*; p ≤ 0.01: *Prf1*; not significant: *Tnf, Ifng*. **(G, H)** Manifestation of overt diabetes.
(G) Cohorts of 16-week-old, initially non-diabetic NOD.DEREG mice were repeatedly injected with 2 doses of DT at 5-day-intervals, as indicated. Blood glucose levels (BGL) were determined at least three times per week. **(H)** Diabetes incidence of female NOD.DEREG mice. Mice were considered diabetic at blood glucose levels above 200 mg/dl on at least two consecutive measurements or with blood glucose levels once above 400 mg/dl. Data are from a single experiment (n = 10) representative of > 8 experiments performed. Note that the diabetes incidence of male NOD.DEREG mice is depicted in **Supplementary Figure S3**.

DT-mediated Treg cell depletion in both sexes of NOD.DEREG mice, and over a wide age range (4 weeks – 12 months).

Massive β Cell Loss and Hyperglycemia Within Days after Acute Treg Cell Ablation

In previous studies on a non-autoimmune-prone background, DT-mediated Treg cell depletion resulted in autoimmune diseases only when injected into newborn DEREG mice (9). Consistently, and despite multiple repeated injections of DT, Treg cell depletion in cohorts of young, 4–5-week-old NOD.DEREG mice caused worsening of initially mild insulitis in both sexes (**Figure 1B**), but the majority of mice (≥ 90%) remained normoglycemic and showed no *scurfy*-like symptoms (scaliness and crusting of eyelids/ears/tail, hepatomegaly, splenomegaly, enlarged lymph nodes, early death) (data not shown). In contrast, the pancreas of adult NOD.DEREG females showed strong pathohistological changes, when only two doses of DT were administered on consecutive days, and histological analysis of the pancreas was performed on day 12 (**Figures 1C–E**). This included massive $CD3^+$ T cell infiltrates throughout the islet space and complete islet disaggregation with only a few, if any, residual insulin-producing β cells in DT-treated NOD. DEREG mice (**Figure 1C**). In the control cohorts, DT-treated DTR^- littermates or sham-injected DTR^+ NOD mice exhibited no or only minimal peri-islet infiltration (**Figures 1C, D**). With regard to the susceptibility to multiple autoimmune diseases in the NOD background, histological analysis of adult, 9-12-week-old females of our NOD.DEREG colony revealed marked thyroid immune infiltrates, as expected (33), but the severity of autoimmune thyroiditis appeared similar between sham- and DT-injected mice, irrespective of whether they remained nondiabetic or progressed to hyperglycemia (**Supplementary Figure S2A**). We observed only very rare cases (<5%) of autoimmune neuropathy (34) among diabetic Treg cell-depleted mice, as indicated by the manifestation of hind limp paralysis with histological evidence for immune infiltration in the peripheral nerves (**Supplementary Figure S2B**).

Overall, the manifestation of destructive β cell autoimmunity was strictly dependent on the NOD genetic predisposition, as the pancreata of DT-treated DEREG females on the C57BL/6 or BALB/c background were devoid of immune infiltration and evidence for β cell death (**Figure 1E**). Notably, DT treatment was found to preserve the age-dependent differences in the severity of spontaneous insulitis that is found in DT-untreated NOD.DEREG females, when comparing different age groups (**Figure 1B**, 4-5 weeks; **Figure 1D**, 8-9 weeks; **Figure 1E**, 16 weeks). Thus, it appears that acute Treg cell ablation in NOD.DEREG mice exacerbates pre-established β cell autoimmunity, while preserving key features of spontaneous diabetes development in the NOD model (35, 36). Consistently, DT treatment of prediabetic NOD.DEREG adults increased mRNA expression of the Th1 cytokines TNF-α and IFN-γ selectively in the pancreas, while up-regulation of other autoimmune effector molecules with known functions in β cell destruction could be observed in both pLN and pancreas, such as Granzyme A, Granzyme B or Perforin (**Figure 1F**). The expression of mRNA encoding pro-inflammatory cytokines, such as innate-derived IL-1β or Th2 and Th17 signature cytokines (*e.g.*, IL-4, IL-13, IL-21, IL-22), remained below the detection limit in DT-treated NOD.DEREG mice, but were readily detectable in adolescent $Foxp3^{sf}$ mice (data not shown). Finally, in cohorts of adult NOD.DEREG mice, ≥ 50% of female (**Figures 1G, H**, *see also* **Figure 3E**) but only ≤ 10% of male (**Supplementary Figure S3**) mice progressed to overt diabetes within 5 days after the administration of two doses of DT. In these experiments, the administration of DT on two consecutive days was required to reproducibly promote overt diabetes at a high incidence. A single dose of DT or the repeated injection of three single doses of DT at 7-day-intervals into cohorts of adult (8-16-week-old) or aged (6-12-months-old) females only sporadically resulted in the induction of diabetes, with an incidence ranging from 0-10% (data not shown).

Mechanisms That Constrain Autoimmunity in DT-Treated NOD.DEREG Mice

In DT-treated NOD.DEREG mice, the manifestation of overt diabetes in the absence of other autoimmune symptoms suggests an intricate balance between diabetogenic and tolerogenic mechanisms, which constrain aggressive autoimmunity primarily to pancreatic β cells. Overall, the efficiency of DT-mediated Treg cell depletion was comparable between different lymphoid tissues and pancreas, reaching its maximum on day 3 after the first of two doses of DT at all anatomical sites (**Figure 2A**). However, the kinetics of Treg cell recovery differed between anatomical sites. Consistent with the thymus as a primary site of Treg cell *de novo* generation, $CD4^+GFP^+$ cells became first detectable in the thymus (day 4, **Figure 2A**), followed by the continuous replenishment of the $CD4^+GFP^+$ Treg cell compartments at peripheral sites, resulting in a recovery rate of 60-70% in spleen and scLN by day 10 (**Figure 2A**). In comparison, the kinetics of GFP^+ Treg cell recovery in pancreas and pLN was somewhat delayed, reaching ≤ 35% at day 10 (**Figure 2A**), which is likely to facilitate local autoimmune responses, while the rapid GFP^+ Treg cell recovery in secondary lymphoid tissues is providing a rather narrow time window for the manifestation of systemic autoimmunity.

Given that the endogenous *Foxp3* gene and the $Foxp3^{BAC\text{-}DTR/GFP}$ transgene are not physically linked, the activity of $Foxp3^+$ Treg cells with a DTR/GFP^- phenotype may represent another mechanism that limits catastrophic autoimmunity in DT-treated NOD.DEREG mice. While the expression of GFP and Foxp3 closely correlates in steady-state DEREG mice, DT administration can result in the proliferative expansion of an initially minute population of DT-resistant DTR/GFP^-Foxp3^+ Treg cells (37). In fact, 43.1 ± 3.5% (mean ± SD, n = 3) of pancreatic $CD4^+CD25^+GFP^-$ cells expressed Foxp3 protein at day 5 after DT administration, as compared to 9.1 ± 1.5% (mean and range of duplicate samples) in DT-untreated NOD.DEREG mice, as judged by the analysis of Foxp3 protein expression using anti-Foxp3 mAb (data not shown). Furthermore, the restoration of a pancreatic GFP^+ Treg cell compartment was preceded by the accumulation of such DTR/GFP^-CD25^+ T cells within 1-2 days after DT administration (**Figure 2B**). DT-resistant DTR/GFP^-CD25^+ T cells

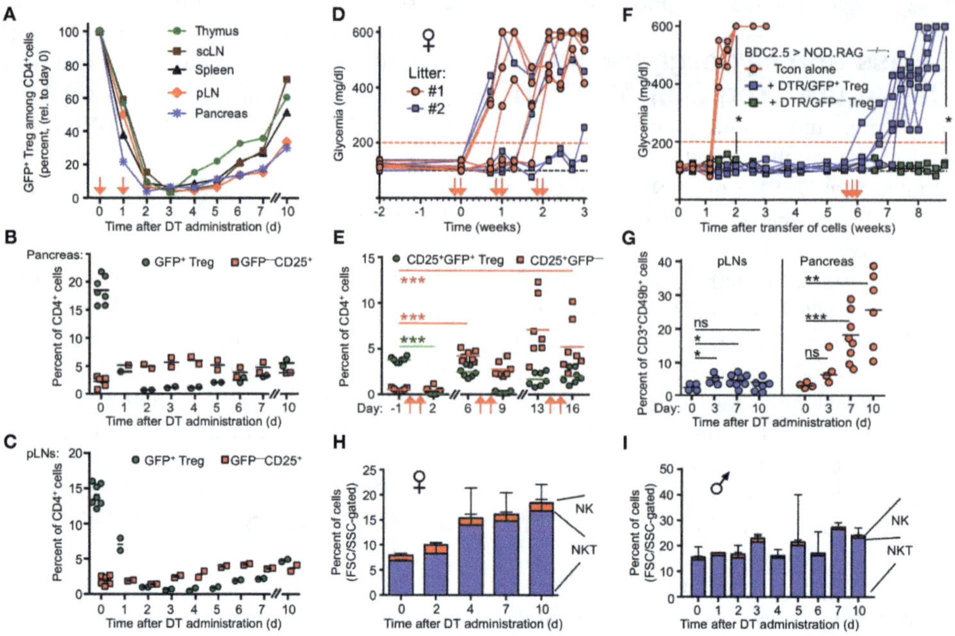

FIGURE 2 | Transient nature of Treg cell ablation in NOD.DEREG mice. **(A)** Kinetics of DT-mediated ablation and subsequent recovery of the CD4$^+$GFP$^+$ Treg cell compartment in pancreas and indicated lymphoid organs of 10-12-week-old NOD.DEREG mice. Data are from a single experiment (2 mice/timepoint) representative of 3 experiments performed. Arrows indicate days of DT injection. **(B, C)** GFP$^+$ Treg cell recovery in **(B)** pancreas and **(C)** pLN is preceded by the rapid accumulation of CD4$^+$CD25$^+$ cells lacking DTR/GFP expression (GFP$^-$). Each symbol corresponds to an individual mouse (10-12-week-old). **(D, E)** Impact of repeated DT administration on glycemic state and Treg cell depletion. **(D)** Blood glucose concentrations of individual NOD.DEREG mice presented in **Figure 1 (H)**. Arrows indicate days of DT injection. **(E)** Kinetics of CD25$^+$GFP$^+$ and CD25$^+$GFP$^-$ cells among CD4-gated cells, as revealed by flow cytometry among peripheral blood-derived CD4$^+$ T cells at different timepoints (Two-way ANOVA in combination with Bonferroni's Multiple Comparison post-test: ***p < 0.001). **(F)** Acute Treg cell ablation in the absence of Treg cell rebound. NOD.RAG1$^{-/-}$ mice were repopulated with diabetogenic BDC2.5 T conventional cells, either alone (red circles) or with GFP$^+$ (blue squares) or DTR/GFP$^-$ (green squares) Treg cells, and blood glucose levels of recipients were routinely assessed at least twice a week for up to 9 weeks. DT was injected at three consecutive days of week 6 (arrows). (Mann-Whitney-U test; two weeks: p = 0.0159, nine weeks: p = 0.0476). **(G–I)** Pancreatic NKT cell accumulation after Treg cell ablation. **(G)** Percentages of CD3$^+$CD49b$^+$ NKT cells among FSC/SSC-gated cells in pLNs (left) and pancreas (right) of 12-16-week-old NOD.DEREG females before (day 0) and at indicated days after DT administration. Symbols and horizontal lines indicate individual mice (4-8 mice per timepoint) and mean values, respectively. Unpaired t-test: ns, not significant; *p ≤ 0.05, **p ≤ 0.01, ***p < 0.001). **(H, I)** Kinetics of pancreas-infiltrating CD3$^+$CD49b$^+$ NKT and CD3$^-$CD49b$^+$ NK cells (FSC/SSC-gated) in **(H)** female and **(I)** male NOD.DEREG mice (10-12-week-old). Shown are mean percentages ± SD (day 0: n = 7) or mean percentages and range of replicate mice (days 1-7, day 10: n = 2).

also accumulated at other anatomical sites of DT-treated NOD.DEREG mice, although with delayed kinetics (**Figure 2C**). The rapid dynamics of Treg cell rebound was further illustrated by longitudinal studies concerned with the impact of prolonged DT administration (**Figures 1H**) on the progression to hyperglycemia (**Figures 2D**) and the GFP$^-$/GFP$^+$ Treg cell compartment size in peripheral blood (**Figure 2E**) of individual mice. Consistent with our data on pancreas (**Figure 2B**) and lymphoid tissues (**Figures 2A, C**), the population size of both GFP$^-$ and GFP$^+$ cells in blood markedly increased by day 6 after the first round of two DT doses (**Figure 2E**). The repeated injection of two doses of DT at 5-day intervals further enhanced the accumulation of DT-resistant CD25$^+$DTR/GFP$^-$ Treg cells, while the depletion efficiency of the CD25$^+$DTR/GFP$^+$ compartment appeared to decrease (**Figure 2E**).

Next, we aimed to assess the impact of DT-mediated Treg cell depletion on β cell autoimmunity mediated by defined numbers of diabetogenic T cells, in the absence of potentially confounding effects of 'rebounding' Treg cells. For this, immunodeficient NOD.Rag1$^{-/-}$ mice (no B and T/NKT cells) were reconstituted with 5 x 10^5 diabetogenic CD4$^+$BDC2.5$^+$ T cells, either alone or with small numbers of DTR/GFP$^+$ Treg cells (5 x 10^4 cells), followed by the injection of DT in week 6 (**Figures 2F**). In this experimental setting, the *de novo* generation of Foxp3$^+$ Treg cells is precluded by the complete block of thymic T cell development in NOD.Rag1$^{-/-}$ recipients, and DT-resistant DTR/GFP$^-$ Treg cells were excluded by FACS-based isolation of GFP$^+$ Treg cells prior to adoptive transfer. While co-transferred Treg cells efficiently interfered with the manifestation of overt diabetes, all recipients of DTR/GFP$^+$ Treg cells nearly synchronously developed severe hyperglycemia within 1 week after DT-mediated depletion (**Figure 2F**). DT-treated NOD.Rag1$^{-/-}$ recipients of diabetogenic CD4$^+$BDC2.5$^+$ T cells and DTR$^-$ Treg cells remained normoglycemic, excluding a major role of DT toxicity on β cell death (**Figure 2F**).

Overall, these data highlight the continuous requirement for Treg cell-mediated suppression in the control of destructive β cell autoimmunity, and suggest Treg cell rebound as plausible mechanism underlying the incomplete diabetes penetrance in

DT-treated NOD.DEREG mice (**Figure 1H**). Additionally, kinetics studies employing flow cytometric immunophenotyping (see Materials and Methods) indicated that $CD3^+CD49b^+$ NKT cells were initially less abundant in the pancreas of female NOD.DEREG mice, but their population size gradually increased after DT administration (**Figures 2G, H**), whereas the pancreatic NKT cell compartment in males remained largely constant (**Figure 2I**). Although their exact role in T1D has been controversially discussed (38–41), these data suggest that NKT cells may exert a tolerogenic function in Treg cell-depleted NOD.DEREG females.

Anti-CD3 mAb Therapy Following Treg Cell Depletion Interferes With Diabetes

With the exception of NKT cells (*see* **Figure 2G, H**), our flow cytometric immunophenotyping revealed no other quantitative changes of major immune cell subsets in the pancreas of NOD.DEREG mice (data not shown). This also holds true for $CD3^-CD49b^+$ NK cells (**Figure 2H**), which have previously been shown to undergo massive proliferative expansion (up to 5-fold) within 48 hours after DT-mediated Treg cell depletion in a $Foxp3^{BAC\text{-}DTR/GFP}$ NOD mouse line carrying the diabetogenic BDC2.5 TCR as additional transgene (30). Additionally, acute Treg cell ablation in adult NOD.DEREG mice had no impact on the population size of pancreatic $CD4^+$ and $CD8^+$ T effector cells (**Supplementary Figure S4**), which are thought to play a major role as physiologic mediators of β cell destruction in the NOD model (2, 35). However, DT administration increased the frequency of $CD8^+$ T cells with an effector/memory phenotype, in pancreas (**Figure 3A**) and pLN (**Figure 3B**), and to a lesser extend in scLN (**Figure 3C**), which could be attributed to an increase in the compartment size of $CD62L^{low}CD44^{high}$ effector/ memory T cells at the expense of $CD62L^{high}CD44^{low}$ naïve T cells. We made similar observations for conventional $CD4^+$ T effector cells (**Supplementary Figure S5**), but anti-CD4 mAb (GK1.5) administration into cohorts of Treg cell-depleted NOD.DEREG mice (n = 10) did not appreciably interfere with the manifestation of overt diabetes, whereas anti-CD8α mAb (53.6.72) administration reduced the diabetes incidence to 10%, as compared to 50% in untreated and 60% in anti-CD4 mAb-treated mice (data not shown). One interpretation of these data is that $CD4^+$ T cells are dispensable at this stage of the disease,

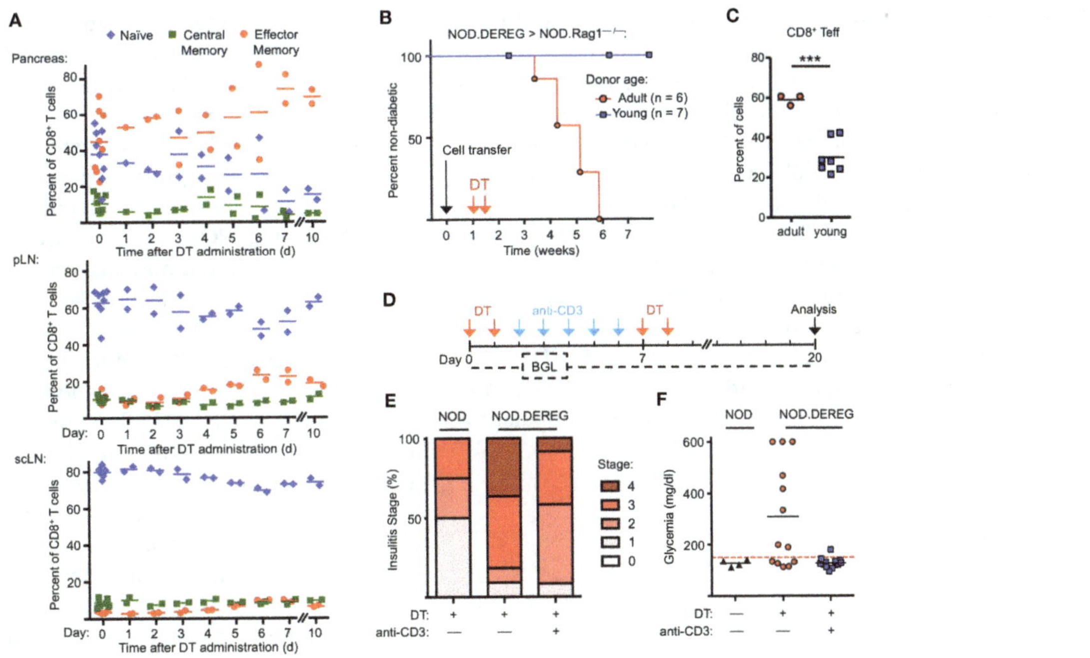

FIGURE 3 | Anti-CD3 mAb therapy after Treg cell ablation ameliorates insulitis and prevents progression to hyperglycemia. **(A)** Kinetics of $CD8^+$ T cells with a naïve ($CD62L^{high}CD44^{low}$), central memory ($CD62L^{int}CD44^{int}$), and effector/memory ($CD62L^{low}CD44^{high}$) phenotype in pancreas (top), pLN (middle), and scLN (bottom) of 10-12-week-old NOD.DEREG mice before (day 0) and at indicated days after DT administration. **(B, C)** Adoptive splenocyte transfer model. **(B)** Splenocytes from adult (16-18-week-old) but not young (4-5-week-old) DTR/GFP^+ NOD.DEREG donors promote overt diabetes in NOD.RAG1$^{-/-}$ recipient mice after DT treatment. Black arrow indicates the day of splenocyte transfer (2×10^6 total cells), and red arrows indicate the days of DT administration. (Log-Rank (Mantel-Cox) test, p = 0.0097). **(C)** Proportions of $CD8^+$ T cells with a $CD62L^{low}CD44^{high}$ effector/memory phenotype in the pLN of NOD.RAG1$^{-/-}$ recipients of splenocytes from young (red circles) or adult (blue squares) NOD.DEREG donors. Unpaired t-test: ***$p < 0.001$. **(D–F)** anti-CD3 mAb treatment of Treg cell-depleted NOD.DEREG mice.
(D) Scheme of experimental design. Cohorts of adult NOD.DEREG females were injected with DT only (n = 13), or were additionally treated with anti-CD3 mAb (n = 13). Untreated DTR/GFP^- NOD.DEREG mice were included for comparison (n = 4). Arrows: red, DT injection; blue, anti-CD3 injection; black, analysis by histology and flow cytometry. Blood glucose concentrations were assessed before (day 0) and every second day after the first injection with DT until the end of the observation period on day 14. **(E)** Histological insulitis score of indicated experimental groups, and **(F)** blood glucose levels of individual mice (one-way ANOVA: $p \leq 0.01$). Each symbol in **(A, C, F)** corresponds to an individual mouse.

while $CD8^+$ T cells represent the final effector cells. As the CD8α chain is not exclusive to αβ T cells, but also expressed on other immune cells (such as NKT or DCs), we next assessed the diabetogenic potential of NOD.DEREG splenocytes after injection into lymphopenic NOD.Rag1$^{-/-}$ mice (**Figure 3D**). In this adoptive transfer model, the manifestation of overt diabetes has been shown to be strictly $CD8^+$ T cell-depend, with numbers of diabetogenic $CD8^+$ T cells closely correlating with the kinetics of β cell destruction (42). Our results show that DT administration into NOD.Rag1$^{-/-}$ recipients of splenocytes from cohorts of adult NOD.DEREG females promotes overt diabetes in all recipients (**Figure 3B**), which correlated with an enrichment of effector/memory-type $CD8^+$ T cells in the pLN (**Figure 3C**) but not scLN (data not shown). In contrast, all NOD.Rag1$^{-/-}$ recipient mice of splenocytes from young NOD.DEREG donors maintained normoglycemia during the entire observation period of 8 weeks (**Figure 3B**). These data further indicate that $CD8^+$ T cells are key mediators of destructive β cell autoimmunity in the NOD.DEREG model, and provide a mechanistic basis for our observation that young, DT-treated NOD.DEREG mice are largely refractory to the manifestation of diabetes (**Figure 1B**).

We also assessed the impact of anti-CD3 mAb therapy on β cell autoimmunity in Treg cell-depleted NOD.DEREG mice (**Figure 3D**). In the NOD model, treatment with anti-CD3 mAb at recent diabetes onset has been shown to restore normoglycemia and long-term immune tolerance, but was ineffective in preventing destructive β cell autoimmunity, when injected at earlier stages of diabetes development (43, 44). Our results show that anti-CD3 mAb administration following DT administration ameliorated the strong pathohistological changes observed in the pancreas of Treg cell-depleted cohorts of adult NOD.DEREG females (**Figure 3E**) and interfered with the manifestation of hyperglycemia in all anti-CD3-treated mice (**Figure 3F**). Normoglycemia was also maintained when DT was repeatedly injected after discontinuation of anti-CD3 mAb treatment (**Figures 3D, F**), indicating that anti-CD3 mAb-mediated β cell protection is independent of repopulating GFP^+ Treg cells.

DISCUSSION

Here, we show that the specific ablation of $Foxp3^+$ Treg cells in DEREG mice can reproducibly precipitate severe insulitis and stable hyperglycemia in the context of a polyclonal TCR repertoire, provided that the autoimmune susceptibility is pre-installed by the NOD genetic background. One of the strengths of the NOD.DEREG model is that it preserves key aspects of the physiologic disease course in Treg cell-proficient NOD mice (*e.g.*, Th1 bias, role of $CD8^+$ T cells, female sex bias), while the transient nature of DT-mediated Treg cell depletion minimizes potentially confounding effects of systemic autoimmunity. The reappearance of $Foxp3^+$ Treg cells shortly after withdrawal of DT has also been observed in other $Foxp3^{DTR}$ lines (8, 45), including $Foxp3^{BAC\text{-}DTR/GFP}$ mice (9), but the apparent differences in the depletion efficiency and recovery kinetics between mouse lines indicate that the DEREG model is particularly suitable for studies on the Treg cell-mediated control of organ-specific autoimmune responses (26).

Overall, our findings indicate that the diabetes incidence in Treg cell-depleted NOD.DEREG mice is largely determined by the extent of preformed pancreatic lesions and numbers of diabetogenic $CD8^+$ T cells at the time of DT administration. This is in line with the observation that $Foxp3^{sf}$ mice (11) and 4-5-week-old, DT-treated NOD.DEREG mice (**Figure 1B**) are refractory to the manifestation of severe insulitis, despite a comparable efficiency in the DT-mediated depletion of the pancreatic Treg cell compartment in young and adult NOD.DEREG mice (data not shown). However, the severity of destructive β cell autoimmunity in DT-treated adult NOD.DEREG females appears rather unexpected, in particular in light of previous studies on $Foxp3^+$ Treg cell targeting using anti-CD25 mAb and the moderate spontaneous diabetes incidence that we observed in the present study in DT-untreated NOD.DEREG mice (**Supplementary Figure S1A**). Importantly, and consistent with strong pancreatic lesions (**Figures 1C–E**), many Treg cell-depleted NOD.DEREG mice nearly synchronously progressed to overt diabetes within 3 days after the administration of only 2 doses of DT (**Figure 2D**). In fact, this rapid kinetics was comparable to previous observations made in BDC2.5 TCR-transgenic DEREG (31)and $NOD^{BAC\text{-}DTR/GFP}$ mice (30). We also addressed the possibility that alleviating the metabolic stress of residual β cells by insulin replacement therapy for the duration of Treg cell recovery may help restoring metabolic homeostasis (*e.g.*, by promoting the regeneration of functional β cells) (46, 47). However, the administration of exogenous insulin into DT-treated NOD.DEREG mice shortly after diagnosis of overt diabetes restored normoglycemia for several weeks, but all mice returned to high blood glucose levels, once insulin therapy was discontinued (data not shown), further illustrating the destructiveness of β cell autoimmunity.

Our data suggest a scenario, in which pancreatic $Foxp3^+$ Treg cells in prediabetic NOD.DEREG mice interfere rather late in the cascade of events ultimately leading to the spontaneous progression of overt diabetes, highlighting the important role of continuous Treg cell activity in constraining terminal β cell destruction by pancreas-infiltrating $CD8^+$ T cells. This interpretation is further supported by our observation that, in contrast to anti-CD4 mAb, anti-CD8 and anti-CD3 mAb (44) administration into DT-treated NOD.DEREG mice interfered with the progression to overt diabetes (**Figure 3F**), despite substantial histopathological changes (**Figure 3E**). In this context, anti-CD3 mAb is of particular interest, as targeting CD3 is a promising approach currently being pursued for the therapy of human T1D (48, 49). Several non-mutually exclusive mechanisms underlying the action of anti-CD3 mAb therapy have been proposed, including the induction of recessive tolerance in pathogenic T effector cells (50), and of dominant tolerance by promoting $Foxp3^+$ Treg cell activity (51, 52). Notably, in the BDC2.5-transgenic NOD^{Rag} model of autoimmune diabetes, anti-CD3 treatment has been shown to induce massive proliferation of an initially constrained population of BDC2.5$^+$Foxp3$^+$ Treg cells and long-term protection from diabetes development, which could be abrogated by subsequent DT-mediated Treg cell depletion (51). Here, we show that anti-CD3 mAb therapy in Treg cell-depleted NOD.DEREG mice potently interfered with diabetes development (**Figures 3E, F**), probably by mechanisms independent of Foxp3$^+$ Treg cells. One plausible explanation of these data is that anti-CD3 mAb can also exert its protective effect by acting on diabetogenic CD8$^+$ T cells (49, 53, 54). Clearly, further studies are warranted to more precisely determine the relative contribution of recessive and dominant tolerance mechanisms to the anti-CD3 mAb-mediated effects on β cell autoimmunity.

In summary, the NOD.DEREG line represents a novel tool to analyze the specific role of Foxp3$^+$ Treg cells in the control of β cell autoimmunity, resolving some of the previous limitations of NOD mice with constitutive Foxp3 deficiency or transgenic expression of a diabetogenic TCR. This includes mechanistic studies on novel Treg cell-based therapies under experimental conditions of synchronized, advanced β cell autoimmunity.

AUTHOR CONTRIBUTIONS

DW designed, performed, and analyzed the experiments, and contributed to the data interpretation and assisted in manuscript preparation. MJan, MJay, FP, MW, CP, AH contributed to the acquisition, analysis, and interpretation of data. TS, EB, and KK conceived the research. KK guided its design, analysis and interpretation, and wrote the manuscript. All authors contributed to the article and approved the submitted version.

ACKNOWLEDGMENTS

The authors would like to thank Marie Boernert and Denise Bärhold for excellent technical assistance, Sonja Schallenberg for helpful discussions and constructive advice, and Katja Bernhardt and Anne Gompf (CMCB Flow cytometry Core Facility) for expert help in flow cytometry and cell sorting.

REFERENCES

1. McDevitt HO, Unanue ER. Autoimmune Diabetes Mellitus–Much Progress, But Many Challenges. *Adv Immunol* (2008) 100:1–12. doi: 10.1016/S0065-2776(08)00801-8
2. Hull CM, Peakman M, Tree TIM. Regulatory T Cell Dysfunction in Type 1 Diabetes: What's Broken and How Can We Fix It? *Diabetologia* (2017) 60 (10):1839–50. doi: 10.1007/s00125-017-4377-1
3. Bacchetta R, Barzaghi F, Roncarolo MG. From IPEX Syndrome to FOXP3 Mutation: A Lesson on Immune Dysregulation. *Ann N Y Acad Sci* (2018) 1417(1):5–22. doi: 10.1111/nyas.13011
4. Bennett CL, Christie J, Ramsdell F, Brunkow ME, Ferguson PJ, Whitesell L, et al. The Immune Dysregulation, Polyendocrinopathy, Enteropathy, X-Linked Syndrome (IPEX) Is Caused by Mutations of FOXP3. *Nat Genet* (2001) 27(1):20–1. doi: 10.1038/83713
5. Wildin RS, Smyk-Pearson S, Filipovich AH. Clinical and Molecular Features of the Immunodysregulation, Polyendocrinopathy, Enteropathy, X Linked (IPEX) Syndrome. *J Med Genet* (2002) 39(8):537–45. doi: 10.1136/jmg.39.8.537
6. Brunkow ME, Jeffery EW, Hjerrild KA, Paeper B, Clark LB, Yasayko SA, et al. Disruption of a New Forkhead/Winged-Helix Protein, Scurfin, Results in the Fatal Lymphoproliferative Disorder of the Scurfy Mouse. *Nat Genet* (2001) 27 (1):68–73. doi: 10.1038/83784
7. Fontenot JD, Gavin MA, Rudensky AY. Foxp3 Programs the Development and Function of CD4+CD25+ Regulatory T Cells. *Nat Immunol* (2003) 4 (4):330–6. doi: 10.1038/ni904
8. Kim JM, Rasmussen JP, Rudensky AY. Regulatory T Cells Prevent Catastrophic Autoimmunity Throughout the Lifespan of Mice. *Nat Immunol* (2007) 8(2):191–7. doi: 10.1038/ni1428
9. Lahl K, Loddenkemper C, Drouin C, Freyer J, Arnason J, Eberl G, et al. Selective Depletion of Foxp3+ Regulatory T Cells Induces a Scurfy-Like Disease. *J Exp Med* (2007) 204(1):57–63. doi: 10.1084/jem.20061852
10. Li X, Kostareli E, Suffner J, Garbi N, Hammerling GJ. Efficient Treg Depletion Induces T-Cell Infiltration and Rejection of Large Tumors. *Eur J Immunol* (2010) 40(12):3325–35. doi: 10.1002/eji.201041093
11. Chen Z, Herman AE, Matos M, Mathis D, Benoist C. Where CD4+CD25+ T Reg Cells Impinge on Autoimmune Diabetes. *J Exp Med* (2005) 202(10):1387–97. doi: 10.1084/jem.20051409
12. Riewaldt J, Duber S, Boernert M, Krey M, Dembinski M, Weiss S, et al. Severe Developmental B Lymphopoietic Defects in Foxp3-Deficient Mice Are Refractory to Adoptive Regulatory T Cell Therapy. *Front Immunol* (2012) 3:141. doi: 10.3389/fimmu.2012.00141
13. Kohm AP, McMahon JS, Podojil JR, Begolka WS, DeGutes M, Kasprowicz DJ, et al. Cutting Edge: Anti-CD25 Monoclonal Antibody Injection Results in the Functional Inactivation, Not Depletion, of CD4+CD25+ T Regulatory Cells. *J Immunol* (2006) 176(6):3301–5. doi: 10.4049/jimmunol.176.6.3301
14. Stephens LA, Anderton SM. Comment on "Cutting Edge: Anti-CD25 Monoclonal Antibody Injection Results in the Functional Inactivation, Not Depletion, of CD4+CD25+ T Regulatory Cells". *J Immunol* (2006) 177 (4):2036; author reply 2037-8. doi: 10.4049/jimmunol.177.4.2037
15. Zelenay S, Demengeot J. Comment on "Cutting Edge: Anti-CD25 Monoclonal Antibody Injection Results in the Functional Inactivation, Not Depletion, of CD4+CD25+ T Regulatory Cells". *J Immunol* (2006) 177(4):2036–7; author reply 2037-8. doi: 10.4049/jimmunol.177.4.2036-a
16. Fukushima K, Abiru N, Nagayama Y, Kobayashi M, Satoh T, Nakahara M, et al. Combined Insulin B:9-23 Self-Peptide and Polyinosinic-Polycytidylic Acid Accelerate Insulitis But Inhibit Development of Diabetes by Increasing the Proportion of CD4+Foxp3+ Regulatory T Cells in the Islets in Non-Obese Diabetic Mice. *Biochem Biophys Res Commun* (2008) 367(4):719–24. doi: 10.1016/j.bbrc.2007.12.191
17. Mellanby RJ, Thomas D, Phillips JM, Cooke A. Diabetes in Non-Obese Diabetic Mice Is Not Associated With Quantitative Changes in CD4+ CD25+ Foxp3+ Regulatory T Cells. *Immunology* (2007) 121(1):15–28. doi: 10.1111/j.1365-2567.2007.02546.x
18. Ly D, Mi QS, Hussain S, Delovitch TL. Protection From Type 1 Diabetes by Invariant NK T Cells Requires the Activity of CD4+CD25+ Regulatory T Cells. *J Immunol* (2006) 177(6):3695–704. doi: 10.4049/jimmunol.177.6.3695
19. Billiard F, Lobry C, Darrasse-Jeze G, Waite J, Liu X, Mouquet H, et al. Dll4-Notch Signaling in Flt3-Independent Dendritic Cell Development and Autoimmunity in Mice. *J Exp Med* (2012) 209(5):1011–28. doi: 10.1084/jem.20111615
20. Marino E, Villanueva J, Walters S, Liuwantara D, Mackay F, Grey ST. CD4(+) CD25(+) T-Cells Control Autoimmunity in the Absence of B-Cells. *Diabetes* (2009) 58(7):1568–77. doi: 10.2337/db08-1504
21. Luo X, Pothoven KL, McCarthy D, DeGutes M, Martin A, Getts DR, et al. ECDI-Fixed Allogeneic Splenocytes Induce Donor-Specific Tolerance for Long-Term Survival of Islet Transplants via Two Distinct Mechanisms. *Proc Natl Acad Sci USA* (2008) 105(38):14527–32. doi: 10.1073/pnas.0805204105
22. Hubner MP, Shi Y, Torrero MN, Mueller E, Larson D, Soloviova K, et al. Helminth Protection Against Autoimmune Diabetes in Nonobese Diabetic Mice Is Independent of a Type 2 Immune Shift and Requires TGF-Beta. *J Immunol* (2012) 188(2):559–68. doi: 10.4049/jimmunol.1100335
23. Liu Q, Sundar K, Mishra PK, Mousavi G, Liu Z, Gaydo A, et al. Helminth Infection Can Reduce Insulitis and Type 1 Diabetes Through CD25- and IL-

10-Independent Mechanisms. *Infect Immun* (2009) 77(12):5347–58. doi: 10.1128/IAI.01170-08
24. Kim J, Lahl K, Hori S, Loddenkemper C, Chaudhry A, deRoos P, et al. Cutting Edge: Depletion of Foxp3+ Cells Leads to Induction of Autoimmunity by Specific Ablation of Regulatory T Cells in Genetically Targeted Mice. *J Immunol* (2009) 183(12):7631–4. doi: 10.4049/jimmunol.0804308
25. Lahl K, Sparwasser T. In Vivo Depletion of FoxP3+ Tregs Using the DEREG Mouse Model. *Methods Mol Biol* (2011) 707:157–72. doi: 10.1007/978-1-61737-979-6_10
26. Mayer CT, Lahl K, Milanez-Almeida P, Watts D, Dittmer U, Fyhrquist N, et al. Advantages of Foxp3(+) Regulatory T Cell Depletion Using DEREG Mice. *Immun Inflammation Dis* (2014) 2(3):162–5. doi: 10.1002/iid3.33
27. Berod L, Stuve P, Varela F, Behrends J, Swallow M, Kruse F, et al. Rapid Rebound of the Treg Compartment in DEREG Mice Limits the Impact of Treg Depletion on Mycobacterial Burden, But Prevents Autoimmunity. *PloS One* (2014) 9(7): e102804. doi: 10.1371/journal.pone.0102804
28. Rausch S, Huehn J, Loddenkemper C, Hepworth MR, Klotz C, Sparwasser T, et al. Establishment of Nematode Infection Despite Increased Th2 Responses and Immunopathology After Selective Depletion of Foxp3+ Cells. *Eur J Immunol* (2009) 39(11):3066–77. doi: 10.1002/eji.200939644
29. You S, Slehoffer G, Barriot S, Bach JF, Chatenoud L. Unique Role of CD4+ CD62L+ Regulatory T Cells in the Control of Autoimmune Diabetes in T Cell Receptor Transgenic Mice. *Proc Natl Acad Sci USA* (2004) 101 Suppl 2:14580–5. doi: 10.1073/pnas.0404870101
30. Feuerer M, Shen Y, Littman DR, Benoist C, Mathis D. How Punctual Ablation of Regulatory T Cells Unleashes an Autoimmune Lesion Within the Pancreatic Islets. *Immunity* (2009) 31(4):654–64. doi: 10.1016/j.immuni.2009.08.023
31. Petzold C, Riewaldt J, Watts D, Sparwasser T, Schallenberg S, Kretschmer K. Foxp3(+) Regulatory T Cells in Mouse Models of Type 1 Diabetes. *J Diabetes Res* (2013) 2013:940710. doi: 10.1155/2013/940710
32. Wang H, Xue Y, Wang B, Zhao J, Yan X, Huang Y, et al. Maternal Obesity Exacerbates Insulitis and Type 1 Diabetes in Non-Obese Diabetic Mice. *Reproduction* (2014) 148(1):73–9. doi: 10.1530/REP-13-0614
33. Bernard NF, Ertug F, Margolese H. High Incidence of Thyroiditis and Anti-Thyroid Autoantibodies in NOD Mice. *Diabetes* (1992) 41(1):40–6. doi: 10.2337/diabetes.41.1.40
34. Bour-Jordan H, Thompson HL, Giampaolo JR, Davini D, Rosenthal W, Bluestone JA. Distinct Genetic Control of Autoimmune Neuropathy and Diabetes in the non-Obese Diabetic Background. *J Autoimmun* (2013) 45:58–67. doi: 10.1016/j.jaut.2013.06.005
35. Anderson MS, Bluestone JA. The NOD Mouse: A Model of Immune Dysregulation. *Annu Rev Immunol* (2005) 23:447–85. doi: 10.1146/annurev.immunol.23.021704.115643
36. Chen YG, Mathews CE, Driver JP. The Role of NOD Mice in Type 1 Diabetes Research: Lessons From the Past and Recommendations for the Future. *Front Endocrinol (Lausanne)* (2018) 9:51. doi: 10.3389/fendo.2018.00051
37. Mayer CT, Ghorbani P, Kuhl AA, Stuve P, Hegemann M, Berod L, et al. Few Foxp3(+) Regulatory T Cells Are Sufficient to Protect Adult Mice From Lethal Autoimmunity. *Eur J Immunol* (2014) 44(10):2990–3002. doi: 10.1002/eji.201344315
38. Novak J, Griseri T, Beaudoin L, Lehuen A. Regulation of Type 1 Diabetes by NKT Cells. *Int Rev Immunol* (2007) 26(1-2):49–72. doi: 10.1080/08830180601070229
39. Novak J, Beaudoin L, Park S, Griseri T, Teyton L, Bendelac A, et al. Prevention of Type 1 Diabetes by Invariant NKT Cells Is Independent of Peripheral CD1d Expression. *J Immunol* (2007) 178(3):1332–40. doi: 10.4049/jimmunol.178.3.1332
40. Griseri T, Beaudoin L, Novak J, Mars LT, Lepault F, Liblau R, et al. Invariant NKT Cells Exacerbate Type 1 Diabetes Induced by CD8 T Cells. *J Immunol* (2005) 175(4):2091–101. doi: 10.4049/jimmunol.175.4.2091
41. Gomez-Diaz RA, Aguilar MV, Meguro EN, Marquez RH, Magana EG, Martinez-Garcia MC, et al. The Role of Natural Killer T (NKT) Cells in the Pathogenesis of Type 1 Diabetes. *Curr Diabetes Rev* (2011) 7(4):278–83. doi: 10.2174/157339911796397839
42. Phillips JM, Parish NM, Raine T, Bland C, Sawyer Y, De La Pena H, et al. Type 1 Diabetes Development Requires Both CD4+ and CD8+ T Cells and can be Reversed by Non-Depleting Antibodies Targeting Both T Cell Populations. *Rev Diabetes Stud* (2009) 6(2):97–103. doi: 10.1900/RDS.2009.6.97
43. Chatenoud L, Thervet E, Primo J, Bach JF. Anti-CD3 Antibody Induces Long-Term Remission of Overt Autoimmunity in Nonobese Diabetic Mice. *Proc Natl Acad Sci USA* (1994) 91(1):123–7. doi: 10.1073/pnas.91.1.123
44. Chatenoud L, Primo J, Bach JF. CD3 Antibody-Induced Dominant Self Tolerance in Overtly Diabetic NOD Mice. *J Immunol* (1997) 158(6):2947–54.
45. Suffner J, Hochweller K, Kuhnle MC, Li X, Kroczek RA, Garbi N, et al. Dendritic Cells Support Homeostatic Expansion of Foxp3+ Regulatory T Cells in Foxp3.LuciDTR Mice. *J Immunol* (2010) 184(4):1810–20. doi: 10.4049/jimmunol.0902420
46. Tang S, Zhang M, Zeng S, Huang Y, Qin M, Nasri U, et al. Reversal of Autoimmunity by Mixed Chimerism Enables Reactivation of Beta Cells and Transdifferentiation of Alpha Cells in Diabetic NOD Mice. *Proc Natl Acad Sci USA* (2020) 117(49):31219–30. doi: 10.1073/pnas.2012389117
47. Rui J, Deng S, Arazi A, Perdigoto AL, Liu Z, Herold KC. Beta Cells That Resist Immunological Attack Develop During Progression of Autoimmune Diabetes in NOD Mice. *Cell Metab* (2017) 25(3):727–38. doi: 10.1016/j.cmet.2017.01.005
48. Herold KC, Hagopian W, Auger JA, Poumian-Ruiz E, Taylor L, Donaldson D, et al. Anti-CD3 Monoclonal Antibody in New-Onset Type 1 Diabetes Mellitus. *N Engl J Med* (2002) 346(22):1692–8. doi: 10.1056/NEJMoa012864
49. Herold KC, Bundy BN, Long SA, Bluestone JA, DiMeglio LA, Dufort MJ, et al. An Anti-CD3 Antibody, Teplizumab, in Relatives at Risk for Type 1 Diabetes. *N Engl J Med* (2019) 381(7):603–13. doi: 10.1056/NEJMc1912500
50. Kuhn C, Weiner HL. Therapeutic Anti-CD3 Monoclonal Antibodies: From Bench to Bedside. *Immunotherapy* (2016) 8(8):889–906. doi: 10.2217/imt-2016-0049
51. Nishio J, Feuerer M, Wong J, Mathis D, Benoist C. Anti-CD3 Therapy Permits Regulatory T Cells to Surmount T Cell Receptor-Specified Peripheral Niche Constraints. *J Exp Med* (2010) 207(9):1879–89. doi: 10.1084/jem.20100205
52. Li L, Nishio J, van Maurik A, Mathis D, Benoist C. Differential Response of Regulatory and Conventional CD4(+) Lymphocytes to CD3 Engagement: Clues to a Possible Mechanism of Anti-CD3 Action? *J Immunol* (2013) 191 (7):3694–704. doi: 10.4049/jimmunol.1300408
53. Tooley JE, Vudattu N, Choi J, Cotsapas C, Devine L, Raddassi K, et al. Changes in T-Cell Subsets Identify Responders to FcR-Nonbinding Anti-CD3 mAb (Teplizumab) in Patients With Type 1 Diabetes. *Eur J Immunol* (2016) 46(1):230–41. doi: 10.1002/eji.201545708
54. Long SA, Thorpe J, DeBerg HA, Gersuk V, Eddy J, Harris KM, et al. Partial Exhaustion of CD8 T Cells and Clinical Response to Teplizumab in New-Onset Type 1 Diabetes. *Sci Immunol* (2016) 1(5):eaai7793. doi: 10.1126/sciimmunol.aai7793

5

Changes in MDA5 and TLR3 Sensing of the Same Diabetogenic Virus Result in Different Autoimmune Disease Outcomes

Pamela J. Lincez[1], *Iryna Shanina*[2] *and Marc S. Horwitz*[2*]

[1] *Michael Smith Laboratories, The University of British Columbia, Vancouver, BC, Canada,* [2] *Department of Microbiology & Immunology, Life Sciences Institute, The University of British Columbia, Vancouver, BC, Canada*

***Correspondence:**
Marc S. Horwitz
mhorwitz@mail.ubc.com

Seemingly redundant in function, melanoma differentiation-associated protein 5 (MDA5) and toll-like receptor- 3 (TLR3) both sense RNA viruses and induce type I interferon (IFN-I). Herein, we demonstrate that changes in sensing of the same virus by MDA5 and TLR3 can lead to distinct signatures of IFN-α and IFN-ß resulting in different disease outcomes. Specifically, infection with a diabetogenic islet β cell-tropic strain of coxsackievirus (CB4) results in diabetes protection under reduced MDA5 signaling conditions while reduced TLR3 function retains diabetes susceptibility. Regulating the induction of IFN-I at the site of virus infection creates a local site of interferonopathy leading to loss of T cell regulation and induction of autoimmune diabetes. We have not demonstrated another way to prevent T1D in the NOD mouse, rather we believe this work has provided compounding evidence for a specific control of IFN-I to drive a myriad of responses ranging from virus clearance to onset of autoimmune diabetes.

Keywords: autoimmunity, diabetes, interferon, MDA5, TLR3, coxsackievirus, interferonopathy

INTRODUCTION

As is commonly described for most autoimmune diseases, type 1 diabetes (T1D) is a disease that results from changes in specific genes, disruption in the balance of immune responses, and exposure to environmental agents like viruses (1–3). With studies and data that continue to emerge from major T1D pancreatic tissue biobanks (4, 5), it is increasingly clear that genetics alone cannot account for the beta cell destruction and insulitis that ensues in the pancreas of people (mostly children) suffering with T1D.

Although not included as type 1 interferonopathies, organ-specific autoimmune diseases such as T1D have been strongly associated with upregulation of the type 1 interferon (IFN-I) response. In children at risk for T1D, an IFN-I transcriptional signature precedes islet autoimmunity (6). In recent onset studies, patients with insulitis-affected islets have an overexpression of interferon-stimulated genes (ISGs), comparable to responses seen in islets infected with virus or treated with inflammatory agents like IFN-α or IFN-γ (7, 8). Included in the overexpressed ISGs identified in

T1D patients, are the genes that express the enterovirus sensors melanoma differentiation-associated protein 5 (MDA5) and toll-like receptor- 3 (TLR3).

And, in a recent study using a reporter cell line infected with enterovirus strains isolated from T1D patients, immune transcriptome data supports the hypothesis of enterovirus-induced immune changes leading to the development of autoimmunity (9).

Infection by enteroviruses, such as coxsackieviruses, has been strongly associated with the autoimmune disease process T1D (2, 10). MDA5 and TLR3 are double-stranded RNA virus sensing proteins that specifically detect and protect from coxsackievirus infection and upon viral RNA detection, MDA5 and TLR3 activate and stimulate a cascade of anti-viral responses leading to the production of IFN-I (11, 12). Depending on their levels of expression and the timing and location of signaling, MDA5 and TLR3 can also protect from the onset of autoimmune diabetes following infection with diabetogenic viruses like coxsackieviruses and the pancreatropic RNA virus encephalomyocarditis virus strain D (EMCV-D) (1, 3, 12–15). In MDA5 heterozygous NOD mice, reduced expression of MDA5 induces a unique IFN-I signature with greater IFN-β and this protects mice from T1D after CB4 infection (13). Further, blocking IFN-α, but not IFN-β prevented T1D in the RIP-LCMV Tg model post LCMV infection (16).

Herein, we will show in greater detail, how changes in sensing of the same virus by MDA5 and TLR3 can lead to distinct signatures of interferon (INF)-α and IFN-ß resulting in different autoimmune diabetes disease outcomes. These findings add to the growing knowledge of interferonopathy as a contributor in enterovirus-driven autoimmunity (2, 3, 17) and highlight further, the importance of the local immune environment at the site of autoimmunity as an indicator of disease susceptibility.

MATERIALS AND METHODS

Mice

NOD/ShiLtJ mice were purchased from The Jackson Laboratory (Bar Harbor, ME). MDA5$^{+/-}$ mice were backcrossed from C57BL/6 MDA5$^{-/-}$ mice onto the NOD background as previously described. We confirmed by SNP analysis (in house and by DartMouse, Lebanon, NH) that they carry the full complement of NOD *idd* alleles. More importantly, we confirmed that littermates to the backcrosses that were either heterozygous or wild-type for the MDA5$^{-/-}$ alleles mice had the ability to develop spontaneous diabetes which is strongly indicative that the required susceptibility loci had crossed over. TLR3$^{-/-}$ mice were obtained from The Jackson Laboratory (Bar Harbor, USA) and were backcrossed and maintained on the NOD/ShiLtJ mouse background. NOD TLR3$^{+/-}$ and TLR3$^{+/+}$ progeny were bred for use in experiments. Mice were maintained in the Modified Barrier Facility (Pharmaceutical Sciences Building, Vancouver, British Columbia) and kept in a pathogen-free environment. Diabetes incidence was monitored by non-fasting blood glucose measurements. Disease onset was determined by two consecutive blood glucose levels exceeding 300 mg/dL. Only pre-diabetic mice were used for experiments. All animal work was performed under strict accordance with the recommendations of the Canadian Council for Animal Care. The protocol was approved by the Animal Care Committee (ACC) of the University of British Columbia.

Western Blotting

Mice were stimulated by intraperitoneal injection with 100μg of polyinosinic:polycytidylic acid (P1530, Sigma, St. Louis, MO). After 24 hours stimulation, spleens were isolated and homogenized by sonication and tissue homogenates were lysed with CellLytic MT Mammalian Tissue Lysis Reagent (Sigma, St. Louis, MO). Samples were separated on 10% sodium dodecyl sulfate-polyacrylamide gels, transferred to polyvinylidene fluoride membranes, blocked with Odyssey Blocking Buffer (LI-COR, Lincoln, NE) probed with monoclonal mouse anti-TLR3 (Novus Biologicals, Littleton CO) and polyclonal goat anti-tubulin Santa Cruz Biotech, Santa Cruz, CA) primary antibodies and IRDye 800CW and IRDye 680 RD secondary antibodies (LI-COR, Lincoln, NE). Membranes were scanned with the LI-COR Odyssey Scanner (LI-COR, Lincoln, NE). Protein was quantified using LI-COR Odyssey 3.0 Software.

Virus

Ten-to 12-week old mice were infected intraperitoneally with sublethal doses of 400 plaque-forming units (PFUs) of CB4 Edwards strain 2 or coxsackievirus group B type 3 (CB3, Nancy Strain) diluted in DMEM. As there is no gender bias in CB4-mediated T1D, equal numbers of male and female mice were infected with CB4. Both male and female mice were infected with CB3. Virus stocks were prepared and free virus particles were detected from tissue homogenates by plaque assay as described previously (13).

Immunohistochemical and Immunofluorescent Staining

Single cell-suspensions from pancreatic lymph nodes and spleens were restimulated for 4 hours at 37°C in Iscove's modified Dulbecco's medium containing 10% fetal bovine serum with 500ng/ml PMA, 10 ng/ml ionomycin and Golgi Plug (BD Biosciences). Cells were stained for surface and intracellular markers (**Table S2**), fixed, permeabilized, stained for inflammatory cytokines like γ-interferon (IFN-γ) and analyzed by flow cytometry. Cytokines IL-2, IL-4, IL-6, IL-10, IL-17, TNF-α, and IFN-γ were measured from serum days 0, 3 and 7 post-CB4 infection in a multiplexed format using a Cytometric Bead Array (mouse Th1/Th2/Th17 cytokine kit; BD Biosciences, Mississauga, ON). IFN-Is, IFN-α and-β were measured from serum by ELISA using VeriKine Mouse Interferon-α and β ELISA kits (PBL Interferon Source, Piscataway, NJ). All mAbs were purchased from eBiosciences (San Diego, CA) with the exception of Helios from BioLegend (San Diego, CA). Stained cells were analyzed by flow cytometry with the BD Biosciences LSR II (San Jose, CA) and Flow Jo vX.0.6 software (TreeStar, Ashland, OR).

Reverse Transcription and Quantitative Real-Time PCR

Organs were removed and immediately snap frozen in TRIzol reagent (Life Technologies Inc, Burlington, ON). Tissues were weighed and organs were homogenized using QIAGEN stainless steel beads and TissueLyser II benchtop homogenizer at 19/s for 10 min. Total RNA was prepared with TRIzol reagent according to the manufacturer's protocol (TRIzol, Life Technologies). RNA was quantified using a NanoDrop-ND-1000 (VERIFY) (Thermo Scientific, Wilmington, DE).

cDNA was prepared for 1μg of RNA using High Capacity cDNA Reverse Transcription Kit (Applied Biosystems, Foster City, CA) according to the manufacturer's instructions. Reverse transcription-PCR was performed with the BioRad T-100 Thermal Cycler. cDNA was diluted with UltraPure™ DNase/RNase-Free Distilled Water (Life Technologies) and a final RNA concentration equivalent to 10μg/μl was used for real time (RT)-PCR. Gene expression for MDA5, IFN-α, IFN-β, TLR3 and GAPDH was quantified using the iQ™ SYBR® Green Supermix (BioRad, Mississauga, ON) PCR amplification was performed in 384-well plates with the ABI 7900HT Fast Real-Time PCR System (Applied Biosystems). All samples from three independent experiments were evaluated in duplicate amplification reactions. mRNA expression was normalized to GAPDH. The comparative C_t method was used as previously described and data is shown as -Δ C_t and fold change of -Δ C_t relative to Wt (NOD) samples (18). Primers used in this study are listed in **Table S2**.

Poly I:C Treatment

At days 3 and 5 post-infection with CB4, mice were stimulated by intraperitoneal injection with 100μg of polyinosinic:polycytidylic acid (P1530, Sigma, St. Louis, MO).

Statistical Analysis

GraphPad Prism 6.0 software (GraphPad, San Diego, CA) using the Student t test (two-tailed distribution) and a P value <0.05 determined statistical significance. Serum cytokine concentrations were determined with FCAP Array Software (BD Biosciences, Mississauga, ON). Data are presented as means ± SEM.

RESULTS

To better understand how immune pathologies like IFN-I responses that result from MDA5 and TLR3 signaling influence T1D development, we challenged heterozygous NOD mice that retained MDA5 and TLR3 function with known diabetes and IFN-I inducers like coxsackievirus B4 (CB4).

Western blots confirmed a 50% reduction in MDA5 (13) and a 30% reduction in TLR3 expression (**Figure 1A**) in the spleens of our MDA5 and TLR3 heterozygous mice who were stimulated with an RNA mimetic polyinosinic:polycytidylic acid (poly I:C). Expression of MDA and TLR3 is below the level of detection in unstimulated mice (not shown). Complete deficiency in TLR3 expression ($TLR3^{-/-}$) inhibits survival after CB4 infection (12), whereas a slight loss in TLR3 expression ($TLR3^{+/-}$) retains sufficient signaling function for protection against CB4 (**Figure 1B**) and another coxsackievirus associated with T1D, coxsackievirus B1 (CB1, not shown). TLR3 expression, at reduced levels in $TLR3^{+/-}$ mice, is not successful in protecting from CB4-induced T1D (**Figure 1B**) as up to 16 days post-infection, $TLR3^{+/-}$ mice show a higher incidence of T1D compared to infected control wild type $TLR3^{+/+}$ mice. Disease incidence in $TLR3^{+/-}$ mice continued to rise to 50% by day 20 post-infection, just under the 60% disease incidence observed in $TLR3^{+/+}$ mice. Though critical for survival, TLR3 expression does not contribute to protection from CB4-induced T1D, contrary to previous observations in $MDA5^{+/-}$ mice, where a reduction in MDA5 increased survival and protected against the development of T1D after CB4 infection [23].

To examine antiviral responses in CB4 infected mice deficient in TLR3, inflammatory cytokines including IFN-I were measured in $TLR3^{+/-}$ and $TLR3^{+/+}$ mice post-infection at multiple time points using ELISA, cytometric bead array and real-time PCR (RT-PCR). Changes in TLR3 signaling induction of IFN-β compared to MDA5 signaling after infection with the same virus are further reflected in the ratio of sera IFN-β *versus* IFN-α levels. $TLR3^{+/-}$ mice have three times the amount of IFN-β than IFN-α in the sera at baseline, prior to CB4 infection, compared to wt mice and by day 3 post infection, $TLR3^{+/-}$ mice dramatically lose IFN-β production *versus* IFN-α in the sera (ratio of 0.14) compared to wt mice (ratio 0.71, **Figure 1C**).

This suggests that changes in TLR3 expression support the systemic production of IFN-α rather than IFN-β after CB4 infection, contrary to what we have previously observed for $MDA5^{+/-}$ mice, where IFN-β responses are more significantly favored (13). Alterations in TLR3 signaling also induces the production of other inflammatory cytokines after CB4 infection (**Figure 1D** unlike negligible responses observed with changes in MDA5 signaling (13). Serum levels of IL-17a at day 2 post-infection and IL-6, and IL-10 at day 3 post-infection are increased in $TLR3^{+/-}$ compared to CB4-infected wt mice (**Figure 1D**). In $TLR3^{+/-}$ mice, IFN-β is significantly reduced and IFN-α is increased in both the pancreas and spleen (**Figure 1E**). The expression of IFN-I stimulators MDA5 and TLR3 is also tissue-specific. In CB4-infected NOD mice heterozygous for MDA5 (13) expression of both MDA5 and TLR3 is increased compared to wt NOD mice at day 3 post-infection, whereas in CB4-infected $TLR3^{+/-}$ mice only TLR3 expression is increased compared to wt mice in the pancreas (**Figure 1E**). CB4 infection in $TLR3^{+/-}$ mice also induces a significant reduction in TLR3 and increased MDA5 expression in the spleen (**Figure 1E**), opposite to infected $MDA5^{+/-}$ mice that have decreased MDA5 and increased TLR3 expression in the spleen (13). Overall $TLR3^{+/-}$ and $MDA5^{+/-}$ mice have distinctive tissue specific expression of IFN-I inducers TLR3 and MDA5 and unique tissue-specific IFN-I responses after infection with the same virus.

Since we know from previous studies (2, 10, 13, 19) that an imbalance in cellular immune responses, especially locally, can

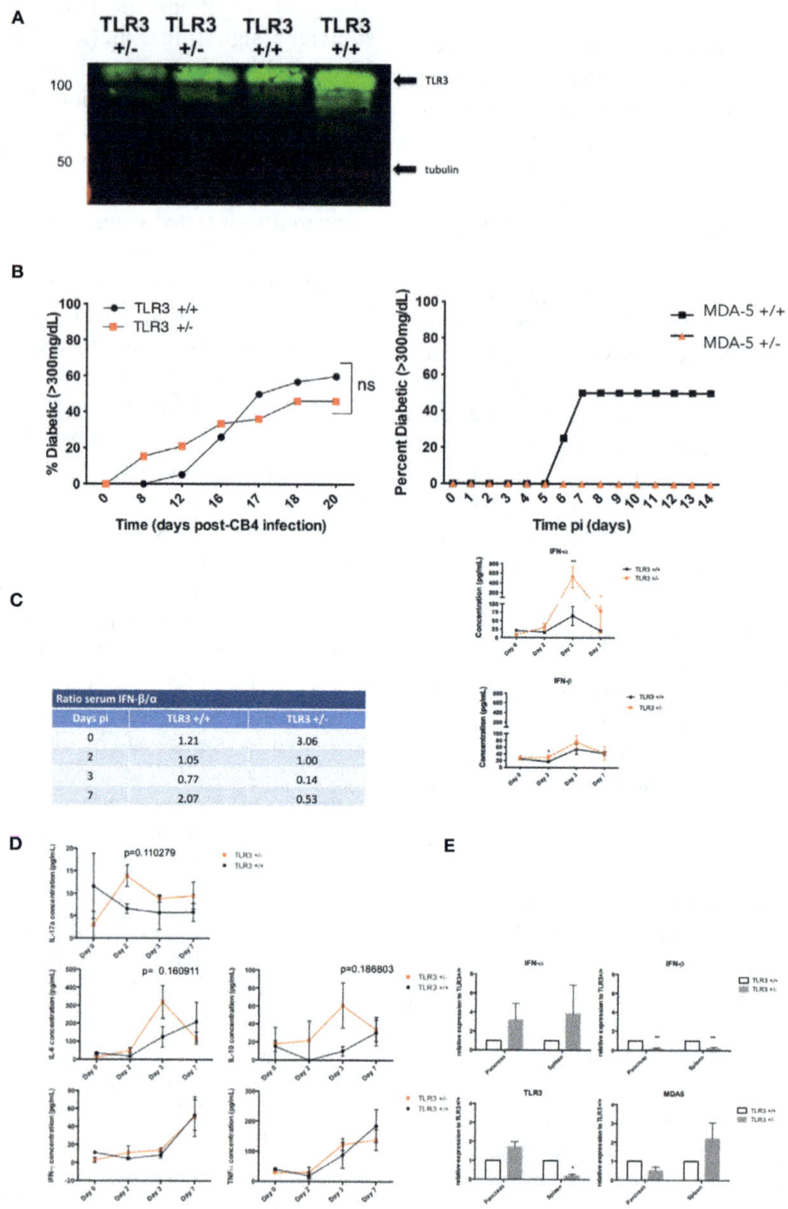

Ratio serum IFN-β/α		
Days pi	TLR3 +/+	TLR3 +/-
0	1.21	3.06
2	1.05	1.00
3	0.77	0.14
7	2.07	0.53

FIGURE 1 | Diabetes incidence in TLR3$^{+/-}$ and TLR3$^{+/+}$ mice post- CB4 infection. **(A)** TLR3 expression in the spleens of TLR3 +/+, TLR3+/-, and TLR3-/- (not shown) mice that were stimulated with poly I:C as described in Materials and Methods. Twenty-four hours after stimulation, a reduction in TLR3 protein from TLR3 +/- spleens compared to TLR3 +/+ was confirmed by Western Blot. **(B)** TLR3 +/- (n = 13) and TLR3 +/+ (n = 20) (left) and MDA5+/- (n = 15) and MDA5 +/+ (n = 20)(right) were infected ip with 400 pfu CB4. Diabetes incidence was monitored up to 20 days post-infection. Two consecutive blood glucose levels greater than 300mg/dL determined diabetes incidence. Systemic and local inflammatory cytokines in TLR3$^{+/-}$ and TLR3$^{+/+}$ mice post-CB4 infection. **(C, D)** TLR3 +/- (n = 4-8) and TLR3 +/+ (n = 4-8) were infected by an intraperitoneal i.p. injection with 400 pfu CB4. IFN-α/β Inflammatory cytokine concentrations (pg/mL) were measured from sera by ELISA and IL-6, IL-10, IL-17a, IFN-γ, and TNF-α by FACS bead array at days 0, 2, 3 and 7 post-infection (pi). Ratios of the average IFN-β concentrations *versus* IFN-α (left) and the individual concentrations (right) **(C)** and averages of inflammatory cytokines **(D)** measured from sera at each time point are shown. **(E)** Relative mRNA expression levels of TLR3, MDA5, IFN-α and β from the spleen and pancreas of TLR3+/+ (n = 4-8) and TLR3+/- mice (n = 4-8) at day 3 post-CB4 infection were quantified by quantitative real time PCR and normalized to GAPDH. The comparative Ct method was used to calculate mean relative expression ± SEM against TLR3+/+ mice as described in *Materials and Methods* section. Data shown are from duplicate samples from two independent experiments. *$p < 0.05$, **$p < 0.01$ and ns, not significant.

lead to the development of T1D following virus challenge, we investigated the regulatory and effector cell responses in the pancreatic lymph nodes and spleen of CB4-challenged mice. Similar to MDA5$^{+/-}$ mice (13), at day 7 following CB4 infection in comparison to wt mice, TLR3$^{+/-}$ mice have significantly increased regulatory Foxp3^{+} T cells in the pancreatic lymph nodes (PLNs) and in the spleen, while statistical significance was not achieved, there was a propensity for increased Tregs

(**Figure 2A**). Though unlike CB4-infected MDA5$^{+/-}$ mice that have a T cell response skewed towards protection from T1D, infected TLR3$^{+/-}$ mice have significantly increased effector T cells in the PLN (IFN-γ- CD4^{+} T cells) and are not protected from T1D.

While statistical signficance was not achieved, in comparison to wt mice at 7 days PI, infected TLR3$^{+/-}$ mice have a tendency for increased CD44^{hi}CD62L^{lo} CD4^{+} effector T cells in the PLNs and spleen(**Figure 2B**). Statistically significant increased levels of IFN-γ-producing CD4^{+} T cells are observed in the PLNs compared to infected wt mice (**Figure 2C**). The increase in IFN-γ and adaptive responses at the site of autoimmunity is thus greatly apparent with changes in TLR3 expression and begs the question whether it is the receptor expression and signaling or the location of viral infection and subsequent interferon and T cell responses rather that influences susceptibility to disease. To address this potential spatial relevance in the function of interferon and T cell responses against viral infection, we turned to our MDA5 model and compared the inflammatory responses from two pancreatropic infections.

To test if MDA5 signaling within the pancreatic islets protects from T1D, we infected MDA5$^{+/-}$ mice with the beta cell tropic-B4 strain and in another set of mice, the non-beta cell tropic virus B3 strain of coxsackievirus. In NOD mice, both the B4 and B3 strains of coxsackievirus infect and cause significant inflammatory pathology in the acinar tissue in the pancreas (19) though CB4 and not CB3 infects the pancreatic beta cells and induces T1D.

Though CB3-infected MDA5$^{+/-}$ mice have similar levels of inflammatory cytokines TNF-α, IFN-γ, IL-6, IL-17a, and IL-10 (data not shown) by day 7 following infection, CB3-infect MDA5$^{+/-}$ mice have greater systemic levels of both IFN-α and IFN-β compared to CB3-infected wt mice (**Figure 3A**). CB4-infected MDA5$^{+/-}$ mice also have increased systemic IFN-α at day 7 post-infection compared to infected wt mice, though they have a significant decrease in IFN-β (**Figure 3A**).

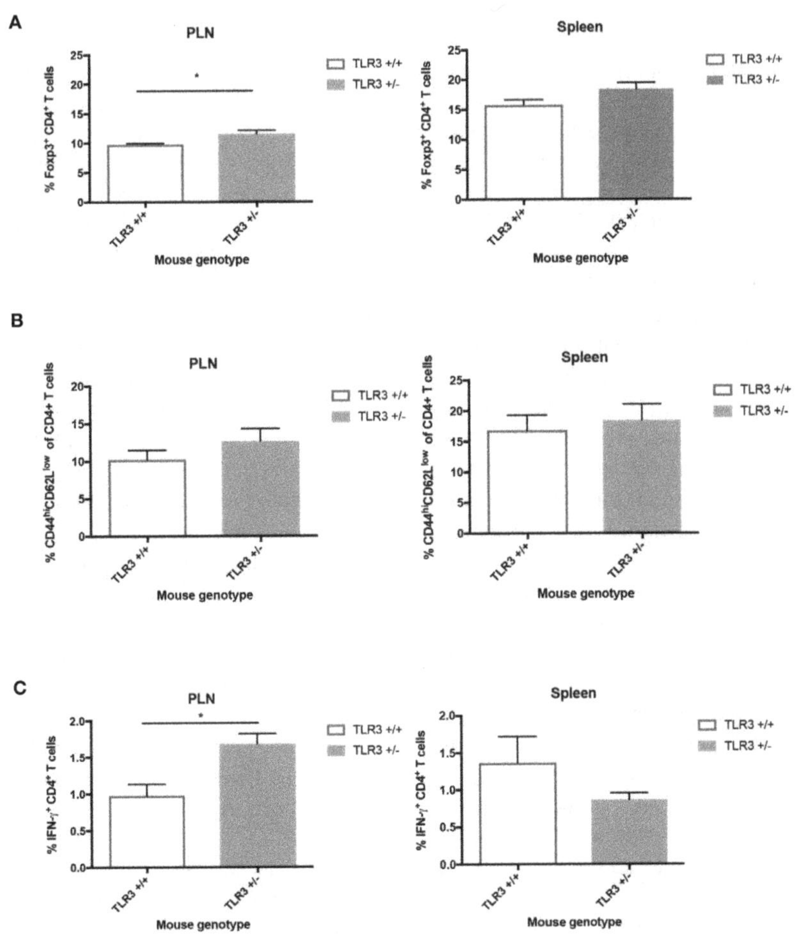

FIGURE 2 | Regulatory and effector CD4+ T cells from the PLNs and spleen of TLR3$^{+/-}$ and TLR3$^{+/+}$ mice post-CB4 infection. **(A)** Regulatory T cells (Foxp3^{+} CD4^{+}) and **(B, C)** effector T cells (CD44^{hi}CD62^{low}CD4^{+} and IFNγ-producing CD4^{+}) were isolated from the pancreatic lymph nodes (PLNs) and spleens of TLR3+/+ (n = 5) and TLR3+/- mice (n = 5) at day 7 post CB4-infection and were stained with classical activation and maturation marker antibodies for FACS analysis. Results are shown as mean ± SEM of a representative from three independent experiments. *$p < 0.05$.

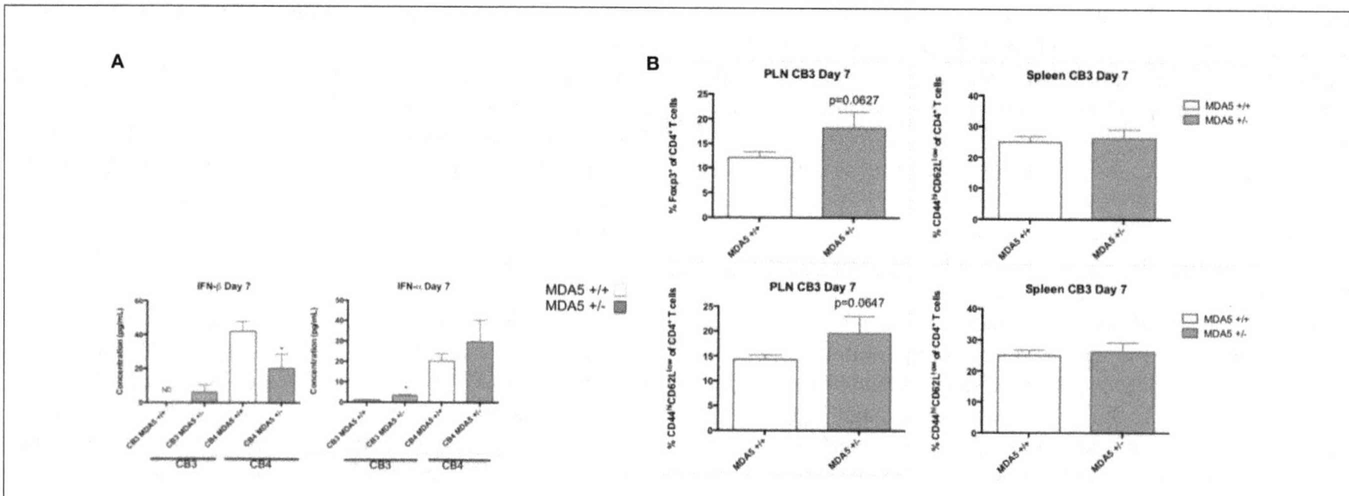

FIGURE 3 | Serum levels of IFN-I and $CD4^+$ T cell responses in $MDA5^{+/-}$ and $MDA5^{+/+}$ mice after CB3 and CB4 infection. **(A)** IFN-α/β Inflammatory cytokine concentrations (pg/mL) were measured from CB4 and CB3 infected $MDA5^{+/-}$ (n = 7) and $MDA5^{+/+}$ (n = 7) mice sera by ELISA. **(B)** Regulatory T cells ($Foxp3^+$ $CD4^+$) and effector T cells ($CD44^{hi}CD62^{low}CD4^+$ and IFNγ-producing $CD4^+$) were isolated from the pancreatic lymph nodes (PLNs) and spleens of CB3 infected $MDA5^{+/-}$ (n = 5) and $MDA5^{+/+}$ (n = 5) mice at day 7 post CB4-infection and were stained with classical activation and maturation marker antibodies for FACS analysis. Results are shown as mean ± SEM of a representative from three independent experiments. *$p < 0.05$.

In $MDA5^{+/-}$ mice, CB4 infection also results in increased regulatory $Foxp3^+$ $CD4^+$ T cells at the site of autoimmunity [23]. Infection with the non-diabetogenic non-beta cell tropic virus CB3 in $MDA5^{+/-}$ mice, however, induces a more inflammatory response with the increased presence of both regulatory $Foxp3^+$ $CD4^+$ T cells and effector $CD44^{hi}CD62L^{lo}$ $CD4^+$ T cells at the site of autoimmunity, in the pancreatic lymph nodes (PLNs) (**Figure 3B**) compared to infected wt mice. And also unlike CB4-infected $MDA5^{+/-}$ mice (13), CB3-infected $MDA5^{+/-}$ mice have similar regulatory and effector $CD4^+$ T cell responses in the spleen compared to infected wt mice (**Figure 3B**). With CB4 infection, effector T cells ($CD4^+$ and $CD8^+$) are significantly reduced in $MDA5^{+/-}$ mice PLNs and spleen (13). These observations demonstrate that infection outside the islets with CB3, leads to systemic, and localized inflammatory responses. Infection within the islets, with CB4, induces regulatory, suppressive responses.

As humans encounter various pathogenic insults from their environment, it is likely that these pathogenic insults induce frequent bursts of IFN-I signaling as a result of innate immune responses. Consequently, innate responses and pathogen clearance may also frequently alter the IFN-I signature in the host and as such, alter immune homeostasis. To simulate alterations in immune homeostasis with frequent IFN-I production and to test whether the IFN-I signature and protective adaptive responses we observe in CB4-infected $MDA5^{+/-}$ mice can be maintained despite additional bursts of IFN-I, we stimulated CB4-infected $MDA5^{+/-}$ and $MDA5^{+/+}$ mice 3 and 5 days post-CB4 infection with the dsRNA mimetic poly I:C.

Contrary to what was expected, a reduction in MDA5 impressively held a unique IFN-I signature despite additional IFN-I stimuli following CB4 infection. At day 7 post-infection, $MDA5^{+/-}$ mice treated with poly I:C at days 3 and 5, maintain lower IFN-β levels similarly to unstimulated $MDA5^{+/-}$ mice. Poly I:C stimulated $MDA5^{+/-}$ mice do, however, show an increase in IFN-α production by day 7 post-infection compared to unstimulated CB4-infected $MDA5^{+/-}$ mice (**Figure 4A**). Poly I:C treatment holds a greater effect on $MDA5^{+/+}$ mice, where both IFN-α and β serum levels are increased at day 7 post-infection compared to untreated CB4-infected wt mice (**Figure 4A**).

To further study the immune consequences of additional IFN-I stimulation in CB4-infected $MDA5^{+/-}$ mice, we examined the expression of significant APC activation markers CD40, CD80 (data not shown) and CD86 in poly I:C treated, CB4-infected $MDA5^{+/-}$ mice. After poly I:C treatment and seven days of CB4 infection, APCs ($CD11b^+CD11c^+$, $CD11b^+CD11c^-$) isolated from PLNs and spleens of $MDA5^{+/-}$ mice express similar levels of CD40 and CD86 compared to untreated CB4-infected $MDA5^{+/-}$ mice (**Figure S2**). With insignificant APC activation, it is also no surprise that pro-inflammatory cytokine production is also insignificant at day 7 infection (data not shown). Further, T cell responses in poly I:C treated and CB4-infected $MDA5^{+/-}$ remain similar with the response in untreated CB4-infected $MDA5^{+/-}$ mice while the number of $Foxp3^+$ $CD4^+$ regulatory T cells remained elevated in the PLNs relative to the number of effector $CD44^{hi}$ $CD62L^{lo}$ $CD4^+$ T cells (**Figure 4B**). This suggests that APC activation and subsequent T cell polarization in $MDA5^{+/-}$ is unaffected by additional IFN-I stimulus.

Injections of poly I:C have a more dramatic effect on CB4-infected $MDA5^{+/+}$ mice. Although CD86 expression remained unchanged in CB4-infected $MDA5^{+/+}$ mice following poly I:C treatment, CD40 expression on $CD11b^+CD11c^+$ cells was decreased (**Figure S2**), regulatory T cells were slightly increased in the spleens (**Figure 4B**) and notably, regulatory T cells were significantly decreased in the PLNs (**Figure 4B**) compared to untreated, infected $MDA5^{+/+}$ mice. These results

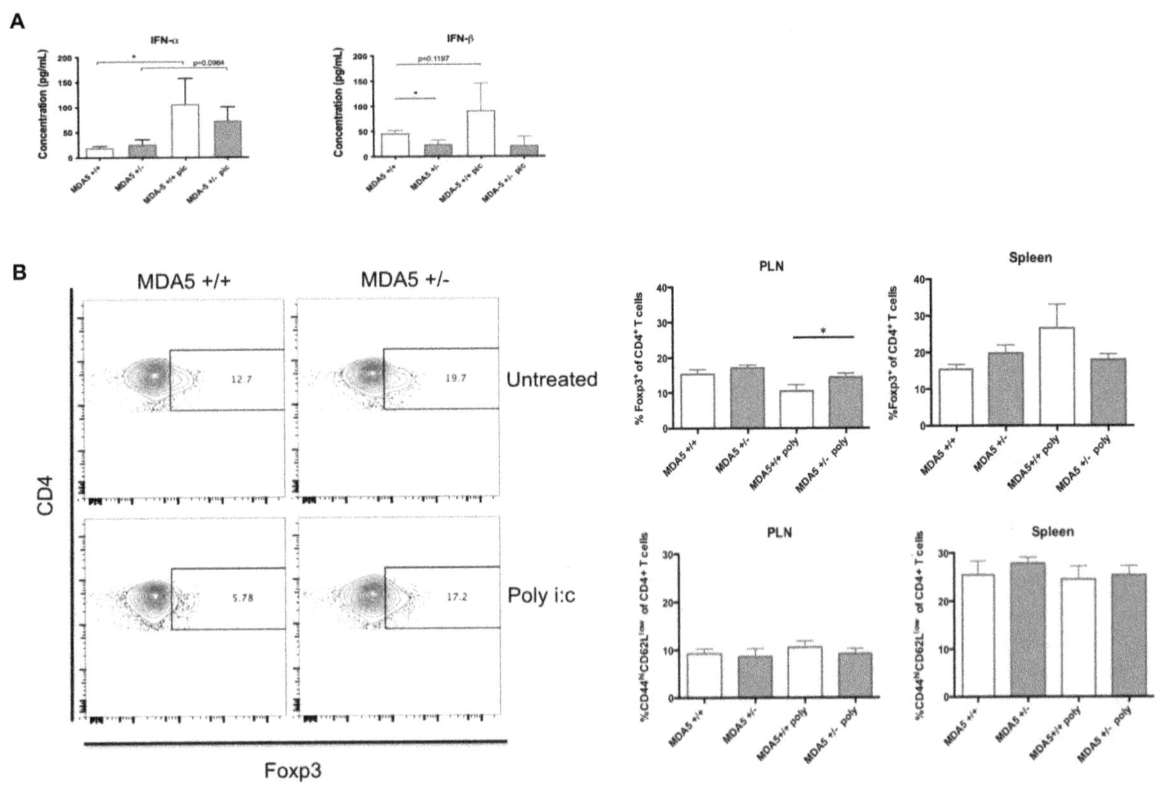

FIGURE 4 | Systemic IFN-I levels, regulatory and effector CD4$^+$ T cell responses in MDA5$^{+/-}$ and MDA5$^{+/+}$ mice after poly I:C stimulation and CB4 infection. **(A)** IFN-α/β Inflammatory cytokine concentrations (pg/mL) were measured from MDA5$^{+/-}$ (n = 7) and MDA5$^{+/+}$ (n = 7) mice sera at day 7 post-infection by ELISA. **(B)** Regulatory T cells (Foxp3$^+$ CD4$^+$) and effector T cells (CD44^{hi}CD62^{low}CD4$^+$ and IFNγ-producing CD4$^+$) were isolated from the pancreatic lymph nodes (PLNs) and spleens of poly I:C treated and untreated MDA5$^{+/-}$ (n = 5) and MDA5$^{+/+}$ (n = 5) mice at day 7 post CB4-infection and were stained with classical activation and maturation marker antibodies for FACS analysis. Results are shown as mean ± SEM of a representative from three independent experiments. GraphPad Prism 6.0 software (GraphPad, San Diego, CA) using the Student t test (two-tailed distribution) and a P value < 0.05 determined statistical significance *p < 0.05.

emphasize the strength of the regulatory protective phenotype observed in MDA5$^{+/-}$ mice to remain at the site of autoimmunity, which is not observed in MDA5$^{+/+}$ mice. Despite the additional poly I:C treatment and potential for greater IFN-I, by day 7 post-infection reduced MDA5 signaling still results in a lower IFN-I level with greater regulatory T cells in the PLNs, at the site of autoimmunity.

DISCUSSION

Establishing a balance between immune activation and immune protection is essential in an already fragile autoimmune-susceptible state. Double stranded RNA sensors like MDA5 and TLR3 are critical in recognizing specific RNA viruses and inducing an inflammatory IFN-I antiviral response to help clear the invading RNA virus. Here, we have provided evidence of a unique and protective IFN-I and regulatory T cell signature induced with a reduction in MDA5 that is specific to changes in MDA5 signaling and not with a reduction in TLR3 signaling. Rather, the two viral sensors signal co-operatively, similar to a thermostat or counter-balance to achieve a range of immune responses.

Although TLR3 signaling is critical for survival against CB4 in NOD mice (12), we observed that IFN-I and adaptive responses produced as a result from TLR3 signaling to clear the virus are not similarly compatible with protection from autoimmunity. CB4-infected TLR3$^{+/-}$ mice have skewed IFN-I responses that favor increases in IFN-α and increases in effector T cells at the site of autoimmunity that ultimately do not protect from T1D.

In diabetes resistant C57BL/6 mice, MDA5 and TLR3 signaling are both required to prevent diabetes following infection with a pancreatropic virus encephalomyocarditis virus strain D (EMCV-D). EMCV-D, however, induces diabetes through the direct destruction of β cells rather than T cell–mediated autoimmunity that we observe with CB4 infection. Interestingly, MDA5 and TLR3 exert different IFN-I response kinetics following EMCV-D infection in C57BL/6 mice, with IFN-I responses detected in MDA5$^{-/-}$ at 15 hours post-infection and at a later time in TLR3$^{-/-}$ mice (15). The potential cooperative role in IFN-I signaling seems to be specific to the

EMCV-D infection model in diabetes resistant C57BL/6 mice. With our CB4-infection model in diabetes susceptible NOD mice we observe distinct IFN-I responses from MDA5 and TLR3 signaling and we do not see a cooperative mechanism from either receptor attempting to compensate for the lack in expression of the other in our heterozygous or knockout (not shown) mice. From what we have demonstrated with our model, TLR3 signaling is more important for anti-viral responses and rather the IFN-I signature and adaptive responses from MDA5 signaling, though still critical for the anti-viral response, are significant in protecting from autoreactive responses.

The location of viral infection and thus the location of MDA5 signaling in response to viral infection is also important in considering anti-viral immune responses such as IFN-I that could exacerbate and activate pre-existing autoreactive responses. IFN-I are primarily produced by the β cells in the pancreas with coxsackievirus infection and intraislet IFN-I production has shown to prevent CB4 replication (20, 21). In T1D patients, a unique IFN-I signature precedes islet autoimmunity and expression of interferon-stimulated genes is exacerbated in insulitic islets (6). The nature of the IFN-I response within the islets is therefore a critical component in the pathology that leads to autoimmunity in T1D.

We previously demonstrated that CB4-infected MDA5$^{+/-}$ mice have tissue-specific and unique systemic IFN-I and adaptive responses that ultimately lead to protection from T1D (13). Here we sought to determine whether MDA5 signaling and anti-viral IFN-I responses within the islets would contribute to the protective phenotype. After challenging MDA5$^{+/-}$ mice with the B3 strain of coxsackievirus that infects and causes significant inflammatory acinar tissue pathology outside of the islets, in comparison to mice challenged with the β- cell tropic virus CB4 we determined whether viral islet tropism could change anti-viral and autoreactive responses. We observed that it is likely that the location of virus infection in MDA5$^{+/-}$ mice that alters IFN-I and adaptive responses. With CB3 infection, we observed in MDA5$^{+/-}$ mice, an increase in systemic IFN-I levels and localized numbers of effector T cells at the site of autoimmunity, similarly to CB3-infected MDA5$^{+/+}$ mice and in contrast to the phenotype observed with CB4 infection.

MDA5 signaling of CB4 and likely other β-cell tropic viruses followed by the presentation of β-cell antigens is therefore necessary to maintain a unique IFN-I signature and regulatory T cell responses at the site of autoimmunity that can ultimately protect from T1D. By regulating the induction of IFN-I at the site of infection, virus infection creates a local site of interferonopathy leading to altered T cell responses, loss of T cell regulation and induction of autoimmune diabetes. As CB4-MDA5$^{+/-}$ mice have a burst in IFN-β shortly after infection that subsides by day 7 post-infection, it is likely that controlled, local, IFN-β signaling at the site of the islet β cell, leads to protection from exacerbated autoreactive responses and ensuing autoimmunity. Studies investigating the role of localized regulation of IFN-I within the islets could establish a new therapeutic avenue for preventing the autoimmune process and susceptibility to T1D.

In addition to considering the localized islet environment, it is also important to consider the environment of the host. As individuals are exposed to multiple environmental factors including viruses, they are exposed to frequent sources of IFN-I stimuli. Frequent bursts of IFN-I, depending on the location and susceptibility of the host, could lead to abrogated immune responses and lead to autoimmunity. To reproduce an environment where the host is exposed to frequent IFN-I stimulation and determine whether additional IFN-I responses are capable in offsetting an existing protective IFN-I signature, we infected MDA5$^{+/-}$ and MDA5$^{+/+}$ controls with CB4 and at days 3 and 5 post-infection, injected CB4-infected mice with the artificial dsRNA mimetic poly I:C.

In NOD mice, at a dose of 5μg/g body weight, poly I:C protects from T1D (22) and in NOD BDC2.5 transgenic mice that do not develop spontaneous diabetes, a similar poly I:C dose is not capable of inducing resting autoreactive memory T cells and diabetes (19). Though poly I:C signals MDA5 and activates IFN-I responses, the dsRNA mimetic does not induce β cell damage directly like β -cell tropic agents such as CB4. In asking whether recurrent IFN-I responses induced by subsequent treatments of poly I:C following CB4 infection could offset an existing IFN-I and immunoregulatory phenotype in MDA5$^{+/-}$ mice, we did not expect and were not surprised to observe that poly I:C treatment did not further accelerate disease onset in our mice following CB4 infection. Instead, it might be expected that in addition to an already existing breakdown in tolerance, a second insult inducing IFN-I, such as poly I:C treatment, could regress tolerogenic mechanisms and progress disease pathogenesis to autoimmunity. As such, we expected that supplemental IFN-I stimulation with poly I:C post-CB4 infection would abrogate the IFN-I signature with higher systemic IFN-I levels and polarized T cell responses typically observed in CB4-infected, untreated MDA5$^{+/-}$ mice would shift to effector rather than regulatory CD4+ T cells dominating in the PLNs. To our delight, we observed that despite the additional IFN-I stimulation with CB4 infection and two doses of poly I:C, MDA5$^{+/-}$ mice maintain IFN-I and immunoregulatory responses similar to the protective phenotype observed in untreated CB4-infected MDA5$^{+/-}$ mice. Though poly I:C is known to stimulate APC maturation and polarize T cell responses in certain susceptible models, we did not observe changes in the expression of classic APC markers CD40, CD80 or CD86 or changes in T cell responses in poly I:C treated CB4-infected MDA5$^{+/-}$ mice from the untreated phenotype.

The reduction and changes in MDA5 signaling at the site of autoimmunity in MDA5$^{+/-}$ mice likely allows for a balanced anti-viral and immunoregulatory adaptive response in the events of exposure to frequent IFN-I stimulation. With low-dose injections (0.05μg/g body weight) in the BioBreeding (BB), diabetes-resistant rat model, poly I:C protects rather than accelerates disease, mostly attributing to the induction of suppressor T cell activity (23). With the B7.1 C57BL/6 model, where the B7.1 costimulatory molecule is expressed in islets, the level of poly I:C–induced IFN-α determines the frequency and timing of diabetes onset, where higher levels of IFN-α coincide with accelerated, earlier onset of T1D (24). These models along with our MDA5$^{+/-}$ model suggest that low level IFN-I signaling, as a result of a reduction in MDA5, can help avoid and regulate rather than activate autoreactive responses in a genetically susceptible host. Local anti-viral IFN-I responses in the pancreas likely create a site of interferonopathy that shifts the balance from immunoprotective to fully regressed immunosusceptible and prone to autoimmunity.

CONCLUSIONS

With our MDA5$^{+/-}$ and TLR3$^{+/-}$ CB4-infection models, we have identified, using a virus clinically linked to T1D, how changes in MDA5 and not TLR3 signaling are critical in producing an IFN-I response and subsequent adaptive responses that protect from T1D. By challenging MDA5$^{+/-}$ mice with different strains of coxsackieviruses we have teased out the location specific importance of IFN-I signaling and the interferonopathy within the pancreas that changes with a reduction in MDA5 and allows for IFN-I and T cell responses in favor of protection from T1D. Conversely, challenging TLR3$^{+/-}$ mice resulted in the opposite effect by retaining an IFN-I response that resolves to T1D. This further dissects the IFNα/β responses to separate sensors demonstrating a need, and not a redundancy, for both TLR3 and MDA5 to sense and respond differentially to infection. Further, in treating MDA5$^{+/-}$ mice with poly I:C, an additional IFN-I inducer, following CB4 infection, we simulated the environmental context in which humans are exposed to multiple IFN-I stimuli, and demonstrated the strength of the protective phenotype that results with a reduction in MDA5 signaling in withstanding additional IFN-I chaos. MDA5 serves as a cellular protector from viral invasion and as such, with inter-individual variability, MDA5 activity will change with variations at the genetic and immunological expression level. Establishing low level IFN-I signaling from MDA5 may be host specific as we see with IFIH1 heterozygous individuals that carry the protective allele. Regulating IFN-I levels to evade interferonopathies whether systemic or organ-specific still remains an effective strategy in evading autoimmunity as we have demonstrated using an autoimmune diabetes model. We have not demonstrated another way to prevent T1D in the NOD mouse, rather we believe this work has provided compounding evidence for a specific control of IFN-I to drive a myriad of responses ranging from virus clearance to onset of autoimmune diabetes.

AUTHOR CONTRIBUTIONS

Conceptualization, PL and MH. Methodology, PL, IS, and MH. Software, X.X. Validation, PL, IS, and MH. Formal analysis, PL and MH. Investigation, PL and MH. Resources, MH. Data curation, PL. Writing—original draft preparation, PL. Writing—review and editing, PL and MH. Supervision, MH. Funding acquisition, MH. All authors contributed to the article and approved the submitted version.

REFERENCES

1. Blum SI, Tse HM. Innate Viral Sensor MDA5 and Coxsackievirus Interplay in Type 1 Diabetes Development. *Microorganisms* (2020) 8:1–23. doi: 10.3390/microorganisms8070993
2. Richardson SJ, Horwitz MS. Is Type 1 Diabetes "Going Viral"? *Diabetes* (2014) 63:2203–05. doi: 10.2337/db14-0510
3. Morse ZJ, Horwitz MS. Innate Viral Receptor Signaling Determines Type 1 Diabetes Onset. *Front Endocrinol* (2017) 8:249. doi: 10.3389/fendo.2017.00249
4. Richardson SJ, Morgan NG. Enteroviral Infections in the Pathogenesis of Type 1 Diabetes: New Insights for Therapeutic Intervention. *Curr Opin Pharmacol* (2018) 43:11–19. doi: 10.1016/j.coph.2018.07.006
5. Rodriguez-Calvo T, Richardson SJ, Pugliese A. Pancreas Pathology During the Natural History of Type 1 Diabetes. *Curr Diabetes Rep* (2018) 18:1–12. doi: 10.1007/s11892-018-1084-3
6. Ferreira RC, Guo H, Coulson RMR, Smyth DJ, Pekalski ML, Burren OS, et al. A Type I Interferon Transcriptional Signature Precedes Autoimmunity in Children Genetically at Risk for Type 1 Diabetes. *Diabetes* (2014) 63:2538–50. doi: 10.2337/db13-1777
7. Lundberg M, Krogvold L, Kuric E, Dahl-Jørgensen K, Skog O. Expression of Interferon-Stimulated Genes in Insulitic Pancreatic Islets of Patients Recently Diagnosed With Type 1 Diabetes. *Diabetes* (2016) 65:3104–10. doi: 10.2337/db16-0616
8. Mostafavi S, Yoshida H, Moodley D, LeBoité H, Rothamel K, Raj T, et al. Parsing the Interferon Transcriptional Network and Its Disease Associations. *Cell* (2016) 164:564–78. doi: 10.1016/j.cell.2015.12.032
9. Poma AM, Genoni A, Broccolo F, Denaro M, Pugliese A, Basolo F, et al. Immune Transcriptome of Cells Infected With Enterovirus Strains Obtained From Cases of Type 1 Diabetes. *Microorganisms* (2020) 8:1–16. doi: 10.3390/microorganisms8071031
10. Horwitz MS, Bradley LM, Harbertson J, Krahl T, Lee J, Sarvennick N. Diabetes Induced by Coxsackie Virus: Initiation by Bystander Damage and Not Molecular Mimicry. *Nat Med* (1998) 4:781–5. doi: 10.1038/nm0798-781
11. Wang JP, Cerny A, Asher DR, Kurt-Jones EA, Bronson RT, Finberg RW. MDA5 and MAVS Mediate Type I Interferon Responses to Coxsackie B Virus. *J Virol* (2010) 84:254–60. doi: 10.1128/JVI.00631-09
12. Richer MJ, Lavallée DJ, Shanina I, Horwitz MS. Toll-Like Receptor 3 Signalling on Macrophages Is Required for Survival Following Coxsackievirus B4 Infection. *PLoS One* (2009) 4:e4127. doi: 10.1371/journal.pone.0004127
13. Lincez PJ, Shanina I, Horwitz MS. Reduced Expression of the MDA5 Gene IFIH1 Prevents Autoimmune Diabetes. *Diabetes* (2015) 64:2184–93. doi: 10.2337/db14-1223
14. Swiecki M, McCartney SA, Wang Y, Colonna M. TLR7/9 *Versus* TLR3/MDA5 Signaling During Virus Infections and Diabetes. *J Leukoc Biol* (2011) 90:691–701. doi: 10.1189/jlb.0311166
15. McCartney SA, Vermi W, Lonardi S, Rossini C, Otero K, Calderon B, et al. RNA Sensor-Induced Type I IFN Prevents Diabetes Caused by A ?? Cell-Tropic Virus in Mice. *J Clin Invest* (2011) 121:1497–507. doi: 10.1172/JCI44005
16. Marro BS, Ware BC, Zak J, de la Torre JC, Rosen H, Oldstone MBA. Progression of Type 1 Diabetes From the Prediabetic Stage Is Controlled by Interferon-α Signaling. *Proc Natl Acad Sci USA* (2017) 114:3708–13. doi: 10.1073/pnas.1700878114
17. De Beeck AO, Eizirik DL. Viral Infections in Type 1 Diabetes Mellitus-Why the β Cells? *Nat Rev Endocrinol* (2016) 12:263–73. doi: 10.1038/nrendo.2016.30
18. Schmittgen TD, Livak KJ. Analyzing Real-Time PCR Data by the Comparative CT Method. *Nat Protoc* (2008) 3:1101–8. doi: 10.1038/nprot.2008.73
19. Horwitz MS, Ilic A, Fine C, Rodriguez E, Sarvetnick N. Presented Antigen From Damaged Pancreatic ?? Cells Activates Autoreactive T Cells in Virus-Mediated Autoimmune Diabetes. *J Clin Invest* (2002) 109:79–87. doi: 10.1172/JCI200211198

20. Flodström M, Maday A, Balakrishna D, Cleary MM, Yoshimura A, Sarvetnick N. Target Cell Defense Prevents the Development of Diabetes After Viral Infection. *Nat Immunol* (2002) 3:373–82. doi: 10.1038/ni771
21. Chehadeh W, Kerr-Conte J, Pattou F, Alm G, Lefebvre J, Wattré P, et al. Persistent Infection of Human Pancreatic Islets by Coxsackievirus B Is Associated With Alpha Interferon Synthesis in β Cells. *J Virol* (2000) 74:10153–64. doi: 10.1128/jvi.74.21.10153-10164.2000
22. Serreze DV, Hamaguchi K, Leiter EH. Immunostimulation Circumvents Diabetes in NOD/Lt Mice. *J Autoimmun* (1989) 2:759–76. doi: 10.1016/0896-8411(89)90003-6
23. Sobel DO, Goyal D, Ahvazi B, Yoon JW, Chung YH, Bagg A, et al. Low Dose Poly I:C Prevents Diabetes in the Diabetes Prone BB Rat. *J Autoimmun* (1998) 11:343–52. doi: 10.1006/jaut.1998.0203
24. Devendra B, Jasinski J, Melanitou E, Nakayama M, Li M, Hensley B, et al. Interferon-α as a Mediator of Polyinosinic : Polycytidylic Acid-Induced Type 1 Diabetes. *Diabetes* (2005) 54:2549–56. doi: 10.2337/diabetes.54.9.2549

Could Age, Sex and Physical Fitness Affect Blood Glucose Responses to Exercise in Type 1 Diabetes?

Jane E. Yardley[1,2,3*], *Nicole K. Brockman*[1] *and Richard M. Bracken*[4]

[1] *Augustana Faculty, University of Alberta, Camrose, AB, Canada,* [2] *Physical Activity and Diabetes Laboratory, Alberta Diabetes Institute, Edmonton, AB, Canada,* [3] *Faculty of Kinesiology, Sport and Recreation, University of Alberta, Edmonton, AB, Canada,* [4] *Diabetes Research Unit and School of Sport and Exercise Science, Swansea University, Swansea, United Kingdom*

Correspondence:
Jane E. Yardley
jane.yardley@ualberta.ca

Closed-loop systems for patients with type 1 diabetes are progressing rapidly. Despite these advances, current systems may struggle in dealing with the acute stress of exercise. Algorithms to predict exercise-induced blood glucose changes in current systems are mostly derived from data involving relatively young, fit males. Little is known about the magnitude of confounding variables such as sex, age, and fitness level—underlying, uncontrollable factors that might influence blood glucose control during exercise. Sex-related differences in hormonal responses to physical exercise exist in studies involving individuals without diabetes, and result in altered fuel metabolism during exercise. Increasing age is associated with attenuated catecholamine responses and lower carbohydrate oxidation during activity. Furthermore, higher fitness levels can alter hormonal and fuel selection responses to exercise. Compounding the limited research on these factors in the metabolic response to exercise in type 1 diabetes is a limited understanding of how these variables affect blood glucose levels during different types, timing and intensities of activity in individuals with type 1 diabetes (T1D). Thus, there is currently insufficient information to model a closed-loop system that can predict them accurately and consistently prevent hypoglycemia. Further, studies involving both sexes, along with a range of ages and fitness levels, are needed to create a closed-loop system that will be more precise in regulating blood glucose during exercise in a wide variety of individuals with T1D.

Keywords: type 1 diabetes, physical activity, closed loop, sex, age, fitness

INTRODUCTION

Type 1 diabetes (T1D) is an autoimmune disorder that destroys an individual's insulin-producing pancreatic β-cells (1). Despite many advances over the years, T1D remains a difficult disorder to manage. Exercise is very beneficial for individuals with T1D, with known improvements in cardiovascular health, insulin sensitivity, and body composition (2). However, fear of low blood glucose, or hypoglycemia, is often a barrier to partaking in exercise in this population (3). Much research has gone into investigating ways to keep blood glucose levels in the target range during and after exercise in individuals with T1D (4), most of which has noted a great deal of variability in responses.

In the past 5 years, there has been impressive progress in the development of a closed-loop system for patients with T1D to better control blood glucose. Improvements in the accuracy of hand-held glucose monitors to meet ISO criteria (5) and continuous glucose monitoring systems (CGM) (6, 7) have made this progress possible. Device development has advanced to a degree such that both single hormone (insulin) and dual hormone (insulin and glucagon) systems show improvements in time spent in target blood glucose ranges compared to continuous subcutaneous insulin infusion (insulin pump) systems when tested in small sample groups under free-living conditions (8).

In spite of these advances, perfecting the system to deal with situations other than rest, namely physical activity/exercise is still recognized as a major challenge (9–11). The need for a smart sensor that is able to detect the onset of exercise, as well as its intensity (which can have substantially different impacts on blood glucose responses) (12), has been identified. Indeed variables such as heart rate, skin temperature, heat flux, accelerometry and galvanic skin response, have been shown to correlate with changes in blood glucose during various types of exercise (13). Simply turning off insulin delivery upon sensing the start of activity, however, may be insufficient to completely prevent declines in blood glucose, and subsequently hypoglycemia (11), unless exercise is performed shortly after a meal (14). It has also been noted that a closed loop system, or artificial pancreas, will have difficulty replicating the multitude of feed-forward and feedback responses related to blood glucose equilibrium (10), in part due to the relatively long half-life of even the shortest acting synthetic insulin.

The variability in exercise responses will also be a major challenge to creating a system that will be able to adapt to all types and durations of activity for a wide variety of individuals, with a broad range of blood glucose levels at the start of exercise. The need for a sensor that not only recognizes changes in blood glucose, but also the onset, type and intensity, of physical activity/exercise has been discussed in detail elsewhere (8, 10). Current algorithms attempting to manage changes in blood glucose during exercise are also lacking information. Acute studies of the effect of different exercise modalities on blood glucose in individuals with T1D are limited in terms of their type, timing (e.g., morning vs. evening), intensity and duration of activity. For the most part, they have small sample sizes of relatively young, fit, male participants, which may obscure some potentially important differences among blood glucose responses to exercise in physiologically different groups. While we know that insulin dosage, carbohydrate intake, time of day, and prior hypoglycemia can impact blood glucose responses to exercise in T1D (**Figure 1**), little is known about the relative impact of underlying physiological factors such as sex, age, and physical fitness, which are beyond the control of the individual.

What we do know about these physiological factors (age, sex, fitness) has, for the most part, only been measured in individuals without diabetes. For example, females (without diabetes) are known to have different hormonal responses to exercise than males (15–28), resulting in differences in fuel selection (15–18, 23, 29–35) that might impact changes in blood glucose during different types of exercise. The same can be said of older individuals compared to younger individuals (36–43), and those of high physical fitness compared to those of low physical fitness (37, 38, 44–50). Where tightly controlled insulin and glucagon responses will help maintain blood glucose levels in a tight range in individuals without diabetes, differences in counter-regulatory responses to exercise depending on age, sex, or physical fitness have the potential to make a greater impact where pancreatic islet function is impaired or absent. Overall, this questions the adequacy of using existing data from acute exercise studies in T1D for modeling these activities in the context of the artificial pancreas, as much of the current research with T1D participants fails to take into account underlying physiological factors that will probably interact to affect blood glucose control. This review aims to summarize the state of knowledge on these factors, and to infer their potential impact on blood glucose responses to exercise in individuals with T1D.

EFFECT OF SEX ON EXERCISE RESPONSES IN INDIVIDUALS WITHOUT DIABETES

A large proportion of studies examining exercise metabolism have been performed uniquely in males. While limited, studies comparing the neuroendocrine and metabolic responses to exercise in healthy men and women have shown clear sex-related differences in the patterns of fuel selection (15–18, 23, 29–35), catecholamine response (15–22) and other hormonal responses such as estrogen (23–25) and growth hormone (16, 26–28). All of these factors have the potential to influence blood glucose concentrations both acutely, and in the hours following exercise (**Table 1**).

Fuel Selection

There is a clear difference between males and females in fuel selection during exercise. While there appears to be no difference between the sexes at rest (51, 52), females exhibit a lower respiratory exchange ratio (RER) during exercise in the fasted state, indicating a greater reliance on lipolysis than males for energy production (15–18, 23, 30–35, 53). This trend has been observed in healthy males and females during endurance exercise (15, 29–32, 34), submaximal exercise (16, 17, 23, 53), high intensity exercise (23) and resistance exercise (34).

The RER measurements are consistent with what has been noted at the cellular level: females use more myocellular triacylglycerol than males, whereas males deplete a greater portion of their glycogen stores during various types of exercise (18, 29, 54). Additionally, it has been observed that men shift to using carbohydrates as the dominant fuel source earlier [at 45 $\pm$ 1% of the participant's maximal aerobic capacity (VO_{2max})] than women (at 52 $\pm$ 1% VO_{2max}, $p < 0.01$) in a graded treadmill exercise test to exhaustion (55). While women still shift to oxidizing carbohydrates with higher intensity exercise, this shift is later and less extreme than in men. Less reliance on carbohydrate oxidation during exercise [53.1 $\pm$ 2.1% in men vs. 45.7 $\pm$ 1.8% ($p < 0.01$) in women during 2 h of cycling at

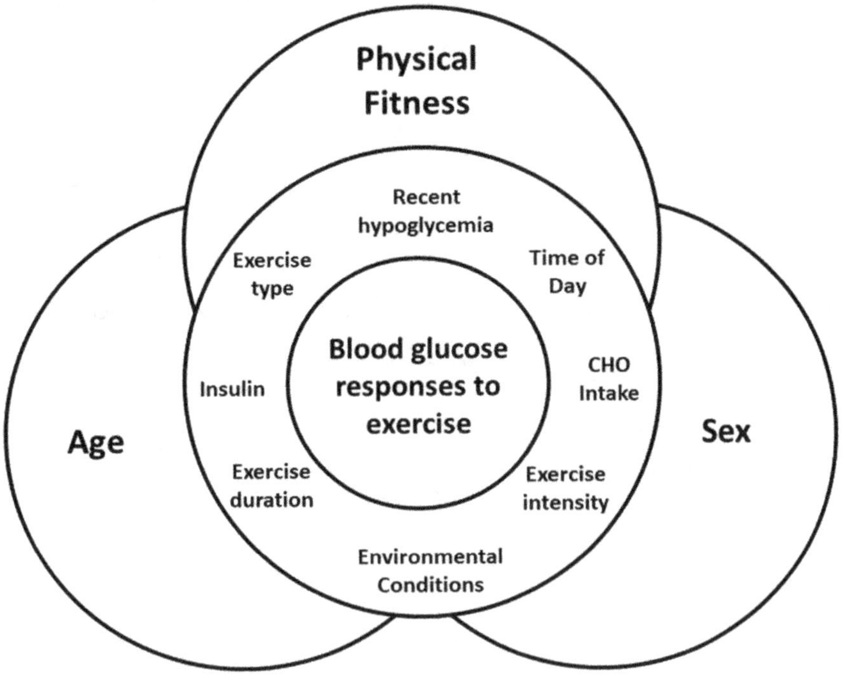

FIGURE 1 | Interaction of factors that can impact blood glucose during exercise, with the physiological factors of age, sex, and physical fitness underlying and interacting with all of them.

40%VO_{2max}] has been related to less depletion of glycogen stores in women (15).

Women also seem to be better able to conserve glycogen stores after extended exercise (90 min at 65% of VO_{2max}) (24), sparing the need for a large uptake of plasma glucose in the recovery period. One study found that women had a more precise defense of homeostasis in the recovery period post-exercise, including the control of blood glucose concentration and fuel selection (56). Due to their greater inherent capacity for lipid oxidation during exercise, women are able to regain control over glycemia and glucose flux in recovery more quickly than men (56). Therefore, men often show an increased rate of lipid mobilization post-exercise compared to women, in order to preserve glucose concentrations when restoring depleted glycogen stores from exercise (15, 33).

Important Hormones Mediating Fuel Selection

Several hormones, in addition to insulin and glucagon, are known to affect blood glucose homeostasis around exercise. Epinephrine and norepinephrine stimulate a substantial increase in hepatic glucose production. Growth hormone is known to promote lipolysis, which may in turn decrease reliance on blood glucose. Levels of estrogen, have also been shown to impact rates of lipolysis. All of these hormones respond differently between the sexes to an acute bout of exercise.

Catecholamines

There is a noticeable sex-related difference in catecholamine response to various forms and intensities of exercise. While a few exceptions exist (57, 58), the majority of studies report a significantly higher catecholamine response to various types of exercise in males compared to females (15–22). This trend has been found during moderate exercise, whether performed in the fasted state (16), or the postprandial state (18). It has also been found to hold during moderate intensity exercise of longer (2 h) duration (15), high intensity resistance exercise (59), and maximal sprints in trained individuals (19). This finding is important in blood glucose regulation, as high catecholamine levels will stimulate hepatic glycogenolysis and gluconeogenesis, increasing blood glucose levels during activity (15, 60–62), but potentially decreasing blood glucose levels post-exercise when glycogen stores are being replenished.

While men have shown an increased catecholamine response to exercise compared to women, there is also an apparent sex-related difference in the adrenergic receptor sensitivity during exercise. Horton et al. (15) found that men had significantly elevated levels of epinephrine, which stimulates lipolysis, at the end of moderate endurance exercise (post-exercise epinephrine: men $= 208 \pm 36$ vs. women $= 121 \pm 15$ pg/ml, $p < 0.007$), but had similar levels of circulating glycerol to women. This finding would suggest a greater sensitivity to the lipolytic action of the catecholamines in women. It is postulated that women may have a higher ß-adrenergic sensitivity, and decreased α-adrenergic sensitivity compared to men (17, 18, 23, 63). ß-adrenoreceptors are known to stimulate, whereas α-adrenoreceptors inhibit lipolysis, and thus a higher sensitivity of ß receptors in women during exercise results in greater net lipolysis (17). Indeed, when epinephrine was kept constant by infusion (63), women showed

TABLE 1 | Summary of hormonal responses to exercise by sex, age, and fitness level and their potential effect on blood glucose responses in type 1 diabetes.

Key factors	Fuel selection	Catecholamine	Growth hormone	Other hormones	Potential blood glucose response in type 1 diabetes
Sex	• Males favor CHO oxidation; Females rely to a greater extent on lipid oxidation.	• Greater E and NE response in males. • Females exhibit greater sensitivity to lipolytic action of E and NE.	• Similar magnitude of response during and after exercise. • Peaks are larger and sooner in females; more prolonged response in males.	• Estrogen: females exhibit greater increase during exercise than males. • Glucagon: no sex differences.	• Potential greater risk of hypoglycemia during and post-exercise in males. Better blood glucose control in post-exercise period in females.
Age	• MOD elicits similar responses. • HI: CHO oxidation decreases with age.	• Lower E response with age. • Blunted lipolytic response to E and NE with age.	• Attenuated GH response in older individuals compared to younger in MOD, HI and RE.	• Glucagon, cortisol and lactate responses decrease with age.	• Suggests higher blood glucose levels with age.
Fitness level	• Greater reliance on lipids during LO-MOD, and increased CHO oxidation during HI with higher fitness levels.	• Increased E response to MOD and HI with higher fitness levels.	• Higher GH responses to HI and RE with higher fitness levels.	• Glucagon: No change in fasting or peak levels with training.	• Improved glucose homeostasis with training. • Potential greater risk of nocturnal hypoglycemia with higher fitness levels.

CHO, carbohydrate; E, epinephrine; NE, norepinephrine; GH, growth hormone; T1D, type 1 diabetes; MOD, moderate intensity exercise; HI, high intensity exercise; RE, resistance exercise; LO, low intensity exercise.

greater lipolytic responses than men, suggesting less activation of the α-adrenergic receptors in women. Overall, this would support the trends seen in fuel selection, where women have relatively greater levels of lipolysis and fat oxidation than men during exercise.

Estrogen

Another factor influencing fuel selection during exercise is the difference in estrogen, between men and women. Estrogen, specifically 17ß-estradiol, has been shown to promote lipid oxidation and glycogen sparing during exercise (15, 23–25). Two separate blinded placebo control studies have shown that intake of 17ß-estradiol in males shifted fuel selection in the direction of lipid oxidation in recreationally-active men so that it was similar to that of women during moderate (65% VO_{2max}) aerobic exercise (25, 64).

While sex has a prominent effect on fuel selection, different phases of the menstrual cycle can also influence metabolism during exercise, and should thus be controlled for in studies involving women. Most studies test women in the early follicular phase, where estrogen concentrations do not differ markedly between men and women (34). This limits the proportion that estrogen contributes to determining fuel selection during exercise. During the luteal phase of the menstrual cycle, there is a higher concentration of estrogen and, consequently, a higher relative rate of fat utilization in females (31). While RER values (and therefore glucose utilization) are uniformly lower in women performing endurance exercise when compared to men, the luteal phase has been shown to produce lower glucose appearance and disappearance rates and less glycogen depletion than when exercise is performed in the follicular phase (24). There is also a greater increase in estradiol during exercise (both aerobic and resistance), which may contribute to greater fat oxidation for energy production in females during the luteal phase (35, 65, 66).

Growth Hormone

There is a lack of consensus regarding differences in growth hormone response to exercise between men and women. While some studies report a significantly increased growth hormone response in men compared to women after sprint (19) or submaximal exercise (67), others report an increased growth hormone response in women following resistance exercise (26, 68) or sprints (28). The majority of studies, however, report a similar response between the sexes in which both men and women experience an increase in growth hormone levels during and following exercise that is >10 min in length (16, 65, 69–71).

Although the majority of studies report similar relative increases in growth hormone during exercise compared to resting controls, there is a sexually dimorphic pattern in the way this occurs. Growth hormone peaks in women are reported to be larger and appear sooner than men, whereas men sustain a more prolonged response (16, 26–28). Sex-related differences in growth hormone levels can be attributed to a lack of testosterone response in women (65). Because women experience little or no increase in testosterone levels in response to exercise, growth hormone appears to compensate for the anabolic requirements stimulated by acute exercise (34, 72). Additionally, women have a higher resting basal level of growth hormone (65, 68, 70), particularly in the early follicular phase of the menstrual cycle (73). Because most exercise studies are performed on women during the early follicular phase of the menstrual cycle due to low levels of estrogen in this phase, there are marked sex differences in basal growth hormone levels (34), and subsequently higher levels of growth hormone during and after exercise. Additionally, increased levels of circulating estradiol are associated with higher growth hormone concentrations (26), as estradiol releases a growth hormone stimulating factor (65).

Increases in growth hormone stimulate lipolysis and lipid oxidation, suppressing glucose oxidation and consequently sparing plasma glucose (74). Higher resting levels of estradiol in women stimulates growth hormone release, which inhibits glucose uptake, thereby enhancing lipolysis, and again, preserving plasma glucose levels in women. The difference in growth hormone response to exercise between the sexes, thus, has the potential to affect blood glucose control directly.

EFFECT OF AGE ON EXERCISE RESPONSES IN INDIVIDUALS WITHOUT DIABETES

While there are clear differences in exercise responses between the sexes, it would seem that declines in functional fitness with age occur evenly in both sexes, and are due mostly to the reduction in upper and lower limb muscle strength, increases in body-fat percentage, and decreases in flexibility, agility and endurance (36). There are also changes in the hormonal response to exercise, which may alter fuel selection patterns during different types of activity, resulting in differences in fuel usage during exercise between younger and older individuals. Aging is also associated with a decrease in cardio-respiratory fitness (reflected by lower maximum oxygen consumption values) (75), which in itself may impact exercise responses (discussed in the section on physical fitness below). There are minimal published data to date examining how these age-related alterations in exercise response affect changes in blood glucose during activity of any type.

Body Composition

Aging is characterized by a decrease in muscle mass and strength (76), and an increase in adiposity (77), which generally translates into declines in physical capacity (78). Older adults also have a decreased resting metabolic rate, which may only be partly due to the changes in body composition (79). A higher level of abdominal adiposity in particular is a significant predictor of insulin sensitivity in older adults (80). With decreases in muscle mass, metabolic rate and aerobic fitness, older individuals will be burning less fuel overall for the same relative intensity of exercise.

Fuel Selection

When exercise is of moderate intensity relative to the individual's peak aerobic rate, the proportion of fuel supplied by carbohydrates is similar among older and younger individuals (37, 76). However, where more intense/anaerobic exercise is concerned, carbohydrate oxidation decreases up to 20% from roughly 20–50 years of age in sedentary (but not trained) men (37). Sedentary men also have a decrease in the lactate threshold during sub-maximal exercise with age (38), however, in spite of this, younger men are able to produce more lactate during activities such as resistance exercise (39), thereby indicating a greater reliance on carbohydrates as a fuel source. This may be part of the reason why one study showed that blood glucose was ~1.0 mmol/L higher before, during and for 30 min after heavy resistance training in older (mean age ~62 years) men without diabetes compared to a younger cohort (mean age ~30 years) (39). Several of these differences between older and younger individuals can be attenuated, however, if a higher level of physical fitness is maintained through the life course. The impact of physical fitness will be discussed in greater detail in the following section.

Important Hormones Mediating Fuel Selection

Catecholamines

A lower reliance on carbohydrate with increasing age may, in part, be due to a lower epinephrine response to exercise of both moderate and high intensity with age. One study showed that men aged 60–70 years old experienced a lower epinephrine response to sub-maximal exercise (~70% VO_{2max}) than 20–32 year old men regardless of fitness level (40). Similarly, ~15 min of exercise at ~78% VO_{2max} resulted in a lower epinephrine response (109 ± 10 vs. 228 ± 29 pg/ml; $p < 0.01$) in a group of older men and women (mean 64 years) compared to younger adults (mean 24 years) (41). Very high intensity exercise (a maximal sprint cycle—Wingate test) also produced lower epinephrine responses in a group of male athletes with a mean age of 34 years (1.86 ± 0.26 mmol/l), compared to a group of athletes with a mean age of 21 years (3.24 ± 0.28 mmol/l; $p < 0.05$) (42). It should also be noted that in older men, there is a blunted lipolytic response to catecholamines compared to younger men, possibly due to decreased sensitivity of the hormone-sensitive lipase complex (43).

Growth Hormone

Older individuals show altered growth hormone responses to several different types and intensities of exercise. Where moderate intensity exercise is concerned, one study found that older men, whether they were trained (10.1 ± 5.5 ng/ml) or untrained (7.7 ± 6.5 ng/ml), had attenuated growth hormone response to 60 min of running at 70% VO_{2max} compared to younger men (trained = 18.1 ± 6.7 vs. untrained = 20.4 ± 11.2 ng/ml) (40). Another study, however, found that responses were similar when exercise was sub-maximal, but that high intensity exercise produced a lower growth hormone response (11.3 ± 3.5 ng/ml vs. 21.9 ± 4.0 ng/ml; $p < 0.05$) in older men (mean ~64 years) compared to younger ones (mean ~23 years) (38). Differences were also found with resistance exercise, where growth hormone levels continued to increase post-exercise in young men (mean ~30 years) while decreasing in older (~62 years) men (39). Attenuated growth hormone responses to heavy resistance exercise have also been observed in older women (~62 years) in comparison to younger women (~24 years) (81), which may impact the fuels that are selected for use both during and after exercise.

Other Hormones

Glucagon and cortisol levels may also be influenced by increasing age. One study showed that glucagon levels were lower at rest in older men (60–70 years) compared to younger men (20–32 years), regardless of training status (older sedentary = 89 ± 28 pg/ml, older trained = 114 ± 34 pg/ml, younger sedentary = 141 ± 73 pg/ml, younger trained = 136 ± 35 pg/ml; $p < 0.05$ for both younger groups compared to both older groups) (40). Changes during exercise, however, were more dependent on physical fitness (discussed below) than age *per se* (40). Finally, lactate and cortisol responses to maximal exercise are also attenuated with age in both men and women (80), which would be consistent with what is known about reliance on carbohydrates as a fuel source being decreased within the same context.

EFFECT OF PHYSICAL FITNESS ON EXERCISE RESPONSES IN INDIVIDUALS WITHOUT DIABETES

While age-related declines in physical activity/exercise and hormonal responses lead to differences in fuel selection between older and younger individuals, some of these changes can be delayed or attenuated by maintaining higher levels of physical fitness (37, 38). In both younger and older men and women, higher levels of physical fitness lead to increases in hormonal responses to exercise fitness (37, 38, 44, 46), and a greater ability to mobilize and use fuels during exercise fitness (37, 38, 45–49) when compared to sedentary counterparts (**Table 1**). Individuals with higher fitness levels are also known to have greater insulin sensitivity than those who are sedentary (44, 50).

Fuel Selection

Improvements in physical fitness are known to change the proportion of fuels oxidized during exercise, with a greater reliance on lipids during low to moderate aerobic activities (37, 38), and an increase in carbohydrate dependence during high intensity exercise (37, 45, 59). At the same relative intensities, trained individuals will burn more calories, with the difference being made up for with fat oxidation (82), while at the same absolute intensities, trained individuals will have a greater reliance on lipid oxidation than untrained individuals (82). Male athletes are also more efficient at using lactate as a gluconeogenic precursor compared to sedentary males when exercising in the fasting state, which may spare endogenous glucose during extended and/or intense exercise (83).

The effects of physical fitness on fuel selection during exercise remain apparent as individuals age. In a study of older (~74 years) individuals, 16 weeks of endurance training caused an increase in whole body fat oxidation (from 166 ± 17 to 221 ± 28 μmol/min; $p = 0.002$) and a decrease in carbohydrate oxidation (from 3937 ± 483 to 3180 ± 461 μmol/min; $p = 0.003$) when exercise was performed at the same absolute intensity post-training (49). Another study of older (~64 years) males noted that carbohydrate oxidation increased with greater exercise intensity, and that trained men experienced a greater increase than untrained men (47). Similar to the case with sex- and age-related differences in metabolism, it is likely that fitness-related differences in hormonal responses to exercise drive these changes in fuel selection.

Important Hormones Mediating Fuel Selection

Catecholamines

As previously discussed, higher levels of epinephrine are associated with a greater amount of hepatic glycogenolysis, and consequently higher levels of blood glucose. Overall, higher levels of physical fitness in men are associated with increased epinephrine responses to both sub-maximal (38, 40) and high intensity exercise (46). In addition, the type of training performed will have an impact on the magnitude of epinephrine responses: male sprinters have a higher sympatho-adrenal output than endurance trained and untrained individuals when faced with supra-maximal exercise. These responses will have a direct impact on glucose metabolism.

Growth Hormone

Growth hormone responses to high intensity exercise can also be affected by the fitness levels of the participant. One study of lean and obese men found that age and physical fitness (and not adiposity) were the strongest predictors of growth hormone responses to a maximal exercise test (84). In spite of the lower response with increasing age, it has also been found that individuals with higher levels of physical fitness maintain higher growth hormone responses to maximal exercise (38, 44). In addition, trained men have demonstrated higher growth hormone responses to heavy resistance exercise, compared to untrained men (from 0.65 ± 0.47 to 5.32 ± 6.67 ng/ml in trained, from 0.50 ± 0.001 to 1.87 ± 3.47 ng/ml in untrained; $p < 0.05$) (85). Where moderate intensity exercise is concerned, one study observed similar growth hormone responses in trained and untrained men, when exercise was performed at the same relative intensity (38), but others have found a significantly higher response in trained men across all age groups (38, 40). There is a paucity of studies to elucidate if these trends hold true for women, or how these differences may impact glucoregulation during exercise.

TYPE 1 DIABETES: EFFECT OF SEX ON EXERCISE RESPONSES

There is currently little exercise research examining differences between men and women with T1D. Many exercise studies involving individuals with T1D have only male participants, or very few female participants. Where studies include both men and women, they generally fail to recognize potential differences between the sexes that may affect the counter-regulatory response to exercise, and affect blood glucose homeostasis. Current studies that do look at sex-related differences are also limited to aerobic exercise, leaving a complete absence of information related to high intensity activities and resistance exercise. In addition, there is currently no information about how fluctuating levels of estrogen throughout the menstrual cycle could affect blood glucose responses to exercise in women with T1D. What we do know about sex-related differences in hormonal responses to exercise in T1D, however, tends to mirror the outcomes of previous studies in individuals without diabetes.

Fuel Selection

Very few studies have examined sex-related differences in fuel selection during exercise in individuals with T1D, and those that do involve small sample sizes (e.g., <10 individuals of each sex). One study that measured RER during 90 min of aerobic exercise (50% VO_{2max} on a cycle ergometer) noted a tendency toward higher carbohydrate oxidation among men during the last 30 min of exercise, although differences were not statistically significant (86). As the study in question used constant dextrose and insulin infusion to maintain blood glucose, it was not possible to examine the impact of sex on changes in blood glucose during this type of activity. From what we know of studies in non-diabetic individuals, however, the greater reliance on glycogen stores in men during exercise compared to women poses a greater risk, in theory, for post-exercise hypoglycemia in men with T1D, as greater uptake of plasma glucose will be needed to replenish depleted glycogen stores during recovery.

Important Hormones Mediating Fuel Selection

While there is a current lack of information regarding sex-related differences in blood glucose responses to exercise in T1D, there is evidence that hormonal responses differ between the sexes. Similar to studies involving individuals without diabetes, Galassetti et al. (86) found that epinephrine (men = 938 ± 104; women = 628 ± 142 pmol/l; post-exercise; $p < 0.05$) and norepinephrine (men = 5.9 ± 0.8; women = 4.0 ± 0.7 nmol/l; post-exercise $p < 0.05$) responses to exercise were greater in men compared to women with T1D after 90 min of exercise on a cycle ergometer at 50% VO_{2max}. The growth hormone response was also significantly lower in women (from 4 ± 2 to 14 ± 3 μg/l) compared to men (from 1 ± 0.4 to 24 ± 9μg/l; $p < 0.05$) (87). However, women still elicited a greater lipolytic response to exercise (glycerol increased from 46 ± 7 to 188 ± 40 μM compared to 31 ± 5 to 131 ± 10 μM in men; $p < 0.05$ area under the curve), with a suggestion of greater tissue sensitivity in women to growth hormone than men (86).

Where glucagon is concerned, sex-related differences seem to exist only where individuals have experienced hypoglycemia prior to exercise. The pancreatic β-cell death that characterizes T1D is accompanied by a progressive loss of α-cell function over time (87), resulting in an impaired glucagon response to falling blood glucose levels (88). The decline in function appears to happen evenly across the sexes, resulting in similar glucagon responses to exercise and to hypoglycemia at rest. Davis et al. (89) found that glucagon responses to hypoglycemia were similar among men and women with T1D (63 ± 18 and 58 ± 12 ng/l respectively). Similarly Galassetti et al. (86) found no sex-related differences in glucagon responses (51 ± 3 ng/l for men vs. 47 ± 7 ng/l for women) to 90 min of cycling at 50% VO_{2max} in participants with T1D who were matched for age, glycemic control, duration of diabetes and exercise fitness.

With the presence of antecedent hypoglycemia, however, Galassetti et al. (90) discovered a greater blunting of counter-regulatory hormonal responses to exercise in men with T1D, compared to women matched for age, fitness, diabetes duration, and glycemic control. The exercise involved 90 min of euglycemic exercise (cycling at 50%VO_{2max}) performed 24 h after a 2 h hypoglycemic period. While both groups had a noticeably blunted response, the differences in counter-regulatory hormones, particularly glucagon (11 ± 2 ng/l lower in men, but only 5 ± 2 ng/l lower in women, $p < 0.05$) led to a higher level of suppression of endogenous glucose production during exercise in the men (90). In the absence of a constant insulin and glucose infusion to maintain blood glucose concentration, this would most likely result in greater declines in blood glucose in males compared to females. Overall, more research in the area of sex and its effects on blood glucose responses to different types, timing, and intensity of exercise in T1D are required.

TYPE 1 DIABETES: EFFECT OF AGE ON EXERCISE RESPONSES

Within the context of T1D, aging is associated with increasing insulin dosage, as resistance to insulin increases with both age (mostly due to decreasing physical activity levels) (91) and disease duration (92). To date, it has yet to be examined whether older adults with T1D have different responses to exercise across various intensities compared to young adults. The differences in fuel selection and hormonal response seen between age groups in individuals without diabetes would indicate that age should be considered as an important factor. As improvements in diabetes care have led to a greater number of individuals with T1D living longer, healthier lives, determining the impact of age on blood glucose responses to different types and durations of exercise will become increasingly important.

TYPE 1 DIABETES: EFFECT OF PHYSICAL FITNESS ON EXERCISE RESPONSES

Where fuel selection is concerned, it would seem that improvements in physical fitness have a similar impact in individuals with T1D as they do in individuals without diabetes. One small study with T1D participants showed that improvements in physical fitness after 7 weeks of sprint training increased the participants' reliance on lipids as a fuel source (as measured by lower RER) during moderate intensity activity (93). This decreased reliance on carbohydrate as a fuel source during exercise, however, does not seem to protect against hypoglycemia: a recent study of 44 participants with T1D found that those who were more fit seemed to be more prone to hypoglycemia during moderate (60% VO_{2max}) aerobic exercise (94).

In individuals with T1D, elevated epinephrine responses can lead to elevations of blood glucose during high intensity exercise that can persist for up to 2 h post-exercise (60). The extent to which fitness levels offer this glucose raising effect in individuals with T1D requires further examination, as current studies of high intensity exercise (either on its own or in the form of high intensity interval exercise) tend to have small sample sizes, of heterogeneous composition. It is also uncertain as to whether higher fitness levels will lead to a greater risk of nocturnal hypoglycemia in trained individuals vs. untrained individuals due to the need to replenish a greater amount of glycogen post-exercise.

CLOSED LOOP/ARTIFICIAL PANCREAS EXERCISE STUDIES TO DATE

A small handful of studies have been completed to assess the performance of existing closed loop systems when faced with the challenge of controlling blood glucose during exercise (95–100). The task of managing blood glucose for different intensities of exercise in individuals with T1D is highlighted in a study by Jayawardene et al. (97) where a high intensity interval exercise protocol of similar energy expenditure to a moderate aerobic exercise protocol resulted in significantly different blood glucose levels 60 min post-exercise (high intensity intermittent exercise: 11.3 ± 0.5 mmol/L vs. aerobic exercise 8.9 ± mmol/L; $p < 0.001$) while using a hybrid closed loop system. This occurred in spite of standardization of exercise timing and food intake. One out of the 12 participants also experienced hypoglycemia (plasma glucose <4.0 mmol/L for more than 15 min) after the moderate exercise session (97).

For hypoglycemia prevention during and after exercise, it has been suggested that closed loop systems should include both insulin and glucagon so that they can more closely replicate the hormonal changes that usually take place. Unfortunately, stable liquid glucagon formulations are currently lacking (101), making the widespread use of bi-hormonal devices impossible at this point. While dual hormone systems have generally been more successful at hypoglycemia prevention during exercise when compared to systems using insulin alone, they still cannot fully prevent hypoglycemia. Taleb et al. (96), for example, examined the performance of dual and single hormone systems in relation to a bout of aerobic exercise (60 min at 60% VO_{2max}) and high intensity intermittent exercise (alternating between 50 and 85% VO_{2max} every 2 min). While the dual hormone system resulted in a trend toward fewer participants experiencing hypoglycemia during the aerobic exercise trial (17.6 vs. 52.9%, $p = 0.07$), it still did not prevent it. Findings were similar for the high intensity intermittent protocol with respect to the number of participants experiencing hypoglycemia during exercise (6.25 for dual vs. 40% for single hormone, $p = 0.07$). Castle et al. (100) also had similar findings for a 45 min exercise session at 60% VO_{2max} where a dual hormone system decreased time spent in hypoglycemia (3.4 ± 4.5% for dual hormone, 8.3 ± 12.6% for single hormone, $p = 0.009$). Hypoglycemia still occurred, albeit in lesser amounts. It is likely that there simply is not enough information available on exercise in T1D for these systems to predict exercise responses accurately.

SUMMARY

Changes in blood glucose during the 24 h after physical activity/exercise (i.e., the recovery period) are likely to be slow enough that a closed loop system will be able to manage them appropriately. The variability in responses to exercise and the magnitude of blood glucose changes over short periods, however, may prove to be a challenging obstacle due to the diversity of responses in a very heterogeneous population. A highly fit, young, female, may have very different responses to various types and intensities of exercise than an older, sedentary male. In the context of how little is currently known about all of the possible variables that might affect blood glucose responses to exercise in individuals with T1D, there may be insufficient information to produce a model that fully predicts it. Additional studies in this area involving participants with a greater range of ages, sexes, and fitness levels are required in order to provide the necessary information to successfully model physical activity/exercise in the context of the artificial pancreas.

AUTHOR CONTRIBUTIONS

All authors JY, NB and RB made equal contributions in the research, drafting and editing of this manuscript.

REFERENCES

1. Bluestone JA, Herold K, Eisenbarth G. Genetics, pathogenesis and clinical interventions in type 1 diabetes. *Nature* (2010) 464:1293–300. doi: 10.1038/nature08933
2. Chimen M, Kennedy A, Nirantharamkumar K, Pang TT, Andrews R, Narendran P. What are the health benefits of physical activity in type 1 diabetes mellitus? A literature review. *Diabetologia* (2012) 55:542–51. doi: 10.1007/s00125-011-2403-2
3. Brazeau AS, Rabasa-Lhoret R, Strychar I, Mircescu H. Barriers to physical activity among patients with type 1 diabetes. *Diabetes Care* (2008) 31:2108–9. doi: 10.2337/dc08-0720
4. Riddell MC, Gallen IW, Smart CE, Taplin CE, Adlofsson P, Lumb AN, et al. Exercise management in type 1 diabetes: a consensus statement. *Lancet Diabetes Endocrinol.* (2017) 5:377–90. doi: 10.1016/S2213-8587(17)30014-1
5. Freckmann G, Schmid C, Baumstark A, Pleus S, Link M, Haug C. System accuracy evaluation of 43 blood glucose monitoring systems for self-monitoring of blood glucose according to DIN EN ISO 15197. *J Diabetes Sci Technol.* (2012) 6:1060–75. doi: 10.1177/193229681200600510
6. Laffel L. Improved accuracy of continuous glucose monitoring systems in pediatric patients with diabetes mellitus: results from two studies. *Diabetes Technol Ther.* (2016) 18:S223–33. doi: 10.1089/dia.2015.0380
7. Bailey TS. Clinical implications of accuracy measurements of continuous glucose sensors. *Diabetes Technol Ther.* (2017) 19:S51–4. doi: 10.1089/dia.2017.0050
8. Weisman A, Bai JW, Cardinez M, Kramer CK, Perkins BA. Effect of artificial pancreas systems on glycaemic control in patients with type 1 diabetes: a systematic review and meta-analysis of outpatient randomised controlled trials. *Lancet Diabetes Endocrinol.* (2017) 5:501–12. doi: 10.1016/S2213-8587(17)30167-5
9. Riddell MC, Zaharieva DP, Yavelberg L, Cinar A, Jamnik VK. Exercise and the development of the artificial pancreas: one of the more

difficult series of hurdles. *J Diabetes Sci Technol.* (2015) 9:1217–26. doi: 10.1177/1932296815609370
10. Colberg SR, Laan R, Dassau E, Kerr D. Physical activity and type 1 diabetes: time for a rewire? *J Diabetes Sci Technol.* (2015) 9:609–18. doi: 10.1177/1932296814566231
11. Zaharieva D, Yavelberg L, Jamnik V, Cinar A, Turksoy K, Riddell MC. The effects of basal insulin suspension at the start of exercise on blood glucose levels during continuous versus circuit-based exercise in individuals with type 1 diabetes on continuous subcutaneous insulin infusion. *Diabetes Technol Ther.* (2017) 19:370–8. doi: 10.1089/dia.2017.0010
12. Colberg SR, Sigal RJ, Yardley JE, Riddell MC, Dunstan DW, Dempsey PC, et al. Physical activity/exercise and diabetes: a position statement of the American Diabetes Association. *Diabetes Care* (2016) 39:2065–79. doi: 10.2337/dc16-1728
13. Turksoy K, Monforti C, Park M, Griffith G, Quinn L, Cinar A. Use of wearable sensors and biometric variables in an artificial pancreas system. *Sensors (Basel).* (2017) 17:E532. doi: 10.3390/s17030532
14. Franc S, Daoudi A, Pochat A, Petit MH, Randazzo C, Petit C, et al. Insulin-based strategies to prevent hypoglycaemia during and after exercise in adult patients with type 1 diabetes on pump therapy: the DIABRASPORT randomized study. *Diabetes Obes Metab.* (2015) 17:1150–7. doi: 10.1111/dom.12552
15. Horton TJ, Pagliassotti MJ, Hobbs K, Hill JO. Fuel metabolism in men and women during and after long-duration exercise. *J. Appl. Physiol (1985)* (1998) 85:1823–32. doi: 10.1152/jappl.1998.85.5.1823
16. Davis SN, Galassetti P, Wasserman DH, Tate D. Effects of gender on neuroendocrine and metabolic counterregulatory responses to exercise in normal man. *J Clin Endocrinol Metab.* (2000) 85:224–30. doi: 10.1210/jcem.85.1.6328
17. Hedrington MS, Davis SN. Sexual dimorphism in glucose and lipid metabolism during fasting, hypoglycemia, and exercise. *Front Endocrinol (Lausanne)* (2015) 6:61. doi: 10.3389/fendo.2015.00061
18. Steffensen CH, Roepstorff C, Madsen M, Kiens B. Myocellular triacylglycerol breakdown in females but not in males during exercise. *Am J Physiol Endocrinol Metab.* (2002) 282:E634–42. doi: 10.1152/ajpendo.00078.2001
19. Justice TD, Hammer GL, Davey RJ, Paramalingam N, Guelfi KJ, Lewis L, et al. Effect of antecedent moderate-intensity exercise on the glycemia-increasing effect of a 30-sec maximal sprint: a sex comparison. *Physiol. Rep.* (2015) 3:e12386. doi: 10.14814/phy2.12386
20. Gratas-Delamarche A, Le Cam R, Delamarche P, Monnier M, Koubi H. Lactate and catecholamine responses in male and female sprinters during a Wingate test. *Eur J Appl Physiol Occup Physiol.* (1994) 68:362–6. doi: 10.1007/BF00571458
21. Amiel SA, Maran A, Powrie JK, Umpleby AM, Macdonald IA. Gender differences in counterregulation to hypoglycaemia. *Diabetologia* (1993) 36:460–4. doi: 10.1007/BF00402284
22. Pullinen T, Nicol C, MacDonald E, Komi PV. Plasma catecholamine responses to four resistance exercise tests in men and women. *Eur J Appl Physiol Occup Physiol.* (1999) 80:125–31. doi: 10.1007/s004210050568
23. Isacco L, Duche P, Boisseau N. Influence of hormonal status on substrate utilization at rest and during exercise in the female population. *Sports Med.* (2012) 42:27–42. doi: 10.2165/11598900-000000000-00000
24. Devries MC, Hamadeh MJ, Phillips SM, Tarnopolsky MA. Menstrual cycle phase and sex influence muscle glycogen utilization and glucose turnover during moderate-intensity endurance exercise. *Am J Physiol Regul Integr Comp Physiol.* (2006) 291:R1120–R1128. doi: 10.1152/ajpregu.00700.2005
25. Hamadeh MJ, Devries MC, Tarnopolsky MA. Estrogen supplementation reduces whole body leucine and carbohydrate oxidation and increases lipid oxidation in men during endurance exercise. *J Clin Endocrinol Metab.* (2005) 90:3592–9. doi: 10.1210/jc.2004-1743
26. Luk HY, Kraemer WJ, Szivak TK, Flanagan SD, Hooper DR, Kupchak BR, et al. Acute resistance exercise stimulates sex-specific dimeric immunoreactive growth hormone responses. *Growth Horm IGF Res.* (2015) 25:136–40. doi: 10.1016/j.ghir.2015.02.002
27. Esbjornsson M, Norman B, Suchdev S, Viru M, Lindghren A, Jansson E. Greater growth hormone and insulin response in women than in men during repeated bouts of sprint exercise. *Acta Physiol (Oxf).* (2009) 197:107–15. doi: 10.1111/j.1748-1716.2009.01994.x
28. Eliakim A, Nemet D, Most G, Rakover N, Pantanowitz M, Meckel Y. Effect of gender on the GH-IGF-I response to anaerobic exercise in young adults. *J Strength Cond Res.* (2014) 28:3411–5. doi: 10.1519/JSC.0000000000000605
29. Devries MC. Sex-based differences in endurance exercise muscle metabolism: impact on exercise and nutritional strategies to optimize health and performance in women. *Exp Physiol.* (2016) 101:243–9. doi: 10.1113/EP085369
30. Tarnopolsky MA. Sex differences in exercise metabolism and the role of 17-beta estradiol. *Med Sci Sports Exerc.* (2008) 40:648–54. doi: 10.1249/MSS.0b013e31816212ff
31. Riddell MC, Partington SL, Stupka N, Armstrong D, Rennie C, Tarnopolsky MA. Substrate utilization during exercise performed with and without glucose ingestion in female and male endurance trained athletes. *Int J Sport Nutr Exerc Metab.* (2003) 13:407–21. doi: 10.1123/ijsnem.13.4.407
32. Mittendorfer B, Horowitz JF, Klein S. Effect of gender on lipid kinetics during endurance exercise of moderate intensity in untrained subjects. *Am J Physiol Endocrinol Metab.* (2002) 283:E58–65. doi: 10.1152/ajpendo.00504.2001
33. Henderson GC, Fattor JA, Horning MA, Faghihnia N, Johnson ML, Mau TL, et al. Lipolysis and fatty acid metabolism in men and women during the postexercise recovery period. *J Physiol.* (2007) 584:963–81. doi: 10.1113/jphysiol.2007.137331
34. Fragala MS, Kraemer WJ, Denegar CR, Maresh CM, Mastro AM, Volek JS. Neuroendocrine-immune interactions and responses to exercise. *Sports Med.* (2011) 41:621–39. doi: 10.2165/11590430-000000000-00000
35. Carter SL, Rennie C, Tarnopolsky MA. Substrate utilization during endurance exercise in men and women after endurance training. *Am J Physiol Endocrinol Metab.* (2001) 280:E898–907. doi: 10.1152/ajpendo.2001.280.6.E898
36. Milanovic Z, Pantelic S, Trajkovic N, Sporis G, Kostic R, James N. Age-related decrease in physical activity and functional fitness among elderly men and women. *Clin Interv Aging* (2013) 8:549–56. doi: 10.2147/CIA.S44112
37. Manetta J, Brun JF, Prefaut C, Mercier J. Substrate oxidation during exercise at moderate and hard intensity in middle-aged and young athletes vs. sedentary men. *Metabolism* (2005) 54:1411–9. doi: 10.1016/j.metabol.2004.12.002
38. Silverman HG, Mazzeo RS. Hormonal responses to maximal and submaximal exercise in trained and untrained men of various ages. *J Gerontol A Biol Sci Med Sci.* (1996) 51:B30–B37.
39. Kraemer WJ, Hakkinen K, Newton RU, McCormick M, Nindl BC, Volek JS, et al. Acute hormonal responses to heavy resistance exercise in younger and older men. *Eur J Appl Physiol Occup Physiol.* (1998) 77:206–11.
40. Hagberg JM, Seals DR, Yerg JE, Gavin J, Gingerich R, Premachandra B, et al. Metabolic responses to exercise in young and older athletes and sedentary men. *J. Appl. Physiol. (1985)* (1988) 65:900–8. doi: 10.1152/jappl.1988.65.2.900
41. Kohrt WM, Spina RJ, Ehsani AA, Cryer PE, Holloszy JO. Effects of age, adiposity, and fitness level on plasma catecholamine responses to standing and exercise. *J. Appl. Physiol. (1985).* (1993) 75, 1828–35. doi: 10.1152/jappl.1993.75.4.1828
42. Zouhal H, Vincent S, Moussa E, Botcazou M, Delamarche P, Gratas-Delamarche A. Early advancing age alters plasma glucose and glucoregulatory hormones in response to supramaximal exercise. *J Sci Med Sport.* (2009) 12:652–6. doi: 10.1016/j.jsams.2008.03.003
43. Lonnqvist F, Nyberg B, Wahrenberg H, Arner P. Catecholamine-induced lipolysis in adipose tissue of the elderly. *J Clin Invest.* (1990) 85:1614–21. doi: 10.1172/JCI114612
44. Manetta J, Brun JF, Maimoun L, Callis A, Prefaut C, Mercier J. Effect of training on the GH/IGF-I axis during exercise in middle-aged men: relationship to glucose homeostasis. *Am J Physiol Endocrinol Metab.* (2002) 283:E929–E936. doi: 10.1152/ajpendo.00539.2001
45. Manetta J, Brun JF, Maimoun L, Galy O, Coste O, Maso F, et al. Carbohydrate dependence during hard-intensity exercise in trained cyclists in the competitive season: importance of training status. *Int J Sports Med.* (2002) 23:516–23. doi: 10.1055/s-2002-35074
46. Manetta J, Brun JF, Perez-Martin A, Callis A, Prefaut C, Mercier J. Fuel oxidation during exercise in middle-aged men: role of training and glucose disposal. *Med Sci Sports Exerc.* (2002) 34:423–9.

47. Bassami M, Ahmadizad S, Doran D, MacLaren DP. Effects of exercise intensity and duration on fat metabolism in trained and untrained older males. *Eur J Appl Physiol.* (2007) 101:525–32. doi: 10.1007/s00421-007-0523-7
48. Boon H, Jonkers RA, Koopman R, Blaak EE, Saris WH, Wagenmakers AJ, et al. Substrate source use in older, trained males after decades of endurance training. *Med Sci Sports Exerc.* (2007) 39:2160–70. doi: 10.1249/mss.0b013e3181572ace
49. Sial S, Coggan AR, Hickner RC, Klein S. Training-induced alterations in fat and carbohydrate metabolism during exercise in elderly subjects. *Am J Physiol.* (1998) 274:E785–E90. doi: 10.1152/ajpendo.1998.274.5.E785
50. Huth C, Pigeon E, Riou ME, St-Onge J, Arguin H, Couillard E, et al. Fitness, adiposopathy, and adiposity are independent predictors of insulin sensitivity in middle-aged men without diabetes. *J Physiol Biochem.* (2016) 72:435–44. doi: 10.1007/s13105-016-0488-2
51. Sarafian D, Schutz Y, Montani JP, Dulloo AG, Miles-Chan JL. Sex difference in substrate oxidation during low-intensity isometric exercise in young adults. *Appl Physiol Nutr Metab.* (2016) 41:977–84. doi: 10.1139/apnm-2016-0127
52. Tremblay J, Peronnet F, Massicotte D, Lavoie D. Carbohydrate supplementation and sex differences in fuel selection during exercise. *Med Sci Sports Exerc.* (2010) 42:1314–23. doi: 10.1249/MSS.0b013e3181cbba0b
53. Wiecek M, Maciejczyk M, Szymura J, Syzgula Z. Sex differences in oxidative stress after eccentric and concentric exercise. *Redox Rep.* (2017) 22:478–85. doi: 10.1080/13510002.2017.1304195
54. Roepstorff C, Steffensen CH, Madsen M, Stallknecht B, Kanstrup IL, Richter EA, et al. Gender differences in substrate utilization during submaximal exercise in endurance-trained subjects. *Am. J. Physiol. Endocrinol. Metab.* (2002) 282:E435–47. doi: 10.1152/ajpendo.00266.2001
55. Venables MC, Achten J, Jeukendrup AE. Determinants of fat oxidation during exercise in healthy men and women: a cross-sectional study. *J. Appl. Physiol (1985)* (2005) 98:160–7. doi: 10.1152/japplphysiol.00662.2003
56. Henderson GC, Fattor JA, Horning MA, Faghihnia N, Johnson ML, Luke-Zeitoun M, et al. Glucoregulation is more precise in women than in men during postexercise recovery. *Am J Clin Nutr.* (2008) 87:1686–94. doi: 10.1093/ajcn/87.6.1686
57. Vincent S, Berthon P, Zouhal H, Moussa E, Catheline M, Bentue-Ferrer D, et al. Plasma glucose, insulin and catecholamine responses to a Wingate test in physically active women and men. *Eur J Appl Physiol.* (2004) 91:15–21. doi: 10.1007/s00421-003-0957-5
58. Marliss EB, Kreisman SH, Manzon A, Halter JB, Vranic M, and Nessim SJ. Gender differences in glucoregulatory responses to intense exercise. *J. Appl. Physiol (1985).* (2000) 88:457–66. doi: 10.1152/jappl.2000.88.2.457
59. Pullinen T, Mero A, Huttunen P, Pakarinen A, Komi PV. Resistance exercise-induced hormonal responses in men, women, and pubescent boys. *Med Sci Sports Exerc.* (2002) 34:806–13. doi: 10.1097/00005768-200205000-00013
60. Mitchell TH, Abraham G, Schiffrin A, Leiter LA, Marliss EB. Hyperglycemia after intense exercise in IDDM subjects during continuous subcutaneous insulin infusion. *Diabetes Care* (1988) 11:311–7. doi: 10.2337/diacare.11.4.311
61. Bussau VA, Ferreira LD, Jones TW, Founier PA. The 10-s maximal sprint: a novel approach to counter an exercise-mediated fall in glycemia in individuals with type 1 diabetes. *Diabetes Care* (2006) 29:601–6. doi: 10.2337/diacare.29.03.06.dc05-1764
62. Bussau VA, Ferreira LD, Jones TW, Founier PA. A 10-s sprint performed prior to moderate-intensity exercise prevents early post-exercise fall in glycaemia in individuals with type 1 diabetes. *Diabetologia* (2007) 50:1815–8. doi: 10.1007/s00125-007-0727-8
63. Schmidt SL, Bessesen DH, Stotz S, Peelor FF, Miller BF, and Horton TJ. Adrenergic control of lipolysis in women compared with men. *J. Appl. Physiol (1985)* (2014) 117:1008–19. doi: 10.1152/japplphysiol.00003.2014
64. Devries MC, Hamadeh MJ, Graham TE, Tarnopolsky MA. 17beta-estradiol supplementation decreases glucose rate of appearance and disappearance with no effect on glycogen utilization during moderate intensity exercise in men. *J Clin Endocrinol Metab.* (2005) 90:6218–25. doi: 10.1210/jc.2005-0926
65. Consitt LA, Copeland JL, Tremblay MS. Endogenous anabolic hormone responses to endurance versus resistance exercise and training in women. *Sports Med.* (2002) 32:1–22. doi: 10.2165/00007256-200232010-00001
66. Copeland JL, Consitt LA, Tremblay MS. Hormonal responses to endurance and resistance exercise in females aged 19-69 years. *J Gerontol A Biol Sci Med Sci.* (2002) 57:B158–B165.
67. Vislocky LM, Gaine PC, Pikosky MA, Martin WF, Rodriguez NR. Gender impacts the post-exercise substrate and endocrine response in trained runners. *J Int Soc Sports Nutr.* (2008) 5:7. doi: 10.1186/1550-2783-5-7
68. Wideman L, Weltman JY, Shah N, Story S, Veldhuis JD, Weltman A. Effects of gender on exercise-induced growth hormone release. *J. Appl. Physiol (1985)* (1999) 87:1154–62. doi: 10.1152/jappl.1999.87.3.1154
69. Benini R, Prado Nunes PR, Orsatti CL, Barcelos LC, Orsatti FL. Effects of acute total body resistance exercise on hormonal and cytokines changes in men and women. *J Sports Med Phys Fitness.* (2015) 55:337–44.
70. Kraemer WJ, Staron RS, Hagerman FC, Hikida RS, Fry AC, Gordon SE, et al. The effects of short-term resistance training on endocrine function in men and women. *Eur J Appl Physiol Occup Physiol.* (1998) 78:69–76.
71. Linnamo V, Pakarinen A, Komi PV, Kraemer WJ, Hakkinen K. Acute hormonal responses to submaximal and maximal heavy resistance and explosive exercises in men and women. *J Strength Cond Res.* (2005) 19:566–71. doi: 10.1519/R-15404.1
72. Kraemer WJ, Fleck SJ, Dziados JE, Harman EA, Marchitelli LJ, Gordon SE, et al. Changes in hormonal concentrations after different heavy-resistance exercise protocols in women. *J. Appl. Physiol (1985)* (1993) 75:594–604. doi: 10.1152/jappl.1993.75.2.594
73. Kraemer WJ, Gordon SE, Fleck SJ, Marchitelli LJ, Mello R, Dziados JE, et al. Endogenous anabolic hormonal and growth factor responses to heavy resistance exercise in males and females. *Int J Sports Med.* (1991) 12:228–35. doi: 10.1055/s-2007-1024673
74. Jorgensen JO, Krag M, Kanaley J, Moller J, Hansen TK, Moller N, et al. Exercise, hormones, and body temperature. Regulation and action of GH during exercise *J Endocrinol Invest.* (2003) 26:838–42. doi: 10.1007/BF03345233
75. Fleg JL, Morrell CH, Bos AG, Brant LJ, Talbot LA, Wright JG, et al. Accelerated longitudinal decline of aerobic capacity in healthy older adults. *Circulation* (2005) 112:674–82. doi: 10.1161/CIRCULATIONAHA.105.545459
76. Doherty TJ. The influence of aging and sex on skeletal muscle mass and strength. *Curr Opin Clin Nutr Metab Care* (2001) 4:503–8. doi: 10.1097/00075197-200111000-00007
77. Poehlman ET, Toth MJ, Bunyard LB, Gardner AW, Donaldson KE, Colman E, et al. Physiological predictors of increasing total and central adiposity in aging men and women. *Arch Intern Med.* (1995) 155:2443–8. doi: 10.1001/archinte.1995.00430220101011
78. Bouchard DR, Beliaeff S, Dionne UK, Brochu M. Fat mass but not fat-free mass is related to physical capacity in well-functioning older individuals: nutrition as a determinant of successful aging (NuAge)–the Quebec Longitudinal Study. *J Gerontol A Biol Sci Med Sci.* (2007) 62:1382–8. doi: 10.1093/gerona/62.12.1382
79. Krems C, Luhrmann PM, Strassburg A, Hartmann B, Neuhauser-Berthold M. Lower resting metabolic rate in the elderly may not be entirely due to changes in body composition. *Eur J Clin Nutr.* (2005) 59:255–62. doi: 10.1038/sj.ejcn.1602066
80. Racette SB, Evans EM, Weiss EP, Hagberg JM, Holloszy JO. Abdominal adiposity is a stronger predictor of insulin resistance than fitness among 50-95 year olds. *Diabetes Care* (2006) 29:673–8. doi: 10.2337/diacare.29.03.06.dc05-1605
81. Gordon SE, Kraemer WJ, Looney DP, Flanagan SD, Comstock BA, Hymer WC. The influence of age and exercise modality on growth hormone bioactivity in women. *Growth Horm IGF Res.* (2014) 24:95–103. doi: 10.1016/j.ghir.2014.03.005
82. van Loon LJ, Jeukendrup AE, Saris WH, Wagenmakers AJ. Effect of training status on fuel selection during submaximal exercise with glucose ingestion. *J. Appl. Physiol (1985)* (1999) 87:1413–20. doi: 10.1152/jappl.1999.87.4.1413
83. Emhoff CA, Messonnier LA, Horning MA, Fattor JA, Carlson TJ, and Brooks GA. Gluconeogenesis and hepatic glycogenolysis during exercise at the lactate threshold. *J. Appl. Physiol (1985)* (2013) 114:297–306. doi: 10.1152/japplphysiol.01202.2012

84. Holt RI, Webb E, Pentecost C, Sonksen PH. Aging and physical fitness are more important than obesity in determining exercise-induced generation of GH. *J Clin Endocrinol Metab.* (2001) 86:5715–20. doi: 10.1210/jcem.86.12.8092
85. Hasani-Ranjbar S, Soleymani Far E, Heshmat R, Rajabi H, Kosari H. Time course responses of serum GH, insulin, IGF-1, IGFBP1, and IGFBP3 concentrations after heavy resistance exercise in trained and untrained men. *Endocrine* (2012) 41:144–51. doi: 10.1007/s12020-011-9537-3
86. Galassetti P, Tate D, Neill RA, Morrey S, Davis SN. Effect of gender on counterregulatory responses to euglycemic exercise in type 1 diabetes. *J Clin Endocrinol Metab.* (2002) 87:5144–50. doi: 10.1210/jc.2002-020757
87. Banarer S, McGregor VP, Cryer PE. Intraislet hyperinsulinemia prevents the glucagon response to hypoglycemia despite an intact autonomic response. *Diabetes* (2002) 51:958–65. doi: 10.2337/diabetes.51.4.958
88. Gerich JE, Langlois M, Noacco C, Karam JH, Forsham PH. Lack of glucagon response to hypoglycemia in diabetes: evidence for an intrinsic pancreatic alpha cell defect. *Science* (1973) 182:171–3. doi: 10.1126/science.182.4108.171
89. Davis SN, Fowler S, Costa F. Hypoglycemic counterregulatory responses differ between men and women with type 1 diabetes. *Diabetes* (2000) 49:65–72. doi: 10.2337/diabetes.49.1.65
90. Galassetti P, Tate D, Neill RA, Morrey S, Wasserman DH, Davis SN. Effect of sex on counterregulatory responses to exercise after antecedent hypoglycemia in type 1 diabetes. *Am J Physiol Endocrinol Metab.* (2004) 287:E16–24. doi: 10.1152/ajpendo.00480.2002
91. Amati F, Dube JJ, Coen PM, Stefanovic-Racic M, Toledo FG, Goodpaster BH. Physical inactivity and obesity underlie the insulin resistance of aging. *Diabetes Care* (2009) 32:1547–9. doi: 10.2337/dc09-0267
92. Bulum T, Duvnjak L. Insulin resistance in patients with type 1 diabetes: relationship with metabolic and inflammatory parameters. *Acta Clin Croat.* (2013) 52:43–51.
93. Harmer AR, Chisholm DJ, McKenna MJ, Hunter SK, Ruell PA, Naylor JM, et al. Sprint training increases muscle oxidative metabolism during high-intensity exercise in patients with type 1 diabetes. *Diabetes Care* (2008) 31:2097–102. doi: 10.2337/dc08-0329
94. Al Khalifah RA, Suppere C, Haidar A, Rabasa-Lhoret R, Ladouceur M, Legault L. Association of aerobic fitness level with exercise-induced hypoglycaemia in Type 1 diabetes. *Diabet Med.* (2016) 33:1686–90. doi: 10.1111/dme.13070
95. Van Bon AC, Jonker LD, Koebrugge R, Koops R, Hoekstra JB, DeVries JH. Feasibility of a bihormonal closed-loop system to control postexercise and postprandial glucose excursions. *J Diabetes Sci Technol.* (2012) 6:1114–22. doi: 10.1177/193229681200600516
96. Taleb N, Emami A, Suppere C, Messier V, Legault L, Ladouceur M, et al. Efficacy of single-hormone and dual-hormone artificial pancreas during continuous and interval exercise in adult patients with type 1 diabetes: randomised controlled crossover trial. *Diabetologia* (2016) 59:2561–71. doi: 10.1007/s00125-016-4107-0
97. Jayawardene DC, McAuley SA, Horsburgh JC, Gerche A, Jenkins AJ, Ward GM, et al. Closed-loop insulin delivery for adults with type 1 diabetes undertaking high-intensity interval exercise versus moderate-intensity exercise: A randomized, crossover study. *Diabetes Technol Ther.* (2017) 19:340–8. doi: 10.1089/dia.2016.0461
98. Abraham MB, Davey R, O'Grady MJ, Ly TT, Paramalingam N, Fournier PA, et al. Effectiveness of a predictive algorithm in the prevention of exercise-induced hypoglycemia in type 1 diabetes. *Diabetes Technol Ther.* (2016) 18:543–50. doi: 10.1089/dia.2016.0141
99. Jacobs PG, El Youssef J, Reddy R, Resalat N, Branigan D, Condon J, et al. Randomized trial of a dual-hormone artificial pancreas with dosing adjustment during exercise compared with no adjustment and sensor-augmented pump therapy. *Diabetes Obes Metab.* (2016) 18:1110–9. doi: 10.1111/dom.12707
100. Castle JR, El Youssef J, Wilson LM, Reddy R, Resalat N, Branigan D, et al. Randomized outpatient trial of single- and dual-hormone closed-loop systems that adapt to exercise using wearable sensors. *Diabetes Care* (2018) 41:1471–7. doi: 10.2337/dc18-0228
101. Wilson LM, Castle JR. Stable Liquid Glucagon: Beyond emergency hypoglycemia rescue. *J Diabetes Sci Technol.* (2018) 12:847–53. doi: 10.1177/1932296818757795

7

Regulatory B Cells: Role in Type 1 Diabetes

Joanne Boldison [1] and F. Susan Wong [2]*

[1] Institute of Biomedical & Clinical Science, University of Exeter, Exeter, United Kingdom, [2] Division of Infection & Immunity, School of Medicine, Cardiff University, Cardiff, United Kingdom

***Correspondence:**
Joanne Boldison
J.Boldison@Exeter.ac.uk

Regulatory B cells (Bregs) have an anti-inflammatory role and can suppress autoimmunity, by employing both cytokine secretion and cell-contact mediated mechanisms. Numerous Breg subsets have been described and have overlapping phenotypes in terms of their immune expression markers or cytokine production. A hallmark feature of Bregs is the secretion of IL-10, although IL-35 and TGFβ–producing B cells have also been identified. To date, few reports have identified an impaired frequency or function of Bregs in individuals with type 1 diabetes; thus our understanding of the role played by these Breg subsets in the pathogenesis of this condition is limited. In this review we will focus on how regulatory B cells are altered in the development of type 1 diabetes, highlighting both frequency and function and discuss both human and animal studies.

Keywords: IL-10, B cell, type 1 diabetes, frequency, function

INTRODUCTION

It is now well-established that regulatory B cells (Bregs) can dampen immune responses and play a role in maintaining immune tolerance. These immunosuppressive Bregs are generally named for the anti-inflammatory cytokines that they produce to exert their regulatory effects, and so a variety of Bregs have been identified. The cytokine most widely associated with Bregs is Interleukin-(IL-)10 (1) and thus has been the major focus of many studies into the failure of Bregs to suppress inflammation in autoimmune conditions. IL-10 independent mechanisms have been identified, including suppression mediated by contact of cell surface molecules (2, 3) or other soluble mediators such as the production of TGFβ (4) and IL-35 (5). However, currently there are no reports of alterations in these IL-10 independent regulatory B cell populations, either in number or function, in human type 1 diabetes; thus their contribution to type 1 diabetes remains an outstanding question.

In type 1 diabetes B cells are typically understood to play a pathogenic role in disease, likely through the production of inflammatory cytokines and presentation of autoantigens to T cells (6). This has been emphasized by the use of Rituximab in clinical trials and the observed temporary delay in the loss of C-peptide (7). However, studies of other autoimmune diseases have highlighted the essential role for regulatory B cells (8) and this has now been reflected in type 1 diabetes, although comparatively with fewer studies. Regulatory B cells in other autoimmune diseases, including diabetes, has recently been reviewed (9). It is imperative that we further understand the balance between effector and regulatory B cells in order to improve immunotherapeutic treatments targeting these lymphocytes, including utilizing Bregs as a therapeutic option. This review will focus on the emerging literature on Bregs and discuss their role in type 1 diabetes.

REGULATORY B CELL PHENOTYPES

Studies in both human and mouse have contributed to identifying numerous IL-10-producing Breg subsets using a variety of immune markers, some of which overlap, to indicate a regulatory population. In humans, several Breg subsets enriched at different stages of B cell maturation, including immature B cells ($CD24^{hi}CD38^{hi}$) (10), memory B cells ($CD24^{hi}CD27^{+}$ [B10]) (11) and plasmablasts ($CD27^{int}CD38^{+}$) (12) have been identified. Similarly, in mice, various subsets have been identified in the transitional (13) and marginal zone (14) B cell compartments, including specific mouse subsets that parallel human B10 cells (11, 15) and human plasmablasts (12).

Other human regulatory B cell subsets have also been described including $CD19^{+}Tim\text{-}1^{+}$ B cells (16) and $CD39^{+}CD73^{+}$ Bregs (17), with equivalent subsets described in mice (18, 19). In addition, human $CD25^{hi}CD71^{hi}$ B cells produce IgG4 and are designated as regulatory Br1 cells (20). However, these subsets have not yet been described in human type 1 diabetes. The diversity and identification of Breg phenotypes has been reviewed extensively (9, 21, 22). The range and variability in methods which induce IL-10-producing B cells, along with a lack of a key definitive marker, makes it difficult to define a Breg cell without assessing IL-10 production, as a key function. Therefore, the evaluation of IL-10-production during the differentiation and developmental stages of B cells is important, as demonstrated by Iwata et al. reporting the distinction between B10 cells and B10-progenitor cells ($B10_{PRO}$) (11). The different subsets of Bregs that have been assessed, specifically in studies of type 1 diabetes, is discussed (in *Impaired Regulatory B Cell Mechanisms in type 1 diabetes*) and **Table 1**.

BREG INDUCTION AND TYPE 1 DIABETES

The heterogeneity of Bregs, both in phenotype and response to stimuli, and the absence of a definitive single marker (so far) has led to the hypothesis that any B cell can differentiate into a Breg depending on their prevailing environment, rather than a subset derived from a distinct lineage (21). Indeed, signals required for the induction or the promotion of regulatory B cells are the result

TABLE 1 | Evidence for numerical defects in Bregs in type 1 diabetes.

Study	Phenotype of B cell	Change in cell frequency (*vs.* healthy donors)	Stimulus for IL-10 induction	Diabetes duration (years)	Age of donors with diabetes (years)	Age of healthy donors (years)
De Filippo., et al. (23)	$CD5^{+}CD19^{+}$	Increase (median 250 *vs.* 95 [cells mm^3])*	NM	<30days diagnosis	Mean ±SD: 6.7±2.5	Age-matched
Deng., et al. (24)	$CD19^{+}CD5^{+}CD1d^{hi}$ (B10 cells)	Decrease (Median, values not described, [B10% of $CD19^{+}$]***	NM	Mean ±SD: 3.1 ± 3.5	Mean ±SD: 28.53 ±16.21	Mean ±SD: 41.37 ± 13.52
Habib., et al. (25)	$CD19^{+}CD27^{-}$ $CD10^{+}CD24^{hi}CD38^{hi}$	Increase (Mean, values not described, [%transitional/$CD19^{+}$]*	NM	Not reported	Range: 19-36	Range: 19-46
Hanley., et al. (26)	$CD24^{hi}CD38^{hi}$	Decrease (Mean ±SD: 1.54± 0.85 *vs.* 2.67 ±1.15 [% of $CD19^{+}$]**	NM	Mean ±SD: 19.25 ± 10.99	Mean ±SD: 34.75 ± 13.13	Mean ±SD: 31.75 ±8.17
Thompson., et al. (27)	$CD19^{+}CD27^{-}$ $CD24^{hi}CD38^{hi}$ (transitional)	No difference (*P*=0.50)	NM	Range: 0.2-31. Median: 1.8	Range: 9-42. Median: 20	Range:18-37. Median: 27
	$IL\text{-}10^{+}$ B cells	No difference (*P*=0.74)	Anti-CD40 + IL-21 (3 days) + CpG + LPS (last 5hrs)			
Kleffel., et al. (28)	$CD19^{+}IL\text{-}10^{+}$ B cells	Decreased (Mean ±SEM, values not described, [IL-10%]**	CD40L + LPS (4 days)	Mean ±SEM: 35 ±2.4	Mean ±SEM: 53.2 ± 2.3	Mean ±SEM: 32.1 ± 2.2
Saxena., et al. (29)	$CD5^{+}IL\text{-}10^{+}$ B cells	No difference (*P*=0.31)	PMA/Ionomycin	Range: 1.5-31.5	Range: 18-49.2	Range: 19.2-46
Wang., et al. (30)	$CD24^{hi}CD38^{hi}$	Decreased (Mean ±SEM, 5.6 ± 3.5 *vs.* 6.9 ± 3.3 [%])*	NM	Mean ±SEM 5.38± 0.72	23.76± 5.89§ (Range 7-29)	24.91± 2.92§ (Range 20-30)
	$CD24^{hi}CD38^{hi}IL\text{-}10^{+}$	Decreased (Mean ±SEM, values not described, [IL-10%])***	CD40L + CpG (3 days)			
El-Mokhtar., et al. (31)	$CD24^{hi}CD38^{hi}IL\text{-}10^{+}$ $CD24^{+}CD27^{+}IL\text{-}10^{+}$	Decreased (% $CD24^{hi}CD38^{hi}IL\text{-}10^{+}$, Mean ±SEM, 0.48 ± 0.54 *vs.* 1.3 ± 0.57)*** (% $CD24^{+}CD27^{+}IL\text{-}10^{+}$, Mean ±SEM, 0.49 ± 0.57 *vs.* 1.3 ± 0.53)***	PMA/Ionomycin	Range 0.1-4.85, Median 1.6	Range 3.4-11, Median 7	Range 2.6-8.5, Median 7

All studies measured IL-10 production by intracytoplasmic staining. NM (not measured). Versus and compared to healthy donors. All studies performed in human peripheral blood. *$p < 0.05$, **$p < 0.01$, ***$p < 0.001$. *§Average age, SEM or SD not stated.*

of an activated inflammatory environment, including pro-inflammatory cytokines, engagement of Toll-like receptors (TLRs) and costimulatory signals (32, 33). This has been reviewed extensively (34). Certainly, evidence from mouse studies show that Bregs are induced in response to inflammation or autoimmunity (13, 35). Moreover, a number of cytokines are involved in promoting Breg responses, many of which have been associated with autoimmune disorders. In autoimmune diabetes a number of cytokines including IL-1β, IL-6 and Interferon (IFN)α, play a role in the development of disease and can contribute to pancreatic β cell death (36). The same cytokines, as well as IL-21, have been shown to activate or expand Breg function (33, 37). IFNα secreted from plasmacytoid DCs (pDCs), in combination with CD40 ligation, can induce IL-10-producing Bregs (37). B cells stimulated with cytosine-phosphate-guanine (CpG) dinucleotides in combination with IL-2, IL-6 and IFNα induced an enhanced IL-10 response (12). Furthermore, IL-1β and IL-6 can drive B cell IL-10-production and Breg differentiation (33). Interestingly, this raises the question of why then in some studies Bregs are numerically or functionally defective in autoimmunity that includes type 1 diabetes (see *Impaired Regulatory B Cell Mechanisms in type 1 diabetes*). One possible reason for this paradox could be explained by other mechanisms required for Breg induction, which are altered in autoimmunity (**Figure 1**).

In a human study of SLE, the failed Breg expansion is attributed to elevated levels of IFNα produced from pDCs during disease, which drives plasmablast differentiation rather than Breg expansion (37). Therefore, it is suggested the concentration levels of cytokine are an important factor in Breg induction, and chronic exposure during inflammation can impair Breg frequency and function (37, 38). Type 1 diabetes, like SLE, is associated with an IFN signature. IFNα expression detected in the pancreatic islets (39) and IFN-associated genes are overexpressed in islets of individuals with type 1 diabetes (40). Additionally, an IFN transcriptional signature has been shown to be increased, even before the onset of human islet autoimmunity (41).

Both IL-21 and CD40 receptor engagement are required for the maturation and function of IL-10-producing B cells, a key

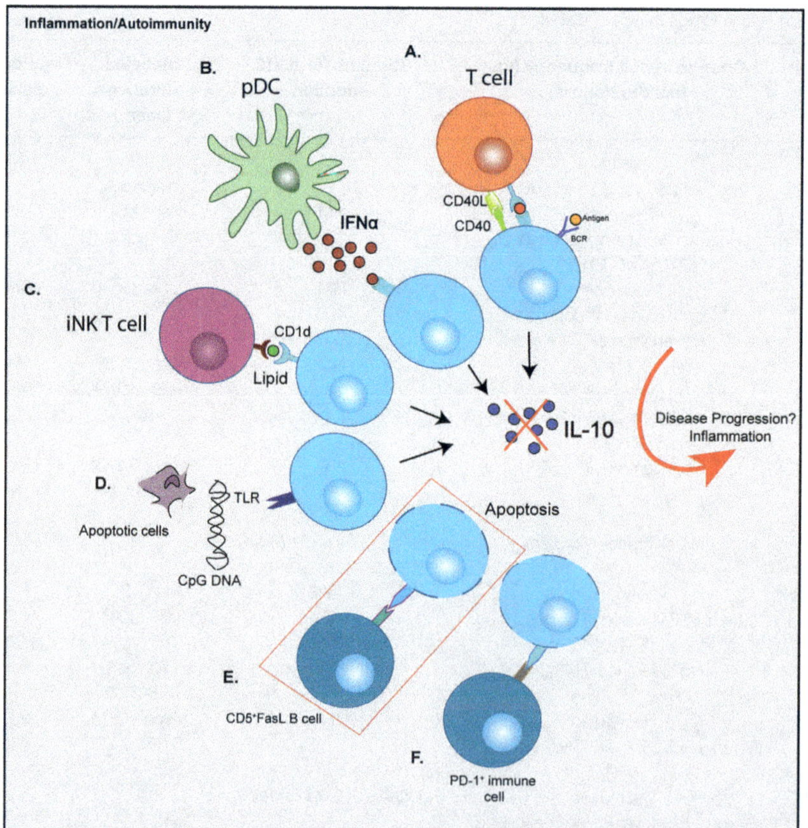

FIGURE 1 | Possible contributions of immune cell crosstalk resulting in dysregulation of regulatory B cells in type 1 diabetes. **(A)** Aberrant CD40:CD40L signalling through T cells **(B)** Elevated IFNα production from pDCs **(C)** Altered iNK T cells and CD1d expression on B cells **(D)** TLR signalling from apoptotic cell debris or the presence of viruses or microbes **(E)** Increased expression of Fas on IL-10$^+$ B cells are targeted by CD5$^+$FasL B cells **(F)** PD-L1: PD-1 engagement resulting in increased Breg apoptosis. Red box depicts a possible mechanism reported in type 1 diabetes. CPG, cytosine-phosphate-guanine; BCR, B cell receptor; IFN, Interferon; iNK, invariant natural killer; pDCs, plasmacytoid dendritic cells; TLR, toll-like receptor; FasL, Fas-ligand; PD-L1, programmed death-ligand 1; PD-1, programmed cell death protein 1.

study demonstrated in mice (42). Interestingly, naïve B cell responses to IL-21 are diminished in established human type 1 diabetes; however this response is enhanced in pre-diabetic individuals with multiple islet autoantibodies (43). Furthermore, CD4 T follicular helper (Tfh) cells in patients with type 1 diabetes have increased IL-21 production, compared to healthy donors (44, 45).

The importance of CD40: CD40L signaling has been noted in autoimmunity. For example, in autoimmune diabetes, the influence of CD40L blockade on the development of diabetes has been demonstrated in the NOD mouse model (46). This fundamental signaling pathway is important in both T and B cells. In people with type 1 diabetes, $CD4^{lo}CD40^{+}$ T cells (T_{CD40}) are expanded in peripheral blood (47). In another autoimmune disease, SLE, aberrant expression of CD40L in circulating B cells, in addition to T cells has been noted (48). Furthermore, reduced numbers of $CD40^{+}$ B cells is observed in individuals with type 1 diabetes, compared to healthy donors; however, the levels of CD40 expression on B cells were not measured in this study (28).

Other mechanisms are necessary for the generation or expansion of Bregs and these include both adaptive and innate immune pathways. B cell receptor (BCR) signaling (32, 49), is diminished in B cells from individuals with established type 1 diabetes (25, 43). Signaling through TLR9 changes the frequency and function of IL-10 producing B cells in NOD mice; TLR9 deficiency specifically in B cells increased IL-10 producing cells and protected against diabetes (50). No direct study has demonstrated a mechanism that drives a Breg defect in type 1 diabetes in humans however, and this remains an outstanding question (see *Discussion and Outstanding Questions*).

IMPAIRED REGULATORY B CELL MECHANISMS IN TYPE 1 DIABETES

Studies on the numerical and functional defects of Bregs have been described in various autoimmune diseases, including SLE, RA and MS and overall an inverse correlation between the frequency of Bregs and disease activity has been observed (10, 51). It should be noted, however, that studies have also reported either no differences or an increased frequency in these cells between autoimmune individuals and healthy donors (11, 25). Others have demonstrated different levels of $CD24^{hi}CD38^{hi}$ Bregs in various autoimmune conditions, compared with healthy controls (52). This theme of contrary results is echoed in studies of type 1 diabetes, which are summarized in **Table 1**.

It still remains unclear whether a defect or an impaired function of Bregs contributes to the development of diabetes or if the observed aberrant frequency and function is a result of chronic inflammation. Studies in the Experimental autoimmune encephalomyelitis (EAE) mouse model of MS has implicated Bregs in disease initiation rather than late-phase progression (53, 54). Moreover, in NOD mice, early treatment (5-6 weeks old) with BCR-activated B cells both delayed and reduced diabetes onset; however later treatment at 9 weeks of age only delayed onset of disease (55). Determining how Bregs contribute to the onset of type 1 diabetes will be of significance when considering immunotherapies targeted at B cells. Future real-time studies of regulatory B cells in islet autoantibody-positive individuals, who have not yet developed overt type 1 diabetes, would improve understanding of this.

Evidence for Numerical Defects in Regulatory B Cells in Type 1 Diabetes

Specific cell subsets that are associated with regulation, and B cells actively producing IL-10 after *ex vivo* stimulation, have been evaluated to ascertain if Breg frequencies are altered in type 1 diabetes. Whether the frequency of Breg-associated populations are altered, which include $CD5^{+}CD1d^{hi}$ and transitional $CD24^{hi}CD38^{hi}$ B cells, has been inconclusive when comparing patients to healthy donors (**Table 1**). A likely contributor to the disparity in these studies is the different sets of immune markers used to distinguish discrete populations or analysis of different Breg subsets. Use of an increased number of immune markers and high-dimensional profiling will help to determine more discrete B cell subsets and may resolve these dichotomies. For example, detailed characterisation has shown that human B cells which readily produce IL-10 are enriched in both T2 ($CD27^{-}IgM^{+}IgD^{+}$) and $CD27^{+}$ B cells in the transitional $CD24^{hi}CD38^{hi}$ compartment (52). Furthermore, stimulation *via* TLR9 resulted in enhanced IL-10 expression in the transitional T3 subset (52).

Direct assessment and evaluation of IL-10 production from B cells requires exogenous stimuli. Targets include either the innate TLRs or other receptors such CD40 or the BCR, either separately or by co-engagement, and if IL-10 is measured by intracytoplasmic staining, the addition of PMA/Ionomycin is also required (56). So far in type 1 diabetes, the studies employing CD40L and TLR stimulants - either LPS [TLR4] or CpG [TLR9] in culture before assessment, or with PMA/ionomycin alone - have shown a decrease in numerical frequency of IL-10-producing B cells from peripheral blood samples (28–30). However, when a combination of LPS and CPG was used, with the addition of IL-21, which can drive IL-10 production from B cells (42), the investigators found no difference in $IL\text{-}10^{+}$ B cells, in either naïve or memory compartments (27). A detailed summary of these studies is described in **Table 1**. It is clear that both the stimulation conditions and the appropriate markers to identify distinct populations are necessary for a more accurate overview on how B cell subsets are altered in type 1 diabetes.

In addition, a key disparity between studies is how accurately healthy donors were age-matched (**Table 1**). It is clear that subsets, such as transitional $CD24^{hi}CD38^{hi}$ B cells, enriched with $IL\text{-}10^{+}$ B cells, decline with age (27, 57), which is an important note for future studies. Recently, in children with type 1 diabetes, a decrease in both the $CD24^{hi}CD27^{+}$ (B10) and transitional $CD24^{hi}CD38^{hi}$ $IL\text{-}10^{+}$ B cells but not in $CD38^{hi}CD27^{+}IL\text{-}10^{+}$ plasmablasts was found (31). This numerical decrease was also negatively correlated with HbA1c levels (31), as was the frequency of $CD24^{hi}CD38^{hi}$ B cells in a study by Wang et al. (30). In view of the recent observation that the frequency of pancreatic $CD20^{+}$ B cells correlates with earlier diagnosis of a rapidly progressing and more aggressive disease (58), considering both age and clinical parameters in studies assessing regulatory B cells will be particularly important.

Currently, very few studies have assessed Breg populations in individuals with multiple islet autoantibodies who are classed as 'at risk' or in 'stage 1' or 'stage 2' (59) of developing diabetes. Kleffel et al. reported that individuals with multiple islet autoantibodies (like individuals with diabetes) had significantly fewer IL-10$^+$ B cells, compared to healthy controls (28). However, Saxena et al. observed that antibody positive individuals had increased CD5$^+$IL-10$^+$ B cells, compared to both healthy and diabetic controls (29). Overall, whether numerical differences exist in IL-10-producing B cells in individuals with islet autoantibodies remains a key outstanding question, which needs to be addressed in order to refine and improve immunotherapy targeted at B cells.

Although evidence has been provided in mouse models that IL-10$^+$ B cells can control autoimmune diabetes (55), few studies have addressed the number of IL-10-producing B cells in mice that have developed overt disease. Recent work from our group has demonstrated that NOD mice that developed diabetes showed a reduced splenic IL-10$^+$ B cell population, measured by intracytoplasmic staining, compared to mice that were long-term normoglycemic or 'naturally-protected' from diabetes (>35 weeks old) (60). Also, the frequency of IL-10$^+$ B cells was dependent on the B cell stimulation used, with anti-CD40 ligation highlighting the greatest loss in frequency of IL-10$^+$ B cells in diabetic NOD mice (60). This again focuses our attention on the need for better understanding and a more comprehensive use of different, combined stimuli. Additionally, we observed either no difference or increased IL-10 secretion in the mice that had developed diabetes, dependent on the stimulus used for study of the B cells (60). To date, type 1 diabetes studies reporting differences in IL-10$^+$ B cells have not evaluated IL-10 secretion. Increased IL-10$^+$ B cell frequency has been demonstrated in long-term normoglycemic or 'naturally protected' NOD mice in pancreatic islets (28, 61), suggesting a Breg-mediated protection against β cell destruction. For further discussion of Bregs related to pancreatic islets see *Regulatory B cells in Pancreatic Islets.*

Impaired Regulatory B Cell Function in Type 1 Diabetes

Functional studies in Bregs have described numerous immunosuppressive mechanisms of IL-10-producing B cells, including inhibiting pro-inflammatory cytokines from immune cells and promoting regulatory T cell differentiation (10, 51, 62), together with dampening of antigen presenting cell (APC) responses (11, 12). In autoimmune conditions, failed mechanisms of Breg immunosuppression are observed. In SLE patients, B cells fail to produce IL-10 in response to CD40 ligation and are unsuccessful in suppressing Th1 responses (10). CD24^{hi}CD38^{hi} Bregs from individuals with active RA are unable to convert CD4$^+$CD25$^-$ into Tregs or suppress Th17 responses (51). Moreover, CD19$^+$CD27$^+$IL-10$^+$ B cells from donors with RA fail to suppress IFNγ from CD4$^+$ T cells, compared to healthy individuals (62).

Evidence for diminished Breg function in human type 1 diabetes studies is limited. A recent study demonstrated that a numerical deficiency of Bregs was coupled with a functional defect in patients (30). Here, IL-10-producing B cells in healthy volunteers were enriched in the CD24^{hi}CD38^{hi} transitional subset, after CD40L and CPG stimulation, as shown previously (10). Furthermore, CD24^{hi}CD38^{hi} B cells inhibited effector cytokines from CD4$^+$ T cells and promoted CD4$^+$FoxP3$^+$ Tregs, in an IL-10-dependent manner (10). However, in patients with type 1 diabetes, CD24^{hi}CD38^{hi} B cells failed to reduce IFNγ, TNFα and IL-17 production from CD4$^+$ T cells (30). Conversely, Kleffel et al. showed that expanded IL-10-producing B cells from individuals with type 1 diabetes could suppress IFNγ production in PBMC cultures, in the presence of IA-2 peptide (28). However, the generation of IL-10$^+$ B cells from both individuals with type 1 diabetes and those with multiple islet autoantibodies was significantly impaired compared to healthy donors (28).

Murine studies have illustrated how regulatory B cells can control autoimmunity (8). Research has focused on how B cells can suppress autoimmune diabetes, demonstrating a role for IL-10-independent (63) and IL-10-dependent (55) mechanisms of B cell-mediated immunosuppression. However, data describing impaired regulatory B cell responses in mice, NOD or otherwise, are limited. TLR4-activated B cells from NOD mice that have developed diabetes suppress insulin-specific CD8 T cells, and in a B cell: DC : CD8 T cell co-culture produced significant amounts of IL-10 (60). This required the presence of the pathogenic CD8 T cells, because without pathogenic CD8 T cells in the cultures, the TLR4-induced B cells produced significantly less IL-10 and were less efficient in reducing DC activation. We also showed, in NOD mice with established diabetes, that CD40-ligation on B cells, followed by co-culture with DCs, the ability to reduce DC activation was decreased and resulted in a contact-dependent increase in IFNγ secretion, compared to NOD mice naturally-protected from autoimmune diabetes (60). In line with these observations, B cells from hyperglycemic NOD mice adoptively transferred into B cell-depleted long-term normoglycemic NOD animals promoted diabetes onset (28).

Other mechanisms of Breg suppression, independent of IL-10 expression and dependent on cell-contact have been noted. For example, PD-L1 and FasL exert suppression *via* apoptosis of target cells upon engagement with their receptors (2, 64). B cells that express FasL can induce apoptosis and suppress proliferation of CD4$^+$ T cells (3, 65). In mice, FasL can be induced by TLR4 activation in CD5$^+$CD1d$^+$ Bregs (65) and in the NOD mouse model can be activated with LPS (TLR4), resulting in TGFβ production, which inhibits Th1 responses and diabetes progression (63). In humans FasL^{hi}CD5$^+$ B cells are increased in frequency in individuals with type 1 diabetes, compared to both islet autoantibody positive and healthy donors (29), although here the levels of TGFβ production with stimulation was not assessed. Interestingly, in this study the frequency of CD5$^+$IL-10$^+$ B cells did not differ between healthy and diabetes donors (described in **Table 1**), but the percentage of Fas-expressing CD5$^+$IL-10$^+$ B cells was elevated in donors with type 1 diabetes (29). This is indicative of Fas-FasL B cell interplay, with elevated CD5$^+$FasL B cells targeting more apoptosis-sensitive $CD5^{+}IL\text{-}10^{+}$ B cells, which results in fewer $IL\text{-}10^{+}$ B cells in individuals with autoimmune diabetes (29) (**Figure 1**, red box).

It remains inconclusive if there is an intrinsic developmental Breg defect that contributes to disease progression in individuals that develop type 1 diabetes, and is complicated by the lack of a definitive Breg marker and their heterogeneity. It is possible the differences in Bregs observed in some studies (described in **Table 1**) results from the inflammatory environment that occurs with the progression of disease, which indirectly impacts the size or function of the Breg compartment (see **Figure 1**). Indeed, IL-10-producing B cells are expanded in mice predisposed to autoimmunity, compared to non-susceptible mice (32). Furthermore, $IL\text{-}10^{+}$ splenic B cells are expanded in 4-week-old NOD mice and $IL\text{-}10^{+}$ B cells from normoglycemic NOD mice are still capable of suppressing T cell-mediated diabetes (28).

Overall, these studies described above in type 1 diabetes suggest that further interrogation is warranted on the defective or dysfunctional Bregs observed, including the autocrine B cell mechanisms and crosstalk with other immune cells (see *Discussion and Outstanding Questions*). Further studies, using both human peripheral blood and tissue sites in different cohorts, taking into account that $IL\text{-}10^{+}$ B cell immune-phenotypes are variable with age (66), will provide insight into Breg defects.

REGULATORY B CELLS IN PANCREATIC ISLETS

B cells residing in pancreatic islets during inflammation contribute to the destruction of β cells, and consequently a loss in the secretion of insulin. Evidence for this direct pathogenic role has been shown by B cell depletion studies in the NOD mouse model, highlighting a reduction in effector T cell function inhibiting tissue-specific inflammation in treated mice (67, 68). In NOD mice, B-1a cells located in the pancreas, early in diabetes, play a role in initiation of disease (69). Furthermore, the observation of different profiles of insulitis in human pancreatic islets, with increased frequency of CD20 B cells correlate with a more progressive earlier diagnosis (58).

Previously, we have alluded to proposed interactions between regulatory B cells and the inflammatory pancreatic islet environment, and how Bregs can control inflammation (70). Islet-specific B cells in naturally-protected normoglycemic NOD mice have increased IL-10 and CD40 expression (28). More recently, we have corroborated this work and demonstrated B cells from naturally-protected NOD mice have an increased frequency of B cells expressing IL-10, CD80 and CD40 (61). In this study we also described an enrichment of $CD19^{int}CD138^{hi}CD44^{hi}Ki67^{+}$ dividing plasmablasts in naturally-protected NOD mice (61) a phenotype attributed to IL-10 production (12). Alongside this increase in regulatory B cells, a significant increase of $CTLA4^{+}FoxP3^{+}$ Tregs was also observed (61), possibly indicating some Breg-Treg crosstalk, which suppresses local pancreatic inflammation. However, it is unknown if this crosstalk is dependent on the expression of IL-10. It is possible that other IL-10-independent Treg induction by B cells may occur, as shown by the requirement for Breg expression of GITR ligand (71). Moreover, it is currently unclear if the altered pancreatic milieu in naturally-protected NOD mice is responsible for the induction of these regulatory immune cells, or a result of expanded $IL\text{-}10^{+}$B cells in the periphery (60). $IL\text{-}10^{+}$ B cells can be detected in the pancreatic islets of younger NOD mice after CD40 ligation along with a PMA/Ionomycin stimulation, albeit the frequency of $IL\text{-}10^{+}$ B cells was very low (28, 61), and it is unknown if they have any role in controlling local β cell damage *in vivo*.

DISCUSSION AND OUTSTANDING QUESTIONS

As discussed above, studies of regulatory B cells in type 1 diabetes are limited in comparison to other autoimmune diseases that include SLE, RA and MS, and thus lessons can be learned in order to extrapolate the findings to direct key research in type 1 diabetes. Finally, we discuss future and outstanding research questions that will advance the treatments of type 1 diabetes.

1. A deeper understanding of the different Breg repertoires that are IL-10-producing or IL-10-competent, together with the altered frequency and function in different stages of autoimmune diabetes development.

The complex picture described, so far, in diabetes and other autoimmune diseases may reflect the divergent role of Breg subsets in various disease settings. Different subsets of Bregs, based on their maturity, may be more influenced by the level of inflammation and disease stage of the individual. As previously shown, different immune profiles for B cell and T cell responses are dependent on disease stage or progression (43). It should also be noted that IL-10-producing B cells can also secrete TNF and IL-6 and so there is heterogeneity in Breg cytokine production (72).

2. Breg interplay and crosstalk with both other B cell populations and different immune cells to dissect the relationships that impact frequency and function (**Figure 1**).

Interrogating Breg: immune cell crosstalk will uncover aberrant regulatory feedback loops. Cell subsets like pDCs (37) or other DC subsets will reveal how Bregs dampen, or fail to dampen APCs. Other Breg studies highlight immunosuppressive mechanisms *via* invariant NKT cells dependent on the surface molecule CD1d (73). Other studies describe a feedback loop between T cells and B cells, *via* CD40:CD40L interactions, to develop regulatory function, which differentially regulate T cell proliferation and Th1 responses (74).

3. Determine the impact of defective Breg frequency and function. Do impaired Bregs contribute to diabetes initiation or progression or both?

Determining if the defect in Breg frequency and/or function is a consequence of chronic inflammation or a contributor to the development of diabetes will have an impact on how B cell depletion therapy is exploited in individuals during various stages of disease progression. Furthermore, understanding if impaired Bregs contribute to disease due to the lack of immunosuppressive action or if Breg plasticity results in a further progression of disease under certain chronic conditions should be addressed.

4. The use of immunotherapies to either selectively expand Bregs or target pathogenic B cells but spare regulatory B cells.

So far, only a pan-B cell depletion approach has been trialed in type 1 diabetes (Rituximab) (7), and therefore we can only discuss preclinical studies that approach expanding Bregs *in vivo* or targeting a specific B cell population. Expansion of $CD73^+$ regulatory B cells after treatment with a small molecule inhibitor that disrupts the *Aicda*-encoded activation-induced cytidine deaminase protein (AID) results in the inhibition of diabetes development in the NOD mouse (75). Conversely, AID deficiency in the NOD mouse model can accelerate type 1 diabetes development (76) and therefore the role of AID in diabetes progression requires further investigation. An additional B cell-targeted therapeutic approach is to selectively deplete effector B cells preserving regulatory B cells; however this is complicated by the lack of a definitive Breg marker. Interestingly, targeting of B cells *via* the blockade of the B cell activating factor (BAFF) induced an increase of $IL\text{-}10^+$ B cells and diabetes protection (77). Furthermore, in this study, anti-CD20 treatment depleted this IL-10-producing B cell population, suggesting that Bregs are more sensitive to deletion during anti-CD20 treatment (77). This Breg sensitivity may have contributed to the limited success of the Rituximab clinical trial (7). However, as discussed above, a deeper understanding of Bregs during the development of type 1 diabetes is needed to harness and develop successful B cell targeted immunotherapies.

Overall, the pathogenesis of type 1 diabetes is complex and multi-stage, and requires a number of pathogenic cell types that give rise to the development of disease. Equally, it is clear that balanced against these pathogenic cells are regulatory cells, that include both T and B cell subsets. Defining the roles of these less-understood Breg subsets will provide important information to be further studied in humans with the aim of increasing therapeutic opportunities.

AUTHOR CONTRIBUTIONS

JB wrote and edited the manuscript. FSW edited the manuscript. All authors contributed to the article and approved the submitted version.

ACKNOWLEDGMENTS

We would like to acknowledge Rebecca C. Wyatt (University of Exeter, UK) for proofreading this article.

REFERENCES

1. Mauri C, Bosma A. Immune Regulatory Function of B Cells. *Annu Rev Immunol* (2012) 30:221–41. doi: 10.1146/annurev-immunol-020711-074934
2. Khan AR, Hams E, Floudas A, Sparwasser T, Weaver CT, Fallon PG. PD-L1hi B Cells are Critical Regulators of Humoral Immunity. *Nat Commun* (2015) 6:5997. doi: 10.1038/ncomms6997
3. Lundy SK, Boros DL. Fas Ligand-Expressing B-1a Lymphocytes Mediate CD4 (+)-T-Cell Apoptosis During Schistosomal Infection: Induction by Interleukin 4 (IL-4) and IL-10. *Infect Immun* (2002) 70(2):812–9. doi: 10.1128/iai.70.2.812-819.2002
4. Lee KM, Stott RT, Zhao G, SooHoo J, Xiong W, Lian MM, et al. TGF-Beta-Producing Regulatory B Cells Induce Regulatory T Cells and Promote Transplantation Tolerance. *Eur J Immunol* (2014) 44(6):1728–36. doi: 10.1002/eji.201344062
5. Shen P, Roch T, Lampropoulou V, O'Connor RA, Stervbo U, Hilgenberg E, et al. IL-35-Producing B Cells are Critical Regulators of Immunity During Autoimmune and Infectious Diseases. *Nature* (2014) 507(7492):366–70. doi: 10.1038/nature12979
6. Wong FS. Wen L. B Cells in Autoimmune Diabetes. *Rev Diabetes Stud* (2005) 2(3):121–35. doi: 10.1900/RDS.2005.2.121
7. Pescovitz MD, Greenbaum CJ, Bundy B, Becker DJ, Gitelman SE, Goland R, et al. B-Lymphocyte Depletion With Rituximab and β-Cell Function: Two-Year Results. *Diabetes Care* (2014) 37(2):453–9. doi: 10.2337/dc13-0626
8. Fillatreau S, Sweenie CH, McGeachy MJ, Gray D, Anderton SM. B Cells Regulate Autoimmunity by Provision of IL-10. *Nat Immunol* (2002) 3 (10):944–50. doi: 10.1038/ni833
9. Ben Nasr M, Usuelli V, Seelam AJ, D'Addio F, Abdi R, Markmann JF, et al. Regulatory B Cells in Autoimmune Diabetes. *J Immunol* (2021) 206(6):1117–25. doi: 10.4049/jimmunol.2001127
10. Blair PA, Noreña LY, Flores-Borja F, Rawlings DJ, Isenberg DA, Ehrenstein MR, et al. CD19(+)CD24(hi)CD38(hi) B Cells Exhibit Regulatory Capacity in Healthy Individuals But are Functionally Impaired in Systemic Lupus Erythematosus Patients. *Immunity* (2010) 32(1):129–40. doi: 10.1016/j.immuni.2009.11.009
11. Iwata Y, Matsushita T, Horikawa M, Dilillo DJ, Yanaba K, Venturi GM, et al. Characterization of a Rare IL-10-Competent B-Cell Subset in Humans That Parallels Mouse Regulatory B10 Cells. *Blood* (2011) 117(2):530–41. doi: 10.1182/blood-2010-07-294249
12. Matsumoto M, Baba A, Yokota T, Nishikawa H, Ohkawa Y, Kayama H, et al. Interleukin-10-Producing Plasmablasts Exert Regulatory Function in Autoimmune Inflammation. *Immunity* (2014) 41(6):1040–51. doi: 10.1016/j.immuni.2014.10.016
13. Evans JG, Chavez-Rueda KA, Eddaoudi A, Meyer-Bahlburg A, Rawlings DJ, Ehrenstein MR, et al. Novel Suppressive Function of Transitional 2 B Cells in Experimental Arthritis. *J Immunol* (2007) 178(12):7868–78. doi: 10.4049/jimmunol.178.12.7868
14. Bankoti R, Gupta K, Levchenko A, Stäger S. Marginal Zone B Cells Regulate Antigen-Specific T Cell Responses During Infection. *J Immunol* (2012) 188 (8):3961–71. doi: 10.4049/jimmunol.1102880
15. Yanaba K, Bouaziz JD, Haas KM, Poe JC, Fujimoto M, Tedder TF. A Regulatory B Cell Subset With a Unique CD1dhiCD5+ Phenotype Controls T Cell-Dependent Inflammatory Responses. *Immunity* (2008) 28:639–50. doi: 10.1016/j.immuni.2008.03.017
16. Aravena O, Ferrier A, Menon M, Mauri C, Aguillon JC, Soto L, et al. TIM-1 Defines a Human Regulatory B Cell Population That is Altered in Frequency and Function in Systemic Sclerosis Patients. *Arthritis Res Ther* (2017) 19(1):8. doi: 10.1186/s13075-016-1213-9
17. Saze Z, Schuler PJ, Hong CS, Cheng D, Jackson EK, Whiteside TL. Adenosine Production by Human B Cells and B Cell-Mediated Suppression of Activated T Cells. *Blood* (2013) 122(1):9–18. doi: 10.1182/blood-2013-02-482406

18. Ding Q, Yeung M, Camirand G, Zeng Q, Akiba H, Yagita H, et al. Regulatory B Cells are Identified by Expression of TIM-1 and can be Induced Through TIM-1 Ligation to Promote Tolerance in Mice. *J Clin Invest* (2011) 121 (9):3645–56. doi: 10.1172/jci46274
19. Kaku H, Cheng KF, Al-Abed Y, Rothstein TL. A Novel Mechanism of B Cell-Mediated Immune Suppression Through CD73 Expression and Adenosine Production. *J Immunol* (2014) 193(12):5904–13. doi: 10.4049/jimmunol.1400336
20. van de Veen W, Stanic B, Yaman G, Wawrzyniak M, Söllner S, Akdis DG, et al. IgG4 Production is Confined to Human IL-10-Producing Regulatory B Cells That Suppress Antigen-Specific Immune Responses. *J Allergy Clin Immunol* (2013) 131(4):1204–12. doi: 10.1016/j.jaci.2013.01.014
21. Rosser EC, Mauri C. Regulatory B Cells: Origin, Phenotype, and Function. *Immunity* (2015) 42(4):607–12. doi: 10.1016/j.immuni.2015.04.005
22. Jansen K, Cevhertas L, Ma S, Satitsuksanoa P, Akdis M, van de Veen W. Regulatory B Cells, A to Z. *Allergy* (2021) 76(9):2699–715. doi: 10.1111/all.14763
23. De Filippo G, Pozzi N, Cosentini E, Cavalcanti M, Carel JC, Tamasi S, et al. Increased CD5+CD19+ B Lymphocytes at the Onset of Type 1 Diabetes in Children. *Acta Diabetol* (1997) 34(4):271–4. doi: 10.1007/s005920050087
24. Deng C, Xiang Y, Tan T, Ren Z, Cao C, Huang G, et al. Altered Peripheral B-Lymphocyte Subsets in Type 1 Diabetes and Latent Autoimmune Diabetes in Adults. *Diabetes Care* (2016) 39(3):434–40. doi: 10.2337/dc15-1765
25. Habib T, Funk A, Rieck M, Brahmandam A, Dai X, Panigrahi AK, et al. Altered B Cell Homeostasis is Associated With Type I Diabetes and Carriers of the PTPN22 Allelic Variant. *J Immunol* (2012) 188(1):487–96. doi: 10.4049/jimmunol.1102176
26. Hanley P, Sutter JA, Goodman NG, Du Y, Sekiguchi DR, Meng W, et al. Circulating B Cells in Type 1 Diabetics Exhibit Fewer Maturation-Associated Phenotypes. *Clin Immunol* (2017) 183:336–43. doi: 10.1016/j.clim.2017.09.021
27. Thompson WS, Pekalski ML, Simons HZ, Smyth DJ, Castro-Dopico X, Guo H, et al. Multi-Parametric Flow Cytometric and Genetic Investigation of the Peripheral B Cell Compartment in Human Type 1 Diabetes. *Clin Exp Immunol* (2014) 177(3):571–85. doi: 10.1111/cei.12362
28. Kleffel S, Vergani A, Tezza S, Ben Nasr M, Niewczas MA, Wong S, et al. Interleukin-10+ Regulatory B Cells Arise Within Antigen-Experienced CD40 + B Cells to Maintain Tolerance to Islet Autoantigens. *Diabetes* (2015) 64 (1):158–71. doi: 10.2337/db13-1639
29. Saxena A, Yagita H, Donner TW, Hamad ARA. Expansion of FasL-Expressing Cd5. *Front Immunol* (2017) 8:402. doi: 10.3389/fimmu.2017.00402
30. Wang Y, Qin Y, Wang X, Zhang L, Wang J, Xu X, et al. Decrease in the Proportion of CD24(hi) CD38(hi) B Cells and Impairment of Their Regulatory Capacity in Type 1 Diabetes Patients. *Clin Exp Immunol* (2020) 200(1):22–32. doi: 10.1111/cei.13408
31. El-Mokhtar MA, Elsherbiny NM, Sayed D, Raafat DM, Askar E, Hussein A, et al. Altered Regulatory B Cell Subsets in Children With Type 1 Diabetes Mellitus. *J Immunol Res* (2020) 2020:8935694. doi: 10.1155/2020/8935694
32. Yanaba K, Bouaziz JD, Matsushita T, Tsubata T, Tedder TF. The Development and Function of Regulatory B Cells Expressing IL-10 (B10 Cells) Requires Antigen Receptor Diversity and TLR Signals. *J Immunol* (2009) 182(12):7459–72. doi: 10.4049/jimmunol.0900270
33. Rosser EC, Oleinika K, Tonon S, Doyle R, Bosma A, Carter NA, et al. Regulatory B Cells are Induced by Gut Microbiota-Driven Interleukin-1β and Interleukin-6 Production. *Nat Med* (2014) 20(11):1334–9. doi: 10.1038/nm.3680
34. Baba Y, Matsumoto M, Kurosaki T. Signals Controlling the Development and Activity of Regulatory B-Lineage Cells. *Int Immunol* (2015) 27(10):487–93. doi: 10.1093/intimm/dxv027
35. Mizoguchi A, Mizoguchi E, Takedatsu H, Blumberg RS, Bhan AK. Chronic Intestinal Inflammatory Condition Generates IL-10-Producing Regulatory B Cell Subset Characterized by CD1d Upregulation. *Immunity* (2002) 16 (2):219–30. doi: 10.1016/S1074-7613(02)00274-1
36. Lu J, Liu J, Li L, Lan Y, Liang Y. Cytokines in Type 1 Diabetes: Mechanisms of Action and Immunotherapeutic Targets. *Clin Transl Immunol* (2020) 9(3): e1122. doi: 10.1002/cti2.1122
37. Menon M, Blair PA, Isenberg DA. Mauri C. A Regulatory Feedback Between Plasmacytoid Dendritic Cells and Regulatory B Cells Is Aberrant in Systemic Lupus Erythematosus. *Immunity* (2016) 44(3):683–97. doi: 10.1016/j.immuni.2016.02.012
38. Mauri C, Menon M. Human Regulatory B Cells in Health and Disease: Therapeutic Potential. *J Clin Invest* (2017) 127(3):772–9. doi: 10.1172/jci85113
39. Foulis AK, Farquharson MA, Meager A. Immunoreactive Alpha-Interferon in Insulin-Secreting Beta Cells in Type 1 Diabetes Mellitus. *Lancet* (1987) 2 (8573):1423–7. doi: 10.1016/s0140-6736(87)91128-7
40. Lundberg M, Krogvold L, Kuric E, Dahl-Jørgensen K, Skog O. Expression of Interferon-Stimulated Genes in Insulitic Pancreatic Islets of Patients Recently Diagnosed With Type 1 Diabetes. *Diabetes* (2016) 65(10):3104–10. doi: 10.2337/db16-0616
41. Ferreira RC, Guo H, Coulson RM, Smyth DJ, Pekalski ML, Burren OS, et al. A Type I Interferon Transcriptional Signature Precedes Autoimmunity in Children Genetically at Risk for Type 1 Diabetes. *Diabetes* (2014) 63 (7):2538–50. doi: 10.2337/db13-1777
42. Yoshizaki A, Miyagaki T, DiLillo DJ, Matsushita T, Horikawa M, Kountikov EI, et al. Regulatory B Cells Control T-Cell Autoimmunity Through IL-21-Dependent Cognate Interactions. *Nature* (2012) 491(7423):264–8. doi: 10.1038/nature11501
43. Habib T, Long SA, Samuels PL, Brahmandam A, Tatum M, Funk A, et al. Dynamic Immune Phenotypes of B and T Helper Cells Mark Distinct Stages of T1D Progression. *Diabetes* (2019) 68(6):1240–50. doi: 10.2337/db18-1081
44. Xu X, Shi Y, Cai Y, Zhang Q, Yang F, Chen H, et al. Inhibition of Increased Circulating Tfh Cell by Anti-CD20 Monoclonal Antibody in Patients With Type 1 Diabetes. *PloS One* (2013) 8(11):e79858. doi: 10.1371/journal.pone.0079858
45. Ferreira RC, Simons HZ, Thompson WS, Cutler AJ, Dopico XC, Smyth DJ, et al. IL-21 Production by CD4+ Effector T Cells and Frequency of Circulating Follicular Helper T Cells Are Increased in Type 1 Diabetes Patients. *Diabetologia* (2015) 58(4):781–90. doi: 10.1007/s00125-015-3509-8
46. Balasa B, Krahl T, Patstone G, Lee J, Tisch R, McDevitt HO, et al. CD40 Ligand-CD40 Interactions are Necessary for the Initiation of Insulitis and Diabetes in Nonobese Diabetic Mice. *J Immunol* (1997) 159(9):4620–7.
47. Waid DM, Wagner RJ, Putnam A, Vaitaitis GM, Pennock ND, Calverley DC, et al. A Unique T Cell Subset Described as CD4loCD40+ T Cells (TCD40) in Human Type 1 Diabetes. *Clin Immunol* (2007) 124(2):138–48. doi: 10.1016/j.clim.2007.05.003
48. Desai-Mehta A, Lu L, Ramsey-Goldman R, Datta SK. Hyperexpression of CD40 Ligand by B and T Cells in Human Lupus and its Role in Pathogenic Autoantibody Production. *J Clin Invest* (1996) 97(9):2063–73. doi: 10.1172/jci118643
49. Matsumoto M, Fujii Y, Baba A, Hikida M, Kurosaki T, Baba Y. The Calcium Sensors STIM1 and STIM2 Control B Cell Regulatory Function Through Interleukin-10 Production. *Immunity* (2011) 34(5):703–14. doi: 10.1016/j.immuni.2011.03.016
50. Huang J, Peng J, Pearson JA, Efthimiou G, Hu Y, Tai N, et al. Toll-Like Receptor 7 Deficiency Suppresses Type 1 Diabetes Development by Modulating B-Cell Differentiation and Function. *Cell Mol Immunol* (2021) 18(2):328–38. doi: 10.1038/s41423-020-00590-8
51. Flores-Borja F, Bosma A, Ng D, Reddy V, Ehrenstein MR, Isenberg DA, et al. CD19+CD24hiCD38hi B Cells Maintain Regulatory T Cells While Limiting TH1 and TH17 Differentiation. *Sci Transl Med* (2013) 5(173):173ra23. doi: 10.1126/scitranslmed.3005407
52. Simon Q, Pers JO, Cornec D, Le Pottier L, Mageed RA, Hillion S. In-Depth Characterization of CD24(high)CD38(high) Transitional Human B Cells Reveals Different Regulatory Profiles. *J Allergy Clin Immunol* (2016) 137 (5):1577–84.e10. doi: 10.1016/j.jaci.2015.09.014
53. Matsushita T, Yanaba K, Bouaziz JD, Fujimoto M, Tedder TF. Regulatory B Cells Inhibit EAE Initiation in Mice While Other B Cells Promote Disease Progression. *J Clin Invest* (2008) 118(10):3420–30. doi: 10.1172/JCI36030
54. Matsushita T, Horikawa M, Iwata Y, Tedder TF. Regulatory B Cells (B10 Cells) and Regulatory T Cells Have Independent Roles in Controlling Experimental Autoimmune Encephalomyelitis Initiation and Late-Phase Immunopathogenesis. *J Immunol* (2010) 185(4):2240–52. doi: 10.4049/jimmunol.1001307
55. Hussain S, Delovitch TL. Intravenous Transfusion of BCR-Activated B Cells Protects NOD Mice From Type 1 Diabetes in an IL-10-Dependent Manner. *J Immunol* (2007) 179(11):7225–32. doi: 10.4049/jimmunol.179.11.7225

56. Tedder TF. B10 Cells: A Functionally Defined Regulatory B Cell Subset. *J Immunol* (2015) 194(4):1395–401. doi: 10.4049/jimmunol.1401329
57. Duggal NA, Upton J, Phillips AC, Sapey E, Lord JM. An Age-Related Numerical and Functional Deficit in CD19(+) CD24(hi) CD38(hi) B Cells is Associated With an Increase in Systemic Autoimmunity. *Aging Cell* (2013) 12(5):873–81. doi: 10.1111/acel.12114
58. Leete P, Willcox A, Krogvold L, Dahl-Jørgensen K, Foulis AK, Richardson SJ, et al. Differential Insulitic Profiles Determine the Extent of β-Cell Destruction and the Age at Onset of Type 1 Diabetes. *Diabetes* (2016) 65(5):1362–9. doi: 10.2337/db15-1615
59. Insel RA, Dunne JL, Atkinson MA, Chiang JL, Dabelea D, Gottlieb PA, et al. Staging Presymptomatic Type 1 Diabetes: A Scientific Statement of JDRF, the Endocrine Society, and the American Diabetes Association. *Diabetes Care* (2015) 38(10):1964–74. doi: 10.2337/dc15-1419
60. Boldison J, Da Rosa LC, Davies J, Wen L, Wong FS. Dendritic Cells License Regulatory B Cells to Produce IL-10 and Mediate Suppression of Antigen-Specific CD8 T Cells. *Cell Mol Immunol* (2020) 17(8):843–55. doi: 10.1038/s41423-019-0324-z
61. Boldison J, Thayer TC, Davies J, Wong FS. Natural Protection From Type 1 Diabetes in NOD Mice Is Characterized by a Unique Pancreatic Islet Phenotype. *Diabetes* (2021) 70(4):955–65. doi: 10.2337/db20-0945
62. Bankó Z, Pozsgay J, Szili D, Tóth M, Gáti T, Nagy G, et al. Induction and Differentiation of IL-10-Producing Regulatory B Cells From Healthy Blood Donors and Rheumatoid Arthritis Patients. *J Immunol* (2017) 198(4):1512–20. doi: 10.4049/jimmunol.1600218
63. Tian J, Zekzer D, Hanssen L, Lu Y, Olcott A, Kaufman DL. Lipopolysaccharide-Activated B Cells Down-Regulate Th1 Immunity and Prevent Autoimmune Diabetes in Nonobese Diabetic Mice. *J Immunol* (2001) 167(2):1081–9. doi: 10.4049/jimmunol.167.2.1081
64. Hahne M, Renno T, Schroeter M, Irmler M, French L, Bornard T, et al. Activated B Cells Express Functional Fas Ligand. *Eur J Immunol* (1996) 26 (3):721–4. doi: 10.1002/eji.1830260332
65. Wang K, Tao L, Su J, Zhang Y, Zou B, Wang Y, et al. TLR4 Supports the Expansion of FasL. *Mol Immunol* (2017) 87:188–99. doi: 10.1016/j.molimm.2017.04.016
66. Kalampokis I, Venturi GM, Poe JC, Dvergsten JA, Sleasman JW, Tedder TF. The Regulatory B Cell Compartment Expands Transiently During Childhood and Is Contracted in Children With Autoimmunity. *Arthritis Rheumatol* (2017) 69(1):225–38. doi: 10.1002/art.39820
67. Brodie GM, Wallberg M, Santamaria P, Wong FS. Green EA. B-Cells Promote Intra-Islet CD8+ Cytotoxic T-Cell Survival to Enhance Type 1 Diabetes. *Diabetes* (2008) 57(4):909–17. doi: 10.2337/db07-1256
68. Da Rosa LC, Boldison J, De Leenheer E, Davies J, Wen L, Wong FS. B Cell Depletion Reduces T Cell Activation in Pancreatic Islets in a Murine Autoimmune Diabetes Model. *Diabetologia* (2018) 61(6):1397–410. doi: 10.1007/s00125-018-4597-z
69. Diana J, Simoni Y, Furio L, Beaudoin L, Agerberth B, Barrat F, et al. Crosstalk Between Neutrophils, B-1a Cells and Plasmacytoid Dendritic Cells Initiates Autoimmune Diabetes. *Nat Med* (2013) 19(1):65–73. doi: 10.1038/nm.3042
70. Boldison J, Wong FS. Immune and Pancreatic β Cell Interactions in Type 1 Diabetes. *Trends Endocrinol Metab* (2016) 27(12):856–67. doi: 10.1016/j.tem.2016.08.007
71. Ray A, Basu S, Williams CB, Salzman NH, Dittel BN. A Novel IL-10-Independent Regulatory Role for B Cells in Suppressing Autoimmunity by Maintenance of Regulatory T Cells via GITR Ligand. *J Immunol* (2012) 188 (7):3188–98. doi: 10.4049/jimmunol.1103354
72. Lighaam LC, Unger PA, Vredevoogd DW, Verhoeven D, Vermeulen E, Turksma AW, et al. In Vitro-Induced Human IL-10(+) B Cells Do Not Show a Subset-Defining Marker Signature and Plastically Co-Express IL-10 With Pro-Inflammatory Cytokines. *Front Immunol* (2018) 9:1913. doi: 10.3389/fimmu.2018.01913
73. Oleinika K, Rosser EC, Matei DE, Nistala K, Bosma A, Drozdov I, et al. CD1d-Dependent Immune Suppression Mediated by Regulatory B Cells Through Modulations of iNKT Cells. *Nat Commun* (2018) 9(1):684. doi: 10.1038/s41467-018-02911-y
74. Lemoine S, Morva A, Youinou P, Jamin C. Human T Cells Induce Their Own Regulation Through Activation of B Cells. *J Autoimmun* (2011) 36(3-4):228–38. doi: 10.1016/j.jaut.2011.01.005
75. Ratiu JJ, Racine JJ, Hasham MG, Wang Q, Branca JA, Chapman HD, et al. Genetic and Small Molecule Disruption of the AID/RAD51 Axis Similarly Protects Nonobese Diabetic Mice From Type 1 Diabetes Through Expansion of Regulatory B Lymphocytes. *J Immunol* (2017) 198(11):4255–67. doi: 10.4049/jimmunol.1700024
76. Tan Q, Tai N, Li Y, Pearson J, Pennetti S, Zhou Z, et al. Activation-Induced Cytidine Deaminase Deficiency Accelerates Autoimmune Diabetes in NOD Mice. *JCI Insight* (2018) 3(1):e95882. doi: 10.1172/jci.insight.95882
77. Wang Q, Racine JJ, Ratiu JJ, Wang S, Ettinger R, Wasserfall C, et al. Transient BAFF Blockade Inhibits Type 1 Diabetes Development in Nonobese Diabetic Mice by Enriching Immunoregulatory B Lymphocytes Sensitive to Deletion by Anti-CD20 Cotherapy. *J Immunol* (2017) 199(11):3757–70. doi: 10.4049/jimmunol.1700822

8

Thymic B Cells as a New Player in the Type 1 Diabetes Response

*Richard B. Greaves, Dawei Chen and E. Allison Green**

Centre for Experimental Medicine and Biomedicine, Hull York Medical School, University of York, York, United Kingdom

***Correspondence:**
E. Allison Green
allison.green@york.ac.uk

Type 1 diabetes (T1d) results from a sustained autoreactive T and B cell response towards insulin-producing β cells in the islets of Langerhans. The autoreactive nature of the condition has led to many investigations addressing the genetic or cellular changes in primary lymphoid tissues that impairs central tolerance- a key process in the deletion of autoreactive T and B cells during their development. For T cells, these studies have largely focused on medullary thymic epithelial cells (mTECs) critical for the effective negative selection of autoreactive T cells in the thymus. Recently, a new cellular player that impacts positively or negatively on the deletion of autoreactive T cells during their development has come to light, thymic B cells. Normally a small population within the thymus of mouse and man, thymic B cells expand in T1d as well as other autoimmune conditions, reside in thymic ectopic germinal centres and secrete autoantibodies that bind selective mTECs precipitating mTEC death. In this review we will discuss the ontogeny, characteristics and functionality of thymic B cells in healthy and autoimmune settings. Furthermore, we explore how *in silico* approaches may help decipher the complex cellular interplay of thymic B cells with other cells within the thymic microenvironment leading to new avenues for therapeutic intervention.

Keywords: type 1 diabetes, thymic B cells, autoimmunity, computational modelling, negative selection

INTRODUCTION

Type 1 diabetes (T1d) is an autoimmune condition characterised by the destruction of the insulin producing beta (β) cells in the islets of Langerhans by co-operative interaction between the innate and adaptive immune systems; the final assault being perpetuated by $CD8^+$ cytotoxic T cells (1–3). The non-obese diabetic (NOD) mouse that spontaneously develops T1d in a manner thought to be similar to man, has been an important resource in analysing the complexity of the T1d immunopathology (4). In line with the important role that the thymus plays in purging thymocytes with autoreactive T cell receptors (TcRs) (5), T1d progression is linked to defects in central tolerance increasing the output of islet-reactive T cells (6, 7), although definitive understanding of why negative selection of islet-reactive T cells occurs remains elusive.

Studies in NOD mice deficient in B cells have revealed an initially unappreciated role for B cells not only in helping the $CD4^+$ T cell response to islet antigens (8–10), but also promoting the survival of islet-reactive $CD8^+$ CTL *in situ* (11). This important role for B cells in the T1d process has been translated to man, where T1d progression risk is determined by the number of serum antibodies to islet antigens (12) and evidence that T1d severity is characterised by increased infiltration of islets letion of B cells in people newly diagnosed with T1d results in transient remission of the condition (14).

Recently, we reported a new role for B cells in the T1d process- mediators of breakdown in thymic central tolerance (15). We showed that thymic B cells, normally a minor constituent of a healthy thymus in both man and mouse (16, 17), rapidly increase following the initiation of islet infiltration with immune cells (termed insulitis) but prior to overt clinical manifestation of T1d. Further, we showed that thymic B cells reside in putative thymic germinal centres, undergo *in situ* class switching and differentiation into plasma cells. Autoantibodies from these plasma cells targeted specific medullary thymic epithelial cells (mTECs) for antibody-mediated apoptosis, leading to increased output of T cells that bypassed negative selection thereby enhancing T1d progression. Our finding was reminiscent of the immunopathology of the autoimmune conditions of myasthenia gravis (18) and systemic lupus erythematosus (19, 20), suggesting that thymic B cell abnormalities may be a common link between certain autoimmune conditions.

Analysis of thymic B cells is challenging; thymic involution as we age necessitates human thymic studies to be largely restricted to foetal or paediatric tissue which, quite rightly, is ethically sensitive to procure. Although it could be argued the availability of murine thymi negates issues of thymic cellularity during the involution process, researchers have an ethical responsibility to minimise the size of murine cohorts undergoing experimental procedures. Systems biology, which incorporates the development of computational models that can recapitulate the complexity of the immune response in defined tissues- offers an attractive approach to evaluate the molecules and signal pathways that contribute to the thymic B cell-mediated progression to T1d.

Examples of existing simulation studies in biology are numerous: granuloma formation (21–23), breast cancer metastasis (24) and lymphoid tissue formation (25, 26). There has also been a considerable body of work on modelling epithelial tissues (27, 28). Following this precedent it will be instructive to create a computer simulation of the early thymic events in T1d development.

This review is, therefore, structured in two parts; first we will discuss our current understanding of the ontogeny, phenotype and function of thymic B cells in health and disease, and secondly, we review the development and challenges of the systems biology approach of generating a computational model of thymic autoimmunity.

ONTOGENY OF THYMIC B CELLS

Thymic B cells were initially discovered during immunohistochemical studies of human thymic tissue (17) and subsequently in mice (29, 30).Thymic B cells, a minor population of cells within the thymic cellular pool, are present from embryonic age through to adulthood, the number of cells remaining stable throughout life, although reports of the ageing murine thymus suggest increasing numbers of thymic B cells are a characteristic of the thymic involution (6, 7, 31). Since the discovery of thymic B cells, the origin of the cells- *in situ* development versus recirculation from the periphery- has been debated. For example, Sato et al., demonstrated that peripheral B cells preferentially migrate to the thymus in response to increasing levels of intrathymic B lymphocyte chemoattractant CXCL13, although it was noted this occurred in aged mice (32). In contrast, parabiosis models argue against peripheral B cell migration to the thymus (33). Our adoptive transfer studies in NOD mice, revealed splenic B cells had minimum capacity to migrate to the thymus even when transferred at the post-insulitic, pre-diabetic phase when thymic B cell numbers rapidly increase (Davis and Green, unpublished observations). Interestingly, B cells isolated from the thymus almost exclusively migrated back to this organ following adoptive transfer into recipient mice. These findings related to peripheral B cell thymic migration, align with others, and suggest that thymic B cells originate from *in situ* development (34, 35). Further support for this hypothesis was provided by studies in NOD-RAG2p-GFP reporter mice (15), that enable monitoring of recombination activating gene (RAG) activity in developing B and T cells (36). Comparison of thymic B cell RAG activity in NOD mice revealed a significant increase in rearrangement of the B cell receptor (BcR) in the post-insulitic, pre-diabetic phase compared to pre-insulitic phase (15). Interestingly, the level of thymic B cell RAG activity was similar between NOD mice in the pre-insulitic phase to the levels seen for control, age-matched mice, and in this latter strain thymic B cell RAG activity remained at a constant level as mice aged. Although it could be speculated that increased RAG activity in thymic B cells may represent aberrant re-ignition of RAG genes in peripheral B cells that migrate to the thymus and potentially undergo receptor editing of the BcR, studies by Gay et al., demonstrating that peripheral RAG^{-} B cells were unable to reactivate RAG following a series of mitogenic and antigenic B cell stimulations, argue against this possibility (37). Similar findings looking at the ability of immunisation to re-ignite RAG activity supports the hypothesis that RAG expression in B cells is restricted to their developmental stages (38, 39). Thus, the thymus of mice *per se* can support B cell development, but in the context of T1d, there is an acceleration in B cell development specifically during the post-insulitis, prediabetic phase, and this coincides with a rapid increase in thymic B cell numbers (15).

If thymic B cells develop *in situ*, what are the progenitor cells and signal pathways involved? Although it is well established that the thymus is seeded with common lymphoid progenitor cells (CLP) that have T, B and NK cell potential (40), it has been challenging to map the thymic B cell development pathway assuming it originates from the CLP population. Several studies have identified B lineage-committing transcription factors and cells within the thymus that have a phenotype akin to B cell committed precursors in their natural developmental habitat, the bone marrow (34). In addition, McKenna et al., demonstrated that addition of bone marrow isolated pro-B cells into thymic organ cultures stimulated with Fms-related receptor tyrosine kinase 3 (FLT3) and IL-7 induced immature B cell development (41). Interestingly, similar culture of pro-B cells with cell-lines derived from bone marrow or thymic stroma cultured did not induce complete B cell development in the presence of FLT3 and IL-7. However, these studies are based on B cell committed progenitors, that is pro-B cells, and it has been far more challenging to identify within the thymus the cell(s) that lie upstream of the pro-B cell that have been identified in the bone marrow (42, 43).

As well as speculation on the definitive progenitor from which intrathymic B cells develop, there also been controversy in the signal pathways that lead to intrathymic B cell development. For example, it has been proposed that intrathymic B cell development may be a default pathway resulting from perturbation of the T cell developmental pathway due to impaired CD3 or T cell receptor β (TcRβ) signalling (44) or inappropriate Notch signalling (45). However, Feyerabend et al., using the cre-lox system to delete Notch in the DN1 population, a population that has both B and T cell potential, did not divert development down the B cell developmental pathway (46). More understanding is required as to both the progenitor and signal pathways that enable the development of thymic B cells. Such studies will be invaluable in determining whether increased thymic B cell development characteristic of T1d progression in NOD mice relates to perturbation of these signal pathways.

PHENOTYPE OF THYMIC B CELLS

B cells can be divided into several classifications: follicular (FO), marginal zone (MZ), peritoneal (B1a) and regulatory (Bregs). Each subgroup of B cells can be identified by their surface markers, and each has particular functions to play in the immune response. Although Bregs have been identified in the thymus (47) Bregs will be discussed elsewhere in this Special Edition and will not be considered here. MZ B cells have received particular attention in the autoimmune setting, due to an aberrant increase in both their numbers and location in murine autoimmune models (48–50) as well as in humans living with certain autoimmune conditions (51, 52). Innate-like MZ B cells express high levels of IgM and low levels of IgD alongside coexpression of CD21 and CD35 (53). They can function to remove apoptotic cell debris impeding autoimmunity (54), or conversely, they may promote autoimmunity *via* their polyreactive receptors (48). Furthermore, weak signalling through the BcR (55, 56) or perturbation of the negative regulators of BcR signalling- including FcγRIIB- promotes expansion of MZ B cells that are more efficient at presenting antigen to T cells (57), including potentially autoreactive T cells. In light of the strong link between mutations in FcγRIIB and T1d in both mouse and man, we assessed whether thymic B cells in NOD mice had a MZ or FO phenotype (15). Our data showed that although MZ-like cells are detectable in the thymus of both NOD and control mice, there are significantly fewer in the NOD mouse thymus compared to control animals. It is intriguing that MZ-like cells are present in the thymus of mice, and it will be interesting to see if they function here as surveillance cells against infection or participate in the removal of apoptotic thymocytes.

Nevertheless, our data overwhelmingly ascribes thymic B cells to have a FO phenotype in the NOD mouse, a finding that is in line with several studies in mice and man (33). In NOD mice, CD5, which has been described as a marker for B1a cells in the peritoneal cavity, is also expressed on the thymic FO B cells, although not as extensively as seen in non-NOD strains (29). Thymic FO B cells, in comparison to splenic FO B cells, express much higher levels of MHC class I and II, as well as costimulatory molecule CD40, signalling through which may regulate expression of CD5 (58). Although the majority of thymic B cells in the NOD mice expressed an $IgM^{+}IgD^{+}$ BcR, class-switched B cells expressing $IgM^{-}IgD^{-}IgG^{+}$ BcRs were readily detectable, although notably control mice also had these class-switched cells too. In contrast to this shared phenotype of NOD thymic B cells with non-NOD strains of mice, the NOD thymus harbours class-switched unusual $IgM^{-}IgD^{+}IgA^{+}$ and $IgM^{-}IgD^{+}IgG^{+}$ FO B cells where such cells were largely absent in control mice (15). Interestingly, human peripheral B cells with this unusual expression of IgD^{+} in the absence of IgM has recently been described in people living with T1d (59). In people with T1d, these IgD^{+} B cells express polyreactive receptors and can interact with insulin. Although we established that insulin-reactive B cells reside in the thymus of NOD mice, similar numbers of insulin-reactive B cells were present in control, non-autoimmune mice (15). Further, our studies focused on the thymic B cell population in its entirety, not this specific subgroup of B cells. Thus, the antigen specificity of these unique thymic $IgD^{+}IgG^{+}$ B cells in NOD mice is yet to be resolved, but potentially harbours an autoreactive BcR repertoire.

ACTIVATION OF THYMIC B CELLS – A ROLE FOR THYMIC GERMINAL CENTRES

B cell activation takes place in specialised germinal centres (GCs) within B cell follicles of secondary lymphoid organs. GCs tend to form in response to infection, although small transient GCs have been seen in non-inflammatory conditions. GC formation requires cross-talk between stromal cells and immune cells, and are integral for the somatic hypermutation, class switching and differentiation of activated B cells into plasma cells and memory B cells reviewed by (60). Aside from conventional GCs, B cell activation can also take place in extrafollicular structures and ectopic GCs. These ectopic GCs occur in non-lymphoid tissue, and result from the remodelling of the tissue stromal cell network in response to inflammation (61). Ectopic GCs are of particular importance in autoimmunity, and several conditions have reported the presence of these structures in the target tissue (62–64), including in the islets of T1d murine models (65), and the presence of ectopic GCs correlates with disease severity. Like conventional GCs, ectopic GCs are compartmentalised into B and T cell areas (64), and several cytokines have been attributed to their localised formation including IL-22 (66) and IL-23 (67). Interferon gamma (IFNγ) seems to be one of the most critical players in ectopic GCs formation (68–70). Despite the remarkable knowledge we now have on conventional and ectopic GCs, little is known about GCs that can form in thymic tissue despite being a characteristic of autoimmune conditions like myasthenia gravis (18, 71), systemic lupus erythematosus (19) and T1d (15). Consistent among the autoimmune conditions where thymic GC occur, the GCs form at the cortical-medullary junction, and in NOD mice, such structures only materialise at the post-insulitic, pre-diabetic phase. Furthermore, the thymus becomes enriched with IL-21 as thymic GCs form, a cytokine that is critical for regulating GC maintenance and promotion of B cell differentiation and proliferation (72). Expression of activation-induced cytidine deaminase (AID) increases, suggesting active somatic hypermutation/class-switching is ongoing. IL-21 has proven a particularly interesting cytokine in promoting T1d both in man (73) and NOD mice (74). At the heart of the link between IL-21 and T1d are the T follicular helper (Tfh) cells (73) and in children at risk of T1d progression, circulating Tfh cell numbers peak around onset of clinical symptoms (75). In man it has been described that Tfh cells within conventional GCs may be identifiable from their recirculating counterpart on the basis of expression of the master transcription factor for Tfh cells- Bcl-6; whereas GC residing Tfh cells express Bcl-6, recirculating Tfh cells may not (76, 77). Nevertheless, circulating Tfh cells are uniquely gifted at entering inflamed tissue, and participating in ectopic GC formation (78) and *in vitro*, can promote B cell class switching retaining characteristics of GC Tfh cells (79, 80). As expected, considering their essential role in GC/ectopic GCs, Tfh cells are enhanced in the thymus of NOD mice at an age when thymic GC formation occurs. These Tfh cells express Bcl-6 and IL-21, as well as other known markers of Tfh cells (15). This suggests that intrathymic Tfh cells may derive from *in situ* CD4 $_+$ T cells, unless circulating Tfh cells that migrate to the thymus take on the phenotype of GC Tfh cells with respect to Bcl-6 expression.

Certain questions remain about the nature of the thymic GCs in T1d; do they contain follicular dendritic cell structures and what is the source of the inflammation to push thymic GC formation? GCs are populated with specialised follicular dendritic cells (FDC) that act as a depot for antigen presentation within the GC (81). However, we have yet to confirm such cells exist in our thymic GCs (Pinto and Green, unpublished observations). Interestingly, it has been postulated that the type of FDC present in a GC/ectopic GC may be unique to the tissue and type of inflammation (67, 82) and markers of conventional GCs may not be present on thymic FDCs. In terms of inflammation, it could be speculated that viral infections linked to T1d development in man may also infect the thymus (83) or endogenous retroviral infection (84) could induce thymic GC formation. Alternatively thymic GC formation may simply be a reflection of an accelerated ageing of the thymus (85). Indeed, others, have documented accelerated thymic involution in NOD mice (6). It will be important to determine if people who develop T1d also have thymic GCs, and potentially accelerated ageing of this tissue.

THYMIC B CELL FUNCTION

The immunohistochemical evidence that thymic B cells form follicles at the cortico-medullary junction, and can form rosette-like structures around T cells in the medulla (86, 87) led to early speculation that thymic B cells were involved in negative selection of autoreactive T cells. Subsequent studies from different groups have substantiated that hypothesis (discussed below), although whether thymic B cells positively or negatively contribute to negative selection seems dependent on the autoimmune nature of the mammal studied. Before we discuss the evidence for the role of thymic B cells in negative selection, let's first consider their antigen specificity.

We earlier touched on the finding that thymic B cells in NOD mice or control animals expressed receptors for insulin i.e. they were autoreactive. In normal B cell development and maturation, efficiency in removing B cells with autoreactive BcRs is high, with approximately 20% of circulating B cells bearing autoreactive BcRs (88). Interestingly, the removal of B cell with autoreactive BcRs occurs in two stages; initially at the immature B cell stage in the bone marrow and subsequently during the transition of immature B cells to mature B cells following their recent egress from the bone marrow, with the early immature to immature B cell development stage exhibiting the largest removal of self-reactive B cells from the repertoire (88). Thus the earliest stages of B cell development in the bone marrow the repertoire of B cells has a high level of self-reactivity. To determine if the thymic B cell repertoire, similar to bone marrow-derived B cells, had self-reactivity, Rother et al. performed comparative sequencing studies of single cell sorted paediatric thymic B cells versus foetal bone marrow B cells (89). Such studies demonstrated that thymic B cells had a greater specificity for self-peptide autoantigens than similar sequenced foetal bone marrow B cells, these latter cells being more specific for dsDNA. Furthermore, thymic B cells had polyreactivity, recognising multiple autoantigens, including insulin. This prevalence of thymic B cells to harbour an autoreactive BcR has been shown by others (90). It can be envisaged that autoreactive thymic B cells may participate in negative selection by presenting 'free' autoreactive antigens- either trafficked to the thymus or captured from dying medullary thymic epithelial cells. Indeed, thymic B cells have been shown to efficiently present antigens their BcR is specific for to developing T cells (91) promoting efficient deletion of autoreactive T cells during T cell development (92–95). However, capture of autoantigens by the thymic B cell autoreactive BcR is not the sole way thymic B cells contribute to negative selection. Yamano et al., using a transgenic autoimmune regulator (AIRE) gene locus encoding a chimeric influenza haemagglutinin protein and human CD2 promoter demonstrated that 50% of thymic B cells express AIRE. In contrast, splenic or bone marrow B cells in the transgenic animal did not (94). Interestingly these AIRE$^+$ thymic B cells resided in the medulla, and comparative studies of tissue restricted antigen (TRA) expression between AIRE$^+$ thymic B cells and AIRE$^+$ medullary thymic epithelial cells found there was no overlap between the two cell types in the TRAs presented. This suggests that thymic B cells may work in concert with medullary thymic epithelial cells to negatively select a greater range of autoreactive T cells. The work of Yamano builds on early reports that thymic B cells deleted superantigen specific T cells and that B cell specific expression of myelin oligodendrocyte glycoprotein enhanced negative selection of MOG-reactive transgenic T cells (16).

This ability of thymic B cells to participate in negative selection is suggested to be linked to their intrathymic class-switching activity (96), autoreactive thymocytes enabling selection and expansion of their cognate autoreactive thymic B cell counterpart. Perera et al., used an AID reporter mouse in a parabiotic model to show that self-antigen can drive class-switching of thymic B cells *in situ*, and the class-switched cells predominantly expressed IgG2b and IgA BcRs (96), and on an autoimmune background, class-switching of autoreactive thymic B cells numbers was enhanced. Further, they showed that impeding class switching of thymic B cells impaired their ability to negatively selective autoreactive T cells.

Others have documented a role for thymic B cells in the development of thymic T regulatory cells (Treg), and animals with expanded thymic B cell compartments have a correlating expanded thymic Treg compartment too (97, 98).

It would appear that there is strong evidence that thymic B cells are important in central tolerance. However, this positive role for thymic B cells in central tolerance is contrasted by the evidence that thymic B cells are key players in mediating tissue damage in myasthenia gravis (18, 63, 71, 99) and more recently systemic lupus erythematosus (19, 100) and T1d (15). Myasthenia gravis is the most documented condition where thymic B cells participate negatively in the autoimmune outcome. In myasthenia gravis, the thymus is the key source for pathogenic acetylcholine receptor antibodies that target this receptor on muscles leading to chronic muscle weakness. The thymus in myasthenia gravis patients have medullary thymic epithelial hyperplasia (18) with autoreactive thymic B cells secreting antibodies to acetylcholine receptors expressed on the medullary thymic epithelial cells triggering their demise *via* Complement-mediated attack (101).

In animal models of systemic lupus erythematosus, thymic B cells have a distinct transcriptome compared to thymic B cells from non-autoimmune prone, with increased prevalence of genes related to B cell survival (19). These increased thymic B cells were shown to promote expansion of the Tfh cells which in turn could enhance the systemic autoantibody response.

Our own studies in NOD mice, suggest that in T1d, thymic B cells may act in a manner similar to that seen in myasthenia gravis. Enhancement of thymic B cell numbers, the formation of thymic germinal centres results in a significant increase in intrathymic antibody levels in contrast to non-autoimmune prone mice. These antibodies are predominantly of the IgG1 and IgA subclass and were unique to the thymic compartment (15). Furthermore, *in situ* binding of these IgG antibodies to thymic medullary epithelial cells correlated with enhanced apoptosis of these antibody-selected cells. We have yet to establish that the antigen recognised by the autoantibodies is insulin, however, we showed that loss of certain medullary thymic epithelial cells resulted in decreased negative selection of autoreactive T cells, and enhanced survival of insulin-reactive thymocytes (15).

These contrasting roles for thymic B cells in negative selection are intriguing. Whether thymic B cells harbour pro-negative selection and anti-negative selection subpopulations, with the latter population having an advantage over the former in the autoimmune setting remains to be established. Alternatively, it may be that as an autoimmune process is ongoing, pro-negative selection thymic B cells switch to an anti-negative selection functionality. The potential mechanisms that promote these divergent properties of thymic B cells is shown in **Figure 1**. Studies that address these hypotheses will be important in understanding the relationship between thymic B cells and central thymic tolerance.

COMPUTATIONAL APPROACHES TO DEVELOP A THYMIC *IN SILICO* MODEL

Many challenges face immunologists studying the thymus; early involution of thymic tissue meaning most human studies are based on procured tissue from foetuses, neonates or young children, and acquiring such tissue is not readily accessible due to, among other issues, ethical reasons. Studies of the thymus, particularly the ageing thymus and its many intricacies in cellular cross-talk, requires large cohorts of mice, again rearing questions of ethics. Recent years have seen a drive towards using computational algorithms and *in silico* models to recapitulate the dynamic environments of immune tissues, and assess the role of candidate molecules in a particular pathway. In this last part of the review, we will discuss the potential of developing *in silico* computational models to identify therapeutic avenues for manipulating thymic B cells in autoimmune disorders like T1d.

IN SILICO APPROACHES TO MODELLING BIOLOGICAL SYSTEMS

Systems biology is the integration of wet-lab experimentation and computational research in order to understand complex biological systems. Computational biology provides tools for the theoretical exploration of biology, permitting scientists to address critical questions directly (102). Simulation is one facet of computational biology that is finding increasing usage (103–106).

The use of simulation would bypass the necessary ethical, financial and practical issues surrounding acquisition of thymic tissue. In addition, the very nature of the system lends itself very precisely to Agent Based Modelling and Simulation (ABMS); consisting as it does of very many heterogeneous individuals of different types e.g. B cells, T cells, thymic medullary epithelial cells. These cell populations can interact with each other in specific ways under specific conditions. The cells will also possess some concept of location (the medulla or the cortico-medullary junction) and state (e.g. some stage of the cellular life cycle). Use of agent-based modelling will permit us to investigate how manipulating cell behaviours will give rise to altered system-wide ('emergent') behaviour. The results will be easily interpretable and so simple to put into words accessible to a wider audience.

MATHEMATICAL VERSUS COMPUTATIONAL MODELS

A simulation is typically either mathematical or computational. Mathematical models are generally based on series of differential equations (107) and cells are modelled as populations rather than as individuals (108). Such models are often seen as opaque to non-mathematicians (109) and the model is typically difficult to extend should further cell types need to be considered. A further perceived disadvantage of mathematical models is that the resulting differential equations tend be complicated to solve

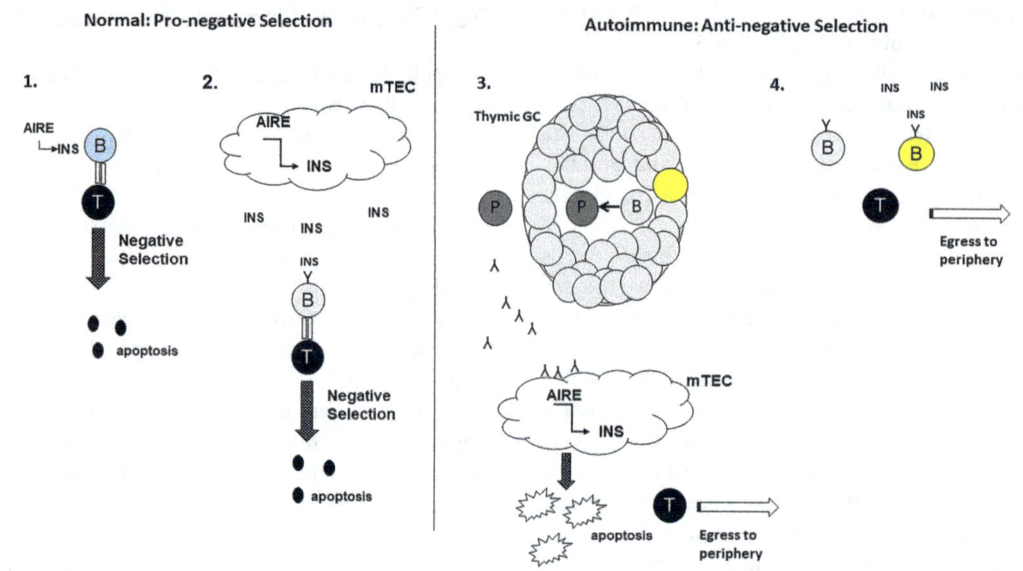

FIGURE 1 | Potential roles for thymic B cells in the thymic negative selection process: a hypothesis. In the normal setting, thymic B cells enhance the negative selection of autoreactive T cells. 1. Aire$^+$ Thymic B cells (blue) express and present self-antigens e.g. insulin (INS) to autoreactive T cells with high affinity TcRs for the self-antigens leading to T cell apoptosis. 2. Self-antigens e.g. INS secreted by Aire$^+$ mTECs are acquired by thymic B cells expressing self-reactive BcRs (light grey). Internalisation, processing and presentation of the self-antigen to autoreactive T cells leads to T cell apoptosis. In the autoimmune setting, thymic B cells impede the negative selection of autoreactive T cells. 3. The emergence of thymic GCs results in thymic B cells receiving signals to develop into plasma cells (dark grey) secreting autoantibodies for self-antigens expressed by mTECs. Binding of the autoantibodies to mTECs leads to mTEC apoptosis, leading to decreased negative selection of autoreactive T cells and increased egress of the T cells to the peripheral tissues. 4. Somatic hypermutated (yellow) thymic B cells egressing from thymic GCs, may outcompete 'normal' thymic B cells for the binding of self-antigen in the thymic milieu impeding negative selection. For this scenario, the sm thymic B cells would either fail to adequately present the self-antigens to autoreactive T cells to support negative selection.

exactly and often require solving *via* numerical methods which entails potentially unacceptable approximations to the model.

On the other hand, computational simulation methodologies such as Agent Based Modelling (ABM) are typically conceptually much simpler (110, 111). Cellular populations are modelled as sets of individuals (112) that share similar behaviours e.g. a population of Single Positive T cells. In this way more descriptive explanations of experimental observations may be proposed from simulation outcomes. Additionally agent-based models are better suited than other modelling techniques to capturing the system-wide, or emergent, behaviour of the system (113). Here, emergent behaviour is understood to be the system behaviour arising from the combined behaviours of the component entities e.g. cells.

An ABM will represent some abstraction of the system created jointly by a scientist, expert in the system of interest, and a software developer. The model should aim to include all factors e.g. cells and signalling molecules, generally held to be essential to system function. It is also important to include any potential roles for the biological environment in the model.

CREATING AN AGENT-BASED MODEL

A number of short tutorials on the creation of agent based models can be found in the literature e.g. Bandini et al., (114). Generally, the principal steps in developing an agent-based simulation are:

i. Identify the agents that are important to what you want to model:

For example in a model of negative selection events in the thymic medulla, we might wish to model the behaviours of Single Positive T cells, B cells and medullary thymic epithelial cells (mTECs).

ii. Identify the environment in which your agents exist:

We might for instance break the thymus into three distinct environments: the cortex, the cortico-medullary junction (CMJ) and the medulla; placing relevant cells in each.

iii. Identify mechanisms whereby the agents interact with each other and with their environment:

We might consider that cells behave differently in different environments. For example, SP T cells will not tend to remain in the cortex, but will rather migrate across the CMJ to the medulla where they will interact with mTECs, *via* recognition of the insulin fragments presented by the mTECs, to facilitate negative selection. Aggressive B cells will also be able to interact directly with mTECs, also *via* recognition of insulin presented by the mTECs.

iv. Consider how best to implement the model as computer code and any assumptions and simplifications necessary in achieving this:

It will be very difficult to exactly replicate precise biological behaviour as computer code. For example, cells are unlikely to be of regular shapes e.g. circular, so the geometry of the system will not be exactly reproducible *in silico* and appropriate approximations will be necessary. In the case of thymic B cells it will be necessary to decide how we will differentiate between those B cells which serve to enhance the negative selective of autoreactive T cells and those that prevent the negative selection of autoaggressive T cells.

CHALLENGES AND LIMITATIONS OF THE APPROACH

Despite the benefits of employing simulation as an investigative tool, it is wise to be mindful of the potential pitfalls in the use of the technique.

As an experiment, a simulation must be reproducible. It is therefore of paramount importance that simulation design be comprehensively documented. The documentation must incorporate all assumptions and design decisions to make them available to the scientific community to assess. The CoSMoS simulation design protocol (115) provides guidance in documentation and development of simulations, in which the user can have confidence.

The first challenge in the design of agent-based models is to correctly capture the relevant entities (cells, signalling molecules etc.) of the system and their behaviours in the model. If a key component of the system (or its behaviour) is omitted from the model then the model will be unfit for the purpose for which it was designed. As an example, two different types of behaviour in the B cell population have been noted. Some cells appear to be essentially quiescent, though may play an active role in sustaining negative selection, whereas others adopt a more aggressive role, apoptosing mTECs and thus triggering the breakdown of negative selection and hence central tolerance. Effective communication between the software developer and the expert biologist will help to mitigate this problem.

Also, simulation outcomes will be determined by the choice of values for the required simulation parameters. Model parameters may represent quantities such as the duration of a particular cell cycle stage or the concentration of cytokine that brings about progression to the next differentiation state. Such values will, in all likelihood, not be available from experiment and must be estimated. Chosen parameter values will ultimately impact on overall system behaviour and simulation output. Calibration is the process of adjusting parameter values so as to align *in silico* simulation results with observed *in vivo* behaviours. The issues surrounding simulation parameterization are discussed briefly below, but are addressed more fully in the relevant literature:

Optimization of parameter values is the subject of numerous widely used techniques such as the Latin Hypercube (116). This technique is based on the random sampling of the entire parameter space and is time and resource intensive to perform for a typical biological system.

The stability of simulation performance with parameter perturbation can be assessed using two different types of analysis. Robustness analysis is used to gauge the impact of simulation parameters on the simulation's ability to execute stably i.e. which parameter values might cause the simulation to crash (117). Sensitivity Analysis can be used to investigate the effects of individual parameters or combinations of parameters on simulation outputs *via* the systematic variation of parameter values and observation of the effect on simulation performance (117). Sensitivity analyses are further discussed in (118, 119).

Recent research has aimed to refine techniques that facilitate calibration of simulations involving large numbers of parameters in a less resource intensive manner than the Latin Hypercube method described above. These novel techniques include the use of Machine Learning and multi-objective calibration (120, 121).

Although the scope and particularly the calibration of computational simulations is potentially limited by the scale of the computational resources available, there is a trend towards easier access to powerful high performance computer clusters which makes these concerns less relevant.

Despite the challenges entailed in employing an ABMS approach to biological simulation, ABMS remains a highly descriptive and powerful methodology for elucidation of cellular and molecular mechanisms of disease and many of the challenges posed by the use of the technique, particularly those relating to parameterization, are becoming more easily addressed using recent developments.

FINAL COMMENTS

Commonalities in autoimmune conditions offer insights into novel therapies that may target multiple autoimmune conditions. Evidence that abnormality in the thymic B cell compartment is a shared characteristic between several autoimmune conditions highlights the need for further studies into this enigmatic cell. Nevertheless, increasing ethical considerations and availability of thymic tissue for analysis makes studies of thymic B cells somewhat challenging, particularly in man. Computational models of the dynamic thymic environment may offer a new approach to address the role of thymic B cells in health and disease, leading to candidate molecules or signal pathways as novel therapeutic targets in autoimmune conditions, including T1d.

AUTHOR CONTRIBUTIONS

DC and EAG wrote the thymic B cell section. RG wrote the computational modelling section. All authors contributed to the article and approved the submitted version.

FUNDING

This work was supported by a Diabetes UK Project Grant 18/0005804 awarded to EAG, and a Daphne Jackson Trust Fellowship awarded to RG. The University of York and the Medical Research Council funded the Fellowship.

REFERENCES

1. Kaufman DL, Clare-Salzler M, Tian J, Forsthuber T, Ting GS, Robinson P, et al. Spontaneous Loss of T-Cell Tolerance to Glutamic Acid Decarboxylase in Murine Insulin-Dependent Diabetes. *Nature* (1993) 366(6450):69–72. doi: 10.1038/366069a0
2. Lieberman SM, DiLorenzo TP. A Comprehensive Guide to Antibody and T-Cell Responses in Type 1 Diabetes. *Tissue Antigens* (2003) 62(5):359–77. doi: 10.1034/j.1399-0039.2003.00152.x
3. Tisch R, Yang XD, Singer SM, Liblau RS, Fugger L, McDevitt HO. Immune Response to Glutamic Acid Decarboxylase Correlates With Insulitis in non-Obese Diabetic Mice. *Nature* (1993) 366(6450):72–5. doi: 10.1038/366072a0
4. Kachapati K, Adams D, Bednar K, Ridgway WM. The non-Obese Diabetic (NOD) Mouse as a Model of Human Type 1 Diabetes. *Methods Mol Biol* (2012) 933:3–16. doi: 10.1007/978-1-62703-068-7_1
5. Takahama Y, Ohigashi I, Baik S, Anderson G. Generation of Diversity in Thymic Epithelial Cells. *Nat Rev Immunol* (2017) 17(5):295–305. doi: 10.1038/nri.2017.12
6. sO'Reilly LA, Healey D, Simpson E, Chandler P, Lund T, Ritter MA, et al. Studies on the Thymus of non-Obese Diabetic (NOD) Mice: Effect of Transgene Expression. *Immunology* (1994) 82(2):275–86.
7. Parish NM, Chandler P, Quartey-Papafio R, Simpson E, Cooke A. The Effect of Bone Marrow and Thymus Chimerism Between non-Obese Diabetic (NOD) and NOD-E Transgenic Mice, on the Expression and Prevention of Diabetes. *Eur J Immunol* (1993) 23(10):2667–75. doi: 10.1002/eji.1830231042
8. Noorchashm H, Lieu YK, Noorchashm N, Rostami SY, Greeley SA, Schlachterman A, et al. I-Ag7-Mediated Antigen Presentation by B Lymphocytes is Critical in Overcoming a Checkpoint in T Cell Tolerance to Islet Beta Cells of Nonobese Diabetic Mice. *J Immunol* (1999) 163 (2):743–50.
9. Serreze DV, Fleming SA, Chapman HD, Richard SD, Leiter EH, Tisch RM. B Lymphocytes are Critical Antigen-Presenting Cells for the Initiation of T Cell-Mediated Autoimmune Diabetes in Nonobese Diabetic Mice. *J Immunol* (1998) 161(8):3912–8.
10. Serreze DV, Gallichan WS, Snider DP, Croitoru K, Rosenthal KL, Leiter EH, et al. MHC Class I-Mediated Antigen Presentation and Induction of CD8(+) Cytotoxic T-Cell Responses in Autoimmune Diabetes-Prone NOD Mice. *Diabetes* (1996) 45(7):902–8. doi: 10.2337/diab.45.7.902
11. Brodie GM, Wallberg M, Santamaria P, Wong FS, Green EA. B-Cells Promote Intra-Islet CD8+ Cytotoxic T-Cell Survival to Enhance Type 1 Diabetes. *Diabetes* (2008) 57(4):909–17. doi: 10.2337/db07-1256
12. Parikka V, Nanto-Salonen K, Saarinen M, Simell T, Ilonen J, Hyoty H, et al. Early Seroconversion and Rapidly Increasing Autoantibody Concentrations Predict Prepubertal Manifestation of Type 1 Diabetes in Children at Genetic Risk. *Diabetologia* (2012) 55(7):1926–36. doi: 10.1007/s00125-012-2523-3
13. Leete P, Willcox A, Krogvold L, Dahl-Jorgensen K, Foulis AK, Richardson SJ, et al. Differential Insulitic Profiles Determine the Extent of Beta-Cell Destruction and the Age at Onset of Type 1 Diabetes. *Diabetes* (2016) 65 (5):1362–9. doi: 10.2337/db15-1615
14. Pescovitz MD, Greenbaum CJ, Krause-Steinrauf H, Becker DJ, Gitelman SE, Goland R, et al. Rituximab, B-Lymphocyte Depletion, and Preservation of Beta-Cell Function. *N Engl J Med* (2009) 361(22):2143–52. doi: 10.1056/NEJMoa0904452
15. Pinto AI, Smith J, Kissack MR, Hogg KG, Green EA. Thymic B Cell-Mediated Attack of Thymic Stroma Precedes Type 1 Diabetes Development. *Front Immunol* (2018) 9:1281. doi: 10.3389/fimmu.2018.01281
16. Inaba M, Inaba K, Hosono M, Kumamoto T, Ishida T, Muramatsu S, et al. Distinct Mechanisms of Neonatal Tolerance Induced by Dendritic Cells and Thymic B Cells. *J Exp Med* (1991) 173(3):549–59. doi: 10.1084/jem.173.3.549
17. Isaacson PG, Norton AJ, Addis BJ. The Human Thymus Contains a Novel Population of B Lymphocytes. *Lancet* (1987) 2(8574):1488–91. doi: 10.1016/S0140-6736(87)92622-5
18. Christensson B, Biberfeld P, Matell G. B-Cell Compartment in the Thymus of Patients With Myasthenia Gravis and Control Subjects. *Ann N Y Acad Sci* (1988) 540:293–7. doi: 10.1111/j.1749-6632.1988.tb27079.x
19. Hidalgo Y, Nunez S, Fuenzalida MJ, Flores-Santibanez F, Saez PJ, Dorner J, et al. Thymic B Cells Promote Germinal Center-Like Structures and the Expansion of Follicular Helper T Cells in Lupus-Prone Mice. *Front Immunol* (2020) 11:696. doi: 10.3389/fimmu.2020.00696
20. Mackay IR, Masel M, Burnet FM. Thymic Abnormality in Systemic Lupus Erythematosus. *Australas Ann Med* (1964) 13:5–14. doi: 10.1111/imj.1964.13.1.5
21. Kirschner D, Pienaar E, Marino S, Linderman JJ. A Review of Computational and Mathematical Modeling Contributions to Our Understanding of Mycobacterium Tuberculosis Within-Host Infection and Treatment. *Curr Opin Syst Biol* (2017) 3:170–85. doi: 10.1016/j.coisb.2017.05.014
22. Segovia-Juarez JL, Ganguli S, Kirschner D. Identifying Control Mechanisms of Granuloma Formation During M. Tuberculosis Infection Using an Agent-Based Model. *J Theor Biol* (2004) 231(3):357–76. doi: 10.1016/j.jtbi.2004.06.031
23. Warsinske HC, DiFazio RM, Linderman JJ, Flynn JL, Kirschner DE. Identifying Mechanisms Driving Formation of Granuloma-Associated Fibrosis During Mycobacterium Tuberculosis Infection. *J Theor Biol* (2017) 429:1–17. doi: 10.1016/j.jtbi.2017.06.017
24. Tang J, Enderling H, Becker-Weimann S, Pham C, Polyzos A, Chen CY, et al. Phenotypic Transition Maps of 3D Breast Acini Obtained by Imaging-Guided Agent-Based Modeling. *Integr Biol (Camb)* (2011) 3(4):408–21. doi: 10.1039/c0ib00092b
25. Butler JA, Cosgrove J, Alden K, Timmis J, Coles MC. Model-Driven Experimentation: A New Approach to Understand Mechanisms of Tertiary Lymphoid Tissue Formation, Function, and Therapeutic Resolution. *Front Immunol* (2017) 7:658. doi: 10.3389/fimmu.2016.00658
26. Cosgrove J, Novkovic M, Albrecht S, Pikor NB, Zhou Z, Onder L, et al. B Cell Zone Reticular Cell Microenvironments Shape CXCL13 Gradient Formation. *Nat Commun* (2020) 11(1):3677. doi: 10.1038/s41467-020-17135-2
27. Walker DC, Hill G, Wood SM, Smallwood RH, Southgate J. Agent-Based Computational Modeling of Wounded Epithelial Cell Monolayers. *IEEE Trans Nanobiosci* (2004) 3(3):153–63. doi: 10.1109/TNB.2004.833680
28. Walker DC, Southgate J, Hill G, Holcombe M, Hose DR, Wood SM, et al. The Epitheliome: Agent-Based Modelling of the Social Behaviour of Cells. *Biosystems* (2004) 76(1-3):89–100. doi: 10.1016/j.biosystems.2004.05.025
29. Miyama-Inaba M, Kuma S, Inaba K, Ogata H, Iwai H, Yasumizu R, et al. Unusual Phenotype of B Cells in the Thymus of Normal Mice. *J Exp Med* (1988) 168(2):811–6. doi: 10.1084/jem.168.2.811
30. Nango K, Inaba M, Inaba K, Adachi Y, Than S, Ishida T, et al. Ontogeny of Thymic B Cells in Normal Mice. *Cell Immunol* (1991) 133(1):109–15. doi: 10.1016/0008-8749(91)90183-C
31. Bredenkamp N, Nowell CS, Blackburn CC. Regeneration of the Aged Thymus by a Single Transcription Factor. *Development* (2014) 141 (8):1627–37. doi: 10.1242/dev.103614
32. Sato T, Ishikawa S, Akadegawa K, Ito T, Yurino H, Kitabatake M, et al. Aberrant B1 Cell Migration Into the Thymus Results in Activation of CD4 T Cells Through its Potent Antigen-Presenting Activity in the Development of Murine Lupus. *Eur J Immunol* (2004) 34(12):3346–58. doi: 10.1002/eji.200425373
33. Perera J, Huang H. The Development and Function of Thymic B Cells. *Cell Mol Life Sci* (2015) 72(14):2657–63. doi: 10.1007/s00018-015-1895-1
34. Akashi K, Richie LI, Miyamoto T, Carr WH, Weissman IL. B Lymphopoiesis in the Thymus. *J Immunol* (2000) 164(10):5221–6. doi: 10.4049/jimmunol.164.10.5221
35. Than S, Inaba M, Inaba K, Fukuba Y, Adachi Y, Ikehara S. Origin of Thymic and Peritoneal Ly-1 B Cells. *Eur J Immunol* (1992) 22(5):1299–303. doi: 10.1002/eji.1830220527
36. McCaughtry TM, Wilken MS, Hogquist KA. Thymic Emigration Revisited. *J Exp Med* (2007) 204(11):2513–20. doi: 10.1084/jem.20070601
37. Gay D, Saunders T, Camper S, Weigert M. Receptor Editing: An Approach by Autoreactive B Cells to Escape Tolerance. *J Exp Med* (1993) 177(4):999–1008. doi: 10.1084/jem.177.4.999
38. Yu W, Nagaoka H, Jankovic M, Misulovin Z, Suh H, Rolink A, et al. Continued RAG Expression in Late Stages of B Cell Development and No Apparent Re-Induction After Immunization. *Nature* (1999) 400(6745):682–7. doi: 10.1038/23287
39. Yu W, Nagaoka H, Misulovin Z, Meffre E, Suh H, Jankovic M, et al. RAG Expression in B Cells in Secondary Lymphoid Tissues. *Cold Spring Harbor Symp Quant Biol* (1999) 64:207–10. doi: 10.1101/sqb.1999.64.207

40. Benz C, Bleul CC. A Multipotent Precursor in the Thymus Maps to the Branching Point of the T Versus B Lineage Decision. *J Exp Med* (2005) 202 (1):21–31. doi: 10.1084/jem.20050146
41. McKenna HJ, Morrissey PJ. Flt3 Ligand Plus IL-7 Supports the Expansion of Murine Thymic B Cell Progenitors That can Mature Intrathymically. *J Immunol* (1998) 160(10):4801–9.
42. Inlay MA, Bhattacharya D, Sahoo D, Serwold T, Seita J, Karsunky H, et al. Ly6d Marks the Earliest Stage of B-Cell Specification and Identifies the Branchpoint Between B-Cell and T-Cell Development. *Genes Dev* (2009) 23 (20):2376–81. doi: 10.1101/gad.1836009
43. Mansson R, Zandi S, Welinder E, Tsapogas P, Sakaguchi N, Bryder D, et al. Single-Cell Analysis of the Common Lymphoid Progenitor Compartment Reveals Functional and Molecular Heterogeneity. *Blood* (2010) 115 (13):2601–9. doi: 10.1182/blood-2009-08-236398
44. Ceredig R. The Ontogeny of B Cells in the Thymus of Normal, CD3 Epsilon Knockout (KO), RAG-2 KO and IL-7 Transgenic Mice. *Int Immunol* (2002) 14(1):87–99. doi: 10.1093/intimm/14.1.87
45. He Y, Pear WS. Notch Signalling in B Cells. *Semin Cell Dev Biol* (2003) 14 (2):135–42. doi: 10.1016/s1084-9521(02)00182.
46. Feyerabend TB, Terszowski G, Tietz A, Blum C, Luche H, Gossler A, et al. Deletion of Notch1 Converts Pro-T Cells to Dendritic Cells and Promotes Thymic B Cells by Cell-Extrinsic and Cell-Intrinsic Mechanisms. *Immunity* (2009) 30(1):67–79. doi: 10.1016/j.immuni.2008.10.016
47. Xing C, Ma N, Xiao H, Wang X, Zheng M, Han G, et al. Critical Role for Thymic CD19+CD5+CD1dhiIL-10+ Regulatory B Cells in Immune Homeostasis. *J Leukoc Biol* (2015) 97(3):547–56. doi: 10.1189/jlb.3A0414-213RR
48. Carnrot C, Prokopec KE, Rasbo K, Karlsson MC, Kleinau S. Marginal Zone B Cells are Naturally Reactive to Collagen Type II and are Involved in the Initiation of the Immune Response in Collagen-Induced Arthritis. *Cell Mol Immunol* (2011) 8(4):296–304. doi: 10.1038/cmi.2011.2
49. Rolf J, Motta V, Duarte N, Lundholm M, Berntman E, Bergman ML, et al. The Enlarged Population of Marginal Zone/CD1d(high) B Lymphocytes in Nonobese Diabetic Mice Maps to Diabetes Susceptibility Region Idd11. *J Immunol* (2005) 174(8):4821–7. doi: 10.4049/jimmunol.174.8.4821
50. Wellmann U, Werner A, Winkler TH. Altered Selection Processes of B Lymphocytes in Autoimmune NZB/W Mice, Despite Intact Central Tolerance Against DNA. *Eur J Immunol* (2001) 31 (9):2800–10. doi: 10.1002/1521-4141(200109)31:9<2800::AID-IMMU2800> 3.0.CO;2-E
51. Daridon C, Pers JO, Devauchelle V, Martins-Carvalho C, Hutin P, Pennec YL, et al. Identification of Transitional Type II B Cells in the Salivary Glands of Patients With Sjogren's Syndrome. *Arthritis Rheum* (2006) 54(7):2280–8. doi: 10.1002/art.21936
52. Segundo C, Rodriguez C, Garcia-Poley A, Aguilar M, Gavilan I, Bellas C, et al. Thyroid-Infiltrating B Lymphocytes in Graves' Disease are Related to Marginal Zone and Memory B Cell Compartments. *Thyroid* (2001) 11 (6):525–30. doi: 10.1089/105072501750302813
53. Palm AE, Kleinau S. Marginal Zone B Cells: From Housekeeping Function to Autoimmunity? *J Autoimmun* (2021) 119:102627. doi: 10.1016/j.jaut.2021.102627
54. Ferguson AR, Youd ME, Corley RB. Marginal Zone B Cells Transport and Deposit IgM-Containing Immune Complexes Onto Follicular Dendritic Cells. *Int Immunol* (2004) 16(10):1411–22. doi: 10.1093/intimm/dxh142
55. Hammad H, Vanderkerken M, Pouliot P, Deswarte K, Toussaint W, Vergote K, et al. Transitional B Cells Commit to Marginal Zone B Cell Fate by Taok3-Mediated Surface Expression of ADAM10. *Nat Immunol* (2017) 18(3):313–20. doi: 10.1038/ni.3657
56. Hampel F, Ehrenberg S, Hojer C, Draeseke A, Marschall-Schroter G, Kuhn R, et al. CD19-Independent Instruction of Murine Marginal Zone B-Cell Development by Constitutive Notch2 Signaling. *Blood* (2011) 118(24):6321–31. doi: 10.1182/blood-2010-12-325944
57. Palm AK, Friedrich HC, Mezger A, Salomonsson M, Myers LK, Kleinau S. Function and Regulation of Self-Reactive Marginal Zone B Cells in Autoimmune Arthritis. *Cell Mol Immunol* (2015) 12(4):493–504. doi: 10.1038/cmi.2015.37
58. Wortis HH, Teutsch M, Higer M, Zheng J, Parker DC. B-Cell Activation by Crosslinking of Surface IgM or Ligation of CD40 Involves Alternative Signal Pathways and Results in Different B-Cell Phenotypes. *Proc Natl Acad Sci U S A* (1995) 92(8):3348–52. doi: 10.1073/pnas.92.8.3348
59. Smith MJ, Packard TA, O'Neill SK, Dunand CJH, Huang M, Fitzgerald-Miller L, et al. Loss of Anergic B Cells in Prediabetic and New-Onset Type 1 Diabetic Patients. *Diabetes* (2015) 64(5):1703–12. doi: 10.2337/db13-1798
60. Elsner RA, Shlomchik MJ. Germinal Center and Extrafollicular B Cell Responses in Vaccination, Immunity, and Autoimmunity. *Immunity* (2020) 53(6):1136–50. doi: 10.1016/j.immuni.2020.11.006
61. Silva-Cayetano A, Linterman MA. Stromal Cell Control of Conventional and Ectopic Germinal Centre Reactions. *Curr Opin Immunol* (2020) 64:26–33. doi: 10.1016/j.coi.2020.03.007
62. Carrillo-Ballesteros FJ, Palafox-Sanchez CA, Franco-Topete RA, Munoz-Valle JF, Orozco-Barocio G, Martinez-Bonilla GE, et al. Expression of BAFF and BAFF Receptors in Primary Sjogren's Syndrome Patients With Ectopic Germinal Center-Like Structures. *Clin Exp Med* (2020) 20(4):615–26. doi: 10.1007/s10238-020-00637-0
63. Zhang X, Liu S, Chang T, Xu J, Zhang C, Tian F, et al. Intrathymic Tfh/B Cells Interaction Leads to Ectopic GCs Formation and Anti-AChR Antibody Production: Central Role in Triggering MG Occurrence. *Mol Neurobiol* (2016) 53(1):120–31. doi: 10.1007/s12035-014-8985-1
64. Zuckerman NS, Howard WA, Bismuth J, Gibson K, Edelman H, Berrih-Aknin S, et al. Ectopic GC in the Thymus of Myasthenia Gravis Patients Show Characteristics of Normal GC. *Eur J Immunol* (2010) 40(4):1150–61. doi: 10.1002/eji.200939914
65. Kendall PL, Yu G, Woodward EJ, Thomas JW. Tertiary Lymphoid Structures in the Pancreas Promote Selection of B Lymphocytes in Autoimmune Diabetes. *J Immunol* (2007) 178(9):5643–51. doi: 10.4049/jimmunol.178.9.5643
66. Barone F, Nayar S, Campos J, Cloake T, Withers DR, Toellner KM, et al. IL-22 Regulates Lymphoid Chemokine Production and Assembly of Tertiary Lymphoid Organs. *Proc Natl Acad Sci U S A* (2015) 112(35):11024–9. doi: 10.1073/pnas.1503315112
67. Canete JD, Celis R, Yeremenko N, Sanmarti R, van Duivenvoorde L, Ramirez J, et al. Ectopic Lymphoid Neogenesis is Strongly Associated With Activation of the IL-23 Pathway in Rheumatoid Synovitis. *Arthritis Res Ther* (2015) 17:173. doi: 10.1186/s13075-015-0688-0
68. Domeier PP, Chodisetti SB, Soni C, Schell SL, Elias MJ, Wong EB, et al. IFN-Gamma Receptor and STAT1 Signaling in B Cells are Central to Spontaneous Germinal Center Formation and Autoimmunity. *J Exp Med* (2016) 213(5):715–32. doi: 10.1084/jem.20151722
69. Jackson SW, Jacobs HM, Arkatkar T, Dam EM, Scharping NE, Kolhatkar NS, et al. B Cell IFN-Gamma Receptor Signaling Promotes Autoimmune Germinal Centers *via* Cell-Intrinsic Induction of BCL-6. *J Exp Med* (2016) 213(5):733–50. doi: 10.1084/jem.20151724
70. Lee SK, Silva DG, Martin JL, Pratama A, Hu X, Chang PP, et al. Interferon-Gamma Excess Leads to Pathogenic Accumulation of Follicular Helper T Cells and Germinal Centers. *Immunity* (2012) 37(5):880–92. doi: 10.1016/j.immuni.2012.10.010
71. Leprince C, Cohen-Kaminsky S, Berrih-Aknin S, Vernet-Der Garabedian B, Treton D, Galanaud P, et al. Thymic B Cells From Myasthenia Gravis Patients are Activated B Cells. Phenotypic and Functional Analysis. *J Immunol* (1990) 145(7):2115–22.
72. Zotos D, Coquet JM, Zhang Y, Light A, D'Costa K, Kallies A, et al. IL-21 Regulates Germinal Center B Cell Differentiation and Proliferation Through a B Cell-Intrinsic Mechanism. *J Exp Med* (2010) 207(2):365–78. doi: 10.1084/jem.20091777
73. Ferreira RC, Simons HZ, Thompson WS, Cutler AJ, Dopico XC, Smyth DJ, et al. IL-21 Production by CD4(+) Effector T Cells and Frequency of Circulating Follicular Helper T Cells are Increased in Type 1 Diabetes Patients. *Diabetologia* (2015) 58(4):781–90. doi: 10.1007/s00125-015-3509-8
74. Sutherland AP, Van Belle T, Wurster AL, Suto A, Michaud M, Zhang D, et al. Interleukin-21 is Required for the Development of Type 1 Diabetes in NOD Mice. *Diabetes* (2009) 58(5):1144–55. doi: 10.2337/db08-0882
75. Viisanen T, Ihantola EL, Nanto-Salonen K, Hyoty H, Nurminen N, Selvenius J, et al. Circulating CXCR5+PD-1+ICOS+ Follicular T Helper Cells Are Increased Close to the Diagnosis of Type 1 Diabetes in Children With Multiple Autoantibodies. *Diabetes* (2017) 66(2):437–47. doi: 10.2337/db16-0714

76. He J, Tsai LM, Leong YA, Hu X, Ma CS, Chevalier N, et al. Circulating Precursor CCR7(lo)PD-1(Hi) CXCR5(+) CD4(+) T Cells Indicate Tfh Cell Activity and Promote Antibody Responses Upon Antigen Reexposure. *Immunity* (2013) 39(4):770–81. doi: 10.1016/j.immuni.2013.09.007
77. Morita R, Schmitt N, Bentebibel SE, Ranganathan R, Bourdery L, Zurawski G, et al. Human Blood CXCR5(+)CD4(+) T Cells are Counterparts of T Follicular Cells and Contain Specific Subsets That Differentially Support Antibody Secretion. *Immunity* (2011) 34(1):108–21. doi: 10.1016/j.immuni.2010.12.012
78. Rao DA. T Cells That Help B Cells in Chronically Inflamed Tissues. *Front Immunol* (2018) 9:1924. doi: 10.3389/fimmu.2018.01924
79. Hill DL, Pierson W, Bolland DJ, Mkindi C, Carr EJ, Wang J, et al. The Adjuvant GLA-SE Promotes Human Tfh Cell Expansion and Emergence of Public TCRbeta Clonotypes. *J Exp Med* (2019) 216(8):1857–73. doi: 10.1084/jem.20190301
80. Vella LA, Buggert M, Manne S, Herati RS, Sayin I, Kuri-Cervantes L, et al. T Follicular Helper Cells in Human Efferent Lymph Retain Lymphoid Characteristics. *J Clin Invest* (2019) 129(8):3185–200. doi: 10.1172/JCI125628
81. Barone F, Gardner DH, Nayar S, Steinthal N, Buckley CD, Luther SA. Stromal Fibroblasts in Tertiary Lymphoid Structures: A Novel Target in Chronic Inflammation. *Front Immunol* (2016) 7:477. doi: 10.3389/fimmu.2016.00477
82. Rangel-Moreno J, Carragher DM, de la Luz Garcia-Hernandez M, Hwang JY, Kusser K, Hartson L, et al. The Development of Inducible Bronchus-Associated Lymphoid Tissue Depends on IL-17. *Nat Immunol* (2011) 12 (7):639–46. doi: 10.1038/ni.2053
83. Michaux H, Martens H, Jaidane H, Halouani A, Hober D, Geenen V. How Does Thymus Infection by Coxsackievirus Contribute to the Pathogenesis of Type 1 Diabetes? *Front Immunol* (2015) 6:338. doi: 10.3389/fimmu.2015.00338
84. Tugnet N, Rylance P, Roden D, Trela M, Nelson P. Human Endogenous Retroviruses (HERVs) and Autoimmune Rheumatic Disease: Is There a Link? *Open Rheumatol J* (2013) 7:13–21. doi: 10.2174/1874312901307010013
85. Domeier PP, Schell SL, Rahman ZS. Spontaneous Germinal Centers and Autoimmunity. *Autoimmunity* (2017) 50(1):4–18. doi: 10.1080/08916934.2017.1280671
86. Spencer J, Choy M, Hussell T, Papadaki L, Kington JP, Isaacson PG. Properties of Human Thymic B-Cells. *Immunology* (1992) 75(4):596–600.
87. Weerkamp F, de Haas EF, Naber BA, Comans-Bitter WM, Bogers AJ, van Dongen JJ, et al. Age-Related Changes in the Cellular Composition of the Thymus in Children. *J Allergy Clin Immunol* (2005) 115(4):834–40. doi: 10.1016/j.jaci.2004.10.031
88. Wardemann H, Yurasov S, Schaefer A, Young JW, Meffre E, Nussenzweig MC. Predominant Autoantibody Production by Early Human B Cell Precursors. *Science* (2003) 301(5638):1374–7. doi: 10.1126/science.1086907
89. Rother MB, Schreurs MWJ, Kroek R, Bartol SJW, van Dongen JJM, van Zelm MC. The Human Thymus Is Enriched for Autoreactive B Cells. *J Immunol* (2016) 197(2):441–8. doi: 10.4049/jimmunol.1501992
90. Tonnelle C, D'Ercole C, Depraetere V, Metras D, Boubli L, Fougereau M. Human Thymic B Cells Largely Overexpress the VH4 Ig Gene Family. A Possible Role in the Control of Tolerance in Situ? *Int Immunol* (1997) 9 (3):407–14. doi: 10.1093/intimm/9.3.407
91. Roche PA, Furuta K. The Ins and Outs of MHC Class II-Mediated Antigen Processing and Presentation. *Nat Rev Immunol* (2015) 15(4):203–16. doi: 10.1038/nri3818
92. Dunn-Walters DK, Howe CJ, Isaacson PG, Spencer J. Location and Sequence of Rearranged Immunoglobulin Genes in Human Thymus. *Eur J Immunol* (1995) 25(2):513–9. doi: 10.1002/eji.1830250231
93. Frommer F, Waisman A. B Cells Participate in Thymic Negative Selection of Murine Auto-Reactive CD4(+) T Cells. *PloS One* (2010) 5(10):e15372. doi: 10.1371/journal.pone.0015372
94. Yamano T, Nedjic J, Hinterberger M, Steinert M, Koser S, Pinto S, et al. Thymic B Cells Are Licensed to Present Self Antigens for Central T Cell Tolerance Induction. *Immunity* (2015) 42(6):1048–61. doi: 10.1016/j.immuni.2015.05.013
95. Yamano T, Steinert M, Klein L. Thymic B Cells and Central T Cell Tolerance. *Front Immunol* (2015) 6:376. doi: 10.3389/fimmu.2015.00376
96. Perera J, Zheng Z, Li S, Gudjonson H, Kalinina O, Benichou JIC, et al. Self-Antigen-Driven Thymic B Cell Class Switching Promotes T Cell Central Tolerance. *Cell Rep* (2016) 17(2):387–98. doi: 10.1016/j.celrep.2016.09.011
97. Walters S, Webster KE, Sutherland A, Gardam S, Groom J, Liuwantara D, et al. Increased CD4+Foxp3+ T Cells in BAFF-Transgenic Mice Suppress T Cell Effector Responses. *J Immunol* (2009) 182(2):793–801. doi: 10.4049/jimmunol.182.2.793
98. Walters SN, Webster KE, Daley S, Grey ST. A Role for Intrathymic B Cells in the Generation of Natural Regulatory T Cells. *J Immunol* (2014) 193(1):170–6. doi: 10.4049/jimmunol.1302519
99. Thangarajh M, Masterman T, Helgeland L, Rot U, Jonsson MV, Eide GE, et al. The Thymus is a Source of B-Cell-Survival Factors-APRIL and BAFF-In Myasthenia Gravis. *J Neuroimmunol* (2006) 178(1-2):161–6. doi: 10.1016/j.jneuroim.2006.05.023
100. Xing C, Zhu G, Xiao H, Fang Y, Liu X, Han G, et al. B Cells Regulate Thymic CD8(+)T Cell Differentiation in Lupus-Prone Mice. *Oncotarget* (2017) 8 (52):89486–99. doi: 10.18632/oncotarget.19002
101. Leite MI, Jones M, Strobel P, Marx A, Gold R, Niks E, et al. Myasthenia Gravis Thymus: Complement Vulnerability of Epithelial and Myoid Cells, Complement Attack on Them, and Correlations With Autoantibody Status. *Am J Pathol* (2007) 171(3):893–905. doi: 10.2353/ajpath.2007.070240
102. Kitano H. Computational Systems Biology. *Nature* (2002) 420(6912):206–10. doi: 10.1038/nature01254
103. An G, Mi Q, Dutta-Moscato J, Vodovotz Y. Agent-Based Models in Translational Systems Biology. *Wiley Interdiscip Rev Syst Biol Med* (2009) 1(2):159–71. doi: 10.1002/wsbm.45
104. Bauer AL, Beauchemin CA, Perelson AS. Agent-Based Modeling of Host-Pathogen Systems: The Successes and Challenges. *Inf Sci (N Y)* (2009) 179 (10):1379–89. doi: 10.1016/j.ins.2008.11.012
105. Forrest S, Beauchemin C. Computer Immunology. *Immunol Rev* (2007) 216:176–97. doi: 10.1111/j.1600-065X.2007.00499.x
106. Vodovotz Y, An G. Agent-Based Models of Inflammation in Translational Systems Biology: A Decade Later. *Wiley Interdiscip Rev Syst Biol Med* (2019) 11(6):e1460. doi: 10.1002/wsbm.1460
107. Perelson AS. Modelling Viral and Immune System Dynamics. *Nat Rev Immunol* (2002) 2(1):28–36. doi: 10.1038/nri700
108. Kleinstein SH, Seiden PE. Simulating the Immune System. *Comput Sci Eng* (2000) 2:69–77. doi: 10.1109/5992.852392
109. Seiden PE, Celada F. A Model for Simulating Cognate Recognition and Response in the Immune System. *J Theor Biol* (1992) 158(3):329–57. doi: 10.1016/S0022-5193(05)80737-4
110. Bonabeau E. Agent-Based Modelling: Methods and Techniques for Simulating Human Systems. *ProcNatlAcadSci* (2002) 99:7280–7. doi: 10.1073/pnas.082080899
111. Kam N, Cohen IR, Harel D. "The Immune System as a Reactive System: Modeling T Cell Activation With Statecharts". In: *Symposium on Human Centric Computing Languages and Environments (HCC)*. Stresa, Italy: IEEE (2001). p. 15–22.
112. Macal CM, North MJ. Tutorial on Agent-Based Modeling and Simulation. *J Simulation* (2010) 4:151–62. doi: 10.1057/jos.2010.3
113. Ghorbani A, Dechesne F, Dignum V, Jonker C. Enhancing ABM Into an Inevitable Tool for Policy Analysis. *Policy Complex Syst* (2014) 1(1). doi: 10.18278/jpcs.1.1.3
114. Bandini S, Manzoni S, Vizzari G. Agent Based Modeling and Simulation: An Informatics Perspective. *J Artif Soc Soc Simulation* (2009) 12(4):4. doi: 10.1007/978-1-0716-0368-0_12
115. Stepney S, Polack FAC, Alden K, Andrews PS, Bown JL, Droop A, et al. *Engineering Simulations as Scientific Instruments: A Pattern Language*. Berlin: Springer (2018).
116. McKay MD, Beckman RJ, Conover WJ. A Comparison of Three Methods for Selecting Values of Input Variables in the Analysis of Output From Computer Code. *Technometrics* (1979) 21(2):239–45. doi: 10.1080/00401706.1979.10489755

117. Alden K, Timmis J, Andrews PS, Veiga-Fernandes H, Coles MC. Pairing Experimentation and Computational Modeling to Understand the Role of Tissue Inducer Cells in the Development of Lymphoid Organs. *Front Immunol* (2012) 3:172. doi: 10.3389/fimmu.2012.00172

118. Marino S, Hogue IB, Ray CJ, Kirschner DE. A Methodology for Performing Global Uncertainty and Sensitivity Analysis in Systems Biology. *J Theor Biol* (2008) 254(1):178–96. doi: 10.1016/j.jtbi.2008.04.011

119. Renardy M, Hult C, Evans S, Linderman JJ, Kirschner DE. Global Sensitivity Analysis of Biological Multi-Scale Models. *Curr Opin BioMed Eng* (2019) 11:109–16. doi: 10.1016/j.cobme.2019.09.012

120. Alden K, Cosgrove J, Coles MC, Timmis J. Using Emulation to Engineer and Understand Simulations of Biological Systems. *IEEE/ACM Trans Comput Biol Bioinform* (2020) 17(1):302–15. doi: 10.1109/TCBB.2018.2843339

121. Read MN, Alden K, Timmis J, Andrews PS. Strategies for Calibrating Models of Biology. *Briefings Bioinf* (2020) 1:24–35. doi: 10.1093/bib/bby092

9

Resistance isn't Futile: The Physiological Basis of the Health Effects of Resistance Exercise in Individuals with Type 1 Diabetes

Olivia McCarthy[1,2], Othmar Moser[1,3], Max L. Eckstein[1,3], Rachel Deere[1,2], Steve C. Bain[2], Jason Pitt[1] and Richard M. Bracken[1,2]*

[1] Applied Sport, Technology, Exercise and Medicine Research Centre (A-STEM), College of Engineering, Swansea University, Swansea, United Kingdom, [2] Diabetes Research Group, Medical School, Swansea University, Swansea, United Kingdom, [3] Cardiovascular Diabetology Research Group, Division of Endocrinology and Diabetology, Department of Internal Medicine, Medical University of Graz, Graz, Austria

***Correspondence:**
Olivia McCarthy
olivia.mccarthy@swansea.ac.uk

The importance of regular exercise for glucose management in individuals with type 1 diabetes is magnified by its acknowledgment as a key adjunct to insulin therapy by several governmental, charitable, and healthcare organisations. However, although actively encouraged, exercise participation rates remain low, with glycaemic disturbances and poor cardiorespiratory fitness cited as barriers to long-term involvement. These fears are perhaps exacerbated by uncertainty in how different forms of exercise can considerably alter several acute and chronic physiological outcomes in those with type 1 diabetes. Thus, understanding the bodily responses to specific forms of exercise is important for the provision of practical guidelines that aim to overcome these exercise barriers. Currently, the majority of existing exercise research in type 1 diabetes has focused on moderate intensity continuous protocols with less work exploring predominately non-oxidative exercise modalities like resistance exercise. This is surprising, considering the known neuro-muscular, osteopathic, metabolic, and vascular benefits associated with resistance exercise in the wider population. Considering that individuals with type 1 diabetes have an elevated susceptibility for complications within these physiological systems, the wider health benefits associated with resistance exercise may help alleviate the prevalence and/or magnitude of pathological manifestation in this population group. This review outlines the health benefits of resistance exercise with reference to evidence in aiding some of the common complications associated with individuals with type 1 diabetes.

Keywords: resistance exercise, type 1 diabetes, physical activity, strength training, weights

INTRODUCTION

Notwithstanding their etiological, pathophysiological, and epidemiological complexities, the severity and incidence of complications associated with type 1 diabetes (T1D) are lower in physically active individuals (1, 2). Conversely, at a population level, sedentariness constitutes the fourth leading risk factor for mortality (3), such that individuals with the highest rates of sedentariness are up three times more likely to suffer premature mortality than their physically active counterparts (4). Therefore, whilst pharmaceutical and technological therapies aid glycaemic management, the utility of simple, holistic approaches such as regular physical activity (PA) constitute attractive adjunct treatment options, that alongside standardised medical care facilitate the improvement of T1D related pathological complications. However, a research and advocatory emphasis has been placed on the implementation of sustainable moderate intensity continuous exercise (MICE) in those with T1D, with less discernible evidence exploring alternative exercise modalities such as resistance exercise (RE). Whilst the health benefits associated with MICE are by no means immaterial, longstanding T1D is often accompanied by complications that impact the ability of participants to comfortably perform their rhythmic and/or pounding nature. Furthermore, MICE often fails to maximise the development of skeletal muscle mass and strength, both of which are features that facilitate improvements in various metabolic, neuroendocrine, and osteopathic processes.

As such, the utility of incorporating RE to assist the functional development of skeletal muscle integrity constitutes an important feature of the current exercise guidelines for those with T1D (5).

METHODS

The authors undertook a detailed PubMed literature search for the following key words: "resistance exercise," "exercise," "physical activity," "strength training," "weight training," "type 1 diabetes," "T1DM." The reference lists of systematic reviews, reviews, and included as well as excluded articles were manually screened for studies considered to be relevant. The literature search was conducted by the corresponding and secondary lead authors with additional suggestions and/or missed literature being provided by co-authors when necessary.

IMPORTANCE OF PHYSICAL ACTIVITY AND EXERCISE IN PEOPLE WITH TYPE 1 DIABETES

Research has consistently demonstrated the inverse relationship between PA and a reduced risk of diabetes-related complications (6, 7), including both mental well-being (8), life-expectancy (4, 7), and health related quality of life (9). In addition to the advocation of frequent PA, there is considerable evidence supporting the inclusion of regular exercise as an adjunct therapeutic strategy in people with T1D (10). Definitively, exercise describes activities completed with a structured and intentional approach to maintaining or attaining improvements in physical fitness (11). The increased metabolic activity of skeletal muscle during exercise evokes an adaptive response of several integrative processes, including the cardio-respiratory, vascular, and metabolic systems. As a reflection of the integrative functions of these physiological systems, cardio-respiratory fitness (CRF) is often used as a barometer for physical fitness and reflects the ability of the circulatory-and-respiratory systems to supply the muscular system with the increasing oxygen (O_2) demand experienced during sustained PA. Although the topic remains controversial, lower CRF has been reported in individuals with-vs.-without T1D (12). However, this finding appears to be closely related to glycaemic control, which can considerably influence acute exercise tolerance (12–14). Whilst considerable shifts in both cellular and tissue homeostasis are observed following most exercise activities, these processes are magnified following higher-intensity exercise, which represents a potent physiological stress. In the long-term, this acute stressor functions to optimise the body for subsequent subjection to bouts of physiological or indeed pathophysiological insults. Therefore, the type and intensity of the exercise stimulus can considerably influence the acute physiological and chronic adaptive responses that occur.

EXERCISE DEFINITION AND CLASSIFICATION

The word "exercise" is often used interchangeably and encompasses several adjustable variables including modality, frequency, intensity, and duration. Metabolically speaking, the energy contribution to a given task is determined by the intensity of effort required for its performance. These metabolic disturbances activate several kinases and phosphatases, necessary not only for the immediate supply of energy to sustain contractional output, but also the synthesis of genetic transcriptions that produce an adaptive phenotype for subsequent functional demands. Generally, the pathways responsible for the provision of adenosine triphosphate (ATP) to skeletal muscle are categorised as aerobic i.e., with the use of O_2 or anaerobic i.e., without the use of O_2. In each pathway, muscle must convert free adenosine diphosphate (ADP) and inorganic phosphate (Pi) to ATP. The regenerated ATP is then made available to the myosin ATPase enzymes that facilitate the contractile processes that enable movement. During low to moderate intensity exercise, the rate of O_2 supply necessary for continued contraction is comfortably met via the oxidative metabolism of carbohydrates and lipids. During intense physical exercise conditions of cellular hypoxia are experienced, as the rate of O_2 demand far exceeds the rate of supply capable via oxidative phosphorylation. Under such circumstances, anaerobic metabolism becomes the predominate means via which ATP is produced. The process involves the degradation of phosphocreatine (PCr) i.e., the ATP-CP system and the production of lactate within the glycolytic pathway i.e., the glycolytic system (**Figure 1**).

Essentially, a continuum exists that enables physical exercise activities to be grouped into low, moderate, and high intensity efforts. However, it should be noted that no exercise is ever considered "exclusively" aerobic or anaerobic, rather both pathways are activated simultaneously with one predominating fuel provision. Nonetheless, the terms provide reference guides that can be used generally to classify exercise intensities. Conventionally speaking, predominately aerobic exercise imposes a high-frequency (repetition), low power output (load) demand on muscular contraction. These characteristics are often observed during MICE including endurance orientated activities.

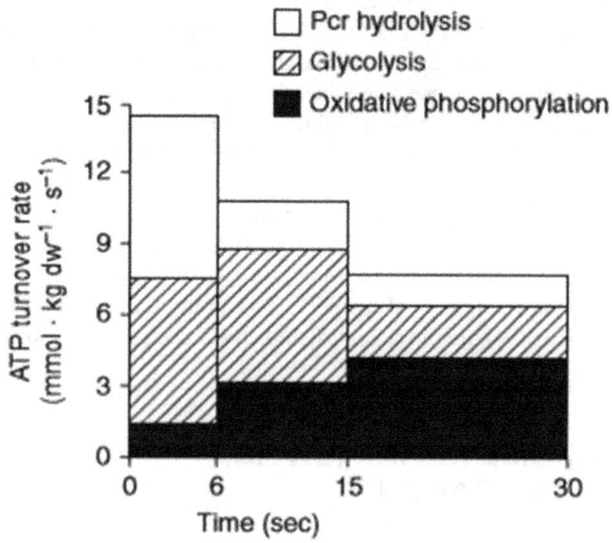

FIGURE 1 | Contributions of the three major energy pathways; phosphocreatine (Pcr), glycolysis, and oxidative phosphorylation to adenosine triphosphate (ATP) turnover during 30 s of maximal isokinetic cycling exercise. Reprinted from Parolin et al. [(15), Figure 7B].

Conversely, predominately anaerobic exercise mandates a low-frequency, high-resistance power output including both high intensity exercise (HIIE) and RE.

Resistance Exercise Definition

Resistance exercise or "strength/weight" exercise is a term used to describe exercise that mandates the body's musculature to move against an opposing force, addressing the functional behaviours mandatory to human movement. Resistance exercise training (RET) is the process of developing strength, flexibility, coordination, and stamina through performing exercises (at self-selected, high-intensity efforts) that involve multiple joints and muscle groups. RE be implemented using a multitude of training modalities, including isokinetic resistance, variable resistance, isometric resistance, and explosive plyometrics. This is important, as the term "resistance exercise" is often strictly associated with the use of equipment-based/external loads placed on the body in a strength orientated fashion. However, it actually reflects the exercise continuum—from which program design allows variable adaptation. Fundamentally the acute program variables (muscle action, intensity and volume, exercise selection and order, rest interval, repetition velocity, and frequency) dictate the specific training outcome (i.e., muscular strength, hypertrophy, maximal strength, or power). As such, there appears to be a specific relationship between the training stimulus and the adaptive response. Due to its malleability RE can be easily adapted to suit the attainment of a specific exercise goal. Indeed, small adjustments in the load, velocity and duration of a typical RE movement can substantially alter the physiological response that occurs.

Resistance Exercise Guidelines

As per the latest position statement by the American Diabetes Association (ADA), the adoption and maintenance of PA are critical foci for blood glucose management and overall health maintenance in individuals with T1D (5). Indeed, as part of their core guidelines, the ADA state that individuals with diabetes should engage in 150 min or more of moderate-to-vigorous intensity activity weekly. Guidelines suggest spreading these minutes over 3 days per week, with no more than 2 consecutive days passing without activity. Shorter durations (minimum 75 min per week) of vigorous-intensity or interval sprint training may be sufficient for younger and more physically fit individuals. Furthermore, the specific advocation of RE is included, and details that adults with T1D should engage in 2–3 sessions per week on non-consecutive days. Encouragingly, this also aligns with the latest position stand by the American College of Sports Medicine, who advocate the implementation of RE for each of the major muscle groups on ≥2 days per week in healthy adults (11). Finally, considering the elevated susceptibility to diabetes related complications, the utility, safety and physiological adaptations associated with RE are increasingly important. Due to its ability to train the peripheral muscles without producing extensive cardiovascular stress, dynamic interval based RE, using loads of 50–60% 1-repetition maximum (1RM), has been established as a safe and effective mode of exercise in high cardiovascular disease (CVD) risk cohorts (16).

Despite these advocatory guidelines, there is currently a lack research comprehensively detailing the physiological responses to RE in individuals with T1D (**Table 1**). Moreover, in what little RE-focused research pertinent to T1D that does exist, there is often a lack of program variability, which may overlook important responses to alterations in acute program variables i.e., time under tension, repetition ranges and exercise selection. Furthermore, existing research has mostly explored acute sessions, with participant numbers failing to exceed 15. Finally, the cohorts used have been relatively homogenous, made up of predominately young, relatively healthy, Caucasian male participants. This not only makes wider generalisation difficult, but also overlooks important gender, ethnic and age-related variables.

MORPHOLOGICAL ADAPTATIONS—SKELETAL MUSCLE MASS: BENEFITS BEYOND SIZE

As an extremely heterogeneous tissue with immense plasticity, skeletal muscle influences locomotion, energy metabolism, thermodynamics, endocrine complexes, and cell signalling.

From a clinical perspective, the morphological adaptations induced by RET are associated with reduced rates of chronic inflammation (29–32), lowered global and central adiposity (31, 33), and a reduced risk of falls and fractures (34). Encouragingly, a recent article highlighted the credibility of RET in augmenting myocyte mitochondrial respiratory capacity and function (35). Considering both skeletal muscle insulin resistance and mitochondrial dysfunction are major features

TABLE 1 | Synopsis of the resistance exercise interventions in human participants with type 1 diabetes.

References	Title	Participant characteristics	Exercise characteristics	Main outcome
Durak et al. (17)	Randomized crossover study of effect of resistance training on glycaemic control, muscular strength, and cholesterol in type I diabetic men	***N*** = Eight adults **Age (years):** 31 ± 3.5 **BMI (kg/m^2):** 25.9 ± 0.48 **Gender:** ♂ 8 ♀ 0 **VO$_{2max}$ (ml·kg·min^{-1}):** **HbA1c (%):** **Diabetes duration:** 12.3 ± 9.8	**Intervention:** Chronic **Intervention duration:** 10 weeks. 3* p/w. **Exercise duration**: 60 min **Exercise Modality**: Whole body RE 6 upper body and 4 lower body exercises Major to minor muscle group sequence **Exercise Intensity**: Heavy, progressive RE designed to reach muscular failure in the latter sets. <12 reps per exercise. Total of 40–50 sets during a typical session. Rests between sets ranged from 30 s to 2 min	Glycaemia
Jimenez et al. (18)	Insulin-sensitivity response to a single bout of resistive exercise in type 1 diabetes mellitus	***N*** = Fourteen adults TG: 7 CG: 7 **Age (years):** TG: 23.4 ± 4.0 CG: 26.3 ± 6.7 **BMI (kg/m^2):** TG: 28.3 CG: 24.2 **Gender:** ♂ 11 ♀ 3 **Co-morbidities: -** **Exercise**: Physically active **VO$_{2max}$ (ml·kg·min^{-1}): -** **HbA1c (%):** 6.8 ± 1.5 **Diabetes duration: -**	**Intervention:** Acute **Exercise duration**: **Exercise Modality**: Lower limb **Exercise Intensity**: 80% 5 sets 6 repetitions **Exercise Classification:** Strength	Glycaemia, CVD biomarkers
D'hooge et al. (19)	Influence of combined aerobic and resistance training on metabolic control, cardiovascular fitness and quality of life in adolescents with type 1 diabetes: a randomized controlled trial	***N*** = Sixteen Children **Age (years):** 10–18 **BMI (kg/m^2):** **Gender:** **VO$_{2max}$ (ml·kg·min^{-1}):** **HbA1c (%):** **Diabetes duration:**	**Intervention:** Chronic **Intervention duration:** 20 weeks 2* p/w **Exercise duration**: 70 min **Exercise Modality**: Combined AE and RE **Exercise Intensity**: RE; - 20 RM 0–6 weeks - 17 RM 6–12 weeks - 12 RM 12–20 weeks	Glycaemia, CRF, Quality of Life
Yardley et al. (20) Yardley et al. (21)	Performing resistance exercise before vs. after aerobic exercise influences growth hormone secretion in type 1 diabetes Effects of performing resistance exercise before vs. after aerobic exercise on glycemia in type 1 diabetes	***N*** = Twelve adults **Age (years):** 31.8 ± 15.3 **BMI (kg/m^2):** 25.3 ± 3.0 **Gender:** Mixed ♂ 10 ♀ 2 **VO$_{2max}$ (ml·kg·min^{-1})** 51.2 ± 10.8 **HbA1c (%):**7.1 ± 1.1 **Diabetes duration:** 12.5 ± 10.0	**Intervention:** Acute **Exercise duration**: 45 min **Exercise Modality**: AE before RE (AR) RE before AE (RA) **Exercise Intensity**: AE 60% VO$_{2peak}$ RE: 67% 1RM. 3 sets 10 reps **RE Classification:** Hypertrophy	Glycaemia
Silveira et al. (22)	Acute effects of different intensities of resistance training on glycaemic fluctuations in patients with type 1 diabetes mellitus	***N*** = Twelve adults **Age (years):** 24.4 ± 6.4 **BMI (kg/m^2): 21.3 ± 2.9** **Gender:** ♂ 6 ♀ 6 **VO$_{2max}$ (ml·kg·min^{-1}):** **HbA1c (%):** **Diabetes duration: 7.3 ± 6.8**	**Intervention:** Acute **Exercise duration**: 70 min **Exercise Modality**: RE **Exercise Intensity**: 60% 1RM vs. 89% 1RM	Glycaemia

(Continued)

TABLE 1 | Continued

References	Title	Participant characteristics	Exercise characteristics	Main outcome
Turner et al. (23)	Reductions in resistance exercise-induced hyperglycaemic episodes are associated with circulating interleukin-6 in Type 1 diabetes	***N*** = Eight adults **Age (years):** 38 **BMI (kg/m^2):** 26.9 ± 4.1 **Gender:** Mixed ♂ 7 ♀ 1 **VO_{2max} (ml·kg·min^{-1}):** **HbA1c (%):** 8.7 ±1.0 **Diabetes duration (years):** 15 ±13	**Intervention:** Acute **Exercise duration**: 42 min **Exercise Modality**: Circuit RE Eight whole body exercises **Exercise Intensity**: RE: 67% 1RM. 3 sets 10 reps **RE Classification:** Hypertrophy	Glycaemia and Inflammation
Turner et al. (24)	Impact of single and multiple sets of resistance exercise in type 1 diabetes	***N*** = Eight adults **Age (years):** 38 **BMI (kg/m^2):** 26.9 ± 4.1 **Gender:** Mixed ♂ 7 ♀ 1 **VO_{2max} (ml·kg·min^{-1}):** **HbA1c (%):** 8.7 ±1.0 **Diabetes duration (years):** 15 ±13	**Intervention:** Acute **Exercise duration**: 42 min Set 1 (14 min) Set 2 (28 min) Set 3 (42 min) **Exercise Modality**: Circuit RE Eight whole body exercises **Exercise Intensity:** RE: 67% 1RM. 3 sets 10 reps **RE Classification:** Hypertrophy	Glycaemia
Waclawovsky et al. (25)	Exercise on progenitor cells in healthy subjects and patients with type 1 diabetes	***N*** = Fourteen adults **Age (years):** 30.3 ± 1.6 **BMI (kg/m^2):** 26.2 ± 0.8 **Gender:** ♂ 14 **VO_{2peak} (ml·kg·min^{-1}):** 37.1 ± 1.4 **HbA1c (%):**7.7% ± 0.2 **Diabetes duration (years):** 30 ± 1.6	**Intervention:** Acute **Exercise duration:** 40 min **Exercise Modality:** Combined AE and RE AE (cycle ergometry) RE (four lower limb exercises) **Exercise Intensity:** AE: 40–60% VO_{2max} RE: 60% 1RM **RE Classification:** Hypertrophy	Microvascular
Turner et al. (26)	Similar magnitude of post-exercise hyperglycaemia despite manipulating resistance exercise intensity in type 1 diabetes individuals	***N*** = Eight adults **Age (years):** 34 ± 7 **BMI (kg/m^2):** 25.7 ± 1.6 **Gender:** Mixed ♂ 7 ♀ 1 **VO_{2max} (ml·kg·min^{-1}):** **HbA1c (%):** 8.7 ±1.0 **Diabetes duration (years):** 15 ±13	**Intervention:** Acute **Exercise duration:** 42 min **Exercise Modality**: Circuit RE Six whole body exercises **Exercise Intensity:** 2 sets of 20 reps @ 30% 1RM (LOW) 2 sets of 10 reps @ 60% 1RM (MOD) **RE Classification:** Muscular endurance vs. Hypertrophy	Glycaemia
Zaharieva et al. (27)	The effects of basal insulin suspension at the start of exercise on blood glucose levels during continuous vs. circuit-based exercise in individuals with type 1 diabetes on continuous subcutaneous insulin infusion	***N*** = Twelve adults **Age (years):** 32 **± 11** **BMI (kg/m^2): 23.5** **Gender:** Mixed ♂ 6 ♀ 6 **VO_{2max} (ml·kg·min^{-1}): 50.1 ± 13.7** **HbA1c (%): 7.0 ± 0.9** **Diabetes duration (years):–2–43**	**Intervention:** Acute **Exercise duration:** 40 min **Exercise Modality**: Mixed AE: Treadmill walk RE: Circuit **Exercise Intensity**: AE: 40–50% VO_{2max} RE: HIIE circuit training **Exercise Classification:** Circuit	Glycaemia
Reddy et al. (28)	Effect of aerobic and resistance exercise on glycemic control in adults with type 1 diabetes	***N*** = Ten adults **Age (years):** 33 ± 6 **BMI (kg/m^2):** 24.4 ± 2.1 **Gender:** ♂ **4** ♀ **6** **Co-morbidities: -** **Exercise:** Physically active **VO_{2max} (ml·kg·min^{-1}):** 46.8 ± 11.55 **HbA1c (%):** 7.4% ± 1% **Diabetes duration:** 18 ± 10	**Intervention:** Acute/Training (1 week) Two sessions of RE. Two sessions of AE. Control (no exercise) **Exercise duration**: 45 min **Exercise Modality**: RE: Whole body (Leg press, bench press, leg extension, leg flexion and seated row) AE: Treadmill running **Exercise Intensity**: RE:60–80% 1RM. 3 sets 8-12 repetitions AE: 60% VO_{2max} **Exercise Classification:** RE: Hypertrophy AE: MICE	Glycaemia

N, number of participants; BMI, body mass index; HbA1c, Glycated haemoglobin; RE, Resistance exercise; AE, aerobic exercise; RM, repetition maximum; VO_2, Volume of oxygen consumed; Reps, repetitions.

in the pathogenesis of T1D (36), interventions aimed at stimulating skeletal muscle growth are increasingly important in a diabetic milieu. The importance of preserved skeletal muscle mass is perhaps most evident in reference to age related muscle wasting or "sarcopenia." This pathological derangement decreases the efficiency of several major metabolic processes, thereby accelerates the development risk of metabolic and mitochondrial abnormalities. Skeletal muscle mass is maintained when there is equilibrium between muscle protein synthesis (MPS) and muscle protein breakdown (37). A disturbance in this finite balance during which MPS exceeds the rate of protein breakdown induces skeletal muscle hypertrophy i.e., an increase in muscle size, whilst the opposite is said for atrophy i.e., a decrease in muscle size. The cellular mechanisms responsible for the initiation of growth involves the activation of various anabolic substrates including the phosphatidylinositol 3-kinase (P13K) signaling substrate mammalian target of rapamycin (mTOR) (38). mTOR is a serine/theronin kinase that integrates nutrient and metabolic stimuli to regulate cell growth and proliferation (39, 40). It's activation is dependent on sequential upregulations of P13K, phosphoinositide-dependent kinase (PDK)-1, 70-kDa ribosomal S6 kinase, and the Akt/PKB isoforms (41). Metabolically, mTOR increases glycolytic flux by activating the transcription and the translation of hypoxia inducible factor 1α (HIF1α) (42), whilst Akt facilitates the stimulation of glycogen synthase and formation by inhibiting glycogen synthase kinase-3 (31). HIF1α is an intermediate of several glycolytic and angiogenic genes including both vascular endothelial growth factor (VEGF) and erythropoietin (EPO) (43). VEGF triggers not only divisional but also phenotypical changes of the vascular endothelial cells to alter their migratory capacity and proliferation potential, whilst EPO stimulates erythropoiesis and therefore systemic O_2 delivery. The hypertrophic potential of RE is not novel and its efficacy in substantially increasing rates of MPS in the many hours after exercise engagement are well-established (44). Biochemically, RE is known to evoke a transient increases in the phosphorylation of several of the aforementioned anabolic signalling molecules including mTOR (41), Akt/PKB (45), and 70-kDa ribosomal S6 kinase (45). Conversely, due to its inhibitory effect on several biochemical mediators of MPS, rates are minimal and/or unapparent following MICE. Encouragingly, recent research has demonstrated significant increases in upstream mediators of mTOR (growth hormone) in a volume dependent manner following acute RE in individuals with T1D (24). Since mTOR deregulation (46) and low CRF (47) are reported features of T1D, the biochemical cascades activated in response to appropriately designed RE are particularly noteworthy.

Skeletal Muscle Strength and Fatigability

The functional significance of hypertrophied skeletal muscle is reflected by the accompanied increase in maximal strength and power (48). Muscular strength describes the amount of force a muscle can produce in a single effort, whilst muscular power describes the ability of the muscle to exert that force rapidly. The development of these two physical attributes extends to beyond enhancements in athletic performance. Strong, powerful muscles are necessary for the completion of simple, everyday tasks, which translate to greater independence and autonomy with aging, lower rates of all-cause mortality, enhanced fluidity of movement, and a decreased risk of injury (49). Beyond its pivotal role in locomotion, the clinical significance of hypertrophied muscle is also noted. The associations between reduced skeletal muscle strength and higher rates of clinical biomarkers of CVD are critically important in those with T1D, who are predisposed to a greater incidence of primary CVD throughout the lifespan (50). Indeed, research has highlighted a significantly lower muscle strength and fatigability in those with-vs.-without T1D (51). A physiological explanation for these declines may be evident within the muscle fibre type, since muscle fibre arrangement and/or type has a functional significance on the rate of force production and contraction velocity. Briefly, there exist two broad classifications of muscle fibres, Type 1, and Type II (the latter of which can be further subdivided to include Type IIa and IIx variations). However, it should be noted that whilst useful, these divisions are overly simplistic and do not reflect the reality of fibre type distribution—which includes a heterogenous mix within the skeletal muscle.

Structurally, there appears to be a reduced number of slow-twitch oxidative fibres (Type 1) coupled with an increased amount of the fast-twitch highly fatigable muscle fibres (Type II) in individuals with T1D. Combined, these increase the development of fatigue during maximal exercise and therefore necessitate earlier exercise cessation (52). Supporting these insights, previous work by Crowther and colleagues evidenced a significantly lower muscle pH at rest and at the end of exercise, indicating a greater reliance on glycolytic metabolism in the muscles of individuals with vs.-those-without T1D (53). Moreover, a significantly slower phosphocreatine (PCr) recovery time has been noted in adolescence with-vs.-without T1D, suggesting a reduced skeletal muscle oxidative profile with impaired recovery capacity (36). Whilst an altered skeletal muscle phenotype has been observed in T1D, the severity of these reductions appears to be magnified by the presence of diabetes-related complications. Recent work by Orlando and colleagues illustrated an impairment in the functionality of skeletal muscle in T1D patients with diabetic polyneuropathy (DPN) vs. those with complication free T1D (T1D) and healthy controls (C) (51). Findings revealed the DNP group had lower knee extensor muscle strength than both the T1D (−19%) and the C groups (−37.5%) as well as an elevated (22 and 45%) rate of lower body fatigability than the T1D and C groups, respectively. Critically, RE induces several neural adaptations, including disinhibition of inhibitory mechanisms, as well as improvements in both intra-and-inter-muscular co-ordination. This enhances the synchronisation of motor unit recruitment and firing capacity to facilitate greater levels of maximal force production. These adaptations are proportional to alteration in muscle morphology as seen by increases in muscle cross-sectional area (CSA) accompanied by increases in Type II muscle fibres and altered muscle architecture (fibre pennation) (37). A large part of this process is mediated by the central nervous system which acts as a highly complex control centre that facilitates movement at the molecular level (54).

METABOLIC RESPONSES TO RESISTANCE EXERCISE

T1D is characterised by the progressive depletion and destruction of pancreatic β-cells accompanied with impaired glucagon-producing α-cell function. The resulting deficiency in endogenous insulin secretion manifests in chronic hyperglycemia, with the sequential need for a lifelong reliance on exogenous insulin therapy (55). On the other hand, hypoglycemia represents a perpetual clinical and conventional worry which independently constitutes a primary patient reported barrier to regular exercise participation (56). Therefore, a key consideration for those with T1D whom partake in any physical exercise is the maintenance of blood glucose (BG) control. However, whilst accounted for with little contemplation in regulatory metabolism, the attainment of this outcome requires a degree of diligent pre-planning in those with T1D, for whom variations in exercise modality, intensity, and duration require specific adjustments in therapeutic and feeding strategies in order to mitigate risk.

Glycaemic Responses to Resistance Exercise

The control of BG during exercise involves the integrative co-ordination of two physiological systems (1) the autonomic nervous system (ANS) with particular emphasis on its sympathetic branch (SNS) and (2) the endocrine system (48). At a simplistic level, biochemical mediators released via these systems provide the feed-forward mechanisms that dictate glucose homeostasis. During moderate-to-high-intensity exercise, this feed-forward mechanism induces a rise in glucose concentrations which is primarily driven by hepatic glucose production (HGP). When glucose concentrations begin to fall as a result of sustained exercise efforts, the body produces a strong counter-regulatory response in an attempt to avoid hypoglycemia. This response is driven by the release of counter-regulatory hormones i.e., those that exert opposing actions to those of insulin. Recent work exploring the impact of single and multiple sets of RE on acute glycemic and glucoregulatory parameters has provided valuable endocrinological information in those with T1D (24). Researchers found significant increases in BG concentrations compared to resting conditions following one (+21%) and two (+29%) but not 3 sets of RE. The increases in BG were concurrent with a significant time*interaction effects in plasma catecholamines (noradrenaline and adrenaline). Indeed, peak catecholamine values were 28% greater under the 2nd set than the 1st set, and 17% greater under the 3rd set than the 2nd set. An increase in these two hormones parallels the idea that sympathoadrenergic activity can modulate HGP during exercise (57). Moreover, peak concentrations in growth hormone (GH) were observed during the 3rd (and final) set, which also agrees with work by Kraemer et al. who support the use of high volume session for maximising potential for hypertrophic outcomes (38). Furthermore, the considerable disturbance in acid-base balance observed during this protocol supports the "anaerobic" classification of RE that utilises predominately non-oxidative fuel metabolism via gluconeogenic pathways. Interestingly, despite the increasing hormonal and BG trajectory during the first two sets, the inclusion of a 3rd set produced BG concentrations similar to that of a non-exercise trial (24). It should also be noted that during recovery from 1 to 3 sets of RE, researchers reported no evidence of either exercise-induced hypoglycaemia or requirement for exogenous carbohydrates (CHO) (24). These findings oppose those commonly associated with AE, which typically reduces BG concentrations to a much greater extent (28, 58). Physiologically, the metabolic consequences of non-oxidative glycolytic activity likely contribute to the associated elevations in BG during the post exercise period, thereby offering protection against the onset of post-exercise hypoglycaemia. As a cautionary note, recent research has illustrated an increase in meal intake and after dinner snacking during the 24 h following both aerobic-and-resistance exercise sessions in order to prevent hypoglycaemia (28). Notably, findings highlighted significant reductions in post RE bolus insulin dosing requirements, which were also accompanied by less severe drops in plasma BG concentrations comparative to those recorded following AE (28). Accordingly, current recommendations are to reduce rapid acting insulin dosages alongside side a CHO rich pre-exercise meal (59, 60). This reductive strategy offsets the degree of hyperinsulinemia in people with T1D, which constitutes an inevitable outcome associated with exogenous insulin administration. Metabolically speaking, hyperinsulinemia exerts an inhibitory effect on fat utilisation during exercise, with the subsequently overreliance on CHO oxidation and therefore glucose dependency by the exercising skeletal muscle. Moreover, irrespective of interventional dose manipulations, insulin concentrations often increase during exercise (61). Mechanistically, this is likely due to an increased absorption rate from the subcutaneous tissue depot, together with a decreased clearance rate from at the systemic level. Combined the elevated degree of concentration of circulating of insulin propagates an increased risk of exercise-induced hypoglycaemia, which unsurprisingly prevails as a major barrier to exercise participation (56). Previous work has shown that postprandial exercise is associated with an increased risk of hypoglycemia if the pre-meal insulin dose is not reduced (62). Physiologically, this dose reduction strategy can augment the clearance rate of BG following the digestion of a CHO rich meal, thereby preserving BG concentrations ahead of exercise (62). The avoidance of in-exercise hyperinsulinemia has also been shown to replicate patterns of substrate oxidation and glucose regulation similar to a non-T1D individual (61). Moreover, a reduction in insulin mediated glucose uptake, in combination with elevations in catecholamine concentrations lessens the uptake and subsequent combustion of BG. Consequently, the major fuel substrates can be provided for both HGP and replenishment of muscle glycogen stores (63), such that a preservation effect is observed (64). Directionally, the cost of a slightly higher plasma glucose level before exercise translates to an improved glycemic profile during-and immediately-post-exercise (62).

It should be noted that when the exercise session is predominately reliant on non-oxidative fuel metabolism, post-exercise hyperglycaemia is common (23). The degree to which BG concentrations rise is dependent on several variables and can differ considerably both within and between individuals. Work by Turner and colleagues noted that when matched for volume, a comparable degree of post exercise hyperglycaemia is experienced in both low-and-high intensity morning RE sessions (26). Subsequent work highlighted the efficacy of administering an individualised dose of post-exercise rapid acting insulin in reducing the magnitude and severity of post-exercise hyperglycaemia, without causing early post-exercise hypoglycaemia in those with T1D (65). However, this protective effect waned thereafter, when prevalence rates of hypoglycaemia ensued during the later hours (65). Research has also demonstrated that the omission of pre-exercise bolus, but continuation of basal insulin dosages offers a protective effect against the occurrence of hypoglycaemia during and soon after a fasted bout of morning RE. A direct comparison between glycaemic responses to evening AE and RE in T1D revealed a decline in plasma glucose during a three-set evening RE session (albeit to a lesser extent than observed in the AE trial). Notably, there was also a tendency towards more frequent nocturnal hypoglycaemia following RE which warrants acknowledgment when considering the implementation of post exercise insulin dosing strategies to avoid acute hyperglycaemia. The differences in methodology between these two studies provides potential clues for contrasting glycaemic responses. Nevertheless, the authors concluded that in comparison to AE, RE may result in greater glycaemic stability both during and after exercise in those with T1D (20). Collectively, these data emphasise the need to account for exercise modality for the governance of appropriate insulin and feeding strategies around physical exercise in people with T1D.

Relationships Between Skeletal Muscle, Obesity, and Insulin Resistance

The fact that skeletal muscle tissue is one of the largest organs in the human body, combined with the discovery that contracting skeletal muscle is a multifactorial control centre for the release of various genetic, cytokine and growth-related factors, supports the reasoning behind it's classification as an endocrine organ (31). Due to its mediatory role in promoting skeletal muscle vitality, integrity, and functionality, the potential of RE in influencing the progression or regression of several pathogenic disease states should not be overlooked. Although not historically a condition associated with obesity, there is an alarming percentage of individuals with T1D now categorised as either overweight or obese (66). Whilst intensive insulin therapy is often advocated to counteract poor glycaemic control, aggressive treatment can lead to weight gain, with the subsequent propensity to develop insulin resistance (IR). Worryingly, IR has become a recognised featured of T1D youth, accompanied by compromised exercise capacity and microvascular derangements (36). Moreover, in a study assessing the hemodynamic parameters to maximal exercise in patients with well-controlled T1D, researchers found IR to be inversely associated with cardiac output (67). IR occurs when an inadequate quantities of glucose transporter molecules (namely GLUT-4) migrate to the cell surface following insulin stimulation (31). The translocation site of GLUT-4 is the T-tubules found within the skeletal muscle, which highlights the potential of contracting skeletal muscle to uptake circulating glucose independently of insulin. Thus, whilst not novel, the "insulin-like" properties of skeletal muscle are extremely important in pathologies with metabolic abnormalities. As a fuel source, fat constitutes the most abundant energy pool in mammals and is stored in three major sites; adipose, skeletal muscle, and liver tissue. Each tissue contains depots of triacylglycerol molecules which are hydrolyzed to form fatty acids (FAs) and used as an energy source (31). However, an excessive accumulation of triacylglycerol leads to conditions of hyperlipidemia, with the subsequent propensity to develop IR (68). Skeletal muscle FA metabolism is acutely sensitive to physical exercise which causes substantial increases in intra and extra-cellular FA utilisation (31). Skeletal muscle is a leading consumer of FA from either lipoprotein-triacylglycerol or plasma non-essential fatty acids, and this consumption process rises exponentially during exercise. Finally, as a metabolically active tissue, skeletal muscle plays a pivotal role in maintaining body composition. Acutely, the prolonged window of increased MPS following RE induces elevations in thermogenesis and energy expenditure. Considering that skeletal muscle accounts for ~40% of total body mass and ~30% of basal metabolic rate (BMR) in adult humans (40), hypertrophied skeletal muscle may elevate resting muscle metabolism due to an increased ratio of skeletal muscle mass relative to body weight. Therefore, appropriately programmed exercise programmes that stimulate skeletal muscle hypertrophy may assist in weight reduction and/or management in those with T1D.

CARDIO-VASCULAR RESPONSES TO RESISTANCE EXERCISE

For individuals with T1D, CVD is a major cause of morbidity and mortality and unsurprisingly constitutes a serious health concern that demands a prevention rather than treatment approach (69–71). Encouragingly, recent research has acknowledged the credibility of RE in reducing several CVD risk factors as well as improving various biomarkers of cardio-metabolic health (albeit it in a non-T1D cohorts) (72, 73). Although sparse, research has emphasised the efficacy of RET in improving traditional indices of CVD in people with T1D, including glycaemic and lipid related parameters (17). Furthermore, increases in heart rate (24, 26) and forearm reactive hyperaemia (25) have been reported following RE in individuals with T1D. Physiologically, the hypertrophic and angiogenic potential of RE is perhaps magnified in importance during circumstances where blood flow maybe compromised due to pathological abnormalities. Supporting this concept, researchers observed greater improvements in blood flow following lower limb RE vs. AE in individuals with T1D (25). However, these peripheral based improvements have thus far failed to correspond with improvements in cellular indices of vascular function. Indeed, a blunted circulating endothelial progenitor cell (cEPC) response has presented regardless of exercise modality, perhaps reflecting derangements in the microvascular domains. Although it should be noted that existing literature has thus far employed mostly MICE (74) and/or submaximal-lower limb RE (25).

SKELETAL MUSCLE: IMPORTANT MICRO-VASCULAR AND ANGIOGENIC POTENTIALS

Prevalence rates of circulatory disease in people with T1D are extensive and at a population level constitute a leading cause of mortality (50). The pathophysiological mechanism responsible for the compromised circulatory system is most evident by the presence of abnormalities in the form and function of the blood vessels (50, 75, 76). Thus, whilst the identification of classical CVD risk factors provides valuable information as to an individual's current CVD vulnerability, they often fail to identify risk in its infancy and/or in those who appear to be asymptomatic. As such, physiological defects can go unrecognised until manifested as irreversible and/or severe acute complications within blood vessels including the presentation of endothelial dysfunction. Whilst the pathogenesis of macro-and-micro-vascular disease is multifactorial, the common recipient of injury is the vascular endothelium; a monolayer of cells that lines the blood vessels. Occupying a strategically important location between circulating blood and the surrounding tissues, the endothelium modulates the tone of the underlying vascular smooth muscle, maintains a non-adhesive luminal surface, mediates homeostasis, evokes cellular proliferation, and modulates inflammatory and immune mechanisms within the vascular wall (77). The functionality of the endothelium is mediated by a tightly regulated balance between the intermediates that induce cell damage i.e., pro-constrictive, pro-inflammatory, pro-thrombotic, and pro-hypertensive factors and the intermediates that support cell vitality i.e., pro-relaxation, anti-inflammatory, anti-thrombotic, and anti-hypertensive factors. Skeletal muscle hosts several sources of these vitality promoting intermediates, including the erythrocytes (which produce ATP and Nitric Oxide [NO]), the endothelial cells (which produce ATP, NO, and Prostacyclin [PGI_2]), the skeletal muscle cells (which produce ATP, NO, and adenosine). Thus, during skeletal muscle contraction, there is an increased turnover of various vasodilatory factors that encourage blood flow and vascular repair processes. Indeed, the co-operative intimacy between skeletal muscle and its surrounding vasculature is made clear by the proximity of capillaries embedded in grooves indenting the sarcolemma and expanding the contact area between myocytes and endothelial cells (78). Muscle fibre mitochondria also appear to cluster along these groves, thereby shortening the travelling distance of O_2 and various nutrients required for diffusion (78). The complex and intermate interaction between the biochemistry of the vascular endothelium, the vascular smooth muscle cells (VSMCs) and the skeletal muscle fibres emphasises the importance of endothelial vitality. Endothelial derangements proposedly contribute to the chronic under perfusion of skeletal muscle, resulting in suboptimal delivery and uptake of various nutrients, hormones and gaseous exchange. Indeed, these findings are somewhat consistent within the literature with research detailing higher rates of leg muscle deoxygenation (79), and altered red blood cell dynamics associated with the T1D milieu (80).

Mechanistically, microvascular abnormalities may be a result of lower skeletal muscle capillary density in individuals with T1D (81) which would agree with the aforementioned muscle fibre phenotype associated with T1D. Collectively, these attributes may contribute to a reduced circulatory ability to increase O_2 delivery to exercising muscle. This may explain the lower rates of regular physical activity (56) as well as the earlier onset of fatigue observed in T1D during exercise testing where O_2 delivery contributes to fatigue (82). Inefficient O_2 and nutrient supply may also impact the vascular tone of skeletal muscle. Vascular responses to light exercise provide insight into the hierarchical regulation of muscle perfusion. With light exercise, vasomotion within the terminal arterioles appears to cease, and the number of perfused capillary increases without significant changes in total muscle blood flow. Thus, during MICE, there is less of an increase in shear stresses traversing over the vessel lumen than during higher intensity exercise. During higher intensity exercise, or following ischemia, under-perfused capillaries are recruited to ensure an increase muscle perfusion. Indeed, in people with T1D, 7 weeks of high-intensity sprint training has been shown reduced metabolic fluctuations and enhance muscle oxidative metabolism (83). Thus, as a major storage site of several nutrients including glucose, amino acids, and free fatty acids, skeletal muscle also plays an integral role in substrate provision during hypoxic or anaerobic conditions.

These insights suggest a credible role for exercise modalities that utilise compound movements performed at high intensity effort as a strategy for re-endothelisation. Perhaps, as a reflection of its capacity to induce ischemia and muscle microtrauma, exhaustive or eccentric exercise protocols including downhill running and RE appear to cause the greatest stress responses. The acute physiological "stress" experienced during these sessions augments the production and release of several mediators of re-endothelisation including stromal cell-derived factor 1 (SDF-1) (84) and VEGF (85). Upon activation, these proteins mediate progenitor cell mobilisation, proliferation, and migration (86). One of the most potent upstream mediators of EPC proliferation is VEGF, which is primarily known for its mediatory role in the (i) sprouting and (ii) intussusceptive splitting of capillary beds to form angiogenesis. Recent research has shown considerable elevations in VEGF concentrations within both skeletal muscle and the peripheral circulation following intense RE (87, 88). As such, the potential of exercise to induce local angiogenesis may assist in the prevention of ischemia within its surrounding tissue (43). Considering the decreased perfusion rates and increased atherosclerotic tendencies associated with T1D, the angiogenic potential of RE in this population is important.

OSTEOPATHIC RESPONSES TO RESISTANCE EXERCISE

The term "osteoporosis" describes inelasticity within the skeletal system when exposed to the habitual subjection of forces experienced during joint movement, locomotion, and loading. Bone mineral density (BMD) is used as a reference of bone mineralisation within bone tissue and is substantially influenced by endocrine activity. The endocrine and metabolic disturbances associated with T1D are hypothesised to contribute to higher rates of poor bone quality noted within the literature (89–91). Biochemically, T1D is associated with reductions in the anabolic agents of bone formation including IGF-1 and transforming growth factor beta 1 (TGFβ1), which initiate a potent stimulatory effect on the synthesis of bone-specific proteins and osteoblastic proliferation potential (92). Moreover, the downstream complications associated with hyperglycaemia including the direct inhibition of osteoblast activity, osmotic damage to osteoblasts, increased peroxisome proliferator-activated receptor activity and low microvascular proliferative capacity, may increase susceptibility to osteoporosis and fracture risk.

Physiologically, bones adapt to loading stimuli by upregulating osteoblast activity in the areas experiencing mechanical strain. With this in mind, the essence of RE may offer support against the poor bone quality sometimes observed in T1D. Supporting this concept, T1D centred paediatric research noted increases in both lean body mass (LBM) and BMD following 9-months of weight bearing activity (93). These physiological adaptations are mutually connected, since there seems to be a stoichiometric relationship between muscle and bone. Indeed, bone architecture depends critically on muscle CSA and tension development (94), whilst muscle immobilization, and/or detraining leads to bone mass loss (95). Moreover, exercises that require large rates of muscular force cause greater bone-related benefits than do isometric or low force exercises (94, 96–98). Conversely, extreme endurance and/or low load bearing activities may exasperate the degradation of bone quality and health (99, 100). Researchers have documented losses in bone mass during the competitive seasons in endurance cycling (100) whilst increases in bone mass are ascertained during the competitive seasons of gymnastics (95). Further research is needed to progress our understanding of the osteopathic responses to RE in individuals with T1D.

RECOMMENDATIONS FOR RESISTANCE EXERCISE IN TYPE 1 DIABETES

There are several acute manipulations which can substantially influence the outcome induced by RE. Indeed, DeLorme's classic work suggested that RET using low repetition/high resistance favoured adaptations for strength, power, and hypertrophy, whereas training with high repetition/low resistance increased muscular endurance and oxidative potential (101). From this, a repetition training continuum (102) or repetition maximum continuum (103) has been hypothesised such that the number of repetitions allowed by the resistance will result in very specific training adaptations. In order to enable a clear outline of program design, early work by Bird et al. (104) collated this information and created a visual representation of RE prescription. A modified version of this template that emphasises the points relevant to this review is included below (**Figure 2**).

Considering the focus of this review has emphasised the importance of skeletal muscle size the practical recommendations to follow will reflect the attainment of muscular hypertrophy. Skeletal muscle experiences the increases in size and strength when forced to contract at maximal or near-maximal efforts. Indeed, the rate of MPS is driven by the intracellular availability of amino acids—a factor which is influenced directly by the intensity and duration of muscle tension. With overall session intensity in mind, early research by Kramer and colleagues concluded that the combined effects of a higher volume, moderate intensity session with shorter rest periods provides a favourable hormonal milieu for promoting skeletal muscle growth (38). Thus, to maximise intensity, rests between exercises and sets should therefore be kept minimal (30–60 s) to maintain an elevated skeletal O_2 demand that requires the use of predominately non-oxidative fuel metabolism.

Furthermore, the duration of muscular contraction significantly contributes to the phenotypic response. This process describes the "*tempo*" or time of the muscular contraction and is typically expressed in seconds. Moderate (2 s CON; 2 s ECC) and fast (1 s CON; 1 s ECC) velocities have been shown to maximise hormonal responses (105) and result in substantial metabolic cost (106). Classically the optimal repetition range for muscular hypertrophy is between 8 and 12. Initially, 2–3 sets may be enough for the untrained individual, however this should progress to >3 sets as with progressive overload. Moreover, programs that demand the simultaneous recruitment of large muscle groups traversing multiple joints in both the lower and upper body segments are advised. In this context, a program that emphasises compound movements towards the start of the session (when the muscle is in a "rested" state so can produce maximal force without fatigue), with isolated work grouped towards the end of a session is advised. In terms of exercise frequency, recommendations provided by the ADA (5) state that RE sessions aimed at skeletal muscle hypertrophy should be performed a minimum of twice but ideally thrice weekly.

Undertaking divergent exercise i.e., RE and MICE in close proximity may cause an "interference" effect on several of the acute molecular responses that orchestrate the adaptive phenotype. For example, activation of AMPK signalling in response to endurance exercise can block or dampen rates of MPS via its inhibitory effect on translation initiation and elongation (107). Moreover, the activation of AMPK is augmented in response to nutrient stress; particularly glycogen depletion; emphasising the need to acknowledge dietary considerations around exercise sessions. Thus, in an attempt to maximise MPS, individuals may wish to avoid both energy stress (increases in carbohydrate and amino acid feeding around exercise) and the concurrent practice of endurance and resistive exercise in close proximity (108).

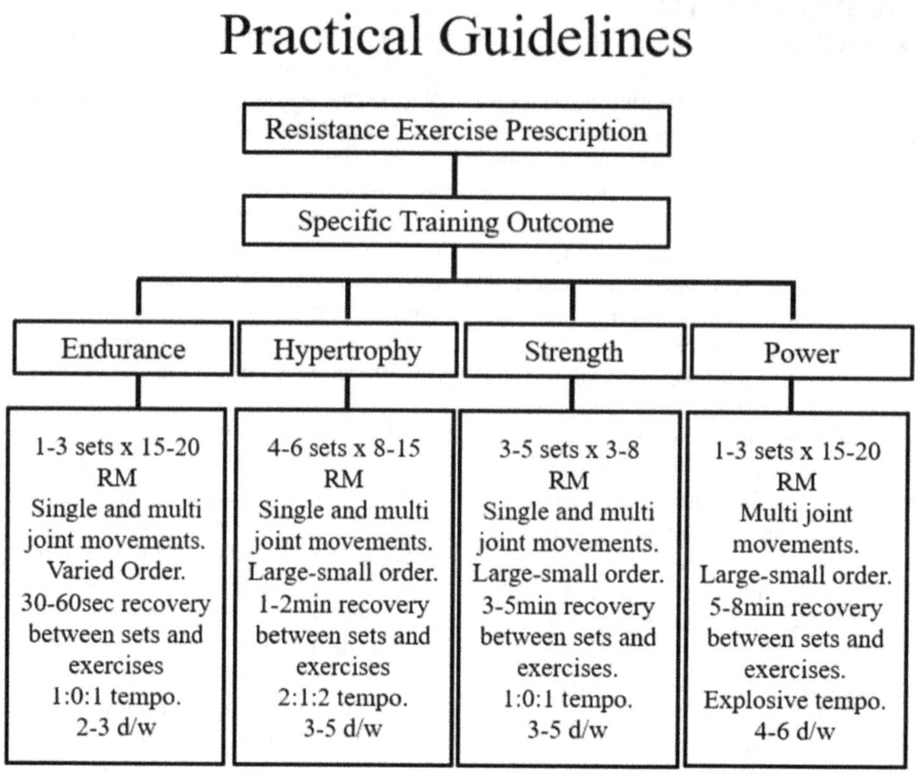

FIGURE 2 | Proper programme design of resistance exercise for specific training outcomes incorporates the acute programme variables and key training principles. ECC, Eccentric; CON, Concentric; ISO, Isometric; Ex, exercise; Sec, seconds; RM, repetition maximum; Btn, Between; d/wk, Days per week. Figure adapted from Bird et al. [(104), Figure 2]. Springer Nature.

Clearly exercise carries impactful glycaemic connotations for individuals with T1D. However, factors including the type, intensity and duration of exercise as well as the level of on-board exogenous insulin can considerably affect the glycemic responses that occur. Due to the pharmacological administration of exogenous insulin therapy, people with T1D frequently engage in exercise under markedly hyperinsulinemic conditions, thus are exposed to a greater risk of hypoglycaemia (62). As such, exercise often poses a glycaemic challenge which must be performed with a degree of contingency planning to both lifestyle and therapeutic strategies. It is prudent to suggest than insulin reductions and/or carbohydrate intake in the pre-and-post exercise periods are important features that need careful consideration with reference to BG values to appropriately manage glycemia. Exercise while fasting may produce a lesser decrease or indeed smaller increase in BG (65). It is advisory that BG is checked frequently in the hours pre, during and post exercise in order to govern safe and effective decisions regarding CHO feeding and insulin administration (5). RE induced hyperglycaemia risk can be abated by interspersing intense lifting efforts with lower intensity aerobic efforts (109) and/or combing RE (completed first) with AE (completed second) to optimize glycaemic stability (110). Further studies are needed to investigate the glycaemic impact of alterations in rapid-acting insulin strategies according to the type, intensity, and duration of the intended RE session.

FUTURE RESEARCH

Intuitively, the implementation of RE, a predominately glycolytic exercise that can be programmed to achieve global conditioning characterises a compelling therapeutic strategy that can be employed to improve several complications associated with T1D. However, despite the wider health merits associated with RE, a clear research emphasis has been placed on MICE with glycemia as its primary outcome.

In the existing RE specific research, program design has orientated around primarily hypertrophy or strength related outcomes, with less work investigating muscular endurance and/or power regimes for raising daily background levels of physical activity. In light of recent research emphasising the angiogenic potential of muscular endurance resistance exercise (MERE); during which healthy participants exercised to-or-near-to muscular failure (88), there presents a compelling rationale to employ these strategies in T1D by means of augmenting skeletal muscle angiogenesis. Indeed, the angiogenic and re-endothelialisation potential of MERE is particularly noted in this patient cohort, for whom circulatory complications are frequently observed (50). Moreover, considering the aforementioned alterations in the bioenergetics of skeletal muscle associated with T1D, the neuromuscular adaptations associated with moderate-to-heavy strength RE which incorporates a mixture of isometric and isokinetic movements i.e., greater motor unit recruitment, increased discharge rate modulation, larger muscle cross section area and changes in muscle architecture, are duly noted. Future research that explores the physiological responses to RE that *varies* in several of the aforementioned acute and chronic training variables would not only deepen our understanding from a research perspective but offer much clinical and patient relevance that may help develop healthcare guidelines specific to those with T1D.

CONCLUSION

The importance of skeletal muscle strength and size extends far beyond it aesthetic and/or athletic performance value. Indeed, skeletal muscle plays an indispensable role in several key physiological processes including locomotion, hemodynamics, thermodynamics, cell signaling, and energy metabolism. Thus, the clinical merit of strategies that assist the maintenance and/or development of skeletal muscle are deserving of wider healthcare attention in patient populations. As a key determinant of muscle size and strength, the rate of MPS is critical for the development and/or preservation of skeletal muscle mass. This review has highlighted the potential of RE in upregulating the activity of several key biochemical and molecular signalling pathways that augment rates of MPS, including the PI3K/Akt/mTOR signalling pathway. Perhaps most importantly, the wider metabolic, vascular and respiratory roles of skeletal muscle each have particular relevance for individuals with T1D, whom are predisposed to greater pathological risk within these systems by virtue of the condition. Thus, the positive, adaptive health benefits associated with the hypertrophic and strength benefits accompanied with RE should be promoted as a necessary adjunct to standard diabetes care.

AUTHOR CONTRIBUTIONS

OlM: investigation and writing—original draft. OtM and RB: validation. OlM, RB, OtM, ME, RD, JP, and SB: writing—review and editing.

REFERENCES

1. Bohn B, Herbst A, Pfeifer M, Krakow D, Zimny S, Kopp F, et al. Impact of physical activity on glycemic control and prevalence of cardiovascular risk factors in adults with type 1 diabetes: a cross-sectional multicenter study of 18,028 patients. *Diabetes Care.* (2015) 38:1536–43. doi: 10.2337/dc15-0030
2. Riddell MC, Perkins BA. Type 1 diabetes and vigorous exercise: applications of exercise physiology to patient management. *Can J Diabetes.* (2006) 30:63–71. doi: 10.1016/S1499-2671(06)01010-0
3. Granata C, Jamnick NA, Bishop DJ. Principles of exercise prescription, and how they influence exercise-induced changes of transcription factors and other regulators of mitochondrial biogenesis. *Sport Med.* (2018) 48:1541–59. doi: 10.1007/s40279-018-0933-1
4. Moy CS, Songer TJ, LaPorte RE, Dorman JS, Kriska AM, Orchard TJ, et al. Insulin-dependent diabetes mellitus, physical activity, and death. *Am J Epidemiol.* (1993) 137:74–81. doi: 10.1093/oxfordjournals.aje.a116604
5. Colberg SR, Sigal RJ, Yardley JE, Riddell MC, Dunstan DW, Dempsey PC, et al. Physical activity/exercise and diabetes: a position statement of the American Diabetes Association. *Diabetes Care.* (2016) 39:2065–79. doi: 10.2337/dc16-1728
6. Kriska AM, LaPorte RE, Patrick SL, Kuller LH, Orchard TJ. The association of physical activity and diabetic complications in individuals with insulin-dependent diabetes mellitus: the Epidemiology of Diabetes Complications Study–VII. *J Clin Epidemiol.* (1991) 44:1207–14. doi: 10.1016/0895-4356(91)90153-Z
7. LaPorte RE, Dorman JS, Tajima N, Cruickshanks KJ, Orchard TJ, Cavender DE, et al. Pittsburgh insulin-dependent diabetes mellitus morbidity and mortality study: physical activity and diabetic complications. *Pediatrics.* (1986) 78:1027–33.
8. Edmunds S, Roche D, Stratton G, Wallymahmed K, Glenn SM. Physical activity and psychological well-being in children with Type 1 diabetes. *Psychol Health Med.* (2007) 12:353–63. doi: 10.1080/13548500600975446
9. Imayama I, Plotnikoff RC, Courneya KS, Johnson JA. Determinants of quality of life in adults with type 1 and type 2 diabetes. *Health Qual Life Outcomes.* (2011) 9:115. doi: 10.1186/1477-7525-9-115
10. Codella R, Terruzzi I, Luzi L. Why should people with type 1 diabetes exercise regularly? *Acta Diabetol.* (2017) 54:615–30. doi: 10.1007/s00592-017-0978-x
11. Garber CE, Blissmer B, Deschenes MR, Franklin BA, Lamonte MJ, Lee IM, et al. Quantity and quality of exercise for developing and maintaining cardiorespiratory, musculoskeletal, and neuromotor fitness in apparently healthy adults. *Med Sci Sport Exerc.* (2011) 43:1334–59. doi: 10.1249/MSS.0b013e318213fefb
12. Baldi JC, Cassuto NA, Foxx-Lupo WT, Wheatley CM, Snyder EM. Glycemic status affects cardiopulmonary exercise response in athletes with type I diabetes. *Med Sci Sport Exerc.* (2010) 42:1454–9. doi: 10.1249/MSS.0b013e3181d1fdb3
13. Moser O, Eckstein ML, McCarthy O, Deere R, Bain SC, Haahr HL, et al. Poor glycaemic control is associated with reduced exercise performance and oxygen economy during cardio-pulmonary exercise testing in people with type 1 diabetes. *Diabetol Metab Syndr.* (2017) 9:93. doi: 10.1186/s13098-017-0294-1
14. Moser O, Eckstein ML, McCarthy O, Deere R, Bain SC, Haahr HL, et al. Heart rate dynamics during cardio-pulmonary exercise testing are associated with glycemic control in individuals with type 1 diabetes. *PLoS ONE.* (2018) 13:e0194750. doi: 10.1371/journal.pone.0194750
15. Parolin ML, Chesley A, Matsos MP, Spriet LL, Jones NL, Heigenhauser GJ. Regulation of skeletal muscle glycogen phosphorylase and PDH during maximal intermittent exercise. *Am. J. Physiol.* (1999) 277:E890-900. doi: 10.1152/ajpendo.1999.277.5.E890
16. Volaklis KA, Tokmakidis SP. Resistance exercise training in patients with heart failure. *Sports Med.* (2005) 35:1085–103. doi: 10.2165/00007256-200535120-00006
17. Durak EP, Jovanovic-Peterson L, Peterson CM. Randomized crossover study of effect of resistance training on glycemic control, muscular strength, and cholesterol in type I diabetic men. *Diabetes Care.* (1990) 13:1039–43. doi: 10.2337/diacare.13.10.1039
18. Jimenez C, Santiago M, Sitler M, Boden G, Homko C. Insulin-sensitivity response to a single bout of resistive exercise in type 1 diabetes. *J Sport Rehabil.* (2009) 18:564–71. doi: 10.1123/jsr.18.4.564
19. D'hooge R, Hellinckx T, Van Laethem C, Stegen S, De Schepper J, Van Aken S, et al. Influence of combined aerobic and resistance training on metabolic control, cardiovascular fitness and quality of life in adolescents with type 1 diabetes: a randomized controlled trial. *Clin Rehabil.* (2011) 25:349–59. doi: 10.1177/0269215510386254
20. Yardley JE, Kenny GP, Perkins BA, Riddell MC, Balaa N, Malcolm J, et al. Resistance vs. aerobic exercise: acute effects on glycemia in type 1 diabetes - ProQuest. *Diabetes Care.* (2013) 36:537–42. doi: 10.2337/dc12-0963
21. Yardley JE, Kenny GP, Perkins BA, Riddell MC, Malcolm J, Boulay P, et al. Effects of performing resistance exercise before vs. after aerobic exercise on glycemia in type 1 diabetes. *Diabetes Care.* (2012) 35:669–75. doi: 10.2337/dc11-1844

22. Silveira AP, Bentes CM, Costa PB, Simão R, Silva FC, Silva RP, et al. Acute effects of different intensities of resistance training on glycemic fluctuations in patients with type 1 diabetes mellitus. *Res Sport Med.* (2014) 22:75–87. doi: 10.1080/15438627.2013.852096
23. Turner D, Luzio S, Kilduff LP, Gray BJ, Dunseath G, Bain SC, et al. Reductions in resistance exercise-induced hyperglycaemic episodes are associated with circulating interleukin-6 in Type 1 diabetes. *Diabet Med.* (2014) 31:1009–13. doi: 10.1111/dme.12462
24. Turner D, Luzio S, Gray BJ, Dunseath G, Rees ED, Kilduff LP, et al. Impact of single and multiple sets of resistance exercise in type 1 diabetes. *Scand J Med Sci Sports.* (2015) 25:e99–e109. doi: 10.1111/sms.12202
25. Waclawovsky G, Umpierre D, Figueira FR, De Lima ES, Alegretti AP, Schneider L, et al. Exercise on progenitor cells in healthy subjects and patients with type 1 diabetes. *Am Coll Sport Med.* (2015) 48:190–9. doi: 10.1249/MSS.0000000000000764
26. Turner D, Gray BJ, Luzio S, Dunseath G, Bain SC, Hanley S, et al. Similar magnitude of post-exercise hyperglycemia despite manipulating resistance exercise intensity in type 1 diabetes individuals. *Scand J Med Sci Sports.* (2016) 26:404–12. doi: 10.1111/sms.12472
27. Zaharieva D, Yavelberg L, Jamnik V, Cinar A, Turksoy K, Riddell MC. The effects of basal insulin suspension at the start of exercise on blood glucose levels during continuous vs. circuit-based exercise in individuals with type 1 diabetes on continuous subcutaneous insulin infusion. *Diabetes Technol Ther.* (2017) 19:370–8. doi: 10.1089/dia.2017.0010
28. Reddy R, Wittenberg A, Castle JR, El Youssef J, Winters-Stone K, Gillingham M, et al. Effect of aerobic and resistance exercise on glycemic control in adults with type 1 diabetes. *Can J Diabetes.* (2018) 43:406–14.e1. doi: 10.1016/j.jcjd.2018.08.193
29. Mccall GE, Byrnes WC, Dickinson A, Pattany PM, Fleck SJ. Muscle fiber hypertrophy, hyperplasia, and capillary density in college men after resistance training. *J Appl Physiol.* (1996) 81:2004–12. doi: 10.1152/jappl.1996.81.5.2004
30. Kemi OJ, Haram PM, Loennechen JP, Osnes JB, Skomedal T, Wisløff U, et al. Moderate vs. high exercise intensity: differential effects on aerobic fitness, cardiomyocyte contractility, and endothelial function. *Cardiovasc Res.* (2005) 67:161–72. doi: 10.1016/j.cardiores.2005.03.010
31. Wagenmakers AJM. *The Biochemical Basis of the Health Effects of Exercise.* London: Portland Press (2006).
32. Morici G, Zangla D, Santoro A, Pelosi E, Petrucci E, Gioia M, et al. Supramaximal exercise mobilizes hematopoietic progenitors and reticulocytes in athletes. *AJP Regul Integr Comp Physiol.* (2005) 289:R1496–R1503. doi: 10.1152/ajpregu.00338.2005
33. Reid CM, Yeater RA, Ullrich IH. Weight training and strength, cardiorespiratory functioning and body composition of men. *Br J Sports Med.* (1987) 21:40–4. doi: 10.1136/bjsm.21.1.40
34. Siegrist M. Role of physical activity in the prevention of osteoporosis. *Med Monatsschr Pharm.* (2008) 31:259–264.
35. Porter C, Reidy PT, Bhattarai N, Sidossis LS, Rasmussen BB. Resistance exercise training alters mitochondrial function in human skeletal muscle. *Med Sci Sports Exerc.* (2015) 47:1922–31. doi: 10.1249/MSS.0000000000000605
36. Cree-Green M, Newcomer BR, Brown MS, Baumgartner AD, Bergman B, Drew B, et al. Delayed skeletal muscle mitochondrial ADP recovery in youth with type 1 diabetes relates to muscle insulin resistance. *Diabetes.* (2015) 64:383–92. doi: 10.2337/db14-0765
37. Cardinale M, Newton RU, Nosaka K. *Strength and Conditioning : Biological Principles and Practical Applications.* Chichester: John Wiley & Sons (2011).
38. Kraemer WJ, Gordon SE, Fleck SJ, Marchitelli LJ, Mello R, Dziados JE, et al. Endogenous anabolic hormonal and growth factor responses to heavy resistance exercise in males and females. *Int J Sports Med.* (1991) 12:228–35. doi: 10.1055/s-2007-1024673
39. Cho H, Mu J, Kim JK, Thorvaldsen JL, Chu Q, Crenshaw EB III, et al. Insulin resistance and a diabetes mellitus-like syndrome in mice lacking the protein kinase Akt2 (PKBbeta). *Science.* (2001) 292:1728–31. doi: 10.1126/science.292.5522.1728
40. Egan B, Zierath JR. Exercise metabolism and the molecular regulation of skeletal muscle adaptation. *Cell Metab.* (2013) 17:162–84. doi: 10.1016/j.cmet.2012.12.012
41. Parkington JD, Siebert AP, LeBrasseur NK, Fielding RA. Differential activation of mTOR signaling by contractile activity in skeletal muscle. *Am J Physiol Integr Comp Physiol.* (2003) 285:R1086–R1090. doi: 10.1152/ajpregu.00324.2003
42. Ribeiro F, Ribeiro IP, Gonçalves AC, Alves AJ, Melo E, Fernandes R, et al. Effects of resistance exercise on endothelial progenitor cell mobilization in women. *Sci Rep.* (2017) 7:17880. doi: 10.1038/s41598-017-18156-6
43. Golbidi S, Laher I. Exercise and the cardiovascular system. *Cardiol Res Pract.* (2012) 2012:1–15. doi: 10.1155/2012/210852
44. Chesley A, MacDougall JD, Tarnopolsky MA, Atkinson SA, Smith K. Changes in human muscle protein synthesis after resistance exercise. *J Appl Physiol.* (1992) 73:1383–8. doi: 10.1152/jappl.1992.73.4.1383
45. Nader GA, Esser KA. Intracellular signaling specificity in skeletal muscle in response to different modes of exercise. *J Appl Physiol.* (2001) 90:1936–42. doi: 10.1152/jappl.2001.90.5.1936
46. Gordon CS, Serino AS, Krause MP, Campbell JE, Cafarelli E, Adegoke OA, et al. Impaired growth and force production in skeletal muscles of young partially pancreatectomized rats: a model of adolescent type 1 diabetic myopathy? *PLoS ONE.* (2010) 5:e14032. doi: 10.1371/journal.pone.0014032
47. Williams BK, Guelfi KJ, Jones TW, Davis EA. Lower cardiorespiratory fitness in children with Type 1 diabetes. *Diabet Med.* (2011) 28:1005–7. doi: 10.1111/j.1464-5491.2011.03271.x
48. Brooks GA, Fahey TD, Baldwin KM. *Exercise Physiology : Human Bioenergetics and Its Applications.* New York, NY: McGraw-Hill (2005).
49. Ruiz JR, Sui X, Lobelo F, Morrow JR, Jackson AW, Sjöström M, et al. Association between muscular strength and mortality in men: prospective cohort study. *BMJ.* (2008) 337:a439. doi: 10.1136/bmj.a439
50. Livingstone SJ, Looker HC, Hothersall EJ, Wild SH, Lindsay RS, Chalmers J, et al. Risk of cardiovascular disease and total mortality in adults with type 1 diabetes: Scottish Registry Linkage Study. *PLoS Med.* (2012) 9:e1001321. doi: 10.1371/journal.pmed.1001321
51. Orlando G, Balducci S, Bazzucchi I, Pugliese G, Sacchetti M. The impact of type 1 diabetes and diabetic polyneuropathy on muscle strength and fatigability. *Acta Diabetol.* (2017) 54:543–50. doi: 10.1007/s00592-017-0979-9
52. Andreassen CS, Jensen JM, Jakobsen J, Ulhøj BP, Andersen H. Striated muscle fiber size, composition, and capillary density in diabetes in relation to neuropathy and muscle strength. *J Diabetes.* (2014) 6:462–71. doi: 10.1111/1753-0407.12124
53. Crowther GJ, Milstein JM, Jubrias SA, Kushmerick MJ, Gronka RK, Conley KE. Altered energetic properties in skeletal muscle of men with well-controlled insulin-dependent (type 1) diabetes. *Am J Physiol Metab.* (2003) 284:E655–E662. doi: 10.1152/ajpendo.00343.2002
54. Carroll TJ, Riek S, Carson RG. Neural adaptations to resistance training. *Sport Med.* (2001) 31:829–40. doi: 10.2165/00007256-200131120-00001
55. Atkinson MA, Eisenbarth GS. Type 1 diabetes: new perspectives on disease pathogenesis and treatment. *Lancet.* (2001) 358:221–9. doi: 10.1016/S0140-6736(01)05415-0
56. Brazeau A-S, Rabasa-Lhoret R, Strychar I, Mircescu H. Barriers to physical activity among patients with type 1 diabetes. *Diabetes Care.* (2008) 31:2108–9. doi: 10.2337/dc08-0720
57. Hargreaves M, Spriet LL. *Exercise Metabolism.* (2006). Available online at: https://uk.humankinetics.com/products/exercise-metabolism-2nd-edition (accessed August 12, 2018).
58. Yardley JE. *The Acute Effects of Aerobic and Resistance Exercise on Blood Glucose Levels in Type 1 Diabetes.* (2011). Available online at: https://ruor.uottawa.ca/bitstream/10393/20031/5/Yardley_Jane_Elizabeth_2011_thesis.pdf (accessed January 8, 2018).
59. West DJ, Stephens JW, Bain SC, Kilduff LP, Luzio S, Still R, et al. A combined insulin reduction and carbohydrate feeding strategy 30 min before running best preserves blood glucose concentration after exercise through improved fuel oxidation in type 1 diabetes mellitus. *J Sports Sci.* (2011) 29:279–89. doi: 10.1080/02640414.2010.531753

60. Campbell MD, Walker M, Trenell MI, Luzio S, Dunseath G, Tuner D, et al. Metabolic implications when employing heavy pre- and post-exercise rapid-acting insulin reductions to prevent hypoglycaemia in type 1 diabetes patients: a randomised clinical trial. *PLoS ONE.* (2014) 9:e97143. doi: 10.1371/journal.pone.0097143
61. Chokkalingam K, Tsintzas K, Norton L, Jewell K, Macdonald IA, Mansell PI. Exercise under hyperinsulinaemic conditions increases whole-body glucose disposal without affecting muscle glycogen utilisation in type 1 diabetes. *Diabetologia.* (2007) 50:414–21. doi: 10.1007/s00125-006-0520-0
62. Rabasa-Lhoret R, Bourque J, Ducros F, Chiasson JL. Guidelines for premeal insulin dose reduction for postprandial exercise of different intensities and durations in type 1 diabetic subjects treated intensively with a basal-bolus insulin regimen (ultralente-lispro). *Diabetes Care.* (2001) 24:625–30. doi: 10.2337/diacare.24.4.625
63. Steppel JH, Horton ES. Exercise in the management of type 1 diabetes mellitus. *Rev Endocr Metab Disord.* (2003) 4:355–60. doi: 10.1023/A:1027302112655
64. Cryer PE, Davis SN, Shamoon H. Hypoglycemia in diabetes. *Diabetes Care.* (2003) 26:1902–12. doi: 10.2337/diacare.26.6.1902
65. Turner D, Luzio S, Gray BJ, Bain SC, Hanley S, Richards A, et al. Algorithm that delivers an individualized rapid-acting insulin dose after morning resistance exercise counters post-exercise hyperglycaemia in people with Type 1 diabetes. *Diabet Med.* (2016) 33:506–10. doi: 10.1111/dme.12870
66. Conway B, Miller RG, Costacou T, Fried L, Kelsey S, Evans RW, et al. Temporal patterns in overweight and obesity in Type 1 diabetes. *Diabet Med.* (2010) 27:398–404. doi: 10.1111/j.1464-5491.2010.02956.x
67. Niedzwiecki P, Naskret D, Pilacinski S, Pempera M, Uruska A, Adamska A, et al. The higher the insulin resistance the lower the cardiac output in men with type 1 diabetes during the maximal exercise test. *Metab Syndr Relat Disord.* (2017) 15:252–257. doi: 10.1089/met.2017.0007
68. Koves TR, Ussher JR, Noland RC, Slentz D, Mosedale M, Ilkayeva O, et al. Mitochondrial overload and incomplete fatty acid oxidation contribute to skeletal muscle insulin resistance. *Cell Metab.* (2008) 7:45–56. doi: 10.1016/j.cmet.2007.10.013
69. Kannel WB, McGee DL. Diabetes and cardiovascular disease. *JAMA.* (1979) 241:2035. doi: 10.1001/jama.1979.03290450033020
70. Vistisen D, Andersen GS, Hansen CS, Hulman A, Henriksen JE, Bech-Nielsen H, et al. Prediction of first cardiovascular disease event in type 1 diabetes: the steno T1 risk engine. *Circulation.* (2016) 133:1058–66. doi: 10.1161/CIRCULATIONAHA.115.018844
71. Rueda SF, Fernández C, Nicolau J, Ricart MJ, Esmatjes E. Prevalence of cardiovascular risk factors in patients with type 1 diabetes in end-stage renal disease: changes in the trend from 1999 to 2006. *J Diabetes Complications.* (2009) 23:317–22. doi: 10.1016/j.jdiacomp.2008.01.003
72. Yang Z, Scott CA, Mao C, Tang J, Farmer AJ. Resistance exercise vs. aerobic exercise for type 2 diabetes: a systematic review and meta-analysis. *Sport Med.* (2014) 44:487–99. doi: 10.1007/s40279-013-0128-8
73. Shiroma EJ, Cook NR, Manson JE, Moorthy MV, Buring JE, Rimm EB, et al. Strength training and the risk of type 2 diabetes and cardiovascular disease. *Med Sci Sport Exerc.* (2017) 49:40–6. doi: 10.1249/MSS.0000000000001063
74. West DJ, Campbell MD, Gonzalez JT, Walker M, Stevenson EJ, Ahmed FW, et al. The inflammation, vascular repair and injury responses to exercise in fit males with and without Type 1 diabetes: an observational study. *Cardiovasc Diabetol.* (2015) 14:71. doi: 10.1186/s12933-015-0235-y
75. Loomans CJM, de Koning EJP, Staal FJT, Rookmaaker MB, Verseyden C, de Boer HC, et al. Endothelial progenitor cell dysfunction: a novel concept in the pathogenesis of vascular complications of type 1 diabetes. *Diabetes.* (2004) 53:195–9. doi: 10.2337/diabetes.53.1.195
76. Gordin D, Wadén J, Forsblom C, Thorn LM, Rosengård-Bärlund M, Heikkilä O, et al. Arterial stiffness and vascular complications in patients with type 1 diabetes: the Finnish Diabetic Nephropathy (FinnDiane) Study. *Ann Med.* (2012) 44:196–204. doi: 10.3109/07853890.2010.530681
77. Rubanyi GM. The role of endothelium in cardiovascular homeostasis and diseases. *J Cardiovasc Pharmacol.* (1993) 22 (Suppl 4):S1–14. doi: 10.1097/00005344-199322004-00002
78. Kusters YHAM, Barrett EJ. Muscle microvasculature's structural and functional specializations facilitate muscle metabolism. *Am J Physiol Endocrinol Metab.* (2016) 310:E379–87. doi: 10.1152/ajpendo.00443.2015
79. Peltonen JE, Koponen AS, Pullinen K, Hägglund H, Aho JM, Kyröläinen H, et al. Alveolar gas exchange and tissue deoxygenation during exercise in type 1 diabetes patients and healthy controls. *Respir Physiol Neurobiol.* (2012) 181:267–76. doi: 10.1016/j.resp.2012.04.002
80. Kindig CA, Sexton WL, Fedde MR, Poole DC. Skeletal muscle microcirculatory structure and hemodynamics in diabetes. *Respir Physiol.* (1998) 111:163–75. doi: 10.1016/S0034-5687(97)00122-9
81. Krause MP, Riddell MC, Hawke TJ. Effects of type 1 diabetes mellitus on skeletal muscle: clinical observations and physiological mechanisms. *Pediatr Diabetes.* (2011) 12(4 Pt 1):345–64. doi: 10.1111/j.1399-5448.2010.00699.x
82. Stubbe B, Schipf S, Schäper C, Felix SB, Steveling A, Nauck M, et al. The influence of type 1 diabetes mellitus on pulmonary function and exercise capacity – results from the study of health in pomerania (SHIP). *Exp Clin Endocrinol Diabetes.* (2016) 125:64–9. doi: 10.1055/s-0042-112219
83. Harmer AR, Chisholm DJ, McKenna MJ, Hunter SK, Ruell PA, Naylor JM, et al. Sprint training increases muscle oxidative metabolism during high-intensity exercise in patients with type 1 diabetes. *Diabetes Care.* (2008) 31:2097–102. doi: 10.2337/dc08-0329
84. Stellos K, Gawaz M. Platelets and stromal cell-derived factor-1 in progenitor cell recruitment. *Semin Thromb Hemost.* (2007) 33:159–64. doi: 10.1055/s-2007-969029
85. Asahara T, Takahashi T, Masuda H, Kalka C, Chen D, Iwaguro H, et al. VEGF contributes to postnatal neovascularization by mobilizing bone marrow-derived endothelial progenitor cells. *EMBO J.* (1999) 18:3964–72. doi: 10.1093/emboj/18.14.3964
86. Sen S, McDonald SP, Coates PTH, Bonder CS. Endothelial progenitor cells: novel biomarker and promising cell therapy for cardiovascular disease. *Clin Sci.* (2011) 120:263–83. doi: 10.1042/CS20100429
87. Gavin TP, Drew JL, Kubik CJ, Pofahl WE, Hickner RC. Acute resistance exercise increases skeletal muscle angiogenic growth factor expression. *Acta Physiol.* (2007) 191:139–46. doi: 10.1111/j.1748-1716.2007.01723.x
88. Ross MD, Wekesa AL, Phelan JP, Harrison M. Resistance exercise increases endothelial progenitor cells and angiogenic factors. *Med Sci Sports Exerc.* (2014) 46:16–23. doi: 10.1249/MSS.0b013e3182a142da
89. Tonoli C, Heyman E, Buyse L, Roelands B, Piacentini MF, Bailey S, et al. Neurotrophins and cognitive functions in T1D compared with healthy controls: effects of a high-intensity exercise. *Appl Physiol Nutr Metab.* (2015) 40:20–7. doi: 10.1139/apnm-2014-0098
90. Maddaloni E, D'Eon S, Hastings S, Tinsley LJ, Napoli N, Khamaisi M, et al. Bone health in subjects with type 1 diabetes for more than 50 years. *Acta Diabetol.* (2017) 54:479–88. doi: 10.1007/s00592-017-0973-2
91. Parajuli A, Liu C, Li W, Gu X, Lai X, Pei S, et al. Bone's responses to mechanical loading are impaired in type 1 diabetes. *Bone.* (2015) 81:152–60. doi: 10.1016/j.bone.2015.07.012
92. de Souza KS, Ururahy MA, da Costa Oliveira YM, Loureiro MB, da Silva HP, Bortolin RH, et al. Low bone mineral density in patients with type 1 diabetes: association with reduced expression of *IGF1*, *IGF1R* and *TGF B 1* in peripheral blood mononuclear cells. *Diabetes Metab Res Rev.* (2016) 32:589–95. doi: 10.1002/dmrr.2772
93. Maggio AB, Rizzoli RR, Marchand LM, Ferrari S, Beghetti M, Farpour-Lambert NJ. Physical activity increases bone mineral density in children with type 1 diabetes. *Med Sci Sport Exerc.* (2012) 44:1206–11. doi: 10.1249/MSS.0b013e3182496a25
94. Rittweger J, Beller G, Ehrig J, Jung C, Koch U, Ramolla J, et al. Bone-muscle strength indices for the human lower leg. *Bone.* (2000) 27:319–26. doi: 10.1016/S8756-3282(00)00327-6
95. Snow CM, Williams DP, LaRiviere J, Fuchs RK, Robinson TL. Bone gains and losses follow seasonal training and detraining in gymnasts. *Calcif Tissue Int.* (2001) 69:7–12. doi: 10.1007/s00223-001-0014-5
96. Gibbs JC, Craven BC, Moore C, Thabane L, Adachi JD, Giangregorio LM. Muscle density and bone quality of the distal lower extremity among individuals with chronic spinal cord injury. *Top Spinal Cord Inj Rehabil.* (2015) 21:282–93. doi: 10.1310/sci2104-282
97. Lang TF. The bone-muscle relationship in men and women. *J Osteoporos.* (2011) 2011:702735. doi: 10.4061/2011/702735
98. Burt LA, Ducher G, Naughton GA, Courteix D, Greene DA. Gymnastics participation is associated with skeletal benefits in the distal forearm: a 6-month study using peripheral Quantitative Computed Tomography. *J Musculoskelet Neuronal Interact.* (2013) 13:395–404.

99. Folscher L-L, Grant CC, Fletcher L, Janse van Rensberg DC. Ultra-marathon athletes at risk for the female athlete triad. *Sport Med Open.* (2015) 1:29. doi: 10.1186/s40798-015-0027-7
100. Barry DW, Kohrt WM. BMD decreases over the course of a year in competitive male cyclists. *J Bone Miner Res.* (2008) 23:484–91. doi: 10.1359/jbmr.071203
101. Todd JS, Shurley JP, Todd TC. Thomas L. DeLorme and the science of progressive resistance exercise. *J Strength Cond Res.* (2012) 26:2913–23. doi: 10.1519/JSC.0b013e31825adcb4
102. Anderson T, Kearney JT. Effects of three resistance training programs on muscular strength and absolute and relative endurance. *Res Q Exerc Sport.* (1982) 53:1–7. doi: 10.1080/02701367.1982.10605218
103. Fleck SJ, Kraemer WJ. Resistance training: basic principles (Part 1 of 4). *Phys Sportsmed.* (1988) 16:160–71. doi: 10.1080/00913847.1988.11709461
104. Bird SP, Tarpenning KM, Marino FE. Designing resistance training programmes to enhance muscular fitness. *Sport Med.* (2005) 35:841–51. doi: 10.2165/00007256-200535100-00002
105. Kraemer RR, Kilgore JL, Kraemer GR, Castracane VD. Growth hormone, IGF-I, and testosterone responses to resistive exercise. *Med Sci Sports Exerc.* (1992) 24:1346–1352. doi: 10.1249/00005768-199212000-00007
106. Hunter GR, Seelhorst D, Snyder S. Comparison of metabolic and heart rate responses to super slow vs. traditional resistance training. *J strength Cond Res.* (2003) 17:76–81. doi: 10.1519/1533-4287(2003)017<0076:COMAHR>2.0.CO;2
107. Coffey VG, Pilegaard H, Garnham AP, O'Brien BJ, Hawley JA. Consecutive bouts of diverse contractile activity alter acute responses in human skeletal muscle. *J Appl Physiol.* (2009) 106:1187–97. doi: 10.1152/japplphysiol.91221.2008
108. Spurway N, Wackerhage H, British Association of Sport and Exercise Sciences. *Genetics and Molecular Biology of Muscle Adaptation.* Amsterdam: Churchill Livingstone/Elsevier (2006).
109. Guelfi KJ, Jones TW, Fournier PA. The decline in blood glucose levels is less with intermittent high-intensity compared with moderate exercise in individuals with type 1 diabetes. *Diabetes Care.* (2005) 28:1289–94. doi: 10.2337/diacare.28.6.1289
110. Yardley JE, Sigal RJ, Riddell MC, Perkins BA, Kenny GP. Performing resistance exercise before vs. vs. after aerobic exercise influences growth hormone secretion in type 1 diabetes. *Appl Physiol Nutr.* (2014) 39:262–5. doi: 10.1139/apnm-2013-0329

10

Partners in Crime: Beta-Cells and Autoimmune Responses Complicit in Type 1 Diabetes Pathogenesis

Eliana Toren[1,2†], KaLia S. Burnette[2,3†], Ronadip R. Banerjee[4], Chad S. Hunter[1,2*] and Hubert M. Tse[2,3*]*

[1] Department of Medicine, Division of Endocrinology Diabetes and Metabolism, University of Alabama at Birmingham, Birmingham, AL, United States, [2] Comprehensive Diabetes Center, University of Alabama at Birmingham, Birmingham, AL, United States, [3] Department of Microbiology, University of Alabama at Birmingham, Birmingham, AL, United States, [4] Division of Endocrinology, Department of Medicine, Johns Hopkins University School of Medicine, Baltimore, MD, United States

***Correspondence:**
Hubert M. Tse
htse@uab.edu
Chad S. Hunter
huntercs@uab.edu
Ronadip R. Banerjee
rrbanerjee@jhmi.edu

†These authors share first authorship

Type 1 diabetes (T1D) is an autoimmune disease characterized by autoreactive T cell-mediated destruction of insulin-producing pancreatic beta-cells. Loss of beta-cells leads to insulin insufficiency and hyperglycemia, with patients eventually requiring lifelong insulin therapy to maintain normal glycemic control. Since T1D has been historically defined as a disease of immune system dysregulation, there has been little focus on the state and response of beta-cells and how they may also contribute to their own demise. Major hurdles to identifying a cure for T1D include a limited understanding of disease etiology and how functional and transcriptional beta-cell heterogeneity may be involved in disease progression. Recent studies indicate that the beta-cell response is not simply a passive aspect of T1D pathogenesis, but rather an interplay between the beta-cell and the immune system actively contributing to disease. Here, we comprehensively review the current literature describing beta-cell vulnerability, heterogeneity, and contributions to pathophysiology of T1D, how these responses are influenced by autoimmunity, and describe pathways that can potentially be exploited to delay T1D.

Keywords: beta-cell, beta-cell heterogeneity, pancreatic islet, autoimmunity, ER stress, oxidative stress, Type 1 Diabetes

INTRODUCTION

Type 1 diabetes (T1D) is a chronic autoimmune disease in which loss of beta-cell mass and subsequent insulin-insufficiency leads to hyperglycemia. T1D is linked to secondary complications including cardiovascular disease, kidney disease, and neuropathy (1). T1D is the most common form of diabetes in children, comprising approximately 75% of new diabetes diagnoses in patients under 19 years of age (2). Nonetheless, T1D is not a disease only of the young. Epidemiological studies now show that the incidence of autoimmune diabetes in adults (age 30 – 49 years) is at least as high as young adults (age 15 – 19 years) (3). Incidence of T1D is between 4 and 41 per 100,000 in the United States, but interestingly there is significant geographic variation in incidence rates worldwide. Asian countries have relatively lower rates of T1D, while Switzerland, Finland, Norway, the UK, and Sardinia have among the highest rates, with values greater than 20 per 100,000 people (4). Even considering the large geographic variability, overall new diagnoses are on the rise in both childhood and adult populations.

T1D is a multifactorial disease; both genetic and environmental factors contribute to risk. While incompletely understood, putative environmental triggers include microbial infections, neonatal nutrition status/weight, and exposure to certain toxins, such as nitrates (5). Following a triggering event in genetically-susceptible individuals, immune effector cells infiltrate the pancreas and activate inflammatory pathways to mediate targeted destruction of insulin-producing beta-cells. Since the early 1970's, when the genetic connection between human leukocyte antigen (HLA) and T1D was first discovered, pathogenesis of T1D was largely defined by autoimmunity and the selective presentation of islet autoantigens. Strictly defining T1D by an immunological mechanism, however, does not acknowledge any potential role for the beta-cell itself in promoting disease pathology. Mounting evidence indicates the beta-cell is more than just a passive target in the development of T1D: the lack of long-term success with immune intervention therapies, the existence of islet autoimmunity without T1D development, and the persistence of beta-cells after diagnosis and T1D progression, all provide evidence that the beta-cell is an active participant along with the immune system in T1D pathogenesis (6, 7).

In this review, we will focus on the beta-cell in both healthy and T1D environments. We will explore inherent beta-cell heterogeneity and vulnerabilities, contributions to the local inflammatory environment, and how the beta-cell response to metabolic stress can perpetuate disease. Shifting focus from the beta-cell as a passive target to an active participant in disease progression will help identify novel therapeutic approaches, potentially leveraging these unique beta-cell responses and susceptibilities for both treatment and prevention of T1D.

THE BETA-CELL: CHARACTERISTICS THAT IMPART VULNERABILITY

In 1985, Dr. Gian Franco Bottazzo's lecture titled "Death of a Beta Cell: Homicide or Suicide?" posed the idea of beta-cell fragility (8). Dr. Bottazzo questioned whether beta-cells were innocent bystanders of immune attack or contributors to their own destruction (9). Beta-cells must rapidly respond to glucose fluctuations by secreting the appropriate amount of insulin to maintain euglycemia, a taxing process that, even in healthy cells, makes them vulnerable to stressors such as inflammation and nutrition excess. The metabolic demand associated with tightly regulated insulin secretion, paired with a highly vascularized environment, reduced antioxidant defense mechanisms, and sensitivity to proinflammatory cytokines, makes beta-cells uniquely susceptible to autoimmune-mediated destruction (**Figure 1**).

Secretory Demand

The beta-cell is responsible for producing and secreting multiple secretory granule proteins including insulin, chromogranin-A (ChgA), and islet amyloid polypeptide (IAPP). The endoplasmic reticulum (ER) is the site of protein production and relies heavily on Ca^{2+} concentrations to maintain the environment needed for proper protein synthesis and folding (**Figure 2A**) (10). Insulin secretory demand makes the beta-cell particularly vulnerable to exceeding ER protein folding capacity, which leads to the accumulation of misfolded proteins and a disruption of ER homeostasis (**Figure 2F**) (11). This physiological state is termed ER stress (12). Prolonged efforts by the cell to correct misfolded proteins can lead to unregulated changes in enzyme activity, reduced beta-cell function, and induction of apoptosis (13–16). To meet the metabolic demands of glucose-stimulated insulin secretion (GSIS), the beta-cell requires a tightly-coupled process with cellular metabolism to properly maintain euglycemia (17). In brief, glucose is transported into the beta-cell *via* the glucose transporter 2 (Glut2) in rodents (GLUT1 and 3 in humans), converted to pyruvate, and shuttled into the mitochondria where it is used for ATP production (18). Changes in the ATP to ADP ratio lead to beta-cell depolarization, Ca^{2+} influx, and insulin release (19–21). *Insulin* mRNA is translated at the ER following nutrient stimulation, which in rodents can signal up to a 10-fold increase in insulin synthesis at a rate of 1 million molecules per minute (22, 23).

To meet these high demands, beta-cells have an extensive ER with multiple chaperones to aid in protein folding, packaging, and secretion. However, high protein synthesis puts a significant amount of stress on the ER. The unfolded protein response (UPR) is triggered when an excessive amount of misfolded proteins accumulate in the ER, which can be caused by overnutrition, increased reactive oxygen species (ROS), or proinflammatory cytokines (24, 25). Three major sensors of the UPR are protein kinase RNA-like endoplasmic reticulum kinase (PERK), inositol-requiring enzyme 1 alpha (IRE1α) and activating transcription factor 6 (ATF6) (13, 26). In an unstressed state, these sensors are bound to the ER chaperone binding immunoglobulin protein (BiP) (**Figure 2A**). Accumulation of misfolded proteins leads to the dissociation of BiP from the three UPR sensors (**Figure 2F**) (27, 28). Together, the UPR sensors alleviate ER stress by attenuating global protein synthesis to reduce the load of unfolded proteins, increasing chaperone synthesis to guide protein degradation or refolding misfolded proteins, and synthesizing lipids to increase ER volume (29).

In addition to protein synthesis, the ER is also responsible for storage of intracellular Ca^{2+} and therefore, regulates calcium-dependent signaling within the cell, such as protein folding and enzymatic function (13). ER stress disrupts intracellular Ca^{2+} balance influencing multiple processes, including activation of cytosolic post-translational modification (PTM) enzymes by facilitating their translocation into subcellular compartments. This imparts downstream changes in gene expression, protein conformation, and enzyme activity (30–33). Dysregulation of PTM enzymes has been linked to the development of rheumatoid arthritis, celiac disease, and T1D (34–38). In T1D, this includes citrullinating peptidyl arginine deiminase (PAD) enzymes and tissue transglutaminase 2 (tTG2) deaminating enzyme (13, 39). PAD, tTG2, and similar enzymes can alter the binding affinity of

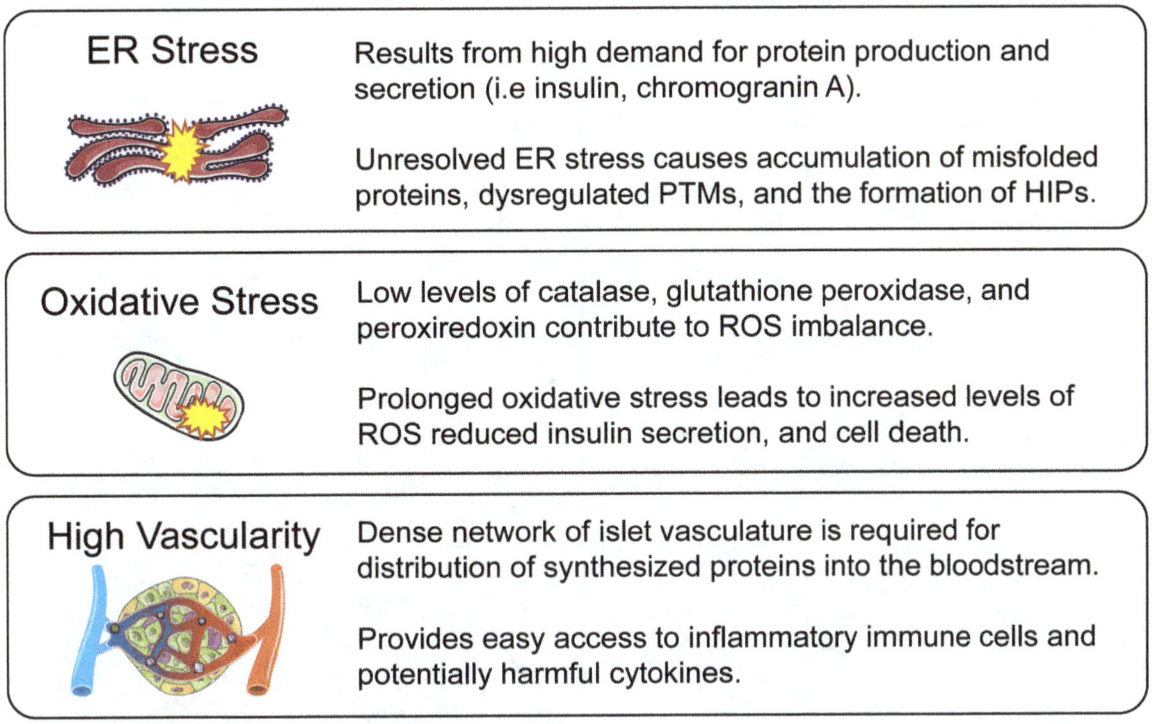

FIGURE 1 | Beta-cell vulnerabilities. While autoimmunity is a major driver of T1D pathogenesis, innate features of beta-cell biology make it a complicit partner in disease progression. These beta-cell characteristics are a result of normal beta-cell function while also active contributors to disease amplification. ER stress is caused by the high protein production and secretory demand of the beta-cell, but in excess leads to misfolded protein response and the generation of HIPs through PTMs. Oxidative stress is caused by an imbalance between the generation of ROS and their detoxification by antioxidants. The reduced antioxidant capabilities of the beta-cell can lead to impaired function and cell death. A densely vascularized environment is required for secretion of insulin and other peptides directly into the bloodstream, but creates a direct dialogue between the beta-cell and potentially harmful immune cells and inflammatory cytokines which may further lead the cell toward stress and apoptosis.

peptide epitopes, such as insulin, to major histocompatibility complex (MHC) class II, resulting in increased CD4 T cell activation (36, 40). Inhibition of systemic PAD enzymes in NOD mice can protect against diabetes progression, suggesting a role in T1D initiation (41).

Stress-induced PTMs can also result in the creation of neo-antigens in peripheral tissues for which the thymus has not established tolerance. Many T1D neo-antigens generated from PTMs have been identified (42). Some PTMs can lead to non-functional protein products resulting from alternately spliced RNA called defective ribosomal products (DRiPs) (43). Increased expression of DRiPs from insulin have been measured in beta-cells in response to ER stress and can be recognized by T cells from patients with T1D (44, 45). Hybrid insulin peptides (HIPs) are another group of neo-antigens generated from transpeptidation, a PTM where insulin peptides are covalently linked to other beta-cell granule peptides including insulin C-peptide, IAPP, and ChgA (**Figure 2G**) (46, 47). HIPs are not only recognized by autoreactive CD4 T cells in mouse models of T1D, but $CD4^+$ T cells from patients with T1D recognized HIPs as well, signifying their potential role in disease initiation and progression (48–50). Our understanding of how neo-antigens are generated and contribute to the development of autoreactivity in T1D is currently unknown. Future studies are warranted to further define how ER stress and subsequent downstream disruptions induced by the secretory demands of the beta-cell can influence autoreactive T cell responses and beta-cell vulnerability in T1D (**Figure 1**).

Oxidative Stress

Oxidative stress occurs when there is an imbalance between ROS generation and antioxidant activity (51). Superoxide is primarily a byproduct of normal cellular metabolism that is generated in the mitochondria and cytoplasm (**Figure 2B**) and is an initiating free radical that can result in the formation of other reactive species such as hydrogen peroxide (H_2O_2), hydroxyl radical, and peroxynitrite (52). Free radicals are highly reactive and can induce cellular damage, but antioxidants including superoxide dismutase (SOD), catalase, glutathione peroxidase (GPx), peroxiredoxins, thioredoxin, and glutathione protect the cell by detoxifying these reactive species (53, 54). SOD dismutates superoxide to molecular oxygen and H_2O_2, a less destructive oxidant and signaling molecule. H_2O_2 regulates insulin secretion by activating the second messenger c-Jun N-terminal Kinase (JNK) (55). This leads to decreased insulin production through the translocation of the transcription factor pancreatic and duodenal homeobox 1 (Pdx1) from the nucleus to the cytoplasm, resulting in decreased *Insulin* transcription (56)

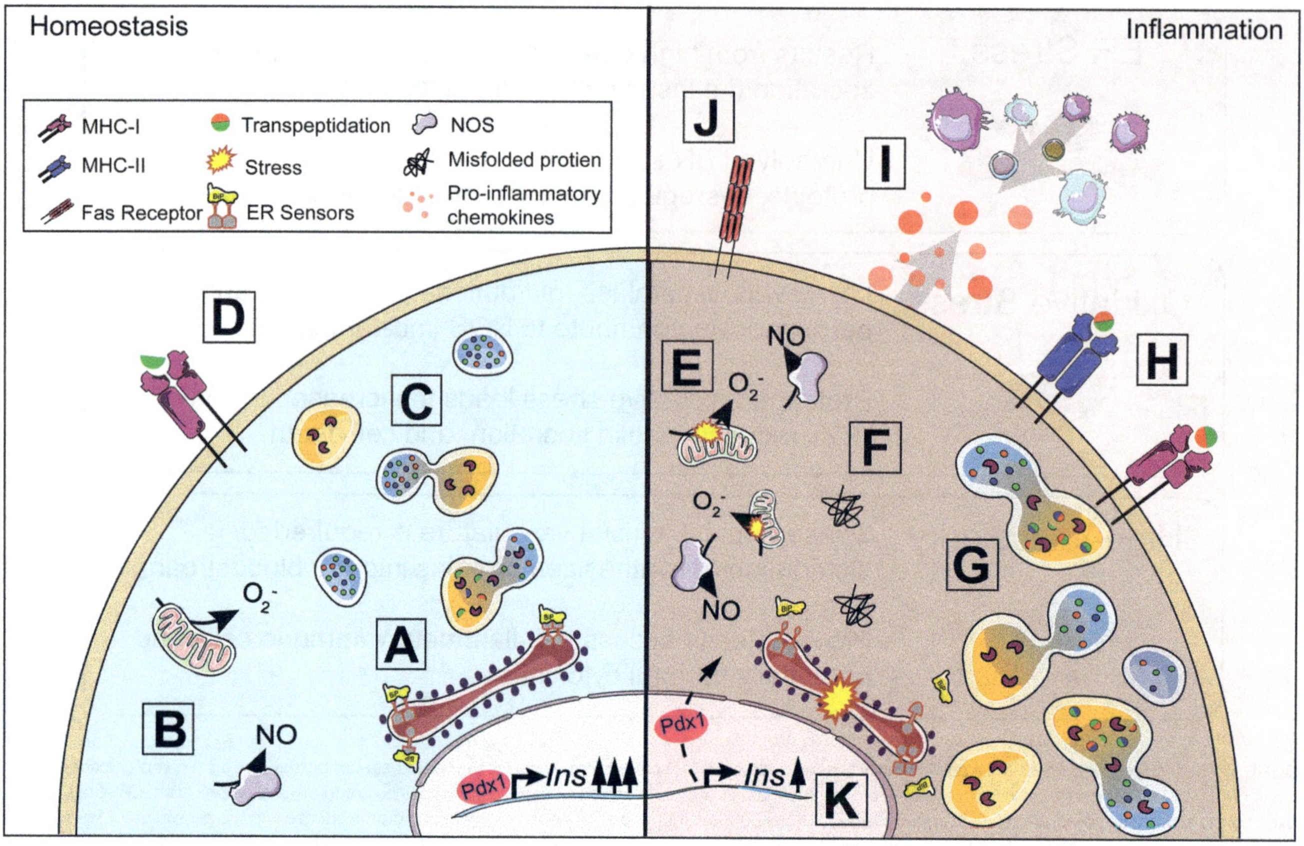

FIGURE 2 | Beta-cell response to inflammation. Under homeostasis conditions, insulin production is tightly coupled with cellular metabolism including protein synthesis in the endoplasmic reticulum (ER) **(A)** and mitochondrial function **(B)**. When insulin secretory granule proteins are in excess, they can be broken down and recycled by crinophagy, a process by which granules fuse with lysosomes **(C)**. Some peptides from this degradation process are presented on MHC-I **(D)** and, in healthy cells, should not lead to activation. A proinflammatory environment around the islet exacerbates ER and oxidative stress **(E)** contributing to the dysregulation of multiple processes in the beta-cell. The accumulation of misfolded proteins can result in the activation of the unfolded protein response **(F)** and increase lysosomal degradation of insulin secretory granule proteins **(G)**. Protein degradation under stress can lead to the production of neo-antigens, such as hybrid insulin peptides, through transpeptidation. ER and oxidative stress results in the upregulation of MHC-I and the unique expression of MHC-II **(H)** by the beta-cell allowing for increased presentation of potential neo-antigens to T cells. Fas receptor expression **(J)** makes the beta-cell vulnerable to Fas-mediated apoptosis. The release of chemokines **(I)** from the beta-cell further contributes to immune cell recruitment and the development of insulitis. Insulin production can be affected as disturbances in cellular homeostasis can lead to the translocation of Pdx1 from the nucleus to the cytoplasm, decreasing insulin production **(K)**.

(**Figure 2K**). H_2O_2 is further converted to oxygen and water by catalase, GPx, and peroxiredoxin. Increased levels of H_2O_2 can form extremely reactive hydroxyl radicals through Fenton reactions with free iron present in the cytoplasm, which has downstream negative effects on intracellular calcium levels, protein synthesis, glycosylation, and redox status (53). Beta-cells, however, have decreased antioxidant levels and therefore, are highly susceptible to free radical-mediated damage (**Figure 2E**). Rodent and human beta-cells have reduced transcriptional and protein levels of cytosolic copper/zinc (Cu/Zn) SOD1, mitochondrial manganese (Mn) SOD2, catalase, and GPx, which can result in exacerbated levels of superoxide, H_2O_2, hydroxyl radical, and peroxynitrite that are implicated in beta-cell death in T1D (57–61). The inability to properly restore cellular homeostasis due to the negative effects of oxidative and ER stress can induce apoptosis in insulin-secreting beta-cells. Increased beta-cell apoptosis has been measured in patients with T1D and NOD mice when compared to healthy controls (14, 62–66). In addition to oxidative stress, the beta-cell is also impacted by the islet microenvironment in which it is closely associated.

Islet Vascularization and Exposure to Cytokines

Importantly for T1D pathology, islets are highly vascularized. This provides an interface by which immune cells, even from distant sites, can gain local access to pancreatic islets (67, 68). Islets contain a glomerular-like network of fenestrated capillaries that comprise about 8-10% of islet volume. Islet capillary density is estimated to be 10 times higher than that of the exocrine pancreas and is driven by high local production of VEGF-A (69, 70). This rich vascularization and high islet blood flow is autonomously regulated through complex interactions between hormones, metabolites, and the nervous system. While islet blood flow is innately required for and coupled to insulin sensing and release, extensive vasculature also makes the beta-cell uniquely poised for interactions with the immune system.

The dense islet vasculature network facilitates activated immune cell trafficking across the vascular endothelium into the islet (**Figure 1**). This causes a local inflammatory microenvironment which in turn, further increases permeability, facilitating access even for naïve T cells (71). Interestingly, this "open" environment remains, even after reversal of diabetes with anti-CD3 treatment. In addition to naïve T cell infiltration, activated immune cells that are primed locally in the pancreatic lymph nodes (pLNs) can also cross the vascular endothelium. pLNs may contribute to T1D pathogenesis as drainage from the pancreas and local gut regions provides a crossroad for the immune cells traveling between these compartments (67, 72). The interplay between the microbiome, the immune system, and a "leaky gut" has been implicated as a key factor in T1D pathogenesis (73, 74). Toll-like receptors (TLRs) are a family of innate pattern recognition receptors important for microbial clearance by the immune system. Many TLRs signal through the MyD88 adapter protein. NOD mice deficient in MyD88 exhibit microbiota-dependent protection from autoimmunity development (75). Specific manipulation of TLR expression and microbiota composition can further regulate disease progression or prevention (76). Sex-specific autoimmune risk can also be influenced by microbiome manipulation (77–79). With new data unveiling the importance of the microbiome for the gut immune environment and shaping peripheral tolerance, the relationship between pLNs, islet vasculature, and immune cell trafficking is increasingly relevant to beta-cell vulnerability and T1D pathogenesis (80, 81). In addition to facilitating interactions between islet cells and immune cells, the islet vasculature also sensitizes the beta-cell to the damaging effects of circulating proinflammatory cytokines.

Beta-cells are sensitive to cytokine-mediated damage. Cytokines can alter crucial beta-cell characteristics including insulin secretion, mitochondrial function, and intracellular calcium stores (82, 83). Inflammatory cytokines including tumor necrosis factor alpha (TNFα), interferon gamma (IFNγ), and interleukin-1 beta (IL-1β), cause beta-cell dysfunction by impairing ATP production, inducing DNA damage, and promoting apoptosis (**Figure 3**) (84, 85). Proinflammatory cytokine exposure inhibits GSIS due to the limited availability of ATP in both rodent and human islets, as well as in beta-cell lines (86–89). Islet exposure to cytokines triggers nuclear factor κB (NFκB) induction of inducible nitric oxide synthase (iNOS), which increases NO formation in the beta-cell (87). NO has temporal effects on beta-cell responses, as early and transient levels of NO (less than 24 hours) facilitate the repair of cytokine-induced DNA damage by inhibiting the activation of the DNA damage response and preventing the induction of apoptosis (90). However, prolonged exposure to NO can induce beta-cell death due to DNA damage, UPR activation, and decreased mitochondrial oxidation (i.e., ATP production) (87, 91). In cultured islets, pre-exposure treatment with NO inhibitors, such as aminoguanidine, attenuates cytokine-mediated beta-cell death (92). Cytokine-mediated beta-cell death becomes exacerbated in an inflammatory microenvironment in the pancreas, creating a positive feedback loop resulting in more inflammation, stress, vulnerability, and eventually cell death (**Figure 3**). Unfortunately, clinical trials with anti-cytokine therapies such as Anakinra, an IL-1 receptor antagonist, were not efficacious in delaying T1D, suggesting a more complex interaction between cytokines and beta-cells *in vivo* (92). Nonetheless, not every beta-cell is lost in T1D, nor do they all respond negatively to ER and/or oxidative stress, indicating an intrinsic beta-cell heterogeneity in response to disease promoting factors.

BETA-CELL HETEROGENEITY

It is challenging to fully understand the response and contribution of the beta-cell to the T1D disease state without understanding beta-cell heterogeneity. Many groups have focused on determining whether different subtypes of beta-cells exist, and if so, how they might differ in functional ways such as proliferative and secretory capacities (93–95). Identifying subpopulations, and then understanding their inter- and intra-islet communication, has uncovered a level of complexity and diversity not previously appreciated. We will briefly explore the recent findings regarding functional and transcriptional heterogeneity of the beta-cell and discuss potential impacts on susceptibility to T1D.

Functional Diversity

Evidence for functional beta-cell heterogeneity in calcium flux, metabolism, ion channel conductance, and insulin secretion has been appreciated for almost 30 years (96, 97). More recently, this functional diversity has been specifically defined by many research groups into beta-cell subpopulations (**Table 1**). Using novel cell surface markers (ST8SIA1 and CD9) identified by immunizing mice with human islets, four human beta-cell subtypes with unique basal and GSIS responses were defined as β1-4 (93). All subtypes contain insulin granules but exhibit variable functionality and abundance; β1 is the most abundant and glucose responsive, while β4 is the rarest and least responsive, with highest basal insulin secretion. Interestingly there are no correlations found between subtype ratios and sex, age, or obesity, but subtype abundance is altered and much more variable in Type 2 diabetes (T2D). For example, β3 and β4 subsets are unusually overrepresented in T2D islets, but abundance of these two subsets varied much more than in control non-diabetic tissue. It is unknown if β1-4 cells exist in unique patterns before or after T1D diagnosis and disease progression.

In 2016, Johnston et al. discovered specialized beta-cells they termed "hub" cells that exert disproportionate control over blood glucose (94). Hub cells, comprising 1-10% of islet beta-cell mass, are metabolically active, exhibit evidence of transcriptional immaturity (low or absent Pdx1 and Nkx6.1 transcription factor levels), and are hypothesized to act as a pacemaker within the islet. Supporting this model, calcium tracing showed that surrounding cells, termed "followers", respond to glucose stimulation slightly after the hub cell. Using optogenetic and pharmacological techniques, silencing hubs caused desynchrony

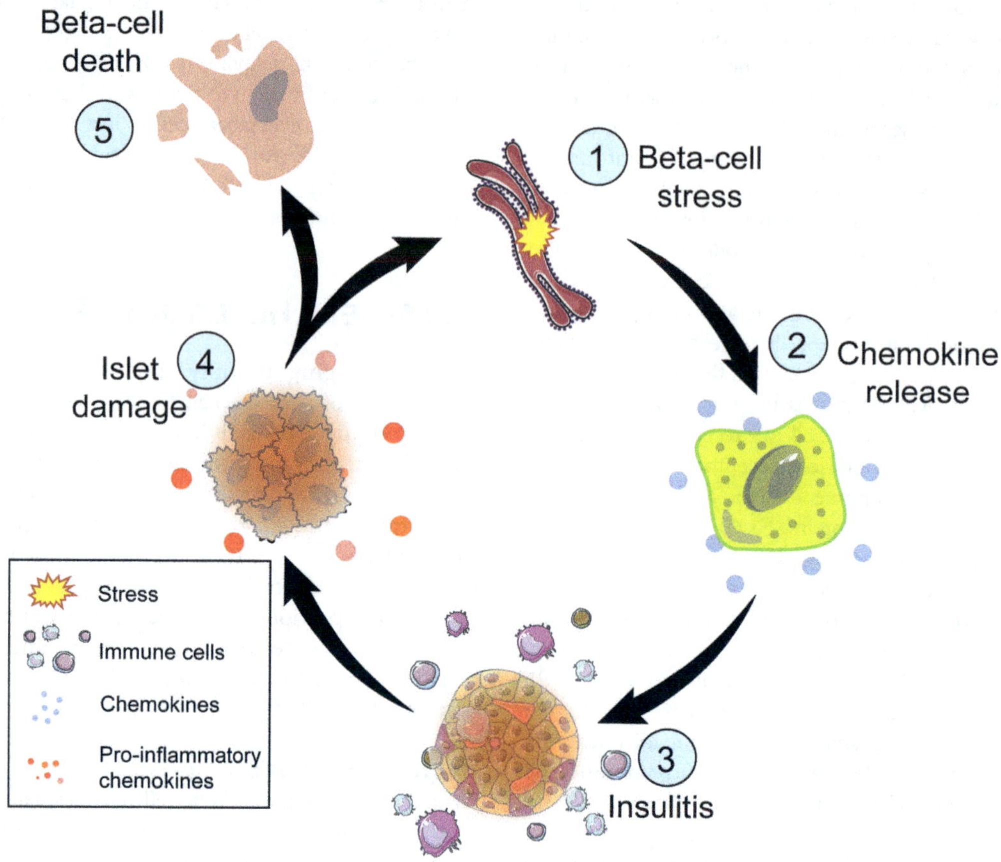

FIGURE 3 | Steps of beta-cell death in T1D. Metabolic demand of nutrient challenge results in ER and oxidative stress (1) followed by chemokine release by the beta-cell (2). Chemokines attract immune cells (3), such as macrophages and T cells, which can damage the islet (4) directly though T cell interactions and indirectly through the release of inflammatory cytokines and reactive oxygen species. Cellular damage exacerbates ER and oxidative stress perpetuating this cycle. The inability to restore cellular homeostasis will result in beta-cell death (5).

in the calcium-induced response of beta-cells. The Huising group reported on a beta-cell subtype located in the islet periphery that is both transcriptionally and functionally immature, called the "virgin" beta-cell (95). Virgin cells lack the maturity marker urocortin 3 (UCN3) and are incapable of sensing glucose or proper calcium influx. Using lineage tracing, they found that these cells are transdifferentiation intermediates between alpha- and beta-cells. This work defined a "neogenic niche" of new beta-cells originating from an alpha-cell lineage, establishing a plasticity between these cell types that had also been suggested by models of extreme beta-cell loss (100). The hub versus virgin subpopulations can be compared to flattop$^+$ and flattop$^-$ populations, where this novel marker differentiates between a mature, functional beta-cell population (flattop$^+$) and an immature and highly proliferative one (flattop$^-$) (101).

In 2020, the Benninger lab defined yet another subpopulation that is functionally distinct from those previously described (102). These cells are termed "first-responder" beta-cells, as defined by calcium dynamics. They found that first-phase response time of beta-cells is spatially organized and dependent on the physical distance from the first-responder cell. How these sub-populations of cells as defined by these specific markers may be unique or overlapping remains to be determined.

Transcriptional Diversity

The implementation of single-cell transcriptomics has allowed exploration of beta-cell heterogeneity on a scale that was not previously possible. The Kubicek lab published the first application of single-cell transcriptomics to human islet cells in 2016 (103); while the number of beta-cells identified was extremely low, they showed transcriptome heterogeneity for genes such as *DLK1*, a T1D associated gene by GWAS (Genome-Wide Association Study) which will be discussed later in more detail. That same year the Kaestner lab published single-cell mass cytometric analysis of human islets and found heterogeneity in markers including Ki67, identifying four distinct beta-cell subpopulations (104). Several groups have since published large-scale single-cell transcriptome analyses of human and mouse beta-cells and identified unique subpopulations. These populations display differential levels of various beta-cell characteristics including maturity (UCN3),

TABLE 1 | Selected pancreatic beta-cell subtypes. Heterogeneity in beta-cell response has led to the identification of beta-cell subtypes. These subtypes may vary in spatial location within the islet, speed of response to a stimulus, and secretory capacity. The names of beta-cell subtypes, description of characteristics, and whether they were identified in mouse or human pancreata are defined below.

Name of Subtype	Description of Characteristics	Mouse or Human	Reference
β1	Highest GSIS, least abundant in T2D tissue	Human	Dorrell et al., 2016 (63)
β2	CD9$^+$, ST8SIA1$^-$, stimulation index second highest after β1	Human	
β3	CD9$^-$, ST8SIA1$^+$, increased in T2D	Human	
β4	Lowest GSIS, high basal secretion, increased in T2D	Human	
Hub	Pacemaker, responds quickly to calcium influx, makes up 1-10% of beta-cell mass	Both	Johnston et al., 2016 (98)
Virgin	Transcriptionally and functionally immature (UCN$^-$), located at islet periphery, incapable of glucosensing	Both	Van der Meulen et al., 2017 (65)
Flattop+	Mature, functional secretory granules, increased with high fat diet	Mouse	Bader et al., 2016 (69)
Flattop-	Immature, highly proliferative, Wnt$^+$ (Become flattop$^+$)	Mouse	
Top	Present in non-T1D setting, glucose responsive, express maturity markers	Mouse	Rui et al., 2017 (99)
Bottom	Population appears in a T1D environment, resistant to immune killing, unresponsive to glucose, express stemness markers	Mouse	
First-Responder	First to respond to calcium influx, other beta-cell response based on distance from these	Mouse	Kravets et al., 2020 (70)
Extreme	High levels of proinsulin and ribosomes, low insulin protein content, increased in *db/db* mice	Mouse	Farack et al., 2019 (78)

aging (IGF1R), and ER stress response (SRXN1, SQSTM1) (105, 106). Genes involved in ER/oxidative stress have been some of the strongest distinguishers of subpopulation clusters in various studies, with ER stress markers also correlating to proliferation and reduced beta-cell function (107–109). As discussed earlier, beta-cell ER stress is extremely relevant to an understanding of T1D contribution and response. Perhaps certain populations of proliferative-ER stressed beta-cells are the first to be lost during T1D pathogenesis.

For years, technical hurdles to interrogating mRNA in islets due to the digestive enzymes present in the surrounding exocrine pancreas limited our understanding of transcriptional dynamics and heterogeneity in the beta-cell. Dr. Shalev Itzkovitz at the Weitzmann Institute developed methods to visualize the dynamics of beta-cell mRNAs. His group designed an optimized single-molecule FISH (fluorescence *in situ* hybridization) protocol that allowed for assessment of transcriptional heterogeneity within the beta-cell population (110). This method revealed a subpopulation of "extreme" beta-cells that contain high levels of *insulin* and secretory factor mRNAs (*IAPP*, *ChgA*), but interestingly, low levels of insulin protein. The investigators suggested this may impart a specialization for basal insulin secretion. Additionally, beta-cell mRNAs displayed a uniquely polarized pattern, with elevated *Insulin* mRNA concentration in apical ER enriched compartments of the cell. The ratio of extreme beta-cells was increased in *db/db* diabetic mice, potentially facilitating increased requirements for basal insulin. This work gives rise to another unappreciated aspect of beta-cell heterogeneity: transcriptional heterogeneity. Future studies are needed to explore the proportion of extreme beta-cells in T1D and how this type of transcriptional variability may affect vulnerability to autoimmune recognition and attack.

The relationship between these different beta-cell subpopulations is still being defined, as the markers discussed above may represent unique or overlapping populations. For example, each of these functional and transcriptional subpopulations represents a unique niche that may have specific susceptibilities or contributions to T1D. Is a hub cell the same as a β1 or flattop$^+$ cell? What are the differences and are they physiologically relevant? What is the relationship between these cell types and how do those relationships change with age and nutrition state? Understanding the relationship between functionality, heterogeneity, and vulnerability will provide a deeper understanding of T1D etiology, potentially setting the stage for more effective therapeutic strategies.

BETA-CELL CONTRIBUTIONS TO INFLAMMATION

Therapeutic strategies for preventing or treating T1D have historically focused on modulating the immune response to the beta-cell. Emerging strategies that instead focus on beta-cell dysfunction through manipulation of ER, oxidative, or cytokine-induced cell stressors may prove to be beneficial, as the beta-cell itself actively contributes to inflammatory responses in T1D. The following section will discuss beta-cell contributions to the T1D inflammatory environment, which may represent optimal targets for future combinatorial therapies.

Chemokine Production

Chemokines are a family of small molecules involved in lymphoid physiology, pathology, and hemopoietic cell migration (111, 112). Chemokines can be broadly separated into two categories: constitutive and inducible (113). Constitutive chemokines perform homeostatic functions involving non-inflammatory leukocyte trafficking, while inducible chemokines are produced in response to inflammation to recruit activated leukocytes to the sites of damage or stress (114). Multiple chemokines, detailed below, are secreted by the beta-cell and contribute to immune infiltration into the islet (**Figure 2I**). These secreted factors make the beta-cell a target for immune invasion and destruction.

CCL2

The chemokine C-C ligand 2 (CCL2) also known as monotype chemoattractant protein (MCP)-1 is an inducible chemokine involved in monocyte, NK cell, and T cell recruitment during inflammation (115–117). Human and NOD islets cultured with proinflammatory cytokines IL-1β and IFNγ can induce CCL2 production (118–120). Beta-cells express *Ccl2* in an NF-κB –dependent manner and can be induced *in vivo* by environmental triggers such as viral infections leading to inflammation and macrophage recruitment (121, 122). Macrophages are the first and most abundant immune cell to infiltrate the islet during the progression of T1D in NOD mice and have also been identified in islets from patients with recent-onset T1D (115, 123, 124). CCL2 may be responsible for this influx in macrophages, as transgenic overexpression of *Ccl2* in murine beta-cells results in increased monocyte recruitment, insulitis, and islet destruction (115). Binding of CCL2 to its receptor C-C chemokine receptor-2 (CCR2) in macrophages leads to the production of proinflammatory cytokines and chemokines such as TNFα, IL-1β, IL-12, and CXCL10 to exacerbate the inflammatory environment of the islet (125). Prolonged exposure to proinflammatory cytokines leads to ER stress, oxidative stress, and cell death (115) (**Figure 3**).

CCL5

CC ligand 5 (CCL5) also called RANTES (regulated on activation, normal T cell expressed and secreted) is a chemoattractant for T cells, eosinophils, and monocytes involved in inflammatory responses. CCL5 has been measured in rodent islets and from cell sorted beta-cells in response to inflammatory cytokines TNFα, IL-1β, and IFNγ (126, 127). Increased expression of CCR5, one of the cognate receptors for CCL5, was detected on T cells from patients with T1D and NOD mice (128, 129). Blocking CCR5 using neutralizing antibodies in 2-month-old NOD mice (after islet infiltration, but before overt diabetes) inhibits future immune infiltration and prevents development of diabetes (126).

CXCL10

C-X-C motif chemokine ligand 10 (CXCL10) also called IP-10 (IFNγ-induced protein 10) is a chemokine secreted by many cell types including monocytes, neutrophils, and endothelial cells (130, 131). CXCL10 is increased in the serum and tissues of patients with various autoimmune diseases including T1D (99, 132). Human islets, murine islets, and NIT-1 NOD beta-cells secrete CXCL10 when cultured with pro-inflammatory cytokines IL-1β and IFNγ (127). CXCL10 binds the seven transmembrane G protein coupled receptor CXC receptor 3 (CXCR3), expressed on both immune and non-immune cells (133, 134). In lymphocytes, CXCR3 mediates chemotaxis, while in non-lymphocytes CXCR3 regulates tissue repair, proliferation, and angiogenesis (135, 136). Mice lacking CXCR3 and infected with lymphocytic choriomeningitis virus-WE strain (LCMV-WE), an established model to study T1D, exhibited a delay in insulitis, while overexpressing CXCL10 in mouse islets accelerated LCMV-induced diabetes (127, 137, 138). As predicted, using neutralizing antibodies to block CXCL10 also decreased T cell trafficking to the islet and abrogated diabetes development (139–141). In culture, the NIT-1 NOD beta-cell line was found to secrete CXCL10 in response to inflammatory cytokines IL-1β, TNFα, and IFNγ (127). These data suggest that elevated CXCL10 secretion by the beta-cell may occur early in T1D progression. CXCL10 not only contributes to immune cell recruitment but is also directly toxic to beta-cells (142). In addition to CXCR3, CXCL10 also binds Toll-like receptor-4 (TLR4), a pattern recognition receptor involved in the immune response to microbial pathogens (143). The CXCL10:TLR4 signaling pathway in beta-cells leads to cleavage and translocation of activated protein activated kinase 2 (PAK-2) into the nucleus, contributing to apoptotic signaling within the cell (144, 145). Islets from C57BL/6 *Tlr4*$^{-/-}$ knockout mice are protected against CXCL10-induced damage. Therefore, CXCL10 released by the beta-cell contributes to cell death by attracting activated immune cells and inducing apoptosis within the beta-cell.

Beta-cells produce proinflammatory CCL2, CCL5, and CXCL10 chemokines when exposed to inflammatory conditions or environmental triggers and can perpetuate the recruitment of immune cells to initiate insulitis. Once present, these immune cells can damage the beta-cell by synthesizing ROS, proinflammatory cytokines, and expressing receptors that can directly mediate beta-cell death (**Figure 2**).

Beta-Cell Promotion of Cellular Death

Of the infiltrating cells causing insulitis in T1D, T cells are the major destroyer of beta-cells, with both CD4 and CD8 T cells being required to effectively transfer disease (146–148). CD4 and CD8 T cells have different roles in disease development (149). When activated, CD4 T cells or T "helper" cells influence the activation of surrounding immune cells through the production of pro- or anti-inflammatory cytokines (149). Human CD4 T cells conventionally recognize peptides presented on HLA-II molecules expressed by antigen-presenting cells (APCs), but the expression of HLA-II has also been detected on beta-cells from patients with T1D (150). CD8 T cells recognize peptides presented on MHC-I on mouse cells and HLA-I on human cells (**Figure 2D**). Islets biopsied from patients with T1D displayed HLA-I hyperexpression, which warrants their susceptibility to CD8 T cell-mediated destruction (151). The activation of CD8 T cells leads to the differentiation of CD8 T cells to become cytolytic T lymphocytes (CTLs) resulting in the directed release of cytotoxic cytokines, cytolytic granules, and Fas ligand (FasL)-mediated death of the target cell. Beta-cells from diabetic patients not only express HLA-I/II molecules, but also the Fas receptor (CD95/Apo-1) (152–154) (**Figure 2J**). Fas/FasL signaling is suggested to play a role in T1D pathology as NOD mice deficient in Fas do not develop inflammation or diabetes (155). Fas-deficient mice are also protected against adoptive transfer of splenocytes from diabetic NOD mice. In rodent and human islets, the expression of Fas receptor in beta-cells is induced by proinflammatory cytokines IL-1α, IL-1β, IFNγ, and the upregulation of iNOS, as sequestering NO in the beta-cell decreases Fas expression (156, 157). Fas/FasL signaling in the beta-cell leads to apoptosis *via* the activation of caspase 8 and the mitochondrial pathway of apoptosis (158). Beta-cell-derived proinflammatory chemokines, HLA-I/II (or MHC-I/II) molecules, and Fas/FasL receptors can perpetuate T1D disease progression by promoting immune cell recruitment, T cell activation, and subsequent beta-cell destruction. Since autoantibodies can be detected in circulation for years prior to disease onset (159) and patients from the Medalist study (discussed below) retain a portion of insulin-secreting beta-cells, these observations provide evidence that at least some beta-cell populations may possess mechanisms to evade the immune response.

THE T1D BETA-CELL

In addition to the intrinsic, "baseline" heterogeneity of beta-cells, heterogeneity of disease progression within islets from individual patients, and heterogeneity of disease progression amongst patients with T1D are becoming apparent through longitudinal clinical studies and new analytical techniques examining T1D animal models. The Joslin Medalist Study of T1D patients with disease duration of 50 years or longer revealed that some insulin producing beta-cells persist, ostensibly even after years in a chronic inflammatory environment (160). This highlights that some level of heterogeneity is present in the T1D islet, supporting that certain beta-cell populations may be protected from autoimmune destruction. The expansion of single-cell transcriptomics has contributed to our understanding of cell populations dynamics, but whether it be mouse or human, almost all published studies have used either healthy or T2D islets.

Exciting work in the past few years has given rise to the idea that disease-specific beta-cell heterogeneity may arise during T1D progression, with certain populations that are more vulnerable than others to autoimmune-mediated death. The Herold lab was one of the first to identify distinct cell populations in T1D with their discovery of a low granularity beta-cell population termed "bottom" cells in the NOD mouse model (161) (**Table 1**). They found that this non-glucose-responsive population emerges prior to hyperglycemia and immune infiltration and expands over time, comprising over 50% of the beta-cell population by 12 weeks of age. The bottom cells express "stemness" markers and were found to be less sensitive to treatment with cytokines and immune infiltrates compared to their "top" counterparts, suggesting they may evade immune attack (161). As we continue to understand disease etiology more deeply, these resistant populations may provide a novel target for treatment.

The discovery of distinct T1D endotypes associated with age of diagnosis has recently contributed to our knowledge of the T1D beta-cell (162). Using immunohistochemical analysis of pancreas samples from patients diagnosed under the age of 30, Leete et al. found a distinct pattern of insulin/proinsulin localization in the beta-cell that is not present in non-T1D controls. Specifically, they found high insulin/proinsulin colocalization in patients who were diagnosed under 13, and even more consistently in patients diagnosed before 7 years of age. Similar subtypes had been described regarding insulitis, with two discrete histological profiles associating strongly with age of diagnosis (163, 164). The authors postulate that discovery of these histologically distinct phenotypes points to disease endotypes that could even be described as T1DE1 and T1DE2 and may require different immunotherapeutic options based on age of diagnosis. While this work is not necessarily beta-cell specific, the heterogenous nature of disease that the field continues to uncover further points to the importance of understanding beta-cell heterogeneity and response to autoimmunity. We propose that an understanding of beta-cell dynamics prior to, during, and after immune-cell infiltration in T1D will be vital to development of therapies that can not only combat T1D development, but perhaps even precede and bypass it.

T1D-ASSOCIATED BETA-CELL SNPs

T1D pathogenesis involves both genetic and environmental triggers and susceptibilities. Thus, examining genetic associations that link specific loci to T1D vulnerability has been a major area of research focus. Surprisingly, the Wellcome Trust Case Control Consortium (WTCCC) established GWAS found relatively few novel risk loci for T1D. It was not until the T1D Genetics Consortium (T1DGC) conducted a meta-analysis that approximately 41 distinct susceptibility loci were identified (165). Fine mapping of these loci using ImmunoChIP established credible sets of single nucleotide polymorphisms (SNPs), most of which are found in non-coding DNA regulatory regions, including tissue-specific enhancers (166). Most of our understanding of the identified SNPs has been centered around the *HLA* loci that are strongly associated with the disease and T cell autoreactivity. While these studies of the immune arm of pathogenesis are invaluable, not only do SNPs in the *INSULIN* (*INS*) gene remain one of the highest risks (167), but approximately 60% of all T1D susceptibility genes are expressed in the islet (168). These data further support the concept that the beta-cell has a larger role in its own destruction than previously appreciated, and that genetic susceptibility is not solely based on the status of the immune system. Below we describe beta-cell-associated SNPs and what is known thus far about their T1D implications.

Insulin

As mentioned above, after the *HLA* locus, the 5' upstream region of the *INS* locus is the genomic region with the strongest association with T1D risk (167). Specifically, it is the INS-VNTR (variable number tandem repeat) locus that confers susceptibility differences. The VNTR alleles are defined by two classes: class I (26-63 repeats) and class III (140-200 repeats). The shorter class I VNTRs confer a 2-5-fold increase in T1D risk while the longer class III allele is protective against T1D, this is thought to be due to effects on proinsulin expression in the thymus (169). Class III VNTRs are associated with increased *INSULIN* transcription in the thymus during induction of central immune tolerance. The authors proposed that these increased thymic insulin levels may promote negative selection of insulin-specific T cells, ultimately leading to a protective effect on T1D susceptibility. Class I VNTRs result in decreased *INSULIN* transcription in the thymus and potentially allow insulin-specific autoreactive T cells to escape from the thymus due to defects in central tolerance and negative selection. This class I versus III allele-specific mechanism illustrates the complexity of T1D risk, and while this susceptibility locus can absolutely be seen as a beta-cell associated SNP, the proposed mechanisms that have been defined thus far are still largely immune system focused. So, despite the 100 years since the discovery of insulin, large gaps in our understanding of how it is involved in the response of the beta-cell itself in T1D remain.

GLIS3

Due to the scarcity of studies of beta-cell contributions to T1D, many associations have been made between beta-cell death and failure in T1D and T2D. Remarkably, GWAS indicates there are very few susceptibility loci associated with both maladies. Variations of the Kruppel-like zinc finger transcription factor *GLIS3* are one of the few that have been strongly associated with both T1 and T2D (170). Also a known MODY (Maturity Onset Diabetes of the Young) gene, *GLIS3* is expressed predominantly in the pancreas, thyroid, and kidney. While there have been some discrepancies in the literature regarding the exact timing of expression, in GLIS3-EGFP knock-in mice, GLIS3 mainly co-expresses with Sox9 in bipotent pancreatic islet progenitor cells and is absent from the acinar progenitors at embryonic day (E) 13.5. This pattern correlates with its importance in development of the pancreatic endocrine lineage and seeming negligibility for the exocrine portion of the pancreas. The association between GLIS3 and T1D was first identified in European populations but has more recently been recapitulated in a Pakistani cohort (171, 172). Interestingly, a GLIS3 variant (A908V) is associated with T1D resistance in Japanese patients (173). Considering the thymic expression of GLIS3, the authors propose that perhaps this variant induces central or peripheral immune tolerance more efficiently than the wild-type variant, but more studies are needed to understand this mechanism. Regarding the molecular mechanisms that underlie the associations of GLIS3 and diabetes, little was known until multiple groups independently generated both global and beta-cell-specific *GLIS3* knockout models (174–176). Not only do *GLIS3*$^{-/-}$ mice die within the first few days of life, but their islet area is approximately 15% that of littermate controls (177). Insulin production was reduced by 80%, making it difficult to assess GSIS in these mice. These groups also found that the endocrine progenitor gene, *Ngn3*, is a GLIS3 target, and that GLIS3 physically and functionally interacts with the beta-cell transcription factor Pdx1 to regulate *insulin* transcription. Interestingly, GLIS3 overexpression leads to an upregulation of *Ngn3* mRNA in ductal cells, further supporting the role of GLIS3 in pancreatic islet progenitor specification. Pancreatic progenitors, as well as the adult acinar compartment, seem to be unperturbed in GLIS3 knockouts showing an islet progenitor specificity to its role during development. These mechanisms do not tie directly to T1D association but understanding the role of GLIS3 in beta-cell identity may help unveil the mechanisms involved in both T1 and T2D disease susceptibility.

CLEC16A

C-type lectin domain family 16, member A (*CLEC16a*) is a gene locus associated with T1D, multiple sclerosis, and adrenal dysfunction (98, 178, 179). Though genetic associations have been long established, until the work of Soleimanpour et al., a molecular basis for how CLEC16A might increase T1D was unknown. Interestingly, these investigators found that mouse Clec16a interacts with Nrdp1 (an E3 ubiquitin ligase) and has roles in normal GSIS in the beta-cell (180). Pancreatic *Clec16a* deletion causes reduced ATP levels and mitochondrial oxygen consumption, establishing the factor as a novel regulator of beta-cell mitophagy. Additionally, patients with the T1D-associated SNP in the *CLEC16A* gene exhibit reductions in CLEC16A expression and perturbed insulin secretion.

These observations of impaired insulin and glucose homeostasis, along with ER-stress in their mouse model, are some of the few providing insight into the non-immune related mechanisms of T1D (180). ER-stress and perturbations in first-phase insulin release are among the earliest signs of T1D, predating immune infiltration and insulitis (181, 182). The role of Clec16a in these processes not only highlights its crucial role in beta-cell function, but also establishes it as a potential player in the first steps of beta-cell vulnerability in T1D.

DLK1

Delta-like 1 (DLK1), also known as DLL1 or Pref-1 (preadipocyte factor 1), is a transmembrane protein that belongs to the Delta-Notch signaling family. Both mouse and human *Dlk1* are known to be subject to genomic imprinting, and Dlk1 is paternally inherited, with the maternal gene being silenced during development. This becomes potentially interesting considering the sexual discordance in inheritance risk in T1DM, as risk of transmission to offspring is 1.7 fold higher from diabetic fathers than mothers (183). However, Wurst et al. found that, in the case of gestational diabetes mellitus (GDM), serum Dlk1 levels were not significantly different between diabetic and control patients (184). Mouse Dlk1 is expressed highly and ubiquitously during development in the embryo and placenta, starting around E11.5, but becomes downregulated in most adult tissues. Adult Dlk1 expression becomes restricted to the beta-cell, bone marrow, pituitary, and adrenal glands. Some evidence suggests that Dlk1 may help undifferentiated cells maintain their pluripotent state, working as a growth factor to maintain proliferation. In preadipocytes, Dlk1 must be downregulated for differentiation to occur (185). Rodent models have remained somewhat controversial, as *Dlk1* null mice have partially penetrant neonatal lethality and complex adult and developmental phenotypes, yet conditional loss of function models in various tissues using floxed mice failed to recapitulate null phenotypes (186, 187). Dlk1 beta-cell knockout mice were found to be fully viable with normal islet architecture up to six weeks of age, though glycemic control was not assessed. More thorough analyses of Dlk1 in the beta-cell, including insulin secretion and glucose tolerance, are required to fully understand if and how it may contribute to both function and potentially pathogenesis of T1D.

The genetic basis of T1D pathogenesis is complicated and still poorly understood. A majority of these studies have been conducted using data exclusively from Caucasian patients, and inclusion of multi-ethnic populations is required for a more complete and accurate understanding of genetic variants. The few studies using African-ancestry participants have already yielded unique haplotypes and signatures (188, 189). Additionally, as mentioned above, non-coding DNA regulatory regions make up a majority of T1D associated SNPs, which suggests that genetic variation may be impacting regulatory functions rather than gene-coding abilities (165, 166). Gene expression can be controlled *via* long-range interactions, with regulatory elements impacting genes that are hundreds of kilobases away. Understanding these potential interactions requires employment of techniques such as chromatin conformation capture, building a more complete picture of how these SNPs may regulate distant genes through physical contact with non-adjacent promoters. Recently, the use of chromatin-accessibility quantitative trait loci (caQTL) and fine mapping analysis expanded the genetic variants and loci associated with T1D and provided novel molecular targets to investigate (190). Whether it be immune or beta-cell related, understanding these "true" gene targets is a vital steppingstone in leveraging this genetic information to develop diagnostic and therapeutic solutions to T1D.

CLINICAL APPLICATIONS: BETA-CELL DIRECTED THERAPEUTICS

Therapeutic strategies for preventing T1D in high-risk patients have often focused on modulating the immune response to the beta-cell. Newer strategies include methods that focus on the beta cell: reduction of beta-cell dysfunction through the manipulation of ER, oxidative, or cytokine induced cell death. Additionally, functional beta-cell mass replacement strategies through alternative sources, such as stem cells, are being exploited in the field. These strategies, however, will likely have limited clinical utility until autoimmune destruction of the beta-cell replacement can be avoided. Therefore, combinatorial therapeutic programs will likely be required to truly prevent or reverse T1D. Here we describe the state of a few current beta-cell focused therapeutics.

Modulation of ER-Induced Beta-Cell Death

Development of compounds targeting ER-stress pathways are being explored to prevent beta-cell death in early onset T1D. The three UPR sensors PERK, ATF6, and IRE1α regulate apoptosis and thus make a promising target for reducing ER stress and subsequent death in the beta-cell (191). Tauroursdoxycholic acid (TUDCA), a naturally occurring bile acid, can reduce ER-stress by inhibiting the dissociation of BiP from PERK, preventing cell death (192). In a multiple low-dose STZ C57BL/6 mouse model of beta-cell death, TUDCA improved glucose tolerance, increased beta-cell mass, and improved glycemia compared to control diabetic mice (193). The benefits of TUDCA and other UPR chaperones continue to be investigated for their ability to prevent ER-stress induced apoptosis in T1D (194).

An ongoing clinical trial using imatinib mesylate (brand name Gleevec), a tyrosine kinase inhibitor, shows promising results in targeting beta-cell ER stress (195). The efficacy of imatinib for the treatment of various immune-mediated diseases is currently being tested. Initially found to abrogate type 2 diabetes in *db/db* mice, imatinib treatment in the NOD mouse was able to reverse autoimmune diabetes (196, 197). By blunting IRE1α RNase hyperactivity, imatinib reduces beta-cell apoptosis and preserves physiological function. In humans, a clinical trial found imatinib preserved beta-cell function at 12 months in adults with recent-onset T1D (195). Ongoing studies will investigate dose and duration of therapy as well as safety and efficacy for use in children.

Targeting Oxidative Stress

Considering the major role of oxidative stress in T1D pathogenesis, therapies designed to improve antioxidant defenses in beta-cells are another promising avenue for clinical use. Thioredoxin interacting protein (TXNIP), a thioredoxin (TRX) inhibitor of the peroxiredoxin/thioredoxin detoxification pathway has demonstrated clinical potential in both animal models and initial clinical trials (198). The binding of TXNIP to TRX promotes oxidative stress by preventing peroxide clearance. TXNIP is elevated in patients with T1D and T2D (199). *In vivo* overexpression of TXNIP in mouse beta-cells induces apoptosis, while inhibition is protective against STZ-induced diabetes (200). Anti-diabetic agents including insulin and metformin, were found to augment TXNIP degradation through activation of adenosine monophosphate activated protein kinase (AMPK), supporting the idea that TXNIP may be a viable clinical target (201). Verapamil, which blocks voltage-gated calcium channels, decreased TXNIP and enhanced beta-cell survival in both human and rodent islets (202). A clinical trial in which Verapamil was administered (along with insulin therapy) promoted patient beta-cell function and lowered exogenous insulin requirements (203). TXNIP is expressed in multiple cell types throughout the body and additional clinical trials (NCT04545151, NCT04233034) are ongoing to explore the efficacy of TXNIP inhibition in protecting beta-cells and affecting autoimmune responses in patients with T1D.

For both imatinib, an FDA approved anti-leukemia drug, and verapamil, a widely used anti-hypertensive, the ability to repurpose drugs already on the market and with established safety profiles for T1D is an attractive way to expedite the often lengthy and costly process of bringing drugs to market.

Stem Cell Derived Beta-Cells and Emerging Technologies

The development of human stem cells for clinical use may provide a long-term solution to T1D without the challenge of organ shortage and HLA mismatch. While for years now, stem cell-derived insulin-producing cells can be generated and studied in the lab, improvements in cell viability, identity, and reproducibility may be needed before they can be applied as a safe and affordable therapy (204). Beta-cell differentiation from multiple cell sources have been attempted, the most promising of which seem to be induced pluripotent stem cell (iPSC)-derived beta-cells (205). Clinical trials are in progress investigating the efficacy of treating T1D with one version of iPSC derived cells designed by Viacyte, Inc. and CRISPR (Clustered Regularly Interspaced Short Palindromic Repeat) Therapeutics (NCT03163511).

Combining iPSC-derived cells with CRISPR gene editing technology allows the potential to correct monoallelic mutations in genes, such as those that cause MODY diabetes. Optimal for T1D treatment, some therapies are also focused on creating "stealthy" beta-cells and islets, that can be specifically engineered to evade immune recognition. One gene of interest is *renalase (Rnls),* which encodes for an FAD-dependent amine oxidase enzyme that was identified in NIT-1 cells. *Rnls* deletion elicits beta-cell protection against autoimmune attack. NIT-1 cells carrying the *Rnls* mutation improved graft survival when transplanted into diabetic NOD mice (206). Using CRISPR, human iPSCs were generated lacking *RNLS.* These $RNLS^{-/-}$ iPSCs could be successfully differentiated and exhibited normal insulin secretion *in vitro.* Thus far, the *in vivo* function of these cells has not been reported. Similarly, some groups have recently generated iPSC lines that are "hypoimmune" by inactivating MHC class I and II genes and overexpressing protective marker CD47 (207, 208). These stem cells evade immune rejection in fully competent recipients, while maintaining their pluripotency. Hypoimmune stem cells have been used to treat pulmonary and cardiovascular disease and have major implications for universal transplantation (209). The widespread availability of techniques such as single-cell RNA sequencing can bolster the design of iPSC derived beta-cells by identifying the gene expression repertoire needed to obtain the appropriate distribution of cell types within the islet (210).

An exciting new technology that may aid in our understanding of the T1D beta-cell is Patch-Seq, a powerful method that can link single-cell transcriptomes with electrophysiology measurements (211). Groups using this technique in the beta-cell may be able to uncover various levels of beta-cell heterogeneity and link it to functionality in both healthy and T1D contexts. The Yoshihara group is also working on combining concepts with their work reproducing disease with 3D organoids engineered to model immune invasion (212). Overexpression of PD-L1 in human islet organoids was able to protect xenografts from immune invasion and restore glucose homeostasis for 50 days in immune competent mice. Similarly, the Melero-Martin group has used a combinatorial approach to incorporate the importance of islet vasculature in their studies. Their "vascular organoids" include microvessels that become perfused during transplantation and even reduce the islet requirement for transplantation, highlighting the importance of vascular cell types for ideal glucose regulation (213). More combinatorial therapies should be explored as we continue to uncover the nuances of the beta-cell and immunological interface of T1D pathology.

CONCLUSIONS

We have highlighted the crosstalk between pancreatic beta-cells and the immune system in T1D and potential mechanisms by which innate beta-cell characteristics contribute to T1D initiation and progression. Beta-cells display an increased vulnerability to destruction and can also perpetuate inflammatory and autoimmune responses in a destructive positive feedback loop. Despite recent advances in technologies such as single-cell sequencing and the optimization of differentiation protocols for stem cell-derived beta-cells, we still have an incomplete understanding regarding the dynamics of beta-cell biology in T1D. In particular, the relationship between the transcription factors involved in beta-cell heterogeneity that can influence immune evasion versus immune susceptibility need to be further defined. Beta-cell vulnerability to oxidative stress needs to be further explored, as redox-dependent signaling pathways influence numerous facets of beta-cell biology including the differentiation of beta-cell subtypes in T1D. Many of the aforementioned emerging technologies have been examined in T2D in the islet but have not been studied in T1D. Despite the challenges, more studies of human islets before, during, and after autoimmunity in T1D should be performed to improve our understanding of beta-cells that can resist immune destruction, and therefore our ability to design more effective treatments. Could an exploitation of beta-cell populations that are less vulnerable prevent or delay T1D onset? Perhaps as we understand these "resistant" populations more fully, therapies can target and pharmacologically expand them.

AUTHOR CONTRIBUTIONS

ET, KB, HT, CH, and RB outlined, wrote, and edited the manuscript. All authors contributed to the article and approved the submitted version.

ACKNOWLEDGMENTS

Our work was supported by the following NIH grant awards R01 DK127497 (HT), R01 DK126456 (HT and CH); R01 DK111483 (CH); F31 DK120217 (ET), T32 GM008111 (KB), and R01 DK120761 (RB). We apologize to any researchers if we inadvertently omitted any of your research articles in this review due to space limitations. Figures created using Servier Medical Art.

REFERENCES

1. Sekercioglu N, Lovblom LE, Bjornstad P, Lovshin JA, Lytvyn Y, Boulet G, et al. Risk Factors for Diabetic Kidney Disease in Adults With Longstanding Type 1 Diabetes: Results From the Canadian Study of Longevity in Diabetes. *Ren Fail* (2019) 41:427–33. doi: 10.1080/0886022X.2019.1614057
2. Patterson CC, Karuranga S, Salpea P, Saeedi P, Dahlquist G, Soltesz G, et al. Worldwide Estimates of Incidence, Prevalence and Mortality of Type 1 Diabetes in Children and Adolescents: Results From the International

Diabetes Federation Diabetes Atlas, 9th Edition. *Diabetes Res Clin Pract* (2019) 157:107842. doi: 10.1016/j.diabres.2019.107842

3. Bruno G, Runzo C, Cavallo-Perin P, Merletti F, Rivetti M, Pinach S, et al. Incidence of Type 1 and Type 2 Diabetes in Adults Aged 30-49 Years: The Population-Based Registry in the Province of Turin, Italy. *Diabetes Care* (2005) 28:2613–9. doi: 10.2337/diacare.28.11.2613
4. Mobasseri M, Shirmohammadi M, Amiri T, Vahed N, Hosseini Fard H, Ghojazadeh M. Prevalence and Incidence of Type 1 Diabetes in the World: A Systematic Review and Meta-Analysis. *Health Promot Perspect* (2020) 10:98–115. doi: 10.34172/hpp.2020.18
5. Rewers M, Ludvigsson J. Environmental Risk Factors for Type 1 Diabetes. *Lancet* (2016) 387:2340–8. doi: 10.1016/S0140-6736(16)30507-4
6. Oram RA, Jones AG, Besser RE, Knight BA, Shields BM, Brown RJ, et al. The Majority of Patients With Long-Duration Type 1 Diabetes Are Insulin Microsecretors and Have Functioning Beta Cells. *Diabetologia* (2014) 57:187–91. doi: 10.1007/s00125-013-3067-x
7. Pugliese A. Insulitis in the Pathogenesis of Type 1 Diabetes. *Pediatr Diabetes* (2016) 17(Suppl 22):31–6. doi: 10.1111/pedi.12388
8. Bottazzo GF. Lawrence Lecture. Death of a Beta Cell: Homicide or Suicide? *Diabetes Med* (1986) 3:119–30. doi: 10.1111/j.1464-5491.1986.tb00722.x
9. Atkinson MA, Bluestone JA, Eisenbarth GS, Hebrok M, Herold KC, Accili D, et al. How Does Type 1 Diabetes Develop?: The Notion of Homicide or Beta-Cell Suicide Revisited. *Diabetes* (2011) 60:1370–9. doi: 10.2337/db10-1797
10. Zhang IX, Raghavan M, Satin LS. The Endoplasmic Reticulum and Calcium Homeostasis in Pancreatic Beta Cells. *Endocrinology* (2020) 161:1–14. doi: 10.1210/endocr/bqz028
11. Lerner AG, Upton JP, Praveen PV, Ghosh R, Nakagawa Y, Igbaria A, et al. IRE1alpha Induces Thioredoxin-Interacting Protein to Activate the NLRP3 Inflammasome and Promote Programmed Cell Death Under Irremediable ER Stress. *Cell Metab* (2012) 16:250–64. doi: 10.1016/j.cmet.2012.07.007
12. Adams CJ, Kopp MC, Larburu N, Nowak PR, Ali MMU. Structure and Molecular Mechanism of ER Stress Signaling by the Unfolded Protein Response Signal Activator Ire1. *Front Mol Biosci* (2019) 6:11. doi: 10.3389/fmolb.2019.00011
13. Marre ML, James EA, Piganelli JD. Beta Cell ER Stress and the Implications for Immunogenicity in Type 1 Diabetes. *Front Cell Dev Biol* (2015) 3:67. doi: 10.3389/fcell.2015.00067
14. Trudeau JD, Dutz JP, Arany E, Hill DJ, Fieldus WE, Finegood DT. Neonatal Beta-Cell Apoptosis: A Trigger for Autoimmune Diabetes? *Diabetes* (2000) 49:1–7. doi: 10.2337/diabetes.49.1.1
15. O'Brien BA, Harmon BV, Cameron DP, Allan DJ. Apoptosis Is the Mode of Beta-Cell Death Responsible for the Development of IDDM in the Nonobese Diabetic (NOD) Mouse. *Diabetes* (1997) 46:750–7. doi: 10.2337/diab.46.5.750
16. Augstein P, Elefanty AG, Allison J, Harrison LC. Apoptosis and Beta-Cell Destruction in Pancreatic Islets of NOD Mice With Spontaneous and Cyclophosphamide-Accelerated Diabetes. *Diabetologia* (1998) 41:1381–8. doi: 10.1007/s001250051080
17. McClenaghan NH. Physiological Regulation of the Pancreatic {Beta}-Cell: Functional Insights for Understanding and Therapy of Diabetes. *Exp Physiol* (2007) 92:481–96. doi: 10.1113/expphysiol.2006.034835
18. Ding L, Han L, Dube J, Billadeau DD. WASH Regulates Glucose Homeostasis by Facilitating Glut2 Receptor Recycling in Pancreatic Beta-Cells. *Diabetes* (2019) 68:377–86. doi: 10.2337/db18-0189
19. Layden BT, Durai V, Lowe WL Jr. G-Protein-Coupled Receptors, Pancreatic Islets, and Diabetes. *Nat Educ* (2010) 3.
20. Klec C, Ziomek G, Pichler M, Malli R, Graier WF. Calcium Signaling in Ss-Cell Physiology and Pathology: A Revisit. *Int J Mol Sci* (2019) 20:1–24. doi: 10.3390/ijms20246110
21. Marasco MR, Linnemann AK. Beta-Cell Autophagy in Diabetes Pathogenesis. *Endocrinology* (2018) 159:2127–41. doi: 10.1210/en.2017-03273
22. Schuit FC, In't Veld PA, Pipeleers DG. Glucose Stimulates Proinsulin Biosynthesis by a Dose-Dependent Recruitment of Pancreatic Beta Cells. *Proc Natl Acad Sci USA* (1988) 85:3865–9. doi: 10.1073/pnas.85.11.3865
23. Scheuner D, Kaufman RJ. The Unfolded Protein Response: A Pathway That Links Insulin Demand With Beta-Cell Failure and Diabetes. *Endocr Rev* (2008) 29:317–33. doi: 10.1210/er.2007-0039
24. Tersey SA, Nishiki Y, Templin AT, Cabrera SM, Stull ND, Colvin SC, et al. Islet Beta-Cell Endoplasmic Reticulum Stress Precedes the Onset of Type 1 Diabetes in the Nonobese Diabetic Mouse Model. *Diabetes* (2012) 61:818–27. doi: 10.2337/db11-1293
25. Cunha DA, Hekerman P, Ladriere L, Bazarra-Castro A, Ortis F, Wakeham MC, et al. Initiation and Execution of Lipotoxic ER Stress in Pancreatic Beta-Cells. *J Cell Sci* (2008) 121:2308–18. doi: 10.1242/jcs.026062
26. Lenghel A, Gheorghita AM, Vacaru AM, Vacaru AM. What Is the Sweetest UPR Flavor for the Beta-Cell? That Is Question. *Front Endocrinol (Lausanne)* (2020) 11:614123. doi: 10.3389/fendo.2020.614123
27. Lee AH, Iwakoshi NN, Glimcher LH. XBP-1 Regulates a Subset of Endoplasmic Reticulum Resident Chaperone Genes in the Unfolded Protein Response. *Mol Cell Biol* (2003) 23:7448–59. doi: 10.1128/MCB.23.21.7448-7459.2003
28. Bertolotti A, Zhang Y, Hendershot LM, Harding HP, Ron D. Dynamic Interaction of BiP and ER Stress Transducers in the Unfolded-Protein Response. *Nat Cell Biol* (2000) 2:326–32. doi: 10.1038/35014014
29. Fonseca SG, Gromada J, Urano F. Endoplasmic Reticulum Stress and Pancreatic Beta-Cell Death. *Trends Endocrinol Metab* (2011) 22:266–74. doi: 10.1016/j.tem.2011.02.008
30. Han JA, Park SC. Transglutaminase-Dependent Modulation of Transcription Factor Sp1 Activity. *Mol Cells* (2000) 10:612–8. doi: 10.1007/s10059-000-0612-5
31. Fok JY, Mehta K. Tissue Transglutaminase Induces the Release of Apoptosis Inducing Factor and Results in Apoptotic Death of Pancreatic Cancer Cells. *Apoptosis* (2007) 12:1455–63. doi: 10.1007/s10495-007-0079-3
32. Jang B, Shin HY, Choi JK, Nguyen du PT, Jeong BH, Ishigami A, et al. Subcellular Localization of Peptidylarginine Deiminase 2 and Citrullinated Proteins in Brains of Scrapie-Infected Mice: Nuclear Localization of PAD2 and Membrane Fraction-Enriched Citrullinated Proteins. *J Neuropathol Exp Neurol* (2011) 70:116–24. doi: 10.1097/NEN.0b013e318207559e
33. Bruggeman Y, Sodre FMC, Buitinga M, Mathieu C, Overbergh L, Kracht MJL. Targeting Citrullination in Autoimmunity: Insights Learned From Preclinical Mouse Models. *Expert Opin Ther Targets* (2021) 25:269–81. doi: 10.1080/14728222.2021.1918104
34. Lee HJ, Joo M, Abdolrasulnia R, Young DG, Choi I, Ware LB, et al. Peptidylarginine Deiminase 2 Suppresses Inhibitory {Kappa}B Kinase Activity in Lipopolysaccharide-Stimulated RAW 264.7 Macrophages. *J Biol Chem* (2010) 285:39655–62. doi: 10.1074/jbc.M110.170290
35. Gundemir S, Colak G, Tucholski J, Johnson GV. Transglutaminase 2: A Molecular Swiss Army Knife. *Biochim Biophys Acta* (2012) 1823:406–19. doi: 10.1016/j.bbamcr.2011.09.012
36. Marre ML, McGinty JW, Chow IT, DeNicola ME, Beck NW, Kent SC, et al. Modifying Enzymes Are Elicited by ER Stress, Generating Epitopes That Are Selectively Recognized by CD4(+) T Cells in Patients With Type 1 Diabetes. *Diabetes* (2018) 67:1356–68. doi: 10.2337/db17-1166
37. Marre ML, Profozich JL, Coneybeer JT, Geng X, Bertera S, Ford MJ, et al. Inherent ER Stress in Pancreatic Islet Beta Cells Causes Self-Recognition by Autoreactive T Cells in Type 1 Diabetes. *J Autoimmun* (2016) 72:33–46. doi: 10.1016/j.jaut.2016.04.009
38. McGinty JW, Marre ML, Bajzik V, Piganelli JD, James EA. T Cell Epitopes and Post-Translationally Modified Epitopes in Type 1 Diabetes. *Curr Diabetes Rep* (2015) 15:90. doi: 10.1007/s11892-015-0657-7
39. Russo L, Marsella C, Nardo G, Massignan T, Alessio M, Piermarini E, et al. Transglutaminase 2 Transamidation Activity During First-Phase Insulin Secretion: Natural Substrates in INS-1e. *Acta Diabetol* (2013) 50:61–72. doi: 10.1007/s00592-012-0381-6
40. Sidney J, Vela JL, Friedrich D, Kolla R, von Herrath M, Wesley JD, et al. Low HLA Binding of Diabetes-Associated CD8+ T-Cell Epitopes Is Increased by Post Translational Modifications. *BMC Immunol* (2018) 19:12. doi: 10.1186/s12865-018-0250-3
41. Sodre FMC, Bissenova S, Bruggeman Y, Tilvawala R, Cook DP, Berthault C, et al. Peptidylarginine Deiminase Inhibition Prevents Diabetes Development in NOD Mice. *Diabetes* (2021) 70:516–28. doi: 10.2337/db20-0421
42. Rodriguez-Calvo T, Johnson JD, Overbergh L, Dunne JL. Neoepitopes in Type 1 Diabetes: Etiological Insights, Biomarkers and Therapeutic Targets. *Front Immunol* (2021) 12:667989. doi: 10.3389/fimmu.2021.667989

43. Pugliese A. Autoreactive T Cells in Type 1 Diabetes. *J Clin Invest* (2017) 127:2881–91. doi: 10.1172/JCI94549
44. Thomaidou S, Zaldumbide A, Roep BO. Islet Stress, Degradation and Autoimmunity. *Diabetes Obes Metab* (2018) 20(Suppl 2):88–94. doi: 10.1111/dom.13387
45. Kracht MJ, van Lummel M, Nikolic T, Joosten AM, Laban S, van der Slik AR, et al. Autoimmunity Against a Defective Ribosomal Insulin Gene Product in Type 1 Diabetes. *Nat Med* (2017) 23:501–7. doi: 10.1038/nm.4289
46. Baker RL, Rihanek M, Hohenstein AC, Nakayama M, Michels A, Gottlieb PA, et al. Hybrid Insulin Peptides Are Autoantigens in Type 1 Diabetes. *Diabetes* (2019) 68:1830–40. doi: 10.2337/db19-0128
47. Delong T, Wiles TA, Baker RL, Bradley B, Barbour G, Reisdorph R, et al. Pathogenic CD4 T Cells in Type 1 Diabetes Recognize Epitopes Formed by Peptide Fusion. *Science* (2016) 351:711–4. doi: 10.1126/science.aad2791
48. Baker RL, Jamison BL, Haskins K. Hybrid Insulin Peptides Are Neo-Epitopes for CD4 T Cells in Autoimmune Diabetes. *Curr Opin Endocrinol diabetes Obes* (2019) 26:195–200. doi: 10.1097/MED.0000000000000490
49. Wiles TA, Powell R, Michel R, Beard KS, Hohenstein A, Bradley B, et al. Identification of Hybrid Insulin Peptides (HIPs) in Mouse and Human Islets by Mass Spectrometry. *J Proteome Res* (2019) 18:814–25. doi: 10.1021/acs.jproteome.8b00875
50. Reed B, Crawford F, Hill RC, Jin N, White J, Krovi SH, et al. Lysosomal Cathepsin Creates Chimeric Epitopes for Diabetogenic CD4 T Cells *via* Transpeptidation. *J Exp Med* (2021) 218:1–17. doi: 10.1084/jem.20192135
51. Betteridge DJ. What Is Oxidative Stress? *Metabolism* (2000) 49:3–8. doi: 10.1016/S0026-0495(00)80077-3
52. Newsholme P, Rebelato E, Abdulkader F, Krause M, Carpinelli A, Curi R. Reactive Oxygen and Nitrogen Species Generation, Antioxidant Defenses, and Beta-Cell Function: A Critical Role for Amino Acids. *J Endocrinol* (2012) 214:11–20. doi: 10.1530/JOE-12-0072
53. Lei XG, Vatamaniuk MZ. Two Tales of Antioxidant Enzymes on Beta Cells and Diabetes. *Antioxid Redox Signal* (2011) 14:489–503. doi: 10.1089/ars.2010.3416
54. Veal EA, Day AM, Morgan BA. Hydrogen Peroxide Sensing and Signaling. *Mol Cell* (2007) 26:1–14. doi: 10.1016/j.molcel.2007.03.016
55. Pi J, Zhang Q, Fu J, Woods CG, Hou Y, Corkey BE, et al. ROS Signaling, Oxidative Stress and Nrf2 in Pancreatic Beta-Cell Function. *Toxicol Appl Pharmacol* (2010) 244:77–83. doi: 10.1016/j.taap.2009.05.025
56. Li Y, Cao X, Li LX, Brubaker PL, Edlund H, Drucker DJ. Beta-Cell Pdx1 Expression Is Essential for the Glucoregulatory, Proliferative, and Cytoprotective Actions of Glucagon-Like Peptide-1. *Diabetes* (2005) 54:482–91. doi: 10.2337/diabetes.54.2.482
57. Elsner M, Gehrmann W, Lenzen S. Peroxisome-Generated Hydrogen Peroxide as Important Mediator of Lipotoxicity in Insulin-Producing Cells. *Diabetes* (2011) 60:200–8. doi: 10.2337/db09-1401
58. Tiedge M, Lortz S, Drinkgern J, Lenzen S. Relation Between Antioxidant Enzyme Gene Expression and Antioxidative Defense Status of Insulin-Producing Cells. *Diabetes* (1997) 46:1733–42. doi: 10.2337/diab.46.11.1733
59. Grankvist K, Marklund SL, Taljedal IB. CuZn-Superoxide Dismutase, Mn-Superoxide Dismutase, Catalase and Glutathione Peroxidase in Pancreatic Islets and Other Tissues in the Mouse. *Biochem J* (1981) 199:393–8. doi: 10.1042/bj1990393
60. Drews G, Krippeit-Drews P, Dufer M. Oxidative Stress and Beta-Cell Dysfunction. *Pflugers Arch* (2010) 460:703–18. doi: 10.1007/s00424-010-0862-9
61. Miki A, Ricordi C, Sakuma Y, Yamamoto T, Misawa R, Mita A, et al. Divergent Antioxidant Capacity of Human Islet Cell Subsets: A Potential Cause of Beta-Cell Vulnerability in Diabetes and Islet Transplantation. *PloS One* (2018) 13:e0196570. doi: 10.1371/journal.pone.0196570
62. Walter U, Franzke A, Sarukhan A, Zober C, von Boehmer H, Buer J, et al. Monitoring Gene Expression of TNFR Family Members by Beta-Cells During Development of Autoimmune Diabetes. *Eur J Immunol* (2000) 30:1224–32. doi: 10.1002/1521-4141(200004)30:4<1224::AID-IMMU1224>3.0.CO;2-B
63. Tomita T. Immunocytochemical Localization of Cleaved Caspase-3 in Pancreatic Islets From Type 1 Diabetic Subjects. *Islets* (2010) 2:24–9. doi: 10.4161/isl.2.1.10041
64. Marroqui L, Dos Santos RS, Floyel T, Grieco FA, Santin I, Op de Beeck A, et al. TYK2, a Candidate Gene for Type 1 Diabetes, Modulates Apoptosis and the Innate Immune Response in Human Pancreatic Beta-Cells. *Diabetes* (2015) 64:3808–17. doi: 10.2337/db15-0362
65. Wilcox NS, Rui J, Hebrok M, Herold KC. Life and Death of Beta Cells in Type 1 Diabetes: A Comprehensive Review. *J Autoimmun* (2016) 71:51–8. doi: 10.1016/j.jaut.2016.02.001
66. Tomita T. Apoptosis of Pancreatic Beta-Cells in Type 1 Diabetes. *Bosn J Basic Med Sci* (2017) 17:183–93. doi: 10.17305/bjbms.2017.1961
67. Mallone R, Eizirik DL. Presumption of Innocence for Beta Cells: Why Are They Vulnerable Autoimmune Targets in Type 1 Diabetes? *Diabetologia* (2020) 63:1999–2006. doi: 10.1007/s00125-020-05176-7
68. Jansson L, Barbu A, Bodin B, Drott CJ, Espes D, Gao X, et al. Pancreatic Islet Blood Flow and Its Measurement. *Ups J Med Sci* (2016) 121:81–95. doi: 10.3109/03009734.2016.1164769
69. Henderson JR, Moss MC. A Morphometric Study of the Endocrine and Exocrine Capillaries of the Pancreas. *Q J Exp Physiol* (1985) 70:347–56. doi: 10.1113/expphysiol.1985.sp002920
70. Kamba T, Tam BY, Hashizume H, Haskell A, Sennino B, Mancuso MR, et al. VEGF-Dependent Plasticity of Fenestrated Capillaries in the Normal Adult Microvasculature. *Am J Physiol Heart Circ Physiol* (2006) 290:H560–76. doi: 10.1152/ajpheart.00133.2005
71. Magnuson AM, Thurber GM, Kohler RH, Weissleder R, Mathis D, Benoist C. Population Dynamics of Islet-Infiltrating Cells in Autoimmune Diabetes. *Proc Natl Acad Sci USA* (2015) 112:1511–6. doi: 10.1073/pnas.1423769112
72. Costa FR, Francozo MC, de Oliveira GG, Ignacio A, Castoldi A, Zamboni DS, et al. Gut Microbiota Translocation to the Pancreatic Lymph Nodes Triggers NOD2 Activation and Contributes to T1D Onset. *J Exp Med* (2016) 213:1223–39. doi: 10.1084/jem.20150744
73. Dedrick S, Sundaresh B, Huang Q, Brady C, Yoo T, Cronin C, et al. The Role of Gut Microbiota and Environmental Factors in Type 1 Diabetes Pathogenesis. *Front Endocrinol (Lausanne)* (2020) 11:78. doi: 10.3389/fendo.2020.00078
74. Bosi E, Molteni L, Radaelli MG, Folini L, Fermo I, Bazzigaluppi E, et al. Increased Intestinal Permeability Precedes Clinical Onset of Type 1 Diabetes. *Diabetologia* (2006) 49:2824–7. doi: 10.1007/s00125-006-0465-3
75. Wen L, Ley RE, Volchkov PY, Stranges PB, Avanesyan L, Stonebraker AC, et al. Innate Immunity and Intestinal Microbiota in the Development of Type 1 Diabetes. *Nature* (2008) 455:1109–13. doi: 10.1038/nature07336
76. Burrows MP, Volchkov P, Kobayashi KS, Chervonsky AV. Microbiota Regulates Type 1 Diabetes Through Toll-Like Receptors. *Proc Natl Acad Sci USA* (2015) 112:9973–7. doi: 10.1073/pnas.1508740112
77. Markle JG, Frank DN, Adeli K, von Bergen M, Danska JS. Microbiome Manipulation Modifies Sex-Specific Risk for Autoimmunity. *Gut Microbes* (2014) 5:485–93. doi: 10.4161/gmic.29795
78. Yurkovetskiy L, Burrows M, Khan AA, Graham L, Volchkov P, Becker L, et al. Gender Bias in Autoimmunity Is Influenced by Microbiota. *Immunity* (2013) 39:400–12. doi: 10.1016/j.immuni.2013.08.013
79. Markle JG, Frank DN, Mortin-Toth S, Robertson CE, Feazel LM, Rolle-Kampczyk U, et al. Sex Differences in the Gut Microbiome Drive Hormone-Dependent Regulation of Autoimmunity. *Science* (2013) 339:1084–8. doi: 10.1126/science.1233521
80. Stewart CJ, Ajami NJ, O'Brien JL, Hutchinson DS, Smith DP, Wong MC, et al. Temporal Development of the Gut Microbiome in Early Childhood From the TEDDY Study. *Nature* (2018) 562:583–8. doi: 10.1038/s41586-018-0617-x
81. Vatanen T, Franzosa EA, Schwager R, Tripathi S, Arthur TD, Vehik K, et al. The Human Gut Microbiome in Early-Onset Type 1 Diabetes From the TEDDY Study. *Nature* (2018) 562:589–94. doi: 10.1038/s41586-018-0620-2
82. Dula SB, Jecmenica M, Wu R, Jahanshahi P, Verrilli GM, Carter JD, et al. Evidence That Low-Grade Systemic Inflammation Can Induce Islet Dysfunction as Measured by Impaired Calcium Handling. *Cell Calcium* (2010) 48:133–42. doi: 10.1016/j.ceca.2010.07.007
83. Ramadan JW, Steiner SR, O'Neill CM, Nunemaker CS. The Central Role of Calcium in the Effects of Cytokines on Beta-Cell Function: Implications for Type 1 and Type 2 Diabetes. *Cell Calcium* (2011) 50:481–90. doi: 10.1016/j.ceca.2011.08.005

84. Miani M, Barthson J, Colli ML, Brozzi F, Cnop M, Eizirik DL. Endoplasmic Reticulum Stress Sensitizes Pancreatic Beta Cells to Interleukin-1beta-Induced Apoptosis *via* Bim/A1 Imbalance. *Cell Death Dis* (2013) 4:e701. doi: 10.1038/cddis.2013.236
85. Gurzov EN, Ortis F, Cunha DA, Gosset G, Li M, Cardozo AK, et al. Signaling by IL-1beta+IFN-Gamma and ER Stress Converge on DP5/Hrk Activation: A Novel Mechanism for Pancreatic Beta-Cell Apoptosis. *Cell Death Differ* (2009) 16:1539–50. doi: 10.1038/cdd.2009.99
86. Zhang S, Kim KH. TNF-Alpha Inhibits Glucose-Induced Insulin Secretion in a Pancreatic Beta-Cell Line (INS-1). *FEBS Lett* (1995) 377:237–9. doi: 10.1016/0014-5793(95)01272-9
87. Collier JJ, Burke SJ, Eisenhauer ME, Lu D, Sapp RC, Frydman CJ, et al. Pancreatic Beta-Cell Death in Response to Pro-Inflammatory Cytokines Is Distinct From Genuine Apoptosis. *PloS One* (2011) 6:e22485. doi: 10.1371/journal.pone.0022485
88. Dickerson MT, Bogart AM, Altman MK, Milian SC, Jordan KL, Dadi PK, et al. Cytokine-Mediated Changes in K(+) Channel Activity Promotes an Adaptive Ca(2+) Response That Sustains Beta-Cell Insulin Secretion During Inflammation. *Sci Rep* (2018) 8:1158. doi: 10.1038/s41598-018-19600-x
89. El Muayed M, Billings LK, Raja MR, Zhang X, Park PJ, Newman MV, et al. Acute Cytokine-Mediated Downregulation of the Zinc Transporter ZnT8 Alters Pancreatic Beta-Cell Function. *J Endocrinol* (2010) 206:159–69. doi: 10.1677/JOE-09-0420
90. Oleson BJ, Corbett JA. Dual Role of Nitric Oxide in Regulating the Response of Beta Cells to DNA Damage. *Antioxid Redox Signal* (2018) 29:1432–45. doi: 10.1089/ars.2017.7351
91. Oleson BJ, Broniowska KA, Naatz A, Hogg N, Tarakanova VL, Corbett JA. Nitric Oxide Suppresses Beta-Cell Apoptosis by Inhibiting the DNA Damage Response. *Mol Cell Biol* (2016) 36:2067–77. doi: 10.1128/MCB.00262-16
92. Akerfeldt MC, Howes J, Chan JY, Stevens VA, Boubenna N, McGuire HM, et al. Cytokine-Induced Beta-Cell Death Is Independent of Endoplasmic Reticulum Stress Signaling. *Diabetes* (2008) 57:3034–44. doi: 10.2337/db07-1802
93. Dorrell C, Schug J, Canaday PS, Russ HA, Tarlow BD, Grompe MT, et al. Human Islets Contain Four Distinct Subtypes of Beta Cells. *Nat Commun* (2016) 7:11756. doi: 10.1038/ncomms11756
94. Johnston NR, Mitchell RK, Haythorne E, Pessoa MP, Semplici F, Ferrer J, et al. Beta Cell Hubs Dictate Pancreatic Islet Responses to Glucose. *Cell Metab* (2016) 24:389–401. doi: 10.1016/j.cmet.2016.06.020
95. van der Meulen T, Mawla AM, DiGruccio MR, Adams MW, Nies V, Dolleman S, et al. Virgin Beta Cells Persist Throughout Life at a Neogenic Niche Within Pancreatic Islets. *Cell Metab* (2017) 25:911–926 e6. doi: 10.1016/j.cmet.2017.03.017
96. Salomon D, Meda P. Heterogeneity and Contact-Dependent Regulation of Hormone Secretion by Individual B Cells. *Exp Cell Res* (1986) 162:507–20. doi: 10.1016/0014-4827(86)90354-X
97. Hiriart M, Ramirez-Medeles MC. Functional Subpopulations of Individual Pancreatic B-Cells in Culture. *Endocrinology* (1991) 128:3193–8. doi: 10.1210/endo-128-6-3193
98. Skinningsrud B, Husebye ES, Pearce SH, McDonald DO, Brandal K, Wolff AB, et al. Polymorphisms in CLEC16A and CIITA at 16p13 Are Associated With Primary Adrenal Insufficiency. *J Clin Endocrinol Metab* (2008) 93:3310–7. doi: 10.1210/jc.2008-0821
99. Lee EY, Lee ZH, Song YW. CXCL10 and Autoimmune Diseases. *Autoimmun Rev* (2009) 8:379–83. doi: 10.1016/j.autrev.2008.12.002
100. Thorel F, Nepote V, Avril I, Kohno K, Desgraz R, Chera S, et al. Conversion of Adult Pancreatic Alpha-Cells to Beta-Cells After Extreme Beta-Cell Loss. *Nature* (2010) 464:1149–54. doi: 10.1038/nature08894
101. Bader E, Migliorini A, Gegg M, Moruzzi N, Gerdes J, Roscioni SS, et al. Identification of Proliferative and Mature Beta-Cells in the Islets of Langerhans. *Nature* (2016) 535:430–4. doi: 10.1038/nature18624
102. Kravets V, Dwulet JM, Schleicher WE, Hodson DJ, Davis AM, Piscopio RA, et al. Functional Architecture of the Pancreatic Islets: First Responder Cells Drive the First-Phase [Ca2+] Response. *bioRxiv* (2020) 2020.12.22.424082. doi: 10.1101/2020.12.22.424082
103. Li J, Klughammer J, Farlik M, Penz T, Spittler A, Barbieux C, et al. Single-Cell Transcriptomes Reveal Characteristic Features of Human Pancreatic Islet Cell Types. *EMBO Rep* (2016) 17:178–87. doi: 10.15252/embr.201540946
104. Wang YJ, Golson ML, Schug J, Traum D, Liu C, Vivek K, et al. Single-Cell Mass Cytometry Analysis of the Human Endocrine Pancreas. *Cell Metab* (2016) 24:616–26. doi: 10.1016/j.cmet.2016.09.007
105. Baron M, Veres A, Wolock SL, Faust AL, Gaujoux R, Vetere A, et al. A Single-Cell Transcriptomic Map of the Human and Mouse Pancreas Reveals Inter- and Intra-Cell Population Structure. *Cell Syst* (2016) 3:346–60.e4. doi: 10.1016/j.cels.2016.08.011
106. Aguayo-Mazzucato C, van Haaren M, Mruk M, Lee TBJr., Crawford C, Hollister-Lock J, et al. Beta Cell Aging Markers Have Heterogeneous Distribution and Are Induced by Insulin Resistance. *Cell Metab* (2017) 25:898–910.e5. doi: 10.1016/j.cmet.2017.03.015
107. Muraro MJ, Dharmadhikari G, Grun D, Groen N, Dielen T, Jansen E, et al. A Single-Cell Transcriptome Atlas of the Human Pancreas. *Cell Syst* (2016) 3:385–94.e3. doi: 10.1016/j.cels.2016.09.002
108. Zeng C, Mulas F, Sui Y, Guan T, Miller N, Tan Y, et al. Pseudotemporal Ordering of Single Cells Reveals Metabolic Control of Postnatal Beta Cell Proliferation. *Cell Metab* (2017) 25:1160–75.e11. doi: 10.1016/j.cmet.2017.04.014
109. Qiu WL, Zhang YW, Feng Y, Li LC, Yang L, Xu CR. Deciphering Pancreatic Islet Beta Cell and Alpha Cell Maturation Pathways and Characteristic Features at the Single-Cell Level. *Cell Metab* (2018) 27:702. doi: 10.1016/j.cmet.2018.01.017
110. Farack L, Golan M, Egozi A, Dezorella N, Bahar Halpern K, Ben-Moshe S, et al. Transcriptional Heterogeneity of Beta Cells in the Intact Pancreas. *Dev Cell* (2019) 48:115–25.e4. doi: 10.1016/j.devcel.2018.11.001
111. Lira SA, Furtado GC. The Biology of Chemokines and Their Receptors. *Immunol Res* (2012) 54:111–20. doi: 10.1007/s12026-012-8313-7
112. Gerard C, Rollins BJ. Chemokines and Disease. *Nat Immunol* (2001) 2:108–15. doi: 10.1038/84209
113. Dangaj D, Bruand M, Grimm AJ, Ronet C, Barras D, Duttagupta PA, et al. Cooperation Between Constitutive and Inducible Chemokines Enables T Cell Engraftment and Immune Attack in Solid Tumors. *Cancer Cell* (2019) 35:885–900.e10. doi: 10.1016/j.ccell.2019.05.004
114. Griffith JW, Sokol CL, Luster AD. Chemokines and Chemokine Receptors: Positioning Cells for Host Defense and Immunity. *Annu Rev Immunol* (2014) 32:659–702. doi: 10.1146/annurev-immunol-032713-120145
115. Martin AP, Rankin S, Pitchford S, Charo IF, Furtado GC, Lira SA. Increased Expression of CCL2 in Insulin-Producing Cells of Transgenic Mice Promotes Mobilization of Myeloid Cells From the Bone Marrow, Marked Insulitis, and Diabetes. *Diabetes* (2008) 57:3025–33. doi: 10.2337/db08-0625
116. Gschwandtner M, Derler R, Midwood KS. More Than Just Attractive: How CCL2 Influences Myeloid Cell Behavior Beyond Chemotaxis. *Front Immunol* (2019) 10:2759. doi: 10.3389/fimmu.2019.02759
117. Daly C, Rollins BJ. Monocyte Chemoattractant Protein-1 (CCL2) in Inflammatory Disease and Adaptive Immunity: Therapeutic Opportunities and Controversies. *Microcirculation* (2003) 10:247–57. doi: 10.1080/mic.10.3-4.247.257
118. Chen MC, Proost P, Gysemans C, Mathieu C, Eizirik DL. Monocyte Chemoattractant Protein-1 Is Expressed in Pancreatic Islets From Prediabetic NOD Mice and in Interleukin-1 Beta-Exposed Human and Rat Islet Cells. *Diabetologia* (2001) 44:325–32. doi: 10.1007/s001250051622
119. Sarkar SA, Lee CE, Victorino F, Nguyen TT, Walters JA, Burrack A, et al. Expression and Regulation of Chemokines in Murine and Human Type 1 Diabetes. *Diabetes* (2012) 61:436–46. doi: 10.2337/db11-0853
120. Cowley MJ, Weinberg A, Zammit NW, Walters SN, Hawthorne WJ, Loudovaris T, et al. Human Islets Express a Marked Proinflammatory Molecular Signature Prior to Transplantation. *Cell Transplant* (2012) 21:2063–78. doi: 10.3727/096368911X627372
121. Burke SJ, Stadler K, Lu D, Gleason E, Han A, Donohoe DR, et al. IL-1beta Reciprocally Regulates Chemokine and Insulin Secretion in Pancreatic Beta-Cells *via* NF-Kappab. *Am J Physiol Endocrinol Metab* (2015) 309:E715–26. doi: 10.1152/ajpendo.00153.2015
122. Burke SJ, Goff MR, Updegraff BL, Lu D, Brown PL, Minkin SCJr., et al. Regulation of the CCL2 Gene in Pancreatic Beta-Cells by IL-1beta and Glucocorticoids: Role of MKP-1. *PloS One* (2012) 7:e46986. doi: 10.1371/journal.pone.0046986
123. Jansen A, Homo-Delarche F, Hooijkaas H, Leenen PJ, Dardenne M, Drexhage HA. Immunohistochemical Characterization of Monocytes-

Macrophages and Dendritic Cells Involved in the Initiation of the Insulitis and Beta-Cell Destruction in NOD Mice. *Diabetes* (1994) 43:667–75. doi: 10.2337/diab.43.5.667

124. Wang YJ, Traum D, Schug J, Gao L, Liu C, Consortium H, et al. Multiplexed *In Situ* Imaging Mass Cytometry Analysis of the Human Endocrine Pancreas and Immune System in Type 1 Diabetes. *Cell Metab* (2019) 29:769–83.e4. doi: 10.1016/j.cmet.2019.01.003
125. Xu R, Li Y, Yan H, Zhang E, Huang X, Chen Q, et al. CCL2 Promotes Macrophages-Associated Chemoresistance *via* MCPIP1 Dual Catalytic Activities in Multiple Myeloma. *Cell Death Dis* (2019) 10:781. doi: 10.1038/s41419-019-2012-4
126. Carvalho-Pinto C, Garcia MI, Gomez L, Ballesteros A, Zaballos A, Flores JM, et al. Leukocyte Attraction Through the CCR5 Receptor Controls Progress From Insulitis to Diabetes in Non-Obese Diabetic Mice. *Eur J Immunol* (2004) 34:548–57. doi: 10.1002/eji.200324285
127. Frigerio S, Junt T, Lu B, Gerard C, Zumsteg U, Hollander GA, et al. Beta Cells Are Responsible for CXCR3-Mediated T-Cell Infiltration in Insulitis. *Nat Med* (2002) 8:1414–20. doi: 10.1038/nm1202-792
128. Hanifi-Moghaddam P, Kappler S, Seissler J, Muller-Scholze S, Martin S, Roep BO, et al. Altered Chemokine Levels in Individuals at Risk of Type 1 Diabetes Mellitus. *Diabetes Med* (2006) 23:156–63. doi: 10.1111/j.1464-5491.2005.01743.x
129. Jamali Z, Nazari M, Khoramdelazad H, Hakimizadeh E, Mahmoodi M, Karimabad MN, et al. Expression of CC Chemokines CCL2, CCL5, and CCL11 Is Associated With Duration of Disease and Complications in Type-1 Diabetes: A Study on Iranian Diabetic Patients. *Clin Lab* (2013) 59:993–1001. doi: 10.7754/Clin.Lab.2012.120810
130. Loetscher M, Loetscher P, Brass N, Meese E, Moser B. Lymphocyte-Specific Chemokine Receptor CXCR3: Regulation, Chemokine Binding and Gene Localization. *Eur J Immunol* (1998) 28:3696–705. doi: 10.1002/(SICI)1521-4141(199811)28:11<3696::AID-IMMU3696>3.0.CO;2-W
131. Vazirinejad R, Ahmadi Z, Kazemi Arababadi M, Hassanshahi G, Kennedy D. The Biological Functions, Structure and Sources of CXCL10 and Its Outstanding Part in the Pathophysiology of Multiple Sclerosis. *Neuroimmunomodulation* (2014) 21:322–30. doi: 10.1159/000357780
132. Nigi L, Brusco N, Grieco GE, Licata G, Krogvold L, Marselli L, et al. Pancreatic Alpha-Cells Contribute Together With Beta-Cells to CXCL10 Expression in Type 1 Diabetes. *Front Endocrinol (Lausanne)* (2020) 11:630. doi: 10.3389/fendo.2020.00630
133. Loetscher M, Gerber B, Loetscher P, Jones SA, Piali L, Clark-Lewis I, et al. Chemokine Receptor Specific for IP10 and Mig: Structure, Function, and Expression in Activated T-Lymphocytes. *J Exp Med* (1996) 184:963–9. doi: 10.1084/jem.184.3.963
134. Luster AD, Ravetch JV. Biochemical Characterization of a Gamma Interferon-Inducible Cytokine (IP-10). *J Exp Med* (1987) 166:1084–97. doi: 10.1084/jem.166.4.1084
135. Nagaoka K, Nojima H, Watanabe F, Chang KT, Christenson RK, Sakai S, et al. Regulation of Blastocyst Migration, Apposition, and Initial Adhesion by a Chemokine, Interferon Gamma-Inducible Protein 10 kDa (IP-10), During Early Gestation. *J Biol Chem* (2003) 278:29048–56. doi: 10.1074/jbc.M300470200
136. Yates-Binder CC, Rodgers M, Jaynes J, Wells A, Bodnar RJ, Turner T. An IP-10 (CXCL10)-Derived Peptide Inhibits Angiogenesis. *PloS One* (2012) 7: e40812. doi: 10.1371/journal.pone.0040812
137. Van Belle TL, Taylor P, von Herrath MG. Mouse Models for Type 1 Diabetes. *Drug Discov Today Dis Models* (2009) 6:41–5. doi: 10.1016/j.ddmod.2009.03.008
138. Christoffersson G, Flodstrom-Tullberg M. Mouse Models of Virus-Induced Type 1 Diabetes. *Methods Mol Biol* (2020) 2128:93–105. doi: 10.1007/978-1-0716-0385-7_7
139. Christen U, McGavern DB, Luster AD, von Herrath MG, Oldstone MB. Among CXCR3 Chemokines, IFN-Gamma-Inducible Protein of 10 kDa (CXC Chemokine Ligand (CXCL) 10) But Not Monokine Induced by IFN-Gamma (CXCL9) Imprints a Pattern for the Subsequent Development of Autoimmune Disease. *J Immunol* (2003) 171:6838–45. doi: 10.4049/jimmunol.171.12.6838
140. Shimada A, Oikawa Y, Yamada Y, Okubo Y, Narumi S. The Role of the CXCL10/CXCR3 System in Type 1 Diabetes. *Rev Diabetes Stud* (2009) 6:81–4. doi: 10.1900/RDS.2009.6.81
141. Morimoto J, Yoneyama H, Shimada A, Shigihara T, Yamada S, Oikawa Y, et al. CXC Chemokine Ligand 10 Neutralization Suppresses the Occurrence of Diabetes in Nonobese Diabetic Mice Through Enhanced Beta Cell Proliferation Without Affecting Insulitis. *J Immunol* (2004) 173:7017–24. doi: 10.4049/jimmunol.173.11.7017
142. Schulthess FT, Paroni F, Sauter NS, Shu L, Ribaux P, Haataja L, et al. CXCL10 Impairs Beta Cell Function and Viability in Diabetes Through TLR4 Signaling. *Cell Metab* (2009) 9:125–39. doi: 10.1016/j.cmet.2009.01.003
143. Lee JH, Kim B, Jin WJ, Kim HH, Ha H, Lee ZH. Pathogenic Roles of CXCL10 Signaling Through CXCR3 and TLR4 in Macrophages and T Cells: Relevance for Arthritis. *Arthritis Res Ther* (2017) 19:163. doi: 10.1186/s13075-017-1353-6
144. Arnush M, Heitmeier MR, Scarim AL, Marino MH, Manning PT, Corbett JA. IL-1 Produced and Released Endogenously Within Human Islets Inhibits Beta Cell Function. *J Clin Invest* (1998) 102:516–26. doi: 10.1172/JCI844
145. Saitoh N, Awaya A, Sakudo A, SungWook S, Saeki K, Matsumoto Y, et al. Serum Thymic Factor Prevents LPS-Induced Pancreatic Cell Damage in Mice *via* Up-Regulation of Bcl-2 Expression in Pancreas. *Microbiol Immunol* (2004) 48:629–38. doi: 10.1111/j.1348-0421.2004.tb03471.x
146. Kanazawa Y, Komeda K, Sato S, Mori S, Akanuma K, Takaku F. Non-Obese-Diabetic Mice: Immune Mechanisms of Pancreatic Beta-Cell Destruction. *Diabetologia* (1984) 27 Suppl:113–5. doi: 10.1007/BF00275663
147. Bottazzo GF, Dean BM, McNally JM, MacKay EH, Swift PG, Gamble DR. In Situ Characterization of Autoimmune Phenomena and Expression of HLA Molecules in the Pancreas in Diabetic Insulitis. *N Engl J Med* (1985) 313:353–60. doi: 10.1056/NEJM198508083130604
148. Slattery R. Transgenic Approaches to Understanding the Role of MHC Genes in Insulin Dependent Diabetes Mellitus. II. The Non-Obese Diabetic (NOD) Mouse. *Baillieres Clin Endocrinol Metab* (1991) 5:449–54. doi: 10.1016/S0950-351X(05)80141-7
149. Roep BO. The Role of T-Cells in the Pathogenesis of Type 1 Diabetes: From Cause to Cure. *Diabetologia* (2003) 46:305–21. doi: 10.1007/s00125-003-1089-5
150. Russell MA, Redick SD, Blodgett DM, Richardson SJ, Leete P, Krogvold L, et al. HLA Class II Antigen Processing And Presentation Pathway Components Demonstrated by Transcriptome and Protein Analyses of Islet Beta-Cells From Donors With Type 1 Diabetes. *Diabetes* (2019) 68:988–1001. doi: 10.2337/db18-0686
151. Richardson SJ, Rodriguez-Calvo T, Gerling IC, Mathews CE, Kaddis JS, Russell MA, et al. Islet Cell Hyperexpression of HLA Class I Antigens: A Defining Feature in Type 1 Diabetes. *Diabetologia* (2016) 59:2448–58. doi: 10.1007/s00125-016-4067-4
152. Leiter EH, Christianson GJ, Serreze DV, Ting AT, Worthen SM. MHC Antigen Induction by Interferon Gamma on Cultured Mouse Pancreatic Beta Cells and Macrophages. Genetic Analysis of Strain Differences and Discovery of an "Occult" Class I-Like Antigen in NOD/Lt Mice. *J Exp Med* (1989) 170:1243–62. doi: 10.1084/jem.170.4.1243
153. Stassi G, De Maria R, Trucco G, Rudert W, Testi R, Galluzzo A, et al. Nitric Oxide Primes Pancreatic Beta Cells for Fas-Mediated Destruction in Insulin-Dependent Diabetes Mellitus. *J Exp Med* (1997) 186:1193–200. doi: 10.1084/jem.186.8.1193
154. Moriwaki M, Itoh N, Miyagawa J, Yamamoto K, Imagawa A, Yamagata K, et al. Fas and Fas Ligand Expression in Inflamed Islets in Pancreas Sections of Patients With Recent-Onset Type I Diabetes Mellitus. *Diabetologia* (1999) 42:1332–40. doi: 10.1007/s001250051446
155. Itoh N, Imagawa A, Hanafusa T, Waguri M, Yamamoto K, Iwahashi H, et al. Requirement of Fas for the Development of Autoimmune Diabetes in Nonobese Diabetic Mice. *J Exp Med* (1997) 186:613–8. doi: 10.1084/jem.186.4.613
156. Sia C, Hanninen A. Apoptosis in Autoimmune Diabetes: The Fate of Beta-Cells in the Cleft Between Life and Death. *Rev Diabetes Stud* (2006) 3:39–46. doi: 10.1900/RDS.2006.3.39
157. Amrani A, Verdaguer J, Thiessen S, Bou S, Santamaria P. IL-1alpha, IL-1beta, and IFN-Gamma Mark Beta Cells for Fas-Dependent Destruction by Diabetogenic CD4(+) T Lymphocytes. *J Clin Invest* (2000) 105:459–68. doi: 10.1172/JCI8185
158. Loweth AC, Williams GT, James RF, Scarpello JH, Morgan NG. Human Islets of Langerhans Express Fas Ligand and Undergo Apoptosis in Response

to Interleukin-1beta and Fas Ligation. *Diabetes* (1998) 47:727–32. doi: 10.2337/diabetes.47.5.727

159. Pihoker C, Gilliam LK, Hampe CS, Lernmark A. Autoantibodies in Diabetes. *Diabetes* (2005) 54 Suppl 2:S52–61. doi: 10.2337/diabetes.54.suppl_2.S52
160. Keenan HA, Sun JK, Levine J, Doria A, Aiello LP, Eisenbarth G, et al. Residual Insulin Production and Pancreatic Ss-Cell Turnover After 50 Years of Diabetes: Joslin Medalist Study. *Diabetes* (2010) 59:2846–53. doi: 10.2337/db10-0676
161. Rui J, Deng S, Arazi A, Perdigoto AL, Liu Z, Herold KC. Beta Cells That Resist Immunological Attack Develop During Progression of Autoimmune Diabetes in NOD Mice. *Cell Metab* (2017) 25:727–38. doi: 10.1016/j.cmet.2017.01.005
162. Leete P, Oram RA, McDonald TJ, Shields BM, Ziller CT.S. TEAM, et al. Studies of Insulin and Proinsulin in Pancreas and Serum Support the Existence of Aetiopathological Endotypes of Type 1 Diabetes Associated With Age at Diagnosis. *Diabetologia* (2020) 63:1258–67. doi: 10.1007/s00125-020-05115-6
163. Leete P, Willcox A, Krogvold L, Dahl-Jorgensen K, Foulis AK, Richardson SJ, et al. Differential Insulitic Profiles Determine the Extent of Beta-Cell Destruction and the Age at Onset of Type 1 Diabetes. *Diabetes* (2016) 65:1362–9. doi: 10.2337/db15-1615
164. Arif S, Leete P, Nguyen V, Marks K, Nor NM, Estorninho M, et al. Blood and Islet Phenotypes Indicate Immunological Heterogeneity in Type 1 Diabetes. *Diabetes* (2014) 63:3835–45. doi: 10.2337/db14-0365
165. Grant SFA, Wells AD, Rich SS. Next Steps in the Identification of Gene Targets for Type 1 Diabetes. *Diabetologia* (2020) 63:2260–9. doi: 10.1007/s00125-020-05248-8
166. Onengut-Gumuscu S, Chen WM, Burren O, Cooper NJ, Quinlan AR, Mychaleckyj JC, et al. Fine Mapping of Type 1 Diabetes Susceptibility Loci and Evidence for Colocalization of Causal Variants With Lymphoid Gene Enhancers. *Nat Genet* (2015) 47:381–6. doi: 10.1038/ng.3245
167. Bell GI, Horita S, Karam JH. A Polymorphic Locus Near the Human Insulin Gene Is Associated With Insulin-Dependent Diabetes Mellitus. *Diabetes* (1984) 33:176–83. doi: 10.2337/diab.33.2.176
168. Eizirik DL, Sammeth M, Bouckenooghe T, Bottu G, Sisino G, Igoillo-Esteve M, et al. The Human Pancreatic Islet Transcriptome: Expression of Candidate Genes for Type 1 Diabetes and the Impact of Pro-Inflammatory Cytokines. *PloS Genet* (2012) 8:e1002552. doi: 10.1371/journal.pgen.1002552
169. Pugliese A, Zeller M, Fernandez AJr., Zalcberg LJ, Bartlett RJ, Ricordi C, et al. The Insulin Gene Is Transcribed in the Human Thymus and Transcription Levels Correlated With Allelic Variation at the INS VNTR-IDDM2 Susceptibility Locus for Type 1 Diabetes. *Nat Genet* (1997) 15:293–7. doi: 10.1038/ng0397-293
170. Wen X, Yang Y. Emerging Roles of GLIS3 in Neonatal Diabetes, Type 1 and Type 2 Diabetes. *J Mol Endocrinol* (2017) 58:R73–85. doi: 10.1530/JME-16-0232
171. Barrett JC, Clayton DG, Concannon P, Akolkar B, Cooper JD, Erlich HA, et al. Genome-Wide Association Study and Meta-Analysis Find That Over 40 Loci Affect Risk of Type 1 Diabetes. *Nat Genet* (2009) 41:703–7. doi: 10.1038/ng.381
172. Kiani AK, John P, Bhatti A, Zia A, Shahid G, Akhtar P, et al. Association of 32 Type 1 Diabetes Risk Loci in Pakistani Patients. *Diabetes Res Clin Pract* (2015) 108:137–42. doi: 10.1016/j.diabres.2015.01.022
173. Awata T, Yamashita H, Kurihara S, Morita-Ohkubo T, Miyashita Y, Katayama S, et al. A Low-Frequency GLIS3 Variant Associated With Resistance to Japanese Type 1 Diabetes. *Biochem Biophys Res Commun* (2013) 437:521–5. doi: 10.1016/j.bbrc.2013.06.102
174. Kang HS, Kim YS, ZeRuth G, Beak JY, Gerrish K, Kilic G, et al. Transcription Factor Glis3, A Novel Critical Player in the Regulation of Pancreatic Beta-Cell Development and Insulin Gene Expression. *Mol Cell Biol* (2009) 29:6366–79. doi: 10.1128/MCB.01259-09
175. Yang Y, Chang BH, Samson SL, Li MV, Chan L. The Kruppel-Like Zinc Finger Protein Glis3 Directly and Indirectly Activates Insulin Gene Transcription. *Nucleic Acids Res* (2009) 37:2529–38. doi: 10.1093/nar/gkp122
176. Watanabe N, Hiramatsu K, Miyamoto R, Yasuda K, Suzuki N, Oshima N, et al. A Murine Model of Neonatal Diabetes Mellitus in Glis3-Deficient Mice. *FEBS Lett* (2009) 583:2108–13. doi: 10.1016/j.febslet.2009.05.039
177. Yang Y, Chang BH, Yechoor V, Chen W, Li L, Tsai MJ, et al. The Kruppel-Like Zinc Finger Protein GLIS3 Transactivates Neurogenin 3 for Proper Fetal Pancreatic Islet Differentiation in Mice. *Diabetologia* (2011) 54:2595–605. doi: 10.1007/s00125-011-2255-9
178. Hakonarson H, Grant SF, Bradfield JP, Marchand L, Kim CE, Glessner JT, et al. A Genome-Wide Association Study Identifies KIAA0350 as a Type 1 Diabetes Gene. *Nature* (2007) 448:591–4. doi: 10.1038/nature06010
179. C. International Multiple Sclerosis Genetics. The Expanding Genetic Overlap Between Multiple Sclerosis and Type I Diabetes. *Genes Immun* (2009) 10:11–4. doi: 10.1038/gene.2008.83
180. Soleimanpour SA, Gupta A, Bakay M, Ferrari AM, Groff DN, Fadista J, et al. The Diabetes Susceptibility Gene Clec16a Regulates Mitophagy. *Cell* (2014) 157:1577–90. doi: 10.1016/j.cell.2014.05.016
181. Chase HP, Cuthbertson DD, Dolan LM, Kaufman F, Krischer JP, Schatz DA, et al. First-Phase Insulin Release During the Intravenous Glucose Tolerance Test as a Risk Factor for Type 1 Diabetes. *J Pediatr* (2001) 138:244–9. doi: 10.1067/mpd.2001.111274
182. In't Veld P, Lievens D, De Grijse J, Ling Z, van der Auwera B, Pipeleers-Marichal M, et al. Screening for Insulitis in Adult Autoantibody-Positive Organ Donors. *Diabetes* (2007) 56:2400–4. doi: 10.2337/db07-0416
183. Harjutsalo V, Reunanen A, Tuomilehto J. Differential Transmission of Type 1 Diabetes From Diabetic Fathers and Mothers to Their Offspring. *Diabetes* (2006) 55:1517–24. doi: 10.2337/db05-1296
184. Wurst U, Ebert T, Kralisch S, Stumvoll M, Fasshauer M. Serum Levels of the Adipokine Pref-1 in Gestational Diabetes Mellitus. *Cytokine* (2015) 71:161–4. doi: 10.1016/j.cyto.2014.10.015
185. Wang Y, Kim KA, Kim JH, Sul HS. Pref-1, a Preadipocyte Secreted Factor That Inhibits Adipogenesis. *J Nutr* (2006) 136:2953–6. doi: 10.1093/jn/136.12.2953
186. Appelbe OK, Yevtodiyenko A, Muniz-Talavera H, Schmidt JV. Conditional Deletions Refine the Embryonic Requirement for Dlk1. *Mech Dev* (2013) 130:143–59. doi: 10.1016/j.mod.2012.09.010
187. Moon YS, Smas CM, Lee K, Villena JA, Kim KH, Yun EJ, et al. Mice Lacking Paternally Expressed Pref-1/Dlk1 Display Growth Retardation and Accelerated Adiposity. *Mol Cell Biol* (2002) 22:5585–92. doi: 10.1128/MCB.22.15.5585-5592.2002
188. Onengut-Gumuscu S, Chen WM, Robertson CC, Bonnie JK, Farber E, Zhu Z, et al. Type 1 Diabetes Risk in African-Ancestry Participants and Utility of an Ancestry-Specific Genetic Risk Score. *Diabetes Care* (2019) 42:406–15. doi: 10.2337/dc18-1727
189. Noble JA, Johnson J, Lane JA, Valdes AM. HLA Class II Genotyping of African American Type 1 Diabetic Patients Reveals Associations Unique to African Haplotypes. *Diabetes* (2013) 62:3292–9. doi: 10.2337/db13-0094
190. Robertson CC, Inshaw JRJ, Onengut-Gumuscu S, Chen WM, Santa Cruz DF, Yang H, et al. Fine-Mapping, Trans-Ancestral and Genomic Analyses Identify Causal Variants, Cells, Genes and Drug Targets for Type 1 Diabetes. *Nat Genet* (2021) 53:962–71. doi: 10.1038/s41588-021-00880-5
191. Moreno JA, Halliday M, Molloy C, Radford H, Verity N, Axten JM, et al. Oral Treatment Targeting the Unfolded Protein Response Prevents Neurodegeneration and Clinical Disease in Prion-Infected Mice. *Sci Transl Med* (2013) 5:206ra138. doi: 10.1126/scitranslmed.3006767
192. Yoon YM, Lee JH, Yun SP, Han YS, Yun CW, Lee HJ, et al. Tauroursodeoxycholic Acid Reduces ER Stress by Regulating of Akt-Dependent Cellular Prion Protein. *Sci Rep* (2016) 6:39838. doi: 10.1038/srep39838
193. Bronczek GA, Vettorazzi JF, Soares GM, Kurauti MA, Santos C, Bonfim MF, et al. The Bile Acid TUDCA Improves Beta-Cell Mass and Reduces Insulin Degradation in Mice With Early-Stage of Type-1 Diabetes. *Front Physiol* (2019) 10:561. doi: 10.3389/fphys.2019.00561
194. Bilekova S, Sachs S, Lickert H. Pharmacological Targeting of Endoplasmic Reticulum Stress in Pancreatic Beta Cells. *Trends Pharmacol Sci* (2021) 42:85–95. doi: 10.1016/j.tips.2020.11.011
195. Gitelman SE, Bundy BN, Ferrannini E, Lim N, Blanchfield JL, DiMeglio LA, et al. Imatinib Therapy for Patients With Recent-Onset Type 1 Diabetes: A Multicentre, Randomised, Double-Blind, Placebo-Controlled, Phase 2 Trial. *Lancet Diabetes Endocrinol* (2021) 9:502–14. doi: 10.1016/S2213-8587(21)00139-X

196. Han MS, Chung KW, Cheon HG, Rhee SD, Yoon CH, Lee MK, et al. Imatinib Mesylate Reduces Endoplasmic Reticulum Stress and Induces Remission of Diabetes in Db/Db Mice. *Diabetes* (2009) 58:329–36. doi: 10.2337/db08-0080
197. Morita S, Villalta SA, Feldman HC, Register AC, Rosenthal W, Hoffmann-Petersen IT, et al. Targeting ABL-IRE1alpha Signaling Spares ER-Stressed Pancreatic Beta Cells to Reverse Autoimmune Diabetes. *Cell Metab* (2017) 25:883–97.e8. doi: 10.1016/j.cmet.2017.03.018
198. Stancill JS, Broniowska KA, Oleson BJ, Naatz A, Corbett JA. Pancreatic Beta-Cells Detoxify H2O2 Through the Peroxiredoxin/Thioredoxin Antioxidant System. *J Biol Chem* (2019) 294:4843–53. doi: 10.1074/jbc.RA118.006219
199. Malone CF, Emerson C, Ingraham R, Barbosa W, Guerra S, Yoon H, et al. mTOR and HDAC Inhibitors Converge on the TXNIP/Thioredoxin Pathway to Cause Catastrophic Oxidative Stress and Regression of RAS-Driven Tumors. *Cancer Discov* (2017) 7:1450–63. doi: 10.1158/2159-8290.CD-17-0177
200. Minn AH, Hafele C, Shalev A. Thioredoxin-Interacting Protein Is Stimulated by Glucose Through a Carbohydrate Response Element and Induces Beta-Cell Apoptosis. *Endocrinology* (2005) 146:2397–405. doi: 10.1210/en.2004-1378
201. Foretz M, Guigas B, Bertrand L, Pollak M, Viollet B. Metformin: From Mechanisms of Action to Therapies. *Cell Metab* (2014) 20:953–66. doi: 10.1016/j.cmet.2014.09.018
202. Xu G, Chen J, Jing G, Shalev A. Preventing Beta-Cell Loss and Diabetes With Calcium Channel Blockers. *Diabetes* (2012) 61:848–56. doi: 10.2337/db11-0955
203. Ovalle F, Grimes T, Xu G, Patel AJ, Grayson TB, Thielen LA, et al. Verapamil and Beta Cell Function in Adults With Recent-Onset Type 1 Diabetes. *Nat Med* (2018) 24:1108–12. doi: 10.1038/s41591-018-0089-4
204. Millman JR, Xie C, Van Dervort A, Gurtler M, Pagliuca FW, Melton DA. Generation of Stem Cell-Derived Beta-Cells From Patients With Type 1 Diabetes. *Nat Commun* (2016) 7:11463. doi: 10.1038/ncomms11463
205. de Klerk E, Hebrok M. Stem Cell-Based Clinical Trials for Diabetes Mellitus. *Front Endocrinol (Lausanne)* (2021) 12:631463. doi: 10.3389/fendo.2021.631463
206. Cai EP, Ishikawa Y, Zhang W, Leite NC, Li J, Hou S, et al. Genome-Scale *In Vivo* CRISPR Screen Identifies RNLS as a Target for Beta Cell Protection in Type 1 Diabetes. *Nat Metab* (2020) 2:934–45. doi: 10.1038/s42255-020-0254-1
207. Han X, Wang M, Duan S, Franco PJ, Kenty JH, Hedrick P, et al. Generation of Hypoimmunogenic Human Pluripotent Stem Cells. *Proc Natl Acad Sci USA* (2019) 116:10441–6. doi: 10.1073/pnas.1902566116
208. Deuse T, Hu X, Gravina A, Wang D, Tediashvili G, De C, et al. Hypoimmunogenic Derivatives of Induced Pluripotent Stem Cells Evade Immune Rejection in Fully Immunocompetent Allogeneic Recipients. *Nat Biotechnol* (2019) 37:252–8. doi: 10.1038/s41587-019-0016-3
209. Deuse T, Tediashvili G, Hu X, Gravina A, Tamenang A, Wang D, et al. Hypoimmune Induced Pluripotent Stem Cell-Derived Cell Therapeutics Treat Cardiovascular and Pulmonary Diseases in Immunocompetent Allogeneic Mice. *Proc Natl Acad Sci USA* (2021) 118:1–11. doi: 10.1073/pnas.2022091118
210. Augsornworawat P, Millman JR. Single-Cell RNA Sequencing for Engineering and Studying Human Islets. *Curr Opin BioMed Eng* (2020) 16:27–33. doi: 10.1016/j.cobme.2020.06.003
211. Camunas-Soler J, Dai XQ, Hang Y, Bautista A, Lyon J, Suzuki K, et al. Patch-Seq Links Single-Cell Transcriptomes to Human Islet Dysfunction in Diabetes. *Cell Metab* (2020) 31:1017–31.e4. doi: 10.1016/j.cmet.2020.04.005
212. Yoshihara E, O'Connor C, Gasser E, Wei Z, Oh TG, Tseng TW, et al. Immune-Evasive Human Islet-Like Organoids Ameliorate Diabetes. *Nature* (2020) 586:606–11. doi: 10.1038/s41586-020-2631-z
213. Wang X, Maxwell KG, Wang K, Bowers DT, Flanders JA, Liu W, et al. A Nanofibrous Encapsulation Device for Safe Delivery of Insulin-Producing Cells to Treat Type 1 Diabetes. *Sci Transl Med* (2021) 13:1–18. doi: 10.1126/scitranslmed.abb4601

GLOSSARY

ATF6	activating transcription factor 6
AMPK	adenosine monophosphate activated protein kinase
APC	antigen-presenting cell
BiP	binding immunoglobulin protein
CCR2	C-C chemokine receptor-2
CCL2	C-C ligand 2
JNK	c-Jun N-terminal Kinase
Clec16A	C-type lectin domain family 16, member A
CXCL10	*C-X-C* motif chemokine ligand 10
Ca^{2+}	calcium
GPx	glutathione peroxidase
CCL5	CC ligand 5
ChgA	chromogranin-A
CRISPR	Clustered Regularly Interspaced Short Palindromic Repeat
CXCR3	CXC receptor 3
DLK1	Delta-like 1
LCMV-WE	diabetogenic lymphocytic choriomeningitis virus-WE strain
E	embryonic day
ER	endoplasmic reticulum
FasL	Fas ligand
FISH	fluorescence *in situ* hybridization
GDM	gestational diabetes mellitus
Glut2	glucose transporter 2
GSIS	glucose-stimulated insulin secretion
Gad65	glutamic acid decarboxylase 65
GWAS	Genome-Wide Association Study
HLA	human leukocyte antigen
HIPs	hybrid insulin peptides
H_2O_2	hydrogen peroxide
iPSC	induced pluripotent stem cell
iNOS	inducible nitric oxide
IRE1a	inositol-requiring enzyme 1 alpha
INS	*INSULIN*

(Continued)

Continued

IFNγ	interferon gamma
IL-1β	interleukin-1 beta
IP-10	IFNγ inducible protein 10
IAPP	islet amyloid polypeptide
LADA	latent autoimmune diabetes in adults
MHC	major histocompatibility chain
MODY	maturity onset diabetes of the young
MCP)-1	monotype chemoattractant protein
NOD	non-obese diabetic
NFκB	nuclear factor κB
Pdx1	pancreatic and duodenal homeobox 1
pLNs	pancreatic lymph nodes
PAD	peptidyl arginine deiminase
PTM	post-translational modification
Pref-1	preadipocyte factor 1
PAK-2	protein activated kinase 2
PERK	protein kinase RNA-like endoplasmic reticulum kinase
RANTES	regulated on activation, normal T cell expressed and secreted
ROS	reactive oxygen species
Rnls	renalase
SNPs	single nucleotide polymorphisms
SOD	superoxide dismutase
T1DGC	T1D Genetics Consortium
TUDCA	tauroursdoxycholic acid
TRX	thioredoxin
TXNIP	thioredoxin interacting protein
tTG2	tissue transglutaminase 2
TLR4	Toll like receptor-4
TNFα	tumor necrosis factor alpha
T1D	Type 1 diabetes
T2D	Type 2 diabetes
UPR	unfolded protein response
UCN-3	urocortin-3
VNTR	variable number tandem repeat
WTCCC	Wellcome Trust Case Control Consortium

11

Modulation of Intestinal ILC3 for the Treatment of Type 1 Diabetes

Ivana Stojanović, Tamara Saksida, Đorđe Miljković and Nada Pejnović*

Department of Immunology, Institute for Biological Research "Siniša Stanković" – National Institute of the Republic of Serbia, University of Belgrade, Belgrade, Serbia

***Correspondence:**
Ivana Stojanović
ivana@ibiss.bg.ac.rs

Gut-associated lymphoid tissue (GALT) is crucial for the maintenance of the intestinal homeostasis, but it is also the potential site of the activation of autoreactive cells and initiation/propagation of autoimmune diseases in the gut and in the distant organs. Type 3 innate lymphoid cells (ILC3) residing in the GALT integrate signals from food ingredients and gut microbiota metabolites in order to control local immunoreactivity. Notably, ILC3 secrete IL-17 and GM-CSF that activate immune cells in combating potentially pathogenic microorganisms. ILC3 also produce IL-22 that potentiates the strength and integrity of epithelial tight junctions, production of mucus and antimicrobial peptides thus enabling the proper function of the intestinal barrier. The newly discovered function of small intestine ILC3 is the secretion of IL-2 and the promotion of regulatory T cell (Treg) generation and function. Since the intestinal barrier dysfunction, together with the reduction in small intestine ILC3 and Treg numbers are associated with the pathogenesis of type 1 diabetes (T1D), the focus of this article is intestinal ILC3 modulation for the therapy of T1D. Of particular interest is free fatty acids receptor 2 (FFAR2), predominantly expressed on intestinal ILC3, that can be stimulated by available selective synthetic agonists. Thus, we propose that FFAR2-based interventions by boosting ILC3 beneficial functions may attenuate autoimmune response against pancreatic β cells during T1D. Also, it is our opinion that treatments based on ILC3 stimulation by functional foods can be used as prophylaxis in individuals that are genetically predisposed to develop T1D.

Keywords: type 3 innate lymphoid cells (ILC3), type 1 diabetes (T1D), gut-associated lymphoid tissue (GALT), regulatory T cells (Treg), interleukin-22 (IL-22), interleukin-2 (IL-2)

INTRODUCTION

Type 1 diabetes (T1D) is an autoimmune disease that is characterized by low insulin concentration and hyperglycemia. The autoimmune process in pancreatic islets can last for years before the clinical signs of the disease appear. This process is initiated by autoreactive effector T cells including $CD4^+$ and $CD8^+$ cells and it is characterized by high levels of proinflammatory cytokines IL-1β, TNF and IFN-γ (1). The described events are accompanied by decreased numbers and/or defective function of regulatory T cells (Treg) that have an immunosuppressive role and maintain immune tolerance by producing IL-10 and TGF-β and by other mechanisms (2). The overall outcome is the destruction of pancreatic β cells that leads to reduced or completely absent insulin production (1, 3).

Many environmental factors including food ingredients (β-casein or bovine insulin from cow's milk, gluten), exposure to infectious agents (enteroviruses), and intestinal microbiota dysbiosis (due to antibiotics, alcohol abuse, inadequate diet or chronic diseases) are believed to be the reason for the dramatic increase in T1D incidence in people under the age of 18, but also in older adults (4–6).

It is becoming increasingly clear that T1D pathogenesis is linked to the complex interaction between the gut-associated lymphoid tissue (GALT) and the gut microbiota (7). Intestinal barrier serves as an integrator of signals coming from the gut lumen and it is comprised of mucus layer leaning on tightly connected epithelial cells (physical border) and mediators secreted by epithelial cells and immune cells (functional border). GALT cells maintain immune tolerance to food constituents and commensal microbes. The reduction or improper function of GALT-residing tolerogenic dendritic cells (DC) and Treg enables the impairment of oral tolerance (8–10), that may lead to T1D initiation mediated by autoreactive T cells present in the intestinal lamina propria (11, 12). In such case, antigens sampled from the gut might activate β cell-reactive immune cells directly *via* molecular mimicry or indirectly by the bystander activation during the immune response towards gut microorganisms (13). The close link between the gut and the pancreas is exemplified in the finding that pancreatic lymph nodes can drain antigens from the duodenum that leads to Treg induction in GALT and development of oral tolerance (14). Therefore, maintaining a balance between effector T cells and Treg in the gut and pancreatic lymph nodes is essential for sustaining tolerance to islet antigens and prevention of autoreactive T lymphocytes activation and migration to the pancreas where they can initiate β-cell destruction.

GUT-PANCREAS AXIS

The impaired function of the intestinal barrier and dysbiosis precede the development of T1D both in humans and mice. The loss of gut barrier integrity and low-grade intestinal inflammation were discovered in first-degree relatives of T1D patients that are at high-risk of disease development (15–17). The same was confirmed in new-onset and long-term T1D patients (17, 18). The altered microbiota content in T1D patients were found in many studies worldwide as reviewed by Marietta et al. (19).

Increased intestinal permeability and the lack of oral tolerance to ovalbumin was found in 4-6 weeks old, insulitis-free nonobese diabetic (NOD) mice that spontaneously develop T1D (10). Also, these mice had diminished mucus production, lower levels of secretory IgA and increased Th17 and type 3 innate lymphoid cells (ILC3) numbers in the small intestine lamina propria. This coincided with the significant reduction of tolerogenic DC and Treg in the gut-draining lymph nodes during prediabetic stage (10).

There are very few studies that address the activation of autoreactive cells in GALT and their causal link to pancreas autoimmunity. Our recent study implies that activation of insulin-specific $CD4^+$ T cells can occur in the GALT as these cells are present in Peyer's patches of prediabetic NOD and healthy C57BL/6 mice (11). Also, a study that used a β cell–specific TCR-transgenic mouse model has shown that islet-specific T cells activated in the intestinal lamina propria migrated to the pancreatic lymph nodes and the islets causing autoimmune diabetes (20). Further, it was demonstrated that the infection with *Fusobacteria* activates β cell-reactive $CD8^+$ T cells by molecular mimicry within GALT of transgenic NOD mice (12). In addition to the possibility of autoreactive cell activation in the GALT, it was shown that gut microbiota can migrate to the pancreatic lymph nodes where it acts through NOD2 receptors to accelerate the onset of streptozotocin-induced T1D in mice (21). Human studies about the autoreactive cells activation within the GALT indirectly suggest that ingested food or bacterial antigens stimulate the production of β cell-specific autoantibodies *via* molecular mimicry. Examples can be found in reports of Auricchio et al. (22) and Niegowska et al. (23) where data about crossreactivity between β cell antigens and antigens derived from gluten or *Mycobacterium avium* subspecies *paratuberculosis*, a bacterium found in cow's milk, were suggested. Also, higher density of intraepithelial $CD3^+$ and γδ cells and activated $CD25^+$ in lamina propria and lower numbers of $FoxP3^+$ cells in the jejunal mucosa of T1D patients were found (22, 24, 25). In general, individuals with T1D exhibit increased markers of inflammation within GALT suggesting its association with disease development (26).

Prevention or treatment of human T1D through diet-based interventions proved to be very difficult (27). However, a forced change in microbiota content through fecal microbiota transplantation from healthy donors to early-onset T1D patients successfully halted a decline in endogenous insulin production and down-regulated colonic $CD4^+$ cell count, thus further confirming the importance of microbiota content for T1D control (28). In contrast to scarce data in humans, numerous studies provide evidence about prevention or treatment of animal T1D through diet or modulation of microbiota (29, 30). To mention a few: NOD mice fed with a fiber-rich diet had decreased T1D incidence and lower proportion of autoantigen-specific $CD8^+$ lymphocytes in the spleen (31), supplementation with bacterial metabolite butyrate decreased severity of insulitis in NOD mice and their offspring by promoting Treg proliferation in GALT and their migration to the pancreas (32, 33), administration of probiotics exerted beneficial effects in T1D in mice (34–36).

The majority of available data point to the importance of intestinal Treg and their suppressive properties in the prevention and/or treatment of T1D (8, 9). ILC3 have recently been identified as cells critical for maintenance and regulation of mucosal homeostasis in mice and humans (37), but their role in the initiation or development of T1D is largely unknown. This Perspective review will specifically discuss ILC3 biology and their hypothetical role in pancreatic autoimmunity along with possibilities of ILC3-targeted therapies.

INTESTINAL ILC3

Immature ILC develop in bone marrow from common lymphoid progenitor and they generally migrate to mucosal tissues, but can also be found in other lymphoid tissues such as spleen and lymph nodes and non-lymphoid organs skin, liver, brain and pancreas (38–41). As reviewed by Guia et al. (42), ILC3 differentiation process is similar in humans and mice. ILC3 can be identified as the innate counterpart of Th17 cells due to their mandatory expression of retinoid-related orphan receptor γt (RORγt). ILC3 exist in at least two subsets that differ developmentally, transcriptionally and functionally: lymphoid tissue inducer cells (LTi)-like ILC3 (characterized by surface expression of CCR6) and natural cytotoxicity receptor $(NCR)^+$ ILC3 that express NKp46 in mice (43) and NKp44 in humans (44). However, human ILC3 can also express NKp46 and their distribution in skin and intestine was found very similar in humans and mice (45). ILC3 are generally sedentary (46, 47), although in some human pathological conditions differentiated ILC3 were found in the bloodstream (48). Therefore, their regular divisions driven by different internal and environmental signals is essential for their maintenance in the tissues. ILC3 proliferation is stimulated by cytokines, such as IL-18 in human tonsils (49), or combination of tumor necrosis factor-like cytokine 1A, IL-1β, IL-23 and IL-2 in both human and mouse intestinal tissue (50, 51). The major environmental stimuli for murine intestinal ILC3 proliferation are short chain free fatty acids (SCFA) and vitamins A and D (52, 53).

Mature ILC3 develop in the lamina propria of the intestine due to specific differentiation factors (retinoic acid, polyphenols and microbiota) (37). Mouse studies indicate that intestinal ILC3 express integrin $\alpha 4\beta 7$. Their specific signature is the expression of GPR183, a receptor for oxysterols that recruits ILC3 to the small intestine and regulates their migration to the cryptopatches and positioning in the mesenteric lymph nodes. The expression of GPR109A (a receptor for butyrate) dictates ILC3 distribution in Peyer's patches, while distinct pattern of chemokine receptors drives their migration to the specific sites in the GALT such as mesenteric lymph nodes (CCR7), microvilli (CXCR6) or lamina propria (CCR9) (reviewed in 54). In addition, intestinal ILC3 exhibit high free fatty acid receptor (FFAR) expression in contrast to spleen ILC3, for example (55).

Intestinal human and mouse ILC3 are critical for the generation of the organized lymphoid tissue in the intestinal wall during development (LTi-like cells) and they regulate microbiota content and the integrity of the intestinal barrier (46, 56). Mouse ILC3 sense environmental cues either coming from the food or microbiota metabolism products by expressing numerous receptors: retinoic acid receptor (RAR) (57), vitamin D receptor (VDR) (58), aryl hydrocarbon receptor (AhR) (56, 59), or FFAR (55). Also, gut ILC3 respond to cytokines predominantly produced by myeloid cells (IL-1β, IL-23, IL-18 and TNF). In response to these triggers, ILC3 produce several cytokines, including IL-22, IL-17A/F, GM-CSF and IL-2.

IL-22 maintains barrier integrity through stimulation of epithelial cells turnover (60, 61), induction of tight junction proteins production, anti-bacterial peptides and mucins (62, 63). Vitamins A or D are potent inducers of IL-22 production by murine ILC3 (57, 58), while human ILC3 produce IL-22 after microbial stimulation of phagocytes (64). AhR activation is mandatory for IL-22 expression in mouse ILC3 due to its protein-protein interaction with RORγt (59). For example, L-kynurenine (produced by gut epithelial cells) after ligation to AhR stimulates the proliferation of $IL\text{-}22^+$ ILC3 (65). Another stimulus for IL-22 production is the activation of G-protein-coupled receptors FFAR on murine ILC3 by the action of SCFA (66, 67). The signaling cues that come from FFAR2 can indirectly affect IL-22 through augmenting expression of the IL-1 receptor and ILC3 responsiveness to IL-1β (66). What is more, IL-23 produced by myeloid cells as a part of an anti-microbial response has the same effect on ILC3 (68).

ILC3-mediated production of IL-17A/F is important for the induction of antimicrobial peptides and tight junction proteins in epithelial cells (69). However, data obtained from both human and murine studies imply that the major role of ILC3-derived IL-17 is to attract neutrophils to the intestinal tissue in response to bacterial (*Mycobacterium tuberculosis* and *Clostridium difficile*) and fungal infections (70–72).

Secretion of GM-CSF and IL-2 from ILC3 is triggered by IL-1β from intestinal macrophages. Mouse ILC3-derived GM-CSF was shown to act upon intestinal macrophages and dendritic cells to promote their production of IL-10 and retinoic acid, that in turn stimulate the induction and enable maintenance of Treg (73). However, ILC3 in the intestine of inflammatory bowel disease patients produce large amounts of GM-CSF that causes a loss in ILC3 and exacerbation of the disease (74). Recently, a very interesting finding was published identifying a population of mouse and human ILC3 that produce IL-2 and are involved in the preservation of oral tolerance through stimulation of Treg differentiation (51). Along with cytokine-mediated activity, ILC3 can modulate adaptive immune response through antigen presentation *via* class II MHC. Namely, ILC3 have the ability to present microbial antigens and to limit $CD4^+$ cell response by inducing their cell death (75). The reduction in the specific $MHCII^+$ ILC3 population in the intestine is associated with Crohn's disease in pediatric patients (76).

ILC3 IN T1D

The precise contribution of intestinal ILC3 to the onset and progression of T1D has not been investigated, so far. However, there are some data that emphasize ILC3 as important players in shaping GALT environment for T1D initiation or progression. First, decreased frequency of ILC3 was found in the duodenum of T1D patients (77). The human data are in contrast to total ILC3 increase found in small intestine lamina propria of prediabetic NOD mice (10) and in 20 weeks old NOD mice (our unpublished data). So, the second key statement for hypothetical ILC3 relation to T1D pathology comes from the investigation of ILC3 function. Namely, our preliminary data show lower numbers of potentially protective IL-2-producing ILC3 in small intestine lamina propria in 20 weeks old NOD mice with insulitis and in diabetic C57BL/6 mice with streptozotocin-induced T1D. This was accompanied by down-regulation of FoxP3$^+$ Treg number and IL-22 and GM-CSF mRNA expression in the intestine suggesting a causal relationship between IL-2$^+$ ILC3 and Treg (unpublished results). Higher number of ILC3 and lower of IL-2-producing ILC3 could point to the pro-inflammatory environment in GALT that is related to T1D pathogenesis. The observed ILC3 reduction in human intestinal biopsies from patients with T1D (77) could be associated with ILC3 ability to convert to IFN-γ-producing ILC1 in the inflammatory environment, a process found both in humans and mice (78, 79). That was surely the case in these T1D patients, as the numbers of ILC1 were significantly increased in the intestinal tissue (77).

The close relationship between gut microbiota and proper function of ILC3 within the pancreas in the prevention of T1D development in mice was identified by Miani et al. (41). T1D in NOD mice was found to be associated with reduced numbers of ILC3 in the pancreas and their down-regulated IL-22 production that led to compromised expression of antimicrobial proteins in the pancreas. In the same study, low IL-22-producing ILC3 were found in pancreatic and mesenteric lymph nodes of diabetic NOD mice. Instead of IL-22, they produced rather significant levels of IFN-γ and TNF. All mentioned findings indicate that the transition from prediabetes to diabetes in NOD mice is associated with impaired ILC3 function that could lead to reduced numbers of Treg and imply the protective role of IL-2$^+$ and IL-22$^+$ ILC3 against T1D. In general, there are many pathological conditions where ILC3 play a role such as inflammatory bowel disease, experimental autoimmune encephalomyelitis, Graves' and Hashimoto's thyroiditis (52, 80–82). Still, further investigation will discriminate whether ILC3 reduction precedes or is the result of ongoing inflammation during T1D pathogenesis.

PERSPECTIVES FOR ILC3 MODULATION IN T1D

There are at least three key ILC3 activities that can counteract initiation and/or progression of T1D: 1. Maintenance of gut barrier integrity; 2. Regulation of gut microbiota homeostasis; 3. Stimulation of Treg proliferation and suppressive function. Therefore, the preserved abundance and function of ILC3 within the intestine could largely aid T1D prevention. The hypothetic model of ILC3 role in protection from autoimmune process during T1D is shown in **Figure 1**.

As previously stated, there is a number of external stimuli that can be used for ILC3 modulation (**Figure 2**). In addition to stimulation of IL-22 production, vitamin A attracts specifically ILC3 to the intestinal tissue in both mouse and humans (83, 84). Although there are no data about the influence of retinoids on ILC3 during T1D pathogenesis, their effect on Treg stimulation and suppression of pro-inflammatory adaptive and innate immune cells both systemically and within the pancreas was firmly established (85, 86). Indeed, the oral or intraperitoneal application of retinoids showed a significant preventive effect in NOD and streptozotocin-treated C57BL/6 mice (85, 86). Similarly, vitamin D3 (calcitriol) supplementation led to reduced T1D incidence in NOD mice through generation of

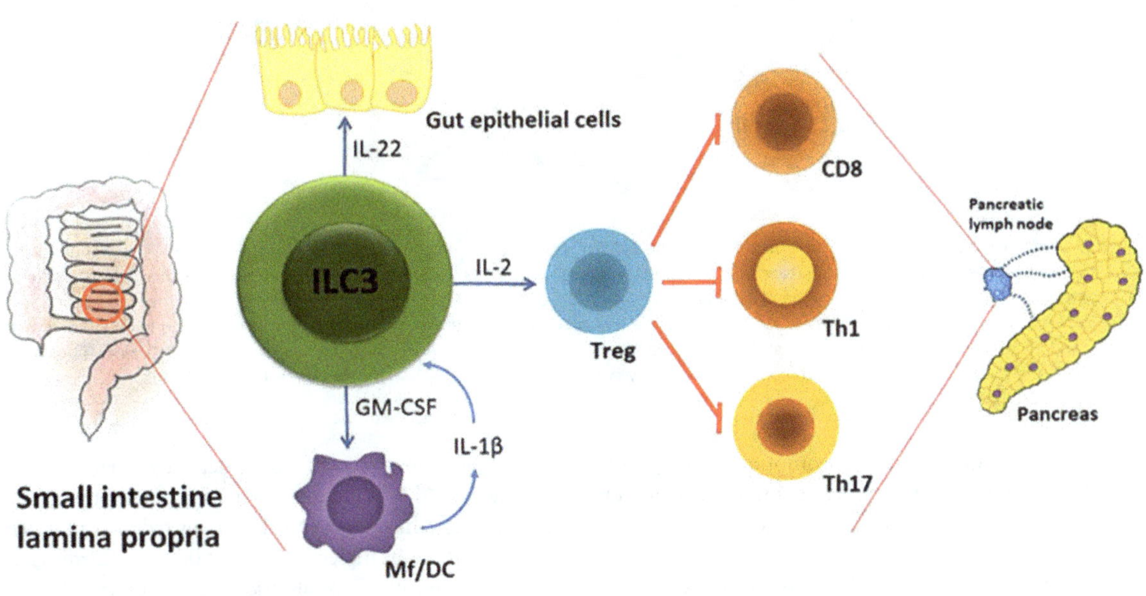

FIGURE 1 | The hypothetical model of ILC3-mediated effects on autoimmune process during T1D. Under the influence of gut microbiota, their metabolites and food ingredients, intestinal ILC3 produce IL-22 that stabilizes the gut barrier and GM-CSF that influences dendritic cells (DC) and macrophages (Mf). Upon activation by microbial cues, Mf produce IL-1β that stimulates ILC3 to increase their production of IL-2 and thus promote intestinal Treg stability and proliferation. Intestinal Treg are able to migrate to the pancreatic lymph nodes and modulate the autoimmune response by providing a suppressive environment in which cytotoxic CD8$^+$ cells, Th1 and Th17 cells are inhibited. The final outcome is the blockade of T cell-mediated autoimmune destruction of pancreatic β cells.

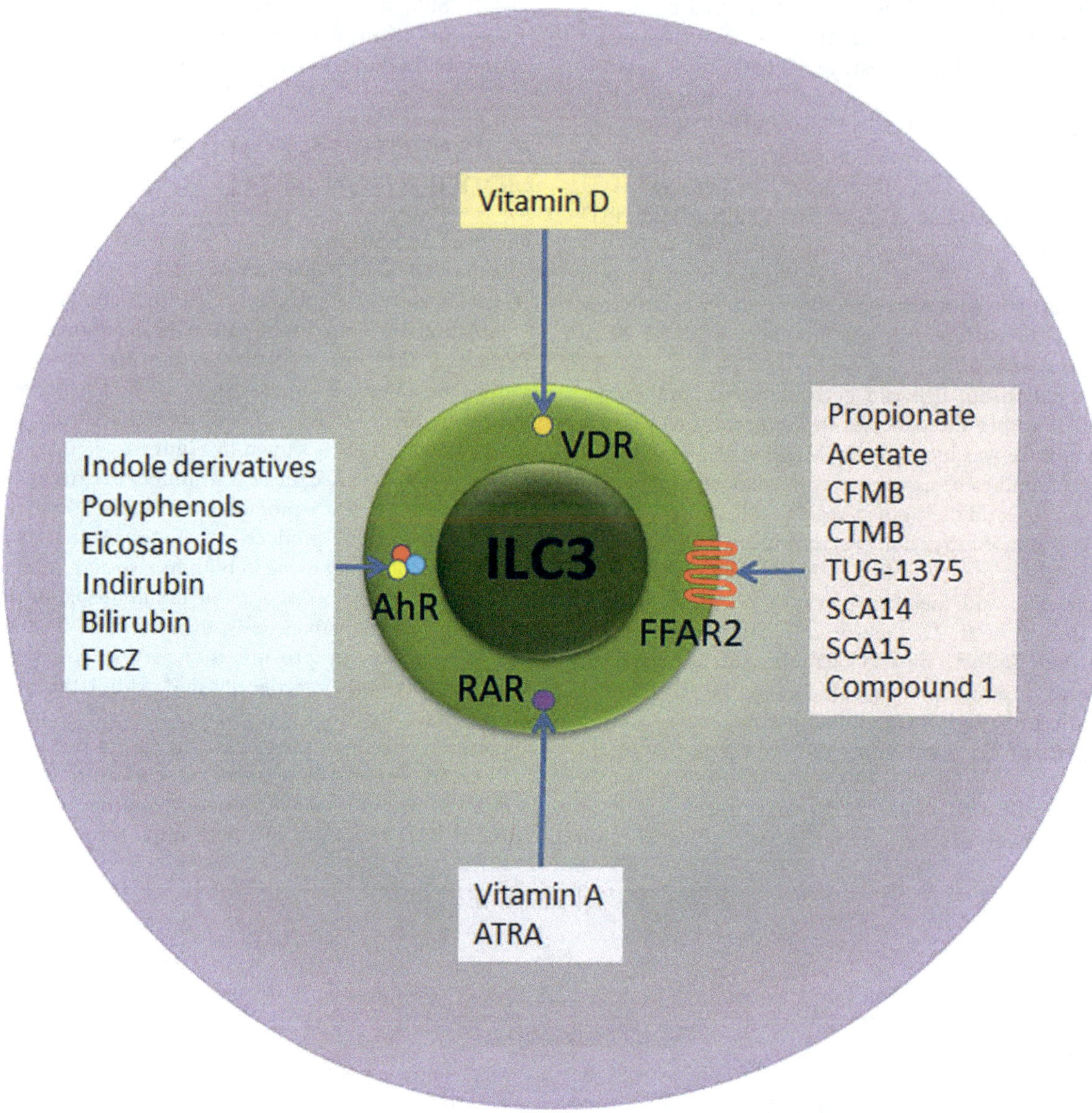

FIGURE 2 | Receptor-ligand interactions relevant for therapeutic targeting of ILC3. ILC3 express receptors for retinoic acid (RAR) and vitamin D (VDR) that upon activation with respective vitamins instigate ILC3 proliferation and/or secretion of IL-22. In addition, ILC3 express AhR transcription factor that can ligate to versatile indol-containing compounds. The activation of AhR is mandatory for the development of mature ILC3 in the intestinal lamina propria, their proliferation and IL-22 secretion. Finally, ILC3 express FFAR2 at very high levels. SCFA (propionate and acetate) as well as several synthetic compounds bind to FFAR2 with high affinity, while Compound 1 and CTMB are selective FFAR2 agonists that promote beneficial ILC3 functions. ATRA, all trans retinoic acid; FICZ, 6-formylindolo[3,2-b] carbazole; CFMB, S)-2-(4-chlorophenyl)-3,3-dimethyl- N-(5-phenylthiazol-2-yl)butamide; 4-CTMB, (S)-2-(4-chlorophenyl)-3- methyl-N-(thiazol-2-yl)butanamide; SCA14, propiolic acid; SCA15, 2-butynoic acid.

suppressive environment, including the promotion of Treg (87, 88). Again, similarly to vitamin A, it remains unknown whether the beneficial effect of vitamin D can be attributed to the modulation of ILC3.

Another way of intestinal ILC3 modulation is the application of AhR ligands. The examples of endogenous AhR ligands are eicosanoids, indirubin, bilirubin, or 6-formylindolo[3,2-b] carbazole (89), while exogenous ligands are mainly derived from cruciferous plants (indole-3-carbinol derivatives) (**Figure 2**). In addition to IL-22 stimulation, AhR ligands promote ILC3 survival and proliferation through Notch-dependent pathways (56, 59). The presence of AhR is mandatory for the development of ILC3 in the intestine as AhR-deficient mice show reduced numbers intestinal ILC3, resulting in increased susceptibility to *Citrobacter rodentium* infection (56, 59). Several studies show that AhR activation can prevent T1D and they point to either Treg-dependent mechanisms (90) or Treg-independent mechanisms (91). Again, the role of ILC3 in AhR-mediated protection from T1D remains unknown.

Finally, SCFA can be potent stimulators of ILC3 function. Acetate, propionate and butyrate, gut microbiota metabolites that are released during the digestion of fibers, bind to FFAR2 and FFAR3 expressed on ILC3 surface. FFAR2 is predominantly expressed on intestinal ILC3, compared to other ILC in the gut (55). FFAR2, unlike FFAR3 exerts higher affinity for acetate and propionate, than for butyrate (92).

To date, there are numerous studies that explored the role of SCFA in the prevention of T1D. Oral intake of fibers or purified SCFA decreased disease severity in animal models of T1D. This specialized diet even prevented T1D initiation in the offspring of treated female NOD mice (31, 32, 93–95). In general, the mechanism of SCFA action is mainly attributed to Treg induction. Although considerably effective in animal models, administration of oral butyrate for one month did not affect autoimmune response in individuals with longstanding T1D (27). This effect might be due to the butyrate higher affinity of binding to FFAR3 (92), and its differential effect on different subsets of ILC3 (96). Specifically, butyrate stimulates NKp46$^-$ ILC3 that, in addition to IL-22, produce pro-inflammatory cytokines IFN-γ and IL-17 (96).

The fact that FFAR2 is predominantly and highly expressed in the small intestine and colon ILC3 (55) suggests that FFAR2 is the most fitted target for the specific modulation of ILC3. As the highest FFAR2 expression was detected in CCR6$^+$ ILC3 subset that predominantly produces IL-22 in response to SCFA (52), the application of FFAR2 ligands implicate even more stringent control of ILC3-mediated immune response within the GALT. The importance of stimulation of ILC3 for autoimmunity prevention or treatment resides in their FFAR2-mediated IL-22 production and proliferation, but also in the fact that this FFAR2-mediated stimulation will not initiate IFN-γ production (97). In addition to natural ligands, several synthetic FFAR2 agonists have been identified so far: class of phenylacetamides that include (S)-2-(4-chlorophenyl)-3,3-dimethyl- N-(5-phenylthiazol-2-yl)butamide (CFMB) and (S)-2-(4-chlorophenyl)-3- methyl-N-(thiazol-2-yl)butanamide (4-CTMB), TUG-1375, propiolic acid (SCA14), 2-butynoic acid (SCA15) and Compound 1 (patent no. WO 2011/076732 A1) (98) (**Figure 2**).

Application of agonists that preferentially bind FFAR2 (such as Compound 1 and 4-CTMB) would increase the probability of beneficial ILC3 activation (52). In contrast to SCFA that activate FFAR2 in such a manner that it couples to either $G_{i/o}$ or G_q proteins, Compound 1-activated FFAR2 on ILC3 binds to both proteins (52). The consequence of such FFAR2 activity is increased AKT and STAT3 phosphorylation that lead to up-regulated IL-22 expression in mouse colonic ILC3 (52). FFAR2 agonists may expand their anti-inflammatory effects by binding to FFAR2 expressed on colonic epithelial cells. Specifically, SCFA administration alleviates colonic inflammation in mice by augmenting inflammasome activation in colon epithelial cells (99). However, FFAR2 is relatively highly expressed on mouse pancreatic β cells where it controls (inhibits) glucose-stimulated insulin secretion (100) implicating the use of selective ILC3 stimulators.

Engagement of two different types of receptors on ILC3 might provide even better output, as for example, signals through AhR and FFAR2 integrate at the level of IL-22 expression (69). Another benefit of this joint treatment may be synergistic activation of Treg as they express AhR and FFAR2 as well (52). The consumption of functional foods that contain vitamins A and D, AhR and FFAR ligands may provide the beneficial activation of ILC3. In addition, some of the synthetic compounds, Compound 1 for example, exert rather selective effects on intestinal ILC3 when applied orally (52). The perspective of such compounds is immense as they can control complex cellular interaction within GALT and intestinal barrier and consolidate the anti-inflammatory environment that can lead to prevention or blockade of autoimmunity in pancreas, as well as at other distant sites.

AUTHOR CONTRIBUTIONS

IS conceptualized the paper. IS, TS and NP drafted the manuscript. DM revised the manuscript and made Figures. All authors contributed to the article and approved the submitted version.

REFERENCES

1. Roep BO, Thomaidou S, van Tienhoven R, Zaldumbide A. Type 1 Diabetes Mellitus as a Disease of the β-Cell (Do Not Blame the Immune System?). *Nat Rev Endocrinol* (2020) 8:1–12. doi: 10.1038/s41574-020-00443-4
2. Hull CM, Peakman M, Tree TIM. Regulatory T Cell Dysfunction in Type 1 Diabetes: What's Broken and How Can We Fix it? *Diabetologia* (2017) 60:1839–50. doi: 10.1007/s00125-017-4377-1
3. Bluestone JA, Herold K, Eisenbarth G. Genetics, Pathogenesis and Clinical Interventions in Typel Diabetes. *Nature* (2010) 464:1293–300. doi: 10.1038/nature08933
4. Vaarala O. Is the Origin of Type 1 Diabetes in the Gut? *Immunol Cell Biol* (2012) 90:271–6. doi: 10.1038/icb.2011.115
5. Mejía-León ME, Barca AM. Diet, Microbiota and Immune System in Type 1 Diabetes Development and Evolution. *Nutrients* (2015) 7:9171–84. doi: 10.3390/nu7115461
6. Geravandi S, Liu H, Maedler K. Enteroviruses and T1D: Is It the Virus, the Genes or Both Which Cause T1d. *Microorganisms* (2020) 8:1017. doi: 10.3390/microorganisms8071017
7. Opazo MC, Ortega-Rocha EM, Coronado-Arrázola I, Bonifaz LC, Boudin H, Neunlist M, et al. Intestinal Microbiota Influences Non-Intestinal Related Autoimmune Diseases. *Front Microbiol* (2018) 9:432. doi: 10.3389/fmicb.2018.00432
8. Round JL, Mazmanian SK. Inducible Foxp3$^+$ Regulatory T-cell Development by a Commensal Bacterium of the Intestinal Microbiota. *Proc Natl Acad Sci U S A* (2010) 107:12204–9. doi: 10.1073/pnas.0909122107
9. Yu H, Gagliani N, Ishigame H, Huber S, Zhu S, Esplugues E, et al. Intestinal Type 1 Regulatory T Cells Migrate to Periphery to Suppress Diabetogenic T Cells and Prevent Diabetes Development. *Proc Natl Acad Sci USA* (2017) 114:10443–8. doi: 10.1073/pnas.1705599114
10. Miranda MCG, Oliveira RP, Torres L, Aguiar SLF, Pinheiro-Rosa N, Lemos L, et al. Frontline Science: Abnormalities in the Gut Mucosa of Non-Obese Diabetic Mice Precede the Onset of Type 1 Diabetes. *J Leukoc Biol* (2019) 106:513–29. doi: 10.1002/JLB.3HI0119-024RR
11. Đedović N, Paunović V, Stojanović I. Isolation and Enrichment of Mouse Insulin-Specific CD4$^+$ T Regulatory Cells. *J Immunol Methods* (2019) 470:46–54. doi: 10.1016/j.jim.2019.04.011
12. Tai N, Peng J, Liu F, Gulden E, Hu Y, Zhang X, et al. Microbial Antigen Mimics Activate Diabetogenic CD8 T Cells in NOD Mice. *J Exp Med* (2016) 213:2129–46. doi: 10.1084/jem.20160526
13. Brown EM, Kenny DJ, Xavier RJ. Gut Microbiota Regulation of T Cells During Inflammation and Autoimmunity. *Annu Rev Immunol* (2019) 37:599–624. doi: 10.1146/annurev-immunol-042718-041841
14. Turley SJ, Lee JW, Dutton-Swain N, Mathis D, Benoist C. Endocrine Self and

Gut non-Self Intersect in the Pancreatic Lymph Nodes. *Proc Natl Acad Sci USA* (2005) 102:17729–33. doi: 10.1073/pnas.0509006102

15. Bosi E, Molteni L, Radaelli MG, Folini L, Fermo I, Bazzigaluppi E, et al. Increased Intestinal Permeability Precedes Clinical Onset of Type 1 Diabetes. *Diabetologia* (2006) 49:2824–7. doi: 10.1007/s00125-006-0465-3
16. Maffeis C, Martina A, Corradi M, Quarella S, Nori N, Torriani S, et al. Association Between Intestinal Permeability and Faecal Microbiota Composition in Italian Children With Beta Cell Autoimmunity at Risk for Type 1 Diabetes. *Diabetes Metab Res Rev* (2016) 32:700–9. doi: 10.1002/dmrr.2790
17. Sapone A, de Magistris L, Pietzak M, Clemente MG, Tripathi A, Cucca F, et al. Zonulin Upregulation Is Associated With Increased Gut Permeability in Subjects With Type 1 Diabetes and Their Relatives. *Diabetes* (2006) 55:1443–9. doi: 10.2337/db05-1593
18. Secondulfo M, Iafusco D, Carratù R, de Magistris L, Sapone A, Generoso M, et al. Ultrastructural Mucosal Alterations and Increased Intestinal Permeability in Mon-Celiac, Type I Diabetic Patients. *Dig Liver Dis* (2004) 36:35–45. doi: 10.1016/j.dld.2003.09.016
19. Marietta E, Mangalam AK, Taneja V, Murray JA. Intestinal Dysbiosis in, and Enteral Bacterial Therapies for, Systemic Autoimmune Diseases. *Front Immunol* (2020) 11:573079. doi: 10.3389/fimmu.2020.573079
20. Sorini C, Cosorich I, Lo Conte M, De Giorgi L, Facciotti F, Lucianò R, et al. Loss of Gut Barrier Integrity Triggers Activation of Islet-Reactive T Cells and Autoimmune Diabetes. *Proc Natl Acad Sci USA* (2019) 116:15140–9. doi: 10.1073/pnas.1814558116
21. Costa FR, Françozo MC, de Oliveira GG, Ignacio A, Castoldi A, Zamboni DS, et al. Gut Microbiota Translocation to the Pancreatic Lymph Nodes Triggers NOD2 Activation and Contributes to T1D Onset. *J Exp Med* (2016) 213:1223–39. doi: 10.1084/jem.20150744
22. Auricchio R, Paparo F, Maglio M, Franzese A, Lombardi F, Valerio G, et al. *In Vitro*-Deranged Intestinal Immune Response to Gliadin in Type 1 Diabetes. *Diabetes* (2004) 53:1680–3. doi: 10.2337/diabetes.53.7.1680
23. Niegowska M, Paccagnini D, Mannu C, Targhetta C, Songini M, Sechi LA. Recognition of ZnT8, Proinsulin, and Homologous Map Peptides in Sardinian Children at Risk of T1D Precedes Detection of Classical Islet Antibodies. *J Diabetes Res* (2016) 2016:5842701. doi: 10.1155/2016/5842701
24. Tiittanen M, Westerholm-Ormio M, Verkasalo M, Savilahti E, Vaarala O. Infiltration of Forkhead Box P3-expressing Cells in Small Intestinal Mucosa in Coeliac Disease But Not in Type 1 Diabetes. *Clin Exp Immunol* (2008) 152:498–507. doi: 10.1111/j.1365-2249.2008.03662.x
25. Badami E, Sorini C, Coccia M, Usuelli V, Molteni L, Bolla AM, et al. Defective Differentiation of Regulatory Foxp3$^+$ T Cells by Small-Intestinal Dendritic Cells in Patients With Type 1 Diabetes. *Diabetes* (2011) 60:2120–4. doi: 10.2337/db10-1201
26. Honkanen J, Vuorela A, Muthas D, Orivuori L, Luopajärvi K, Tejesvi MVG, et al. Fungal Dysbiosis and Intestinal Inflammation in Children With Beta-Cell Autoimmunity. *Front Immunol* (2020) 11:468. doi: 10.3389/fimmu.2020.00468
27. de Groot PF, Nikolic T, Imangaliyev S, Bekkering S, Duinkerken G, Keij FM, et al. Oral Butyrate Does Not Affect Innate Immunity and Islet Autoimmunity in Individuals With Longstanding Type 1 Diabetes: A Randomised Controlled Trial. *Diabetologia* (2020) 63:597–610. doi: 10.1007/s00125-019-05073-8
28. de Groot P, Nikolic T, Pellegrini S, Sordi V, Imangaliyev S, Rampanelli E, et al. Faecal Microbiota Transplantation Halts Progression of Human New-Onset Type 1 Diabetes in a Randomised Controlled Trial. *Gut* (2021) 70:92–105. doi: 10.1136/gutjnl-2020-322630
29. Mishra SP, Wang S, Nagpal R, Miller B, Singh R, Taraphder S, et al. Probiotics and Prebiotics for the Amelioration of Type 1 Diabetes: Present and Future Perspectives. *Microorganisms* (2019) 7:67. doi: 10.3390/microorganisms7030067
30. Gavin PG, Hamilton-Williams EE. The Gut Microbiota in Type 1 Diabetes: Friend or Foe? *Curr Opin Endocrinol Diabetes Obes* (2019) 26:207–12. doi: 10.1097/MED.0000000000000483
31. Mariño E, Richards JL, McLeod KH, Stanley D, Yap YA, Knight J, et al. Gut Microbial Metabolites Limit the Frequency of Autoimmune T Cells and Protect Against Type 1 Diabetes. *Nat Immunol* (2017) 18:552–62. doi: 10.1038/ni.3713
32. Huang J, Pearson JA, Peng J, Hu Y, Sha S, Xing Y, et al. Gut Microbial Metabolites Alter IgA Immunity in Type 1 Diabetes. *JCI Insight* (2020) 5: e135718. doi: 10.1172/jci.insight.135718
33. Jacob N, Jaiswal S, Maheshwari D, Nallabelli N, Khatri N, Bhatia A, et al. Butyrate Induced Tregs are Capable of Migration From the GALT to the Pancreas to Restore Immunological Tolerance During Type-1 Diabetes. *Sci Rep* (2020) 10:19120. doi: 10.1038/s41598-020-76109-y
34. Kim TK, Lee JC, Im SH, Lee MS. Amelioration of Autoimmune Diabetes of NOD Mice by Immunomodulating Probiotics. *Front Immunol* (2020) 11:1832. doi: 10.3389/fimmu.2020.01832
35. Valladares R, Sankar D, Li N, Williams E, Lai KK, Abdelgeliel AS, et al. *Lactobacillus Johnsonii* N6.2 Mitigates the Development of Type 1 Diabetes in BB-DP Rats. *PLoS One* (2010) 5:e10507. doi: 10.1371/journal.pone.0010507
36. Dolpady J, Sorini C, Di Pietro C, Cosorich I, Ferrarese R, Saita D, et al. Oral Probiotic Vsl3 Prevents Autoimmune Diabetes by Modulating Microbiota and Promoting Indoleamine 2,3-Dioxygenase-Enriched Tolerogenic Intestinal Environment. *J Diabetes Res* (2016) 2016:7569431. doi: 10.1155/2016/7569431
37. Domingues RG, Hepworth MR. Immunoregulatory Sensory Circuits in Group 3 Innate Lymphoid Cell (Ilc3) Function and Tissue Homeostasis. *Front Immunol* (2020) 11:116. doi: 10.3389/fimmu.2020.00116
38. Serafini N, Klein Wolterink RG, Satoh-Takayama N, Xu W, Vosshenrich CA, Hendriks RW, et al. Gata3 Drives Development of RORgammat+ Group 3 Innate Lymphoid Cells. *J Exp Med* (2014) 211:199–208. doi: 10.1084/jem.20131038
39. Robinette ML, Fuchs A, Cortez VS, Lee JS, Wang Y, Durum SK, et al. Immunological Genome Consortium. Transcriptional Programs Define Molecular Characteristics of Innate Lymphoid Cell Classes and Subsets. *Nat Immunol* (2015) 16:306–17. doi: 10.1038/ni.3094
40. Wang S, Li J, Wu S, Cheng L, Shen Y, Ma W, et al. Type 3 Innate Lymphoid Cell: A New Player in Liver Fibrosis Progression. *Clin Sci (Lond)* (2018) 132:2565–82. doi: 10.1042/CS20180482
41. Miani M, Le Naour J, Waeckel-Enée E, Verma SC, Straube M, Emond P, et al. Gut Microbiota-Stimulated Innate Lymphoid Cells Support β-Defensin 14 Expression in Pancreatic Endocrine Cells, Preventing Autoimmune Diabetes. *Cell Metab* (2018) 28:557–72.e6. doi: 10.1016/j.cmet.2018.06.012
42. Guia S, Narni-Mancinelli E. Helper-Like Innate Lymphoid Cells in Humans and Mice. *Trends Immunol* (2020) 41:436–52. doi: 10.1016/j.it.2020.03.002
43. Vonarbourg C, Mortha A, Bui VL, Hernandez PP, Kiss EA, Hoyler T, et al. Regulated Expression of Nuclear Receptor Rorγt Confers Distinct Functional Fates to NK Cell Receptor-Expressing Rorγt$^+$ Innate Lymphocytes. *Immunity* (2010) 33:736–51. doi: 10.1016/j.immuni.2010.10.017
44. Hughes T, Becknell B, McClory S, Briercheck E, Freud AG, Zhang X, et al. Stage 3 Immature Human Natural Killer Cells Found in Secondary Lymphoid Tissue Constitutively and Selectively Express the TH17 Cytokine Interleukin-22. *Blood* (2009) 113:4008–10. doi: 10.1182/blood-2008-12-192443
45. Luci C, Reynders A, Ivanov II, Cognet C, Chiche L, Chasson L, et al. Influence of the Transcription Factor Rorγt on the Development of NKp46$^+$ Cell Populations in Gut and Skin. *Nat Immunol* (2009) 10:75–82. doi: 10.1038/ni.1681
46. Kim CH, Hashimoto-Hill S, Kim M. Migration and Tissue Tropism of Innate Lymphoid Cells. *Trends Immunol* (2016) 37:68–79. doi: 10.1016/j.it.2015.11.003
47. Dutton EE, Gajdasik DW, Willis C, Fiancette R, Bishop EL, Camelo A, et al. Peripheral Lymph Nodes Contain Migratory and Resident Innate Lymphoid Cell Populations. *Sci Immunol* (2019) 4:eaau8082. doi: 10.1126/sciimmunol.aau8082
48. Teunissen MBM, Munneke JM, Bernink JH, Spuls PI, Res PCM, Te Velde A, et al. Composition of Innate Lymphoid Cell Subsets in the Human Skin: Enrichment of NCR(+) ILC3 in Lesional Skin and Blood of Psoriasis Patients. *J Invest Dermatol* (2014) 134:2351–60. doi: 10.1038/jid.2014.146
49. Victor AR, Nalin AP, Dong W, McClory S, Wei M, Mao C, et al. Il-18 Drives Ilc3 Proliferation and Promotes Il-22 Production Via NF-κb. *J Immunol* (2017) 199:2333–42. doi: 10.4049/jimmunol.1601554
50. Ahn YO, Weeres MA, Neulen ML, Choi J, Kang SH, Heo DS, et al. Human Group3 Innate Lymphoid Cells Express DR3 and Respond to TL1A With

Enhanced IL-22 Production and IL-2-dependent Proliferation. *Eur J Immunol* (2015) 45:2335–42. doi: 10.1002/eji.201445213
51. Zhou L, Chu C, Teng F, Bessman NJ, Goc J, Santosa EK, et al. Innate Lymphoid Cells Support Regulatory T Cells in the Intestine Through Interleukin-2. *Nature* (2019) 568:405–9. doi: 10.1038/s41586-019-1082-x
52. Chun E, Lavoie S, Fonseca-Pereira D, Bae S, Michaud M, Hoveyda HR, et al. Metabolite-Sensing Receptor Ffar2 Regulates Colonic Group 3 Innate Lymphoid Cells and Gut Immunity. *Immunity* (2019) 51:871–84.e6. doi: 10.1016/j.immuni.2019.09.014
53. He L, Zhou M, Li YC. Vitamin D/Vitamin D Receptor Signaling is Required for Normal Development and Function of Group 3 Innate Lymphoid Cells in the Gut. *iScience* (2019) 17:119–31. doi: 10.1016/j.isci.2019.06.026
54. Willinger T. Metabolic Control of Innate Lymphoid Cell Migration. *Front Immunol* (2019) 10:2010. doi: 10.3389/fimmu.2019.02010
55. Sepahi A, Liu Q, Friesen L, Kim CH. Dietary Fiber Metabolites Regulate Innate Lymphoid Cell Responses. *Mucosal Immunol* (2020) 14:317–30. doi: 10.1038/s41385-020-0312-8
56. Kiss EA, Vonarbourg C, Kopfmann S, Hobeika E, Finke D, Esser C, et al. Natural Aryl Hydrocarbon Receptor Ligands Control Organogenesis of Intestinal Lymphoid Follicles. *Science* (2011) 334:1561–5. doi: 10.1126/science.1214914
57. Goverse G, Labao-Almeida C, Ferreira M, Molenaar R, Wahlen S, Konijn T, et al. Vitamin A Controls the Presence of Rorγ+ Innate Lymphoid Cells and Lymphoid Tissue in the Small Intestine. *J Immunol* (2016) 196:5148–55. doi: 10.4049/jimmunol.1501106
58. Lin YD, Arora J, Diehl K, Bora SA, Cantorna MT. Vitamin D is Required for ILC3 Derived IL-22 and Protection From. *Citrobacter Rodentium Infect Front Immunol* (2019) 10:1. doi: 10.3389/fimmu.2019.00001
59. Qiu J, Heller JJ, Guo X, Chen ZM, Fish K, Fu YX, et al. The Aryl Hydrocarbon Receptor Regulates Gut Immunity Through Modulation of Innate Lymphoid Cells. *Immunity* (2012) 36:92–104. doi: 10.1016/j.immuni.2011.11.011
60. Aparicio-Domingo P, Romera-Hernandez M, Karrich JJ, Cornelissen F, Papazian N, Lindenbergh-Kortleve DJ, et al. Type 3 Innate Lymphoid Cells Maintain Intestinal Epithelial Stem Cells After Tissue Damage. *J Exp Med* (2015) 212:1783–91. doi: 10.1084/jem.20150318
61. Lindemans CA, Calafiore M, Mertelsmann AM, O'Connor MH, Dudakov JA, Jenq RR, et al. Interleukin-22 Promotes Intestinal-Stem-Cell-Mediatedepithelial Regeneration. *Nature* (2015) 528:560–4. doi: 10.1038/nature16460
62. Guo X, Qiu J, Tu T, Yang X, Deng L, Anders RA, et al. Induction of Innate Lymphoid Cell-Derived Interleukin-22 by the Transcription Factor STAT3mediates Protection Against Intestinal Infection. *Immunity* (2014) 40:25–39. doi: 10.1016/j.immuni.2013.10.021
63. Sonnenberg GF, Monticelli LA, Alenghat T, Fung TC, Hutnick NA, Kunisawa J, et al. Innate Lymphoid Cells Promote Anatomical Containment of Lymphoid-Resident Commensal Bacteria. *Science* (2012) 336:1321–5. doi: 10.1126/science.1222551
64. Longman RS, Diehl GE, Victorio DA, Huh JR, Galan C, Miraldi ER, et al. CX_3CR1^+ Mononuclear Phagocytes Support Colitis-Associated Innate Lymphoid Cell Production of IL-22. *J Exp Med* (2014) 211:1571–83. doi: 10.1084/jem.20140678
65. Qi H, Li Y, Yun H, Zhang T, Huang Y, Zhou J, et al. *Lactobacillus* Maintains Healthy Gut Mucosa by Producing L-Ornithine. *Commun Biol* (2019) 2:171. doi: 10.1038/s42003-019-0424-4
66. Fachi JL, Sécca C, Rodrigues PB, Mato FCP, Di Luccia B, Felipe JS, et al. Acetate Coordinates Neutrophil and ILC3 Responses Against C. Difficile Through FFAR2. *J Exp Med* (2020) 217:jem.20190489. doi: 10.1084/jem.20190489
67. Yang W, Yu T, Huang X, Bilotta AJ, Xu L, Lu Y, et al. Intestinal Microbiota-Derived Short-Chain Fatty Acids Regulation of Immune Cell IL-22 Production and Gut Immunity. *Nat Commun* (2020) 11:4457. doi: 10.1038/s41467-020-18262-6
68. Cella M, Fuchs A, Vermi W, Facchetti F, Otero K, Lennerz JK, et al. A Human Natural Killer Cell Subset Provides an Innate Source of IL-22 for Mucosal Immunity. *Nature* (2009) 457:722–5. doi: 10.1038/nature07537
69. Liang SC, Tan XY, Luxenberg DP, Karim R, Dunussi-Joannopoulos K, Collins M, et al. Interleukin (IL)-22 and IL-17 are Coexpressed by Th17 Cells and Cooperatively Enhance Expression of Antimicrobial Peptides. *J Exp Med* (2006) 203:2271–9. doi: 10.1084/jem.20061308
70. Nakagawa T, Mori N, Kajiwara C, Kimura S, Akasaka Y, Ishii Y, et al. Endogenous IL-17 as a Factor Determining the Severity of *Clostridium Difficile* Infection in Mice. *J Med Microbiol* (2016) 65:821–7. doi: 10.1099/jmm.0.000273
71. Ardain A, Domingo-Gonzalez R, Das S, Kazer SW, Howard NC, Singh A, et al. Group 3 Innate Lymphoid Cells Mediate Early Protective Immunity Against Tuberculosis. *Nature* (2019) 570:528–32. doi: 10.1038/s41586-019-1276-2
72. Gladiator A, Wangler N, Trautwein-Weidner K, Leibund Gut-Landmann S. Cutting Edge: Il-17secreting Innate Lymphoid Cells are Essential for Host Defense Against Fungal Infection. *J Immunol* (2013) 190:521–5. doi: 10.4049/jimmunol.1202924
73. Mortha A, Chudnovskiy A, Hashimoto D, Bogunovic M, Spencer SP, Belkaid Y, et al. Microbiota-Dependent Crosstalk Between Macrophages and ILC3 Promotes Intestinal Homeostasis. *Science* (2014) 343:1249288. doi: 10.1126/science.1249288
74. Li J, Shi W, Sun H, Ji Y, Chen Y, Guo X, et al. Activation of DR3 Signaling Causes Loss of ILC3s and Exacerbates Intestinal Inflammation. *Nat Commun* (2019) 10:3371. doi: 10.1038/s41467-019-11304-8
75. Hepworth MR, Monticelli LA, Fung TC, Ziegler CG, Grunberg S, Sinha R, et al. Innate Lymphoid Cells Regulate $CD4^+$ T-Cell Responses to Intestinal Commensal Bacteria. *Nature* (2013) 498:113–7. doi: 10.1038/nature12240
76. Hepworth MR, Fung TC, Masur SH, Kelsen JR, McConnell FM, Dubrot J, et al. Immune Tolerance. Group 3 Innate Lymphoid Cells Mediate Intestinal Selection of Commensal Bacteria-Specific $CD4^+$ T Cells. *Science* (2015) 348:1031–5. doi: 10.1126/science.aaa4812
77. Graves CL, Li J, LaPato M, Shapiro MR, Glover SC, Wallet MA, et al. Intestinal Epithelial Cell Regulation of Adaptive Immune Dysfunction in Human Type 1 Diabetes. *Front Immunol* (2017) 7:679. doi: 10.3389/fimmu.2016.00679
78. Bernink JH, Peters CP, Munneke M, te Velde AA, Meijer SL, Weijer K, et al. Human Type 1 Innate Lymphoid Cells Accumulate in Inflamed Mucosal Tissues. *Nat Immunol* (2013) 14:221–9. doi: 10.1038/ni.2534
79. Klose CS, Kiss EA, Schwierzeck V, Ebert K, Hoyler T, d'Hargues Y, et al. A T-bet Gradient Controls the Fate and Function of $CCR6^-Ror\gamma t^+$ Innate Lymphoid Cells. *Nature* (2013) 494:261–5. doi: 10.1038/nature11813
80. Aguiar SLF, Miranda MCG, Guimarães MAF, Santiago HC, Queiroz CP, Cunha PDS, et al. High-Salt Diet Induces IL-17-Dependent Gut Inflammation and Exacerbates Colitis in Mice. *Front Immunol* (2018) 8:1969. doi: 10.3389/fimmu.2017.01969
81. Hatfield JK, Brown MA. Group 3 Innate Lymphoid Cells Accumulate and Exhibit Disease-Induced Activation in the Meninges in EAE. *Cell Immunol* (2015) 297:69–79. doi: 10.1016/j.cellimm.2015.06.006
82. Mohr A, Trésallet C, Monot N, Bauvois A, Abiven D, Atif M, et al. Tissue Infiltrating Lti-Like Group 3 Innate Lymphoid Cells and T Follicular Helper Cells in Graves' and Hashimoto's Thyroiditis. *Front Immunol* (2020) 11:601. doi: 10.3389/fimmu.2020.00601
83. Kim MH, Taparowsky EJ, Kim CH. Retinoic Acid Differentially Regulates the Migration of Innate Lymphoid Cell Subsets to the Gut. *Immunity* (2015) 43:107–19. doi: 10.1016/j.immuni.2015.06.009
84. Ruiter B, Patil SU, Shreffler WG. Vitamins A and D Have Antagonistic Effects on Expression of Effector Cytokines and Gut-Homing Integrin in Human Innate Lymphoid Cells. *Clin Exp Allergy* (2015) 45:1214–25. doi: 10.1111/cea.12568
85. Stošić-Grujičić S, Cvjetićanin T, Stojanović I. Retinoids Differentially Regulate the Progression of Autoimmune Diabetes in Three Preclinical Models in Mice. *Mol Immunol* (2009) 47:79–86. doi: 10.1016/j.molimm.2008.12.028
86. Koprivica I, Gajic D, Saksida T, Cavalli E, Auci D, Despotovic S, et al. Orally Delivered All-Trans-Retinoic Acid- and Transforming Growth Factor-β-Loaded Microparticles Ameliorate Type 1 Diabetes in Mice. *Eur J Pharmacol* (2019) 864:172721. doi: 10.1016/j.ejphar.2019.172721
87. Giulietti A, Gysemans C, Stoffels K, van Etten E, Decallonne B, Overbergh L, et al. Vitamin D Deficiency in Early Life Accelerates Type 1 Diabetes in non-Obese Diabetic Mice. *Diabetologia* (2004) 47:451–62. doi: 10.1007/s00125-004-1329-3
88. Mathieu C, Waer M, Laureys J, Rutgeerts O, Bouillon R. Prevention of

Autoimmune Diabetes in NOD Mice by 1,25 Dihydroxyvitamin D3. *Diabetologia* (1994) 37:552–8. doi: 10.1007/BF00403372

89. Dvořák Z, Sokol H, Mani S. Drug Mimicry: Promiscuous Receptors PXR and AhR, and Microbial Metabolite Interactions in the Intestine. *Trends Pharmacol Sci* (2020) 41:900–8. doi: 10.1016/j.tips.2020.09.013
90. Kerkvliet NI, Steppan LB, Vorachek W, Oda S, Farrer D, Wong CP, et al. Activation of Aryl Hydrocarbon Receptor by TCDD Prevents Diabetes in NOD Mice and Increases Foxp3^{+} T Cells in Pancreatic Lymph Nodes. *Immunotherapy* (2009) 1:539–47. doi: 10.2217/imt.09.24
91. Ehrlich AK, Pennington JM, Wang X, Rohlman D, Punj S, Löhr CV, et al. Activation of the Aryl Hydrocarbon Receptor by 10-Cl-BBQ Prevents Insulitis and Effector T Cell Development Independently of Foxp3^{+} Regulatory T Cells in Nonobese Diabetic Mice. *J Immunol* (2016) 196:264–73. doi: 10.4049/jimmunol.1501789
92. Bolognini D, Tobin AB, Milligan G, Moss CE. The Pharmacology and Function of Receptors for Short-Chain Fatty Acids. *Mol Pharmacol* (2016) 89:388–98. doi: 10.1124/mol.115.102301
93. Jia L, Cao M, Chen H, Zhang M, Dong X, Ren Z, et al. Butyrate Ameliorates Antibiotic-Driven Type 1 Diabetes in the Female Offspring of Nonobese Diabetic Mice. *J Agric Food Chem* (2020) 68:3112–20. doi: 10.1021/acs.jafc.9b07701
94. Sun J, Furio L, Mecheri R, van der Does AM, Lundeberg E, Saveanu L, et al. Pancreatic β-Cells Limit Autoimmune Diabetes Via an Immunoregulatory Antimicrobial Peptide Expressed Under the Influence of the Gut Microbiota. *Immunity* (2015) 43:304–17. doi: 10.1016/j.immuni.2015.07.013
95. Needell JC, Ir D, Robertson CE, Kroehl ME, Frank DN, Zipris D. Maternal Treatment With Short-Chain Fatty Acids Modulates the Intestinal Microbiota and Immunity and Ameliorates Type 1 Diabetes in the Offspring. *PLoS One* (2017) 12:e0183786. doi: 10.1371/journal.pone.0183786
96. Kim SH, Cho BH, Kiyono H, Jang YS. Microbiota-Derived Butyrate Suppresses Group 3 Innate Lymphoid Cells in Terminal Ileal Peyer's Patches. *Sci Rep* (2017) 7:3980. doi: 10.1038/s41598-017-02729-6
97. Luu M, Weigand K, Wedi F, Breidenbend C, Leister H, Pautz S, et al. Regulation of the Effector Function of CD8^{+} T Cells by Gut Microbiota-Derived Metabolite Butyrate. *Sci Rep* (2018) 8:14430. doi: 10.1038/s41598-018-32860-x
98. Kimura I, Ichimura A, Ohue-Kitano R, Igarashi M. Free Fatty Acid Receptors in Health and Disease. *Physiol Rev* (2020) 100:171–210. doi: 10.1152/physrev.00041.2018
99. Macia L, Tan J, Vieira AT, Leach K, Stanley D, Luong S, et al. Metabolite-Sensing Receptors GPR43 and GPR109A Facilitate Dietary Fibre-Induced Gut Homeostasis Through Regulation of the Inflammasome. *Nat Commun* (2015) 6:6734. doi: 10.1038/ncomms7734
100. Lorza-Gil E, Kaiser G, Rexen Ulven E, König GM, Gerst F, Oquendo MB, et al. FFA2-, But Not FFA3-agonists Inhibit GSIS of Human Pseudoislets: A Comparative Study With Mouse Islets and Rat INS-1E Cells. *Sci Rep* (2020) 10:16497. doi: 10.1038/s41598-020-73467-5

12

Elevated Biomarkers of NETosis in the Serum of Pediatric Patients with Type 1 Diabetes and their First-Degree Relatives

Adam Klocperk[1], *Jana Vcelakova*[2], *Petra Vrabcova*[1], *Irena Zentsova*[1], *Lenka Petruzelkova*[2], *Zdenek Sumnik*[2], *Stepanka Pruhova*[2], *Anna Sediva*[1] *and Zuzana Parackova*[1*]

[1] *Department of Immunology, 2nd Faculty of Medicine Charles University, University Hospital in Motol, Prague, Czechia,*
[2] *Department of Pediatrics, 2nd Faculty of Medicine, Charles University and Motol University Hospital, Prague, Czechia*

Correspondence:
Zuzana Parackova
zuzana.parackova@fnmotol.cz

Type 1 diabetes (T1D) is an autoimmune disorder with unambiguous involvement of both innate and adaptive immune mechanisms in the destruction of pancreatic beta cells. Recent evidence demonstrated that neutrophils infiltrate the pancreas prior to disease onset and therein extrude neutrophil extracellular traps (NETs), web-like structures of DNA and nuclear proteins with a strong pro-inflammatory biologic activity. Our previous work showed that T1D NETs activate dendritic cells, which consequently induce IFNγ-producing Th1 lymphocytes. The aim of this study was to assess direct *ex vivo* biomarkers of NETosis in the serum of recent onset and long-term pediatric T1D patients, their first-degree relatives and healthy controls. To this end we evaluated serum levels of myeloperoxidase (MPO), neutrophil elastase (NE), proteinase 3 (PR3), protein arginine deiminase 4 (PAD4), LL37 and cell-free DNA-histone complexes in sex- and age-matched cohorts of T1D first-degree relatives, recent-onset T1D patients, and in patients 12 months after clinical manifestation of the disease. Our data shows that disease onset is accompanied by peripheral neutrophilia and significant elevation of MPO, NE, PR3, PAD4 and cell-free DNA-histone complexes. Most biomarkers subsequently decrease but do not always normalize in long-term patients. First-degree relatives displayed an intermediate phenotype, except for remarkably high levels of LL37. Together, this report provides evidence for the presence of ongoing NETosis in pediatric patients with T1D at time of clinical manifestation of the disease, which partly subsides in subsequent years.

Keywords: type 1 diabetes, neutrophils, NETosis, PAD4, pediatric, neutrophil extracellular trap, NET, ELISA

INTRODUCTION

Type 1 diabetes (T1D) is an autoimmune disease resulting from the destruction of insulin-producing beta cells in the pancreas, which involves both innate and adaptive immunity. Neutrophils in particular enjoy the interest of the scientific community, with both reduced (1–3) and elevated (4, 5) neutrophil counts being reported in T1D patients. While it has been shown that neutrophils can infiltrate the pancreas and initiate the autoimmune response driving its destruction in mice (6), their precise role in the pathogenesis of T1D is still under debate.

Neutrophils are able to extrude web-like structures called neutrophil extracellular traps (NET) in a process of specific cell death called NETosis (7). Even though NETosis is an essential part of host defense against infection, it can also be involved in the pathogenesis of autoimmune diseases. We and others have shown the involvement of NETs in the pathogenesis of autoimmune diabetes (6, 8–10), where neutrophils and NET-related products act as drivers of inflammation (11), Th1 polarization and type II interferon production (10). Conversely, the inhibition of NET formation is able to attenuate the development of T1D (6).

In previous studies, increased circulating levels of neutrophil elastase (NE) and proteinase 3 (PR3), both serine proteinases produced by neutrophils and stored in their primary azurophilic granules, as well as increased levels of myeloperoxidase (MPO)-DNA complexes, were reported in patients with T1D (12), suggesting enhanced NET formation. However, another study refuted this observation and documented significantly decreased levels of NE and PR3 (9) in patients within 3 years of diagnosis, a finding possibly related to the previously shown gradual decrease of neutrophil counts after clinical onset of the disease (13).

In this study we aim to expand the spectrum of investigated NETosis related products to NE, PR3, MPO, peptidyl arginine deiminase 4 (PAD4) – an enzyme which facilitates chromatin decondensation vital for NET formation, LL37 – an antimicrobial cathelicidin, and DNA-histone complexes and assess their levels in the serum of a cohort of patients at the onset of T1D, with well-established disease and in their first-degree relatives, both autoantibody positive and negative.

METHODS

Cohort Description

Peripheral blood neutrophil counts were measured as part of complete blood count with differential, using routine in-house methods in 333 patients with long-term T1D at an average of 5.73 ± 3.82 years since clinical manifestation of T1D, 172 patients with newly diagnosed T1D sampled within 7 days of manifestation, 51 antibody positive [at least one of the following: anti-glutamic acid decarboxylase 65 (anti-GAD65), anti-tyrosine phosphatase-like insulinoma antigen 2 (anti-IA2), anti-indole-3-acetic acid (anti-IAA), anti-zinc transporter protein 8 (anti-ZNT8)] first-degree relatives of T1D patients, 122 antibody negative first-degree relatives of T1D patients and 17 healthy children.

Serum neutrophil products were measured in a subset of 31 patients with newly diagnosed T1D [8 who presented with diabetic ketoacidosis (DKA, pH < 7.3)], 32 patients at one year since clinical manifestation of T1D. Additionally, we investigated 32 antibody negative and 32 antibody positive healthy first-degree relatives. The control group with no personal history of autoimmune disease comprised 32 age and sex-matched healthy children.

Detailed cohort description data can be inspected in **Tables 1** and **2**.

Legal guardians of all study participants signed a written informed consent prior to entering the study. The study was approved by the institutional Ethics Committees of the University Hospital Motol and 2nd Faculty of Medicine, Charles University in Prague, Czech Republic and was conducted in accordance with the Declaration of Helsinki.

Neutrophil Counts and Autoantibody Determination

Anti-GAD65, -IA2, -IAA autoantibodies were measured using radioimmunoassay (RIA) based on 125I-labelled antigens (Medipan GmbH, Berlin, Germany). All three assays were evaluated using the Islet Autoantibody Standardization Program 2015. The following assay cut-offs were determined with receiver operating characteristic (ROC) plots using all the samples: 0.4 U/ml for anti-IAA, 1.0 U/ml for anti-GAD65 and 0.9 U/mL for anti-IA2. Anti-ZnT8 were examined by ELISA (RSR Limited, Wales, UK) as

TABLE 1 | Cohort description – neutrophil counts.

	Number (n)	Age (years, mean ± SD) (range)	Sex (n)	Time since diagnosis of T1D (years, mean ± SD) (range)	HbA1c (mmol/mol, mean ± SD) (range)
Healthy	17	14.29 ± 1.87 (11.81-17.37)	5 male, 12 female	NA	NA
Ab- relatives	122	9.11 ± 4.48 (0.3-20.7)	61 male, 61 female	NA	34.77 ± 2.76 (27–39)
Ab+ relatives	51	9.07 ± 4.37 (2.7-25.6)	29 male, 22 female	NA	32.83 ± 3.57 (25-40)
Recent onset	172	9.19 ± 4.44 (1.1-18.27)	85 male, 87 female	NA	97.63 ± 29.83 (33-172)
Long-term T1D	333	12.61 ± 4.21 (2.28-24.58)	168 male, 165 female	5.73 ± 3.82 (0.71-17.5)	64.48 ± 15.42 (35-143)

TABLE 2 | Cohort description – serum neutrophil products.

	Number (n)	Age (years, mean ± SD)	Sex (n)	HbA1c (mmol/mol, mean ± SD) (range)
Healthy	32	9.6 ± 4.2 (3.8-17.9)	16 male, 16 female	NA
Ab- relatives	32	9.5 ± 4.1 (2.0-17.4)	16 male, 16 female	33 ± 4.1 (28-43)
Ab+ relatives	32	9.9 ± 4.2 (3.2-17.6)	16 male, 16 female	33 ± 4.8 (27-40)
Recent onset	31	9.6 ± 4.2 (3.3-17.5)	15 male, 16 female	106.5 ± 25.5 (59-156)
Long-term T1D	32	10.1 ± 4.3 (3.2-17.5)	16 male, 16 female	50 ± 22.8 (32-125)

described previously (14). Complete blood count with differential was analysed on the Sysmex XN-3000 platform (Sysmex Europe, Norderstedt, Germany).

NET Components

Commercially available ELISA kits were used to quantify myeloperoxidase, neutrophil elastase, proteinase 3 (Abcam, Cambridge, USA), LL37 (Hycult Biotech, Wayne, USA), DNA-histone complexes (Sigma-Aldrich, St. Luis, USA) and PAD4 (LSBio, Seattle, USA) according to manufacturer's instructions.

Statistics

Statistical analyses were performed using Brown-Forsythe and Welch one-way analysis of variance (ANOVA), unpaired t-tests with Welch's correction and linear regression using GraphPad PRISM 8.0 (San Diego, CA, USA). Values of p=0.01-0.05 (*), p=0.001-0.01 (**), p<0.001 (***) and p<0.0001 (****) were considered statistically significant.

RESULTS

T1D Onset Is Accompanied by Transient Neutrophilia

In this study we observed substantial changes in absolute circulating neutrophil counts between healthy controls, first-degree relatives of T1D patients both negative and positive for T1D-specific autoantibodies, patients at clinical onset of the disease and patients with long-term disease (**Figure 1A**, Brown-Forsythe and Welch ANOVA $p < 0.0001$, summary data for other leukocyte populations shown in **Supplementary Table 1**).

In particular, we saw a modest but statistically insignificant decrease of neutrophils in relatives regardless of seropositivity and in patients with long-term disease, compared to healthy controls (**Figure 1A**), which was independent from age (**Figure 1B**). In contrast, patients at the onset of clinical disease had elevated absolute neutrophil counts compared to first-degree relatives ($p < 0.0001$ for antibody negative and $p = 0.001$ for antibody positive, unpaired t-test with Welch's

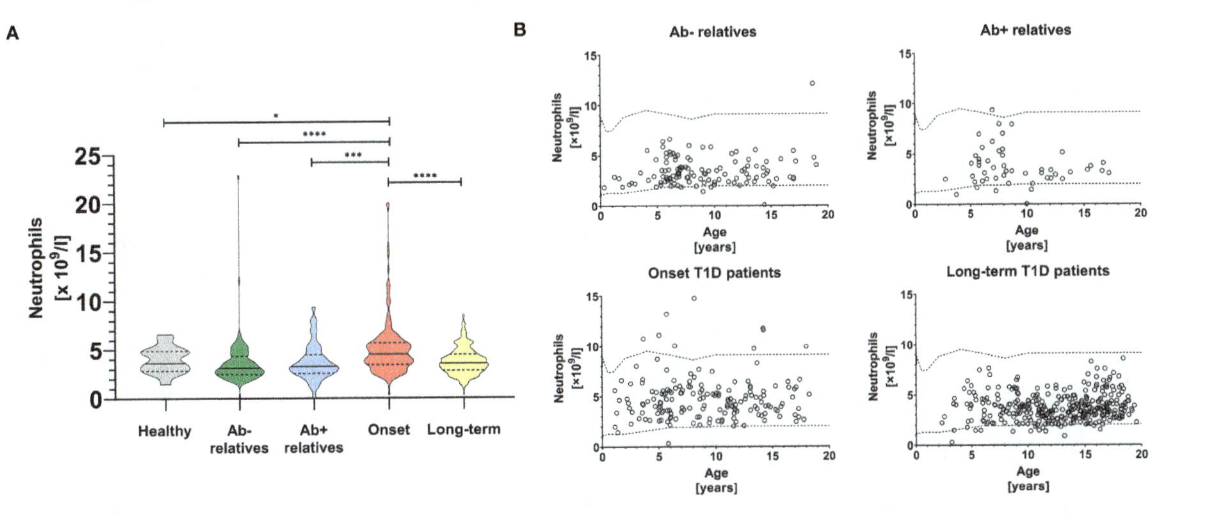

FIGURE 1 | Peripheral blood neutrophils. Absolute neutrophil counts in the peripheral blood of healthy controls, antibody negative and antibody positive first-degree relatives of T1D patients, T1D patients at the clinical onset of the disease and T1D patients with long-term, well-established disease **(A)**. Temporal development of absolute neutrophil counts in the peripheral blood of healthy controls, antibody negative and antibody positive first-degree relatives of T1D patients, T1D patients at the clinical onset of the disease and T1D patients with long-term, well-established disease **(B)**. Healthy in-house reference range visualized with dashed line. Unpaired t-test with Welch's correction p-values shown, p=0.01-0.05 (*), p=0.001-0.01 (**), p<0.001 (***), p<0.0001 (****).

correction), long-term T1D patients ($p < 0.0001$) and healthy controls ($p = 0.014$).

Increased Circulating Levels of NET-Associated Biomarkers Are a Hallmark of Recent Onset T1D Patients

Since the process of NETosis has previously been implicated in the pathogenesis of T1D and our patients displayed a discrete transient neutrophilia upon reaching clinical onset of T1D, we hypothesized that NET-associated biomarkers should be elevated in the serum of T1D patients, especially at the time of clinical manifestation of the disease.

Indeed, we were able to detect high levels of myeloperoxidase (MPO) (**Figure 2A**, Brown-Forsythe and Welch ANOVA $p = 0.0024$), neutrophils elastase (NE) (**Figure 2B**, $p = 0.0005$) and proteinase 3 (PR3) (**Figure 2C**, $p < 0.0001$), enzymes widely present in NET structures and released during the degranulation process, in the sera of T1D patients and their relatives, compared to healthy controls.

Antibody positive relatives (Ab+) also exhibited significantly elevated levels of LL37 (cathelicidin), an antimicrobial peptide commonly present in NET structures (**Figure 2D**, $p = 0.0058$). There was no relationship between a number of autoantibodies and NET-related products (**Supplementary Figure 1**).

Patients at the clinical onset of T1D displayed increased levels of cell-free DNA-histone complexes (**Figure 2E**, $p = 0.0031$) and peptidyl arginine deiminase 4 (PAD4), an enzyme which facilitates protein citrullination and has been intricately linked to NET formation (**Figure 2F**, $p < 0.0001$).

We did not observe significant difference in serum levels of any of the analytes and absolute circulating neutrophil counts in recent onset patients who presented with and without diabetic ketoacidosis (DKA), defined as $pH < 7.3$ (**Supplementary Figure 2**). MPO and DNA-histones levels significantly correlated with blood pH and MPO was slightly higher in patients with DKA but showed high variance (unpaired t-test with Welch's correction $p = 0.046$).

None of the NET-associated biomarkers was significantly associated with age (**Supplementary Figure 3**) or sex (**Supplementary Figure 4**). There was also no significant correlation between their serum levels and absolute counts of circulating neutrophils (**Supplementary Figure 5**).

Residual beta-cell activity was not directly quantified through the measurement of fasting or stimulated C-peptide, however there was no correlation between the metabolic control of T1D measured as glycated hemoglobin fraction HbA1c (**Supplementary Figure 6**) and NET-associated biomarkers in either recent onset or long-term patients.

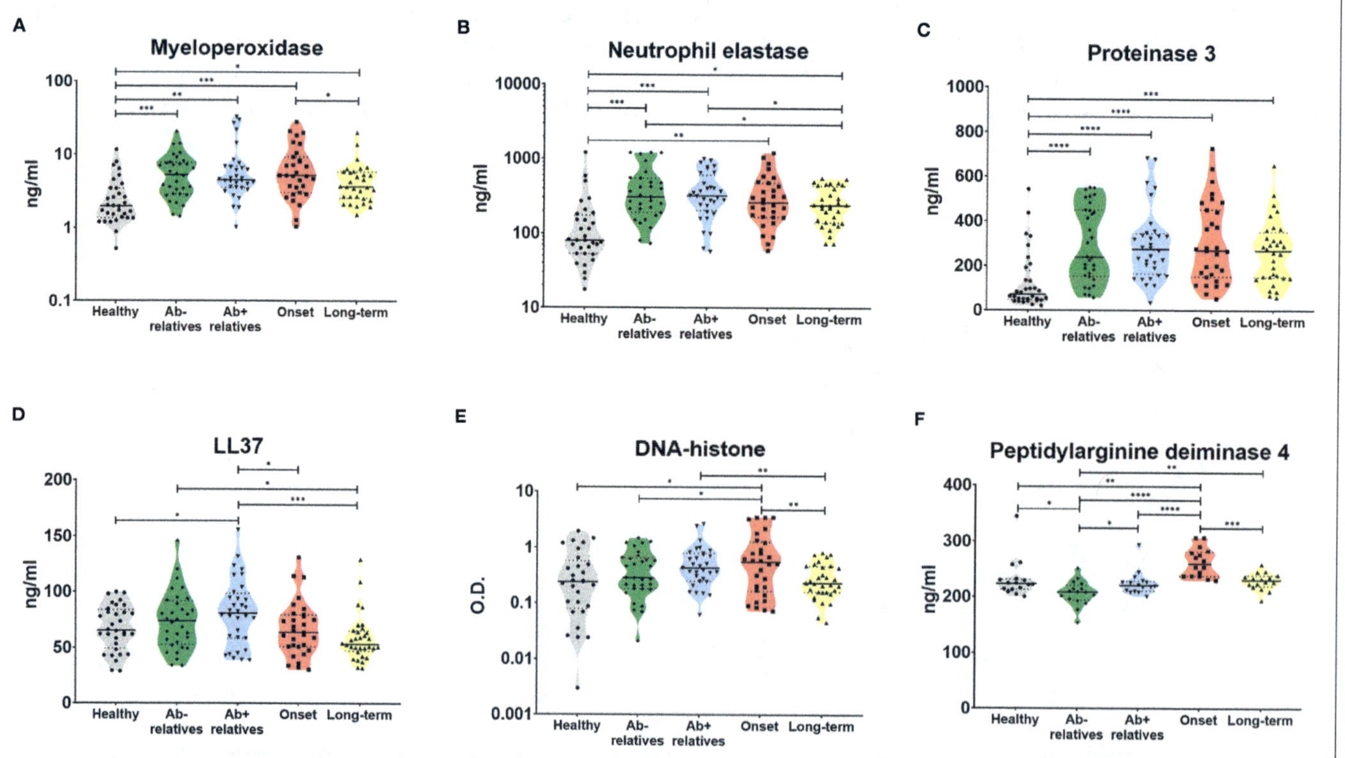

FIGURE 2 | Serum products of NETosis. Products of NETosis **(A)** myeloperoxidase, **(B)** neutrophil elastase, **(C)** proteinase 3, **(D)** LL37, **(E)** DNA-histone complexes and **(F)** peptidyl arginine deiminase 4) in the serum of healthy controls, antibody negative and antibody positive first-degree relatives of T1D patients, T1D patients at the clinical onset of the disease and T1D patients with long-term, well-established disease. Unpaired t-test with Welch's correction p-values shown, p=0.01-0.05 (*), p=0.001-0.01 (**), p<0.001 (***), p<0.0001 (****). O.D. = optical density.

DISCUSSION

In this brief report we demonstrate the elevation of neutrophils and indirect serum biomarkers of neutrophil NETosis – the enzymes myeloperoxidase (MPO), proteinase 3 (PR3), neutrophil elastase (NE) and protein arginine deiminase 4 (PAD4), the active form of the antimicrobial peptide cathelicidin, LL37, and cell-free DNA-histone complexes – in the blood of pediatric patients with recent onset type 1 diabetes.

Our study builds on and expands the previous works by Wang et al., who have shown similar results, but whose analysis was limited to PR3 and NE (12). We show for the first-time elevated serum levels of cell-free DNA and MPO. At the same time, the elevated concentration of PAD4 provides mechanistic insight into the process of NETosis in diabetic patients, as PAD4 citrullinates arginine residues on histones, reducing their positive charge and allowing chromatin decondensation vital for NET formation (15). LL37, which apart from its antimicrobial activity can suppress neutrophil apoptosis (16), was highest in antibody positive relatives, but quite normal in recent onset patients, suggesting concurrent activity of several pathways involving neutrophils.

The data concerning neutrophils and NETosis-biomarkers in T1D are not homogeneous. A study by Qin et al. (9) reported reduced NE and PR3 in T1D patients, which was associated with decreased neutrophils. While we too observed some correlation between MPO, NE, LL37 and neutrophil counts in T1D patients, this was not apparent in first-degree relatives and was driven by a single data point in each cohort. A possible explanation for these diverging results are the different inclusion criteria, as Qin's "recent-onset" cohort included patients up to 3 years after disease manifestation and featured mainly adults, whereas our recent onset cohort was sampled within 7 days of the clinical manifestation of the disease and comprised chiefly children under 10 years of age. A closer comparison may be drawn to the study by Valle et al., which reported decreased neutrophil counts in newly diagnosed pediatric T1D patients (1). The potential effect of recent metabolic stress on circulating neutrophils and NETosis cannot be discounted and presents a unique and currently unresolved challenge in determining which of these two is the initial driving factor, which will require further study. The slight neutropenia we reported in first-degree relatives is in agreement with previous observations by Vecchio et al. (2), suggesting that despite the absence of overt endocrinopathy, abnormalities in neutrophil biology are already present in at risk subjects. Further work on neutrophil phenotype in recent onset patients and at-risk relatives is warranted and could elucidate their activation status, maturity and more.

While we have already previously shown that T1D NETs activate dendritic cells and drive T cell polarization towards the IFN-γ Th1 response in a series of *in vitro* studies performed on material from patients with well-established disease (10), here for the first time we show NETosis biomarkers directly *ex vivo* and expand the studied cohorts to include recent onset patients and their relatives. As the current literature lacks any data analyzing the enzymatic activity of MPO, PAD4 and other enzymes, or the serum concentration of NET-derived citrullinated proteins in T1D patients, this report provides first indirect evidence of their role in T1D pathogenesis.

The double-edged role of NETosis in driving not only antimicrobial host defense, but also pathological inflammation, remains highly topical and has recently been shown in COVID-19, where elevated neutrophil counts predicted worse clinical outcome and serum MPO and cell-free DNA were elevated in patients requiring mechanical ventilation (17). The mass egress of proteolytic enzymes from neutrophils into circulation can trigger a proteolytic storm, drive activation of pro-enzymes and result in proinflammatory cytokine release and host damage (18).

We thus hypothesize that a yet unidentified trigger, perhaps a subclinical viral infection (19), contributes to the ongoing neutrophil activation and low-grade NETosis that we show already in antibody-positive relatives. The biological activity of NETs may then result in further accentuation of the inflammation, egress of neutrophils from the bone marrow – reflected in the transient neutrophilia we show – and neutrophil infiltration into the pancreas as documented by Diana et al. Ultimately, this vicious cycle leads to the destruction of insulin-producing beta-cells and clinical manifestation of diabetes mellitus.

AUTHOR CONTRIBUTIONS

AK gathered and analyzed longitudinal data mapping peripheral neutrophil counts and co-wrote the article. PV and IZ performed experiments. JV, LP, ZS, and SP provided patient information and primary biomaterial and reviewed the manuscript. AS co-conceived the study, provided support and reviewed the manuscript. ZP conceived the article, designed experiments evaluating the serum concentration of NETosis products, analyzed the data and co-wrote the article. All authors contributed to the article and approved the submitted version.

ACKNOWLEDGMENTS

The authors wish to thank the patients and their families for their consent with inclusion in this study.

REFERENCES

1. Valle A, Giamporcaro GM, Scavini M, Stabilini A, Grogan P, Bianconi E, et al. Reduction of Circulating Neutrophils Precedes and Accompanies Type 1 Diabetes. *Diabetes* (2013) 62:2072–7. doi: 10.2337/DB12-1345
2. Vecchio F, Lo Buono N, Stabilini A, Nigi L, Dufort MJ, Geyer S, et al. Abnormal Neutrophil Signature in the Blood and Pancreas of Presymptomatic and Symptomatic Type 1 Diabetes. *JCI Insight* (2018) 3:1–17. doi: 10.1172/jci.insight.122146
3. Harsunen M, Puff R, D'Orlando O, Giannopoulou E, Lachmann L, Beyerlein A,

et al. Reduced Blood Leukocyte and Neutrophil Numbers in the Pathogenesis of Type 1 Diabetes. *Horm Metab Res* (2013) 45:467–70. doi: 10.1055/s-0032-1331226

4. Jackson MH, Collier A, Nicoll JJ, Muir AL, Dawes J, Clarke BF, et al. Neutrophil Count and Activation in Vascular Disease. *Scott Med J* (1992) 37:41–3. doi: 10.1177/003693309203700205
5. Yu Y, Lin Q, Ye D, Wang Y, He B, Li Y, et al. Neutrophil Count as a Reliable Marker for Diabetic Kidney Disease in Autoimmune Diabetes. *BMC Endocr Disord* (2020) 20:158. doi: 10.1186/s12902-020-00597-2
6. Diana J, Simoni Y, Furio L, Beaudoin L, Agerberth B, Barrat F, et al. Crosstalk Between Neutrophils, B-1a Cells and Plasmacytoid Dendritic Cells Initiates Autoimmune Diabetes. *Nat Med* (2012) 19:65–73. doi: 10.1038/nm.3042
7. Brinkmann V, Reichard U, Goosmann C, Fauler B, Uhlemann Y, Weiss DS, et al. Neutrophil Extracellular Traps Kill Bacteria. *Science* (2004) 303:1532–5. doi: 10.1126/science.1092385
8. Wong SL, Demers M, Martinod K, Gallant M, Wang Y, Goldfine AB, et al. Diabetes Primes Neutrophils to Undergo NETosis, Which Impairs Wound Healing. *Nat Med* (2015) 21:815–9. doi: 10.1038/nm.3887
9. Qin J, Fu S, Speake C, Greenbaum CJ, Odegard JM. Netosis-Associated Serum Biomarkers Are Reduced in Type 1 Diabetes in Association With Neutrophil Count. *Clin Exp Immunol* (2016) 184:318–22. doi: 10.1111/cei.12783
10. Parackova Z, Zentsova I, Vrabcova P, Klocperk A, Sumnik Z, Pruhova S, et al. Neutrophil Extracellular Trap Induced Dendritic Cell Activation Leads to Th1 Polarization in Type 1 Diabetes. *Front Immunol* (2020) 11:661. doi: 10.3389/fimmu.2020.00661
11. Njeim R, Azar WS, Fares AH, Azar ST, Kassouf HK, Eid AA. Netosis Contributes to the Pathogenesis of Diabetes and Its Complications. *J Mol Endocrinol* (2020) 65:R65–76. doi: 10.1530/JME-20-0128
12. Wang Y, Xiao Y, Zhong L, Ye D, Zhang J, Tu Y, et al. Increased Neutrophil Elastase and Proteinase 3 and Augmented NETosis Are Closely Associated With β-Cell Autoimmunity in Patients With Type 1 Diabetes. *Diabetes* (2014) 63:4239–48. doi: 10.2337/db14-0480
13. Klocperk A, Petruzelkova L, Pavlikova M, Rataj M, Kayserova J, Pruhova S, et al. Changes in Innate and Adaptive Immunity Over the First Year After the Onset of Type 1 Diabetes. *Acta Diabetol* (2019) 57(3). doi: 10.1007/s00592-019-01427-1
14. Petruzelkova L, Ananieva-Jordanova R, Vcelakova J, Vesely Z, Stechova K, Lebl J, et al. The Dynamic Changes of Zinc Transporter 8 Autoantibodies in Czech Children From the Onset of Type 1 Diabetes Mellitus. *Diabetes Med* (2014) 31:165–71. doi: 10.1111/dme.12308
15. Wang Y, Li M, Stadler S, Correll S, Li P, Wang D, et al. Histone Hypercitrullination Mediates Chromatin Decondensation and Neutrophil Extracellular Trap Formation. *J Cell Biol* (2009) 184:205–13. doi: 10.1083/jcb.200806072
16. Nagaoka I, Suzuki K, Niyonsaba F, Tamura H, Hirata M. Modulation of Neutrophil Apoptosis by Antimicrobial Peptides. *ISRN Microbiol* (2012) 2012:1–12. doi: 10.5402/2012/345791
17. Zuo Y, Yalavarthi S, Shi H, Gockman K, Zuo M, Madison JA, et al. Neutrophil Extracellular Traps in COVID-19. *JCI Insight* (2020) 5(11). doi: 10.1172/JCI.INSIGHT.138999
18. Fornasari PM. SARS-Cov-2 Protease-Dependent Human Cell Infection Induces Immunological Response Imbalance and Neutrophils "Proteolytic Storm". Proteolysis Inhibitors Can Prevent and Treat Covid-19. *J Cardiol Res Rev Rep* (2021) 2:1–10. doi: 10.47363/jcrrr/2021(2)135
19. De Beeck AO, Eizirik DL. Viral Infections in Type 1 Diabetes Mellitus-Why the β Cells? *Nat Rev Endocrinol* (2016) 12:263–73. doi: 10.1038/nrendo.2016.30

13

The Benefits and Limits of Technological Advances in Glucose Management Around Physical Activity in Patients Type 1 Diabetes

Sémah Tagougui [1,2†], Nadine Taleb [1,3†] and Rémi Rabasa-Lhoret [1,2,3,4,5]*

[1] Institut de Recherches Cliniques de Montréal, Montreal, QC, Canada, [2] Département de Nutrition, Faculté de Médicine, Université de Montréal, Montreal, QC, Canada, [3] Département des Sciences Biomédicales, Faculté de Médicine, Université de Montréal, Montreal, QC, Canada, [4] Division of Endocrinology, McGill University, Montreal, QC, Canada, [5] Endocrinology Division, Montreal Diabetes Research Center, Montreal, QC, Canada

***Correspondence:**
Rémi Rabasa-Lhoret
remi.rabasa-lhoret@ircm.qc.ca

† These authors have contributed equally to this work

Physical activity is highly recommended for patients living with type 1 diabetes (T1D) due to its varied health benefits. Nevertheless, glucose management, during and in the hours following exercise, represents a great challenge for these patients who most often end up leading a sedentary life style. Important technological advances in insulin delivery devices and glucose monitoring are now available and continue to progress. These technologies could be used to alleviate glucose management related to physical activity in T1D. Continuous glucose monitoring (CGM) helps patients observe the trends of glycemic fluctuations when exercising and in the following night to deal pre-emptively with hypoglycemic risks and treat hypoglycemic episodes in a timely manner. Insulin pumps offer the flexibility of adjusting insulin basal rates and boluses according to patient's specific needs around exercise. The artificial pancreas links CGM to pump through an intelligent hormone dosing algorithm to close the loop of glucose control and has thus the potential to ease the burden of exercise in T1D. This review will examine and discuss the literature related to physical activity practice using each of these technologies. The aim is to discuss their benefits as well as their limitations and finally the additional research needed in the future to optimize their use in T1D.

Keywords: type 1 diabetes, exercise, continuous subcutaneous insulin infusion, continuous subcutaneous glucose monitoring, artificial pancreas, single-hormone, dual-hormone, closed-loop

INTRODUCTION

Regular physical activity (PA) offers many potential health benefits for individuals with type 1 diabetes (T1D) including improvements in insulin sensitivity and requirements, reduced risk of cardiovascular diseases and increased overall life expectancy (1). Despite these benefits, physical activity is practiced at a much lower frequency than recommended by patients with T1D (2) who may adopt unhealthy lifestyles worsening their cardiometabolic risk profile (3). The principal barrier for PA is the fear of hypoglycemia that is mainly driven by the inability to identify and/or implement effective strategies for hypoglycemia avoidance (2).

As compared to people without T1D, the inability to reduce circulating insulin during and after exercise restricts hepatic glucose production concurrently to an enhanced glucose disposal rate into skeletal muscle. Skeletal muscle plays a considerable role in maintaining homeostasis of blood glucose. It uses glucose as a source of energy during dynamic exercise, and represents the major site for insulin-stimulated glucose uptake. Glucose is transported from blood into muscle fibers by the glucose transporter-4. This process is regulated by the translocation of glucose transporters-4 to the plasma membrane and transverse tubules under insulin and exercise-stimulated conditions (4) (**Figure 1**). Because of the disparity between glucose production and utilization (e.g., combined exercise and relative hyperinsulinemic conditions), hypoglycemia can occur during and in the hours following exercise (5). The type, intensity, duration, and distance to meals of exercise as well as the aerobic fitness are all important factors influencing glucose homeostasis (6, 7) (**Figure 2**). Therefore, aerobic, sprint, and resistance training can be responsible for wide variations in blood glucose responses (8, 9). While low to moderate aerobic exercise usually induces progressive glucose lowering, high intensity activities can trigger significant release of counter regulatory hormones (e.g., epinephrine and glucagon) causing rapid elevations in blood glucose levels (**Figure 2**). Exercise duration also affects glucose control for example, extended periods of exercise results in a higher rate of glucose disposal and thus increased risk of hypoglycemia. Hormonal counter-regulatory response (e.g., catecholamines, glucagon, etc.) to different types of prolonged exercise could be highly variable inter- and intra- individuals as shown in well-controlled T1D (10, 11). For very intense exercise it can trigger a short but large hepatic glucose output exceeding glucose utilization ability by other tissues resulting in transient but significant hyperglycemia (5) (**Figure 2**). Even with low intensity and realtively short duration exercise practiced during the day, an increase in insulin sensitivity can last up to 11–16 h post-exercise which combined with glycogen store replacement can increase the risk of late-onset or nocturnal hypoglycemia (**Figure 2**).

Guidelines for minimizing exercise-related hypo- and hyperglycemic risks exist but remain general (12). In practice, 3 main adjustments may be considered (13, 14): **1/** carbohydrate (CHO) supplementation (15, 16), particularly for unanticipated exercise and for prolonged exercise; **2/** premeal insulin-dose reduction (17, 18) provided exercise can be anticipated and undertaken within meal bolus insulin action and for patients using continuous subcutaneous insulin infusion (CSII: pump) for both post-prandial and post-absorptive periods using temporary basal insulin reduction; **3/** adding high intensity sprints in intervals, or resistance training at beginning or end of exercise sessions (9). However, even when one or combinations of these strategies are used, the right combination for a specific exercise is complex to establish and most patients still have wide exercise-related glucose fluctuations.

Remarkable progress has been achieved in technologies to improve and facilitate diabetes management including insulin pumps, continuous glucose monitoring (CGM), and external artificial pancreas systems. This review aims to discuss how technological advances could be used to alleviate the burden of glucose management during exercise in patients with T1D. Each of these technologies is reviewed to examine its benefits as well as limitations around exercise.

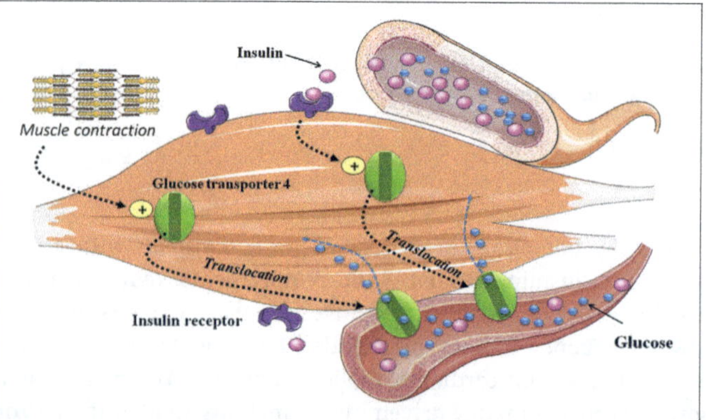

FIGURE 1 | Skeletal muscle glucose uptake during exercise. Exercise increases insulin-stimulated glucose uptake in skeletal muscle. This process is regulated by the translocation of glucose transporter-4 glucose to the plasma membrane and transverse tubules. Both exercise and insulin utilize different signaling pathways, both of which lead to the activation of glucose transport.

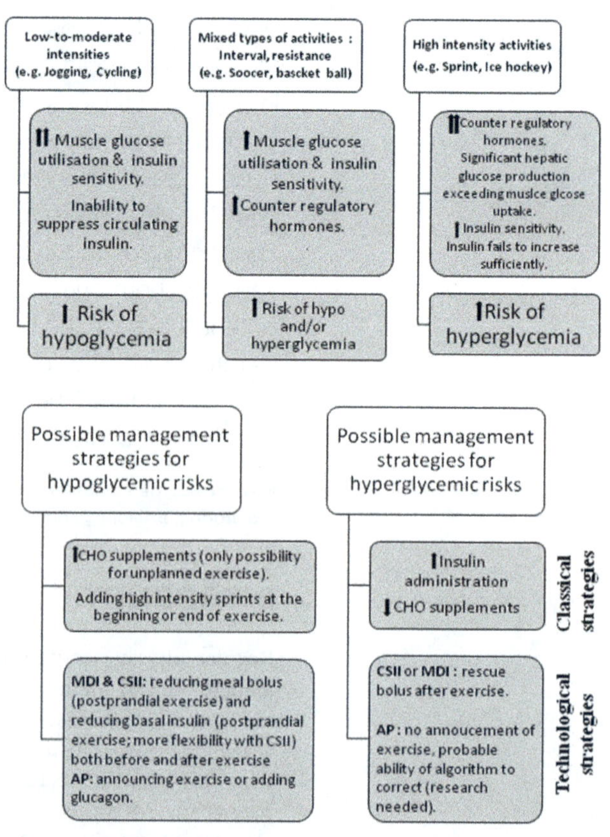

FIGURE 2 | Physiological mechanisms related to hypo and hyperglycemia & strategies to limit exercise-induced hypo and hyperglycaemia in patients with type 1 diabete. CHO, carbohydrate; CSII, continuous subcutaneous insulin infusion; MDI, Multiple dose injection; AP, artificial pancreas.

CONTINUOUS SUBCUTANEOUS INSULIN INFUSION (CSII: INSULIN PUMPS)

In this section we aim to present an update of practical management strategies during exercise in patients using insulin pump therapy. The introduction in the 1980's of CSII therapy in the form of pump systems was an important landmark in technological advances in insulin delivery (19). Insulin pumps provides a flexibility in an attempt to mimic physiologic insulin delivery, infusing rapid acting insulin subcutaneously at preselected basal rates to cover a 24 h period in addition to insulin boluses at mealtimes or to correct hyperglycemia that are activated on demand by the patient (20).

New insulin pumps are small in size and endowed with many programming options that facilitate their use. Insulin pumps exist in various designs the main difference being patch or tubeless pump vs. using an external catheter. In patch pumps, a container housing the insulin ampoule attaches directly to the skin with a catheter directly under the patch and a controller communicates wirelessly with the patch pump. In contrast, with the conventional design, the pump holds the insulin reservoir and connects to the body through a tubule up to a subcutaneous insulin catheter (21). While for aquatic physical activity patch pump since it is waterproof and does not require disconnection, the ability to transiently disconnect the pump with offered by conventional pumps can be useful for some other activities with contact (judo, hockey, etc.).

CSII therapy is proven to improve glucose control in many patients with diabetes resulting in lower HbA_{1c} levels and frequency of hypoglycemia, it is however associated with higher treatment cost and require to be continuously worn (22–24). Furthermore, a change in basal insulin delivery rate around the time of exercise is only possible with insulin pumps; an approach that cannot be used in multiple dose insulin injections (MDI) regimens where basal insulin is injected once or twice daily at preset timings. Indeed, for physically active patients with T1D, CSII can be a preferred option to facilitate glucose regulation.

Mild to moderate intensity aerobic exercise is probably the most chosen type of physical activity by patients and entails a high risk of hypoglycemia as discussed above. Therefore, this type of exercise was included in most of the conducted studies that have looked up ways to reduce hypoglycemia in patients with T1D (5). When exercise is planned within 90–120 min post meal, a pre-meal insulin bolus reduction that is proportional to exercise duration and intensity has been backed-up by a couple of studies and thus endorsed consensus statements (5, 17, 18, 25). When an exercise session is practiced in close proximity to a meal without anticipation, which is very frequent in adolescents and children, or when a longer than expected activity occurs then the consumption of carbohydrates (CHO) is usually required (15, 16). The CHO rescue could be an effective strategy to improve performance for certain patients who wish to improve their performance but could be counter-productive for those who wish to lose weight.

A third approach that can be applied in insulin pumps users consists of reducing temporarily basal insulin rate. Franc et al. (26) have tested the efficacy of reducing hypoglycemia by decreasing or stopping basal insulin rate at exercise onset. Adult patients with T1D performed 30 min of either moderate or high intensity aerobic in a post-absorptive state (>3 h post-meal). No hypoglycemia events (glucose <3.3 mmol/l) were recorded: when basal insulin was reduced: **1/** by 50% or 80% during moderate exercise (50% VO_{2peak}) or **2/** by 80% or pump stopped for the intense exercise sessions (75%VO_{2peak}). Another relevant observation from this study is that late post-exercise hypoglycemia risk was similar to rest interventions with the implementation of an 80% basal insulin reduction for moderate exercise and with pump suspension for the intense exercise (26). Another study conducted in an adult population with T1D looked at the effects of basal insulin suspension at exercise onset on blood glucose levels during 40-min continuous (40–50% VO_{2peak}) vs. circuit-based exercise. The authors reported that basal insulin suspension at the onset of exercise leads to a greater drop in glycemia during Continuous vs. Circuit-Based Exercise (27). Currently, studies comparing the effects of basal rate reduction during continuous exercise vs. interval exercise remain uncommon. Considering that these type of exercise have a different impact the blood glucose level in T1D patients, it will be important to test strategies to determine the optimal approach to reduce hypoglycemia during these 2 types of exercise.

The studies cited above (26, 27) showed that as compared to no action, significant reduction in insulin infusion at exercise onset is generally helpful in improving time spent with blood glucose levels in target ranges during exercise, but the risk of hypoglycemia remains largely present. Thus, other studies have thereafter focused on completely suspending insulin infusion. In a pediatric study ($n = 10$), hypoglycemia episodes and the drop in glycemia during a 40–45-min exercise sessions were similar between a pump-on vs. pump-off strategies (28). In 49 children and adolescents (8–17 years old) with T1D, the DirecNet Study Group were able to bring down the risk of hypoglycemia from 43 to 16% by a pump-off design at exercise onset; 60-min aerobic exercise performed 4 h after lunch (29). The drawback in this study was an increased risk of post-exercise hyperglycemia.

Although reducing insulin basal rate at exercise onset seems could help in attenuating the hypoglycemia risk, earlier timings might be needed for a better effect. This is mostly supported by the pharmacokinetics of available rapid acting insulin analogs; suggesting that decreasing insulin rates up to 90 min prior to exercise onset might be needed to sufficiently reduce circulating insulin levels during a post-absorptive activity (26, 30). Practically speaking, though, such early anticipation is not practical for a large fraction of patients. A recent study compared 3 more practical timings of 80% basal insulin reduction: 40 min, 20 min prior and at exercise onset (31). This study reiterated the fact that exercise-induced hypoglycemia is frequent (close to 50% of exercise sessions). Moreover, although some favorable trends were observed with the reduction at 40 min prior to exercise, hypoglycemia remained a frequent event with that timing. Similarly, McAuley et al. (32) reported that reducing insulin infusion by 50% 1 h prior to a 30-min exercise at moderate intensity did not reduce plasma insulin levels at exercise onset and did not fully prevent exercise-induced hypoglycemia. An earlier basal rate reduction is thus probably needed to have a more significant impact on hypoglycemic risk.

It should be noted that practicing physical activity does not increase the risk of hypoglycemia only during exercise but also in the following hours frequently including overnight a time at which hypoglycemia prevention, detection and treatment is harder. To mitigate post-exercise hypoglycemia, very few evidence-based data is available. We have reviewed the impact of bedtime snack on nocturnal hypoglycemic risk and highlighted the very low level of evidence of this widely recommended practice (33). Taplin et al. (34) showed that children on CSII could significantly reduce their nocturnal hypoglycemia risk by stopping insulin infusion during exercise and reducing its rate by 20% over the following night (between 21 h:00 and 03 h:00).

The available studies are generally of a small scale (summarized in **Table 1**) and mostly conducted in laboratory settings, but could still help shaping some guidelines for glucose management around exercise for patients using insulin pumps. For anticipated exercise, if exercise occur during meal bolus action a reduction of this bolus proportional to exercise intensity and duration is a reasonably well-validated strategy; for exercise undertaken in the post-absorptive period in patients using CSII, the best timing and amount of insulin reduction prior to exercise onset is still a pending question. In all situations (post-meal vs. post absorptive as well as CSII vs. MDI) different timings and percentages need to be tested in different types of exercise (e.g., aerobic vs. resistance vs. interval; duration; intensity; etc.). In the case of unanticipated exercise, although insulin suspension at exercise onset seems the best solution for the time being, related studies have tackled mainly continuous moderate intensity exercise sessions. An increased risk of hyperglycemia could be speculated for intense continuous or interval exercise with pump suspension and evidence-based data is lacking. In that situation, to correct post exercise hyperglycemia, a recent study validated the efficacy and safety of a correction bolus based on usual correction factor (35). Finally to prevent late post-exercise hypoglycemic risk a nighttime basal rate reduction could be useful strategy.

Further studies are clearly warranted to guide insulin dose adjustments with CSII use. Because of the large inter- and intra-individual variability in glycemic responses to exercise, recommendations can only serve as general starting points that will need to be individualized.

CONTINUOUS GLUCOSE MONITORING

With the difficulty of glucose management during and post exercise in patients with T1D due to rapidly changing levels and hypoglycemia risks, individuals must increase the frequency of glucose monitoring during exercise and the following recovery period. This can be very cumbersome and undesired by many patients, especially when based on capillary glucose measurements. However, the introduction of continuous glucose monitoring in the early 2,000 has had a great impact on facilitating glucose profiling and helping with diabetes management. With CGM, interstitial glucose is measured repeatedly (e.g., each 10 min) via a subcutaneous sensor linked to a skin applied transmitter that relays these readings wirelessly either to a matched insulin pump or to a separate receiver which can be a cell-phone. CGM provides detailed glucose profiling in contrast to the readings that are possible with capillary measurements and has proved its efficacy in improving diabetes management and reducing hypoglycemia rates (36–38).

For physical activity, CGM has helped in gaining better understanding of changing glucose levels during and particularly in the hours following different types and conditions of exercise [an aspect reviewed recently by Houlder et al. (39).

One of the first reports to demonstrate the utility of CGM during exercise was an observational study conducted in 25 adolescents (8–17 years old) during a 2-week sports camp (40). An algorithm of CHO consumption (8–20 g) was followed according to CGM alerts, tendencies and rates of glucose change. Out of 22 uses of the CHO intake algorithm after CGM trend arrows indicated rapidly dropping glucose levels, only 2 hypoglycemia (3–3.9 mmol/l) events occurred (9%). The rate of hypoglycemia was higher (38%) though when glucose was lower than 5 mmol/l at the time of the alert despite consuming 16 g CHO (40). A recent study has also shed the light on the efficacy of combining CGM with a decision support system (DSS) in managing diabetes (41). The CGM+DSS helped patients adjust their insulin and CHO intake through insulin bolus, exercise and automated insulin titration advice. In a cross-over design with a wash-out period, 24 adults (on CSII or insulin injections) spent 48 h at a research clinic using CGM+DSS vs. usual care (41). The protocol included 2 sessions of 45 min (three 15 min exercise with 5 min rest in between) of mild to moderate aerobic exercise. Less time was spent in hypoglycemia (<3.9 mmol/l) with CGM+DSS during exercise (1.8 ± 2 vs. $3.8 \pm 4.6\%$, $p = 0.018$). This improvement with CGM+DSS was observed despite significantly lower consumption of CHO before initiating and during exercise and reduced glucose variability in comparison to usual care (41).

Interestingly, patients with T1D and health professionals who attended a boot camp that included real time CGM, in-class teaching and supervised exercise sessions have identified real time CGM as the best learning tool about glucose changes during exercise (42). Patients reported that CGM helped improve glucose control by keeping it in target ranges during sports without needing extra capillary measurements (e.g., less fear of hypoglycemia as well as decreased intake of unnecessary CHO with CGM use) (42).

One possible limitation to CGM usage is a lower accuracy during exercise. This has been recognized in the literature and needs to be understood by patients and healthcare professionals. Among factors involved to explain this lower accuracy rapid blood glucose changes that accompany physical activity is probably a dominant factor. Such situations increase the lag time between blood and interstitial glucose values due to delay to reach equilibration between compartments (5). This CGM delay has been estimated to reach up to 15 min during exercise and could result in either over- or most frequently underestimation of blood glucose. For example, mean difference between CGM

TABLE 1 | Main continuous subcutaneous insulin infusion studies with reported exercise related conclusions.

References	Participants, *n*	Design, insulin adjustments	Exercise description	Study conclusion
Franc et al. (26)	Adults, 20	Randomized, single-blind, single-center, crossover study: 1/Moderate-intensity exercise: 50% BRR at start of exercise (+2 h in recovery) vs. 80% BRR at start of exercise (+2 h during recovery) 2/ Intense exercise: Pump suspended during exercise vs. 80% BRR	1/30 min aerobic cycling (50% of VO_{2peak}) 2/30 min intense cycling (75% of VO_{2peak})	To limit the hypoglycaemic risk associated with 30 min of exercise 3 h after lunch, without CHO supplements, the best strategy seem to be to reduce BR by 80% or to stop the pump for moderate or intense exercise, or for moderate exercise 90 min after lunch, to reduce the prandial bolus (~50%) rather than the basal rate
McAuley et al. (32)	Adults, 14	Prospective, open-label, two-stage randomized crossover study: 50% BRR 1 h prior exercise after single insulin BRR overnight vs. Rest condition (T1D maintained a constant BR)	30 min aerobic cycling (65–70% of maximum heart rate)	Halving the BR 1 h prior to exercise did not significantly reduce circulating free insulin when BG is in low-normal range When BG<7.0 mmol/L before exercise, consider carbohydrate snack and BR >50%
Zaharieva et al. (27)	Adults, 12	Randomized and counterbalanced study: Suspended BR during aerobic exercise vs. Suspended BR during circuit exercise	40 min aerobic exercise of treadmill walking (~50% of VO_{2max}) 40 min circuit exercise (mean intensity ~55% of VO_{2max})	With BR suspension, aerobic exercise is associated with a greater drop in BG compared with circuit-based exercise
Roy-Fleming et al. (31)	Adults, 22	Randomized, 3-way crossover study: 80% BBR 40 min before exercise vs. 80% BBR, 20 min before exercise vs. BRR at the start of exercise	45 min submaximal cycling (~60% of VO_{2max})	Decreasing BR by 80% up to 40 min before exercise onset is insufficient to reduce exercise-induced hypoglycaemia.
Admon et al. (28)	Children and adolescents, 10	Randomized, single-blind, crossover study: Pump on (50% BRR) during exercise. vs. Pump off (Suspended BR) during exercise.	40–45 min submaximal cycling (~60% of VO_{2max})	No difference in hypoglycemia episodes between pump on vs. pump off and no significant difference in the drop in glycemia.
DirecNet Trial group. (29)	Children and adolescents, 49	Randomized crossover study: Pump on (normal BR) during exercise vs. Pump off (suspended BR) during exercise.	Four 15-min intervals on the treadmill at a target heart rate of 140 bpm (interspersed with three 5-min rest breaks over 75 min), followed by a 45-min observation period	Discontinuing BR during exercise is an effective strategy for reducing hypoglycemia in children with T1D, but the risk of hyperglycemia is increased.
Taplin et al. (34)	Children and adolescents, 16	Randomized crossover study: Suspended BR during exercise flowed by 50% BRR for 45 min during the 3 conditions: 20% basal rate reduction for 6 h vs. 2.5 mg oral terbutaline vs. No treatment	Four 15-min intervals on the treadmill a target heart rate of 140 bpm (interspersed with three 5-min rest)	The authors speculate that suspending BR during exercise and reducing BR for 45 min post-exercise, reduce the frequency of afternoon hypoglycemia was well as delayed hypoglycemia during the night. BRR was safe and effective in raising post-exercise nocturnal BG nadir and in reducing hypoglycemia

BR, basal rate; BRR, basal rate reduction; BG, blood glucose.

(Medtronic Guardian Real-Time system) and plasma glucose was 1.4 ± 0.8 mmol/L during continuous aerobic exercise implicating an overestimation of plasma glucose (43). On the other hand, an underestimation of blood glucose by CGM has been reported with resistance type of exercise (44).

Most manufacturers and studies report CGM accuracy with median absolute relative difference (MARD) of CGM relative to blood glucose (capillary or venous); reflecting an average deviation from the reference in either direction. MARD of two CGM devices Dexcom G4 Platinum and Enlite in reference to plasma glucose was evaluated at rest vs. exercise (continuous and interval) (45). MARD was increased from 13.3 (6.1–12.2)% at rest to 15.1 (9.4–26.8 %; $p = 0,02$) during exercise for Dexcom and from 11.9 (7.8–14.2)% to 14.1 (8.5–22.7%, $p = 0.02$) for Enlite (45). In this cross-over trial design, no significant differences in MARD were observed between continuous vs. interval exercise that were notably matched in total energy expenditure per patient (45), this is in congruence with another study comparing continuous moderate intensity and high intensity interval exercise sessions (46). On the other hand, significant differences in accuracy by MARD during continuous vs. interval exercise was reported by another group despite comparing the two types of exercise at similar intensities (47). Contrasting conclusions from these reports about CGM accuracy per distinct exercise types could be related to the respective studies design and small sample size. For example, including a pre-exercise snack (slower decline in blood glucose) or hypoglycemia correction with CHO are all factors that could affect the interpretation and comparison of MARD across different studies.

The overall accuracy of CGM devices during exercise is lower but still remains acceptable under exercising conditions. Patients are encouraged to follow the arrow trends in their GCM devices and set their hypoglycemia alarms to higher values to anticipate events (5). Future research efforts should thus consider more comprehensive analysis of CGM biases over the course of different types of exercise and not only reporting average over the whole exercise session. Studies should also report clear analysis of CGM accuracy during hypoglycemic episodes (onset to reduce occurrence and following correction to reduce possible overcorrection) preferably in comparison to capillary or venous reference values. The results of such analyses could then be translated into clinical messages to help patients choose thresholds when setting their alarms to optimize the use of this option while concurrently following CGM arrow trends.

In summary, CGM technology eases the challenge of glucose management during and after physical activity in patients with T1D but patients need to be educated about the lower accuracy of these devices during exercise.

ARTIFICIAL PANCREAS SYSTEMS:

Further technological progress has been achieved by linking CGM to insulin pumps (48, 49) including sensor-augmented pumps (SAP), low suspend and predictive-suspend pump systems. In order to reduce hypoglycemia frequency, importance and length these technologies helps patients adjust their insulin treatment based on real-time feedback from the CGM function (50). These systems are technological steps along the way to closing the loop of glucose control with the artificial pancreas systems targeting both hypo and hyperglycemia.

The artificial pancreas (AP), equally referred to as closed-loop system, constitute to date the most advanced, and promising technology for insulin delivery in T1D (51). Readings from CGM are communicated every few minutes to hormonal dosing algorithm which dynamically commands changes in hormonal basal rates or boluses administered by subcutaneous infusion pumps. Clinical studies investigating artificial pancreas systems are increasing exponentially. These clinical trials mainly cover research on two AP versions; single-hormone AP (SH-AP) which delivers only insulin and dual-hormone AP (DH-AP) which delivers besides insulin mini-boluses of glucagon. Two approaches govern the addition of glucagon to AP, either to allow more aggressive insulin delivery while avoiding hypoglycemia and generally aiming for lower glucoses targets or a more conservative approach which uses glucagon only after suspending insulin for low blood glucose in attempt to prevent pre-emptive hypoglycemia (51). Around two-thirds to one-third is the proportion of SH-AP to DH-AP in the published literature with a lot of heterogeneity in terms of design, reported parameters, types of algorithms used and patient populations tested.

Two recent meta-analyses have clearly shown the clinical efficacy of AP systems in comparison to conventional or sensor-augmented insulin pumps (52, 53). Time spent with glucose levels in-target-range (most used definition is 3.9–10 mmol/l) was increased in both analysis by means of 10–15% which are equivalent to 2.5 and 3 additional hours in target per 24 h (52, 53). The percentage of time spent in hypoglycemia (<3.09 mmol/l) was decreased by means of 1.5–2.5 %, equivalent to a decrease by 20 and 35 min over 24 h (52, 53). *Post-hoc* analyses showed an added benefit of DH-AP with an increase by +8.4 and +8.6% in time-in-target and a further decrease by 1.9 and 1.6% over 24 h in hypoglycemia (52, 53). Some of these studies included exercise in their protocol but their designs and outcomes were not primarily centered around exercise and/or did not specifically present data during exercise limiting the conclusions that can be drawn in relation to physical activity practice. For this reason, we will limit the discussions in the following sections to the clinical trials that specifically reported exercise related outcomes.

Clinical research in AP examining exercise span a spectrum from SH-AP studies adopting fully closed loop systems to those testing hybrid systems with required input from patients/research team to guide the algorithm. Ideally, fully closed loop AP would be the easiest especially in the case of unplanned exercise. The algorithm would then be expected to adjust insulin delivery solely based on changing glucose readings. On the other end of the spectrum, hybrid systems involve exercise announcement by the patient to the algorithm to adjust glucose target ranges (higher targets) and adopt a more cautious insulin delivery. In between the two ends, trials include addition of glucagon in DH-AP, use of exercise detectors (such as heart rate or movement) to guide the algorithm to self-adjust or combinations of these approaches.

The aim behind investigating these different strategies is to account for exercise-induced: 1-increases in insulin sensitivity and absorption from subcutaneous depot due to skin heat and movement, 2- delays in CGM due to rapid changes in blood glucose levels (5, 6). As discussed in the previous sections, the effect on glucose of different types, duration, intensity and timing of exercise need to be taken into consideration when examining AP studies around physical activity (6).

Good overall results were observed in a study conducted with unannounced 40 min exercise performed in a postprandial state as moderate and interval sessions in children and adolescents with T1D (54). Median time of glucose-in-target (3.9–10 mmol/l) was improved during exercise with SH-AP vs. standard insulin

TABLE 2 | Main artificial pancreas studies with reported exercise related outcomes.

References	Participants, *n*	Design, comparators	Exercise description	Main outcomes
Dovc et al. (54)	Chidren and adolescents, 20	Cross-over randomized SH-AP vs. CSII CSII: pump stopped during exercise and basal rate reduced by 20% for 4 h post exercise AP: exercise unannounced	Two exercise types of 40 min, postabsorptive Cycle ergometer Moderate 55% VO_2 max Interval 55%/85% VO_2 max	No difference in time spent in hypoglycemia range during exercise Better median time-in-target (3.9–10 mmol/l) with AP for interval: 75.3 (IQR: 66.6–92.9) % vs. 68.4 (52.1–77.2) %, $p = 0.02$ and for moderate 80.9 (64.3–92.2)% vs. 68.1(59.1–83.6)%, $p = 0.09$ No difference in hypoglycemia events requiring CHO correction over the whole study period 22 h (7 AP vs. 8 CSII)
Breton et al. (55)	Adolescents, 32 (16 per group)	Controlled randomized SH-AP vs. SAP AP: exercise unannounced	5 days skiing camp Two skiing sessions/day 9 h:30 to 12h:00 13 h:00 to 16h:00	No difference in mean time-in-target (3.9–10 mmol/l) between AP and SAP during skiing sessions: 63.2 ± 31.1% vs. 62.8 ± 31.4%, $p = 0.60$ less time spent below 3.9 mmol/l in AP: 1.4 ± 1.6% vs. 2.3 ± 6.4%, $p = 0.04$ No difference in hypoglycemia events or CHO requiring incidences
Patel et al. (56)	Adolescents and adults, 12	Cross-over randomized SH-AP vs. SH-AP + snack Snack: 15–30 g CHO before and midway during exercise for PG <8.3 and > 8.3 mmol/l respectively AP: exercise unannounced	Four 15 min 60–75% of maximal heart rate, with three 5 min in between rest and 30 min recovery Treadmill ergometer	15 g CHO were given to 75% of participants prior to exercise and to all of them midway through exercise Hypoglycemia events requiring CHO were 3 in AP vs. 0 in AP+snack Mean PG at end of session was 10 ± 0.5 vs. 6.1 ± 0.9 mmol/l in AP+snack vs. AP, $p = 0.004$
Jacobs et al. (57)	Adults, 21	Cross-over randomized DH-AP with adjustments vs. DH-AP without adjustments vs. SAP(with allowed adjustment per patient) Adjustment description at start of exercise: Insulin suspended for 30 min then reduced by 50% for 1 hr Glucagon doubled for 90 min AP: exercise announced at start	45 min exercise at 60% of maximal heart rate 2 h post breakfast Treadmill ergometer	Mean time in hypoglycemia (<3.9 mmol/L) was 0.3 (95%CI: −0.1%,0.7)% with adjustment, 3.1 (0.8–5.3)% with no adjustment and 0.8 (0.1–1.4)% with SAP, adjustment vs. no adjustment $p = 0.001$, adjustment vs. AP $p = 0.16$ No difference for time spent in target among the three trial arms
Taleb et al. (58)	Adults, 17	Cross-over, randomized, 4 arms SH-AP vs. DH-AP during continuous and interval exercise AP: exercise announced 20 min prior to start	60 min exercise, postabsorptive continuous session: 60% VO_2 max Interval session: 2 min interval alternating 50%/85% Cycle ergometer	Benefit of DH-AP vs. SH-AP seen with both types of exercise, more glucagon used during continuous than interval For pooled exercise sessions, DH-AP vs. SH-AP: median time PG in target was 100 (IQR: 100–100)% vs. 71.4 (53.2–100)%, $p = 0.003$ and in hypoglycemia (< 3.9 mmol/l) was 0% vs. 11 (0–46.7)%, $p = 0.0001$ 3 vs. 15 hypoglycemia events corrected with CHO in DH-ap vs. SH-AP
Breton at al. (59)	Adults, 12	Cross-over, randomized, 2 arms SH-AP+heart rate vs. SH-AP AP: exercise detected	mild intensity exercise reaching 9–10 on exhaustion borg scale Postprandial Cycle ergometer	less glucose decline in SH-AP with heart rate at −0.3 vs. −1.6 mmol/l, $p = 0.02$ less hypoglycemia events with heart monitoring but not significant (0 vs. 2)

(Continued)

TABLE 2 | Continued

References	Participants, *n*	Design, comparators	Exercise description	Main outcomes
Jacobs et al. (60)	Adolescents, 18	Cross-over, randomized, 2 arms SH-AP+heart rate vs. SH-AP AP: exercise detected	45 min exercise, postabsorptive Three 15 min episodes of exercise with HR reaching 140 beats/min separated with 5 min rest Cycle ergometer	Mean time spent in hypoglycemia (< 3.9 mmol/l) was 0.5 ± 2.1 % in SH-AP+HR. vs. SH-AP 7.4 ± 12% (p = 0.03) No difference in hypoglycemia events which were overall low in both arms
Castle et al. (61)	Adults, 20	Cross-over, randomized, 4 arms DH-AP, SH-AP, Predictive low glucose suspend and Current care (pre-exercise insulin adjustments were allowed) Both DH-AP and DH-AP had exercise detection algorithms with inputs from heart rate and accelerometer (ZephyrLife BioPatch) AP: exercise detected then confirmed to algorithm	45 min exercise 2 h post lunch at 60% of VO_2 max performed on days 1 and 4 in research lab while the rest was free living at home	Time in hypoglycemia (< 3.9 mmol/l) during exercise was lowest with DH-AP 3.4 ± 4.5 % vs. 8.3 ± 12.6% with SH-AP (P = 0.009) vs.7.6% ± 8.0% with predictive low glucose suspend (P < 0.001) vs. 4.3 ± 6.8% with current care (P = 0.49), (p-values are DH-AP against the other arms) lower hypoglycemia events requiring CHO correction was seen with DH-AP over the 4 day period

DH-AP, dual-hormone artificial pancreas; SH-AP, single-hormone artificial pancreas; CSII, continuous subcutaneous insulin infusion; SAP, sensor-augmented pump, CHO, carbohydrates.

pump therapy; however, there were no differences in percentage of time in hypoglycemia ranges or in events requiring CHO replacement (54). In another study, unannounced exercise to SH-AP algorithm was examined during prolonged skiing activity (two sessions per day, 5 day camp) in a group of adolescents and compared to another matched group under sensor augmented pump (SAP) control (55). Although an overall benefit was seen with SH-AP vs. SAP per 24 h and overnight for time spent with glucose-in-target, this was not maintained during the pooled skiing sessions and the hypoglycemia events requiring CHO correction (**Table 2**) (55).

With unannounced exercise to SH-AP, adding a snack (15 or 30 g CHO for PG <8.3 mmol/l and > 8.3 mmol/l, respectively) prior and midway through moderate intensity aerobic exercise could prevent drops in plasma glucose and hypoglycemia requiring correction (0 in AP with snack vs. 3 in AP without snack) (56). Authors in this study did not report percentages of time-in-target, hypo- or hyperglycemia, but around half of the participants ended up with plasma glucose between 10 and 13 mmol/l in SH-AP+snack. These results support the use of a simple snacking strategy to avoid exercise-induced lowering of PG while on AP (56). However, snack consumption may be undesired given the increased prevalence of the metabolic syndrome in patients with T1D who frequently practice exercise with in weight loss or maintenance objectives (3).

Other strategies to improve AP performance around physical activity consisted of examining the effect of glucagon addition through DH-AP systems and exercise announcement to the algorithm. Jacobs et al. tested if announcing physical activity to their DH-AP algorithm by adjusting its insulin and glucagon dosing at the start of a 45 min aerobic moderate intensity exercise could improve glucose management in the following hours (57). Insulin was suspended for 30 min and reduced by 50% for the following 60 min while glucagon was doubled for 90 min from start of exercise (57). Less time was spent in hypoglycemia with adjustment to DH-AP by 2.8% vs. no adjustment ($p = 0.001$) and no difference vs. sensor augmented pump ($p = 0.16$). The authors observed a similar time spent with glucose-in-target between the three arms (57).

Another head-to-head SH-AP to DH-AP comparison in which insulin dosing algorithm is similar in order to specifically investigate the additional benefit of glucagon incorporation in AP during exercise (58). Two types of exercise sessions consisting of 60 min of continuous and interval exercise were performed in the postprandial state under both SH-AP and DH-AP on 4 separate visits (58). Exercise was announced 20 min prior to its start which resulted in changing the target glucose level from 5.3 to 8.3 mmol/l till the end of the 60 min session. Overall, with DH-AP, median time spent with glucose-in-target was increased by 28.6% ($p = 0.003$) and time in hypoglycemia (PG < 3.9 mmol/l) was decreased by 11% ($p = 0.0001$) in comparison to SH-AP. The number of hypoglycemia events requiring CHO treatment were also reduced (3 in DH-AP vs. 15 in SH-AP), all showing an added benefit of glucagon in AP during exercise (58).

An alternative to directly announcing exercise sessions to an AP algorithm was sought by some groups using exercise detectors such as heart rate monitors or accelerometers. The idea behind exercise detection and indirect announcement is to relieve patients from active inputs especially during unplanned and unknown activity intensities. Such systems would be particularly interesting to investigate in youngsters whose activity level is often unpredictable making them at high risk for both hypo- and hyperglycemia. Breton et al. were among the first to study the feasibility of adding heart rate monitoring to a SH-AP in 12 adults performing mild 30 min exercise sessions (exhaustion at 9–10 on Borg scale) (59). Whenever the heart rate exceeded 125% of its resting value, the algorithm was informed manually which would result in less aggressive insulin delivery and modification of hypoglycemia risk (59). A significant decrease in glucose decline during exercise was noticed when adding HR monitoring (-0.3 vs. -1.6 mmol/l, $p = 0.02$), but only a mild non-significant effect was observed in terms of hypoglycemia events (59). Similar results were observed by Jacobs et al. with their SH-AP with a heart rate monitor connected via blue tooth which informed the algorithm of exercise of physical activity when heart rate exceeded 125% of resting levels (60). This triggered a change in glucose target from 6.2 to 7.8 mmol/l and subsequent insulin delivery by the algorithm. A decrease in time spent in hypoglycemia (<3.9 mmol/l) was significantly reduced with heart rate signal integration to SH-AP $0.5 \pm 2.1\%$ vs. $7.4 \pm 12.5\%$ ($p = 0.028$) without an effect on the incidence of hypoglycemic events which was however low in both arms (60).

A combination of different strategies was also tested. Recently, an interesting study was performed in adults comparing DH-AP and SH-AP that adapt to exercise using wearable sensors with predictive low glucose suspend and current care during and after exercise (61). Both AP systems had an integrated algorithm for exercise detection that receives input from heart rate monitor and accelerometer (the ZephyrLife BioPatch). Once exercise was detected, the participant was asked by the algorithm to confirm it and the changes to insulin and glucagon were similar to what is described above for the study by Jacobs et al. (57). Additionally the DH-AP was adaptive with adjustments to glucagon delivery at earlier timings and higher glucose levels on subsequent days 2–4 in comparison to day 1. Day 1 and 4 were partly spent at research clinic and the rest at home, formal 45 min exercise sessions 2 h post lunch were performed at 60% VO_{2max} during clinic stay (day 1 and day 4) (61). The lowest time spent in hypoglycemia (< 3.9 mmol/l) during exercise till next meal was with DH-AP 3.4 ± 4.5 vs. $8.3 \pm 12.6\%$ with SH-AP ($p = 0.009$) vs. $7.6 \pm 8.0\%$ with predictive low glucose suspend pump ($p < 0.001$) vs. $4.3 \pm 6.8\%$ during usual care ($p = 0.49$) (61). Number of hypoglycemia events requiring CHO consumption was also lowest with DH-AP over the whole study period with a mean of 0.8 ± 0.7 treatments per day vs. 1.7 ± 1.4 with SH-AP ($p = 0.004$), 1.3 ± 1.3 with the predictive low glucose suspend pump ($p = 0.065$), and 1.5 ± 1.2 with usual care ($p = 0.10$) (61).

The AP studies that specifically tackled glucose control in relation to exercise are still heterogeneous, small in size and do not cover all exercise scenarios (**Table 2** summarizes the discussed trials). Most to date cover moderate intensity exercise performed in the post-absorptive state (**Table 2**). Nevertheless, they highlight the positive impact of artificial pancreas systems around exercise. AP is still an emerging technology and many future trials at large scale and in outpatient settings are needed in general and around exercise in particular.

Directly announcing exercise seems to still be needed for optimized results but the timing of the announcement from the start of exercise maybe an area to explore in future studies particularly for postprandial exercise when meal insulin boluses are active. Exercise detection by sensors is an interesting avenue particularly for children and adolescents living with T1D but adds the burden of wearing additional devices necessitating active research efforts in the future to develop small sensors integrated to the artificial pancreas itself.

Glucagon clearly shows an added benefit but the complexity of adding an additional chamber and material needs to be weighed against the additional hypoglycemia benefit. Therefore, future research trails should be designed to carefully identify patients who are most in need of glucagon and show high rates of exercise-induced hypoglycemia. While SH-AP currently reach the market in various countries, DH-AP are not expected to be commercialized in the near future since stable glucagon formulations are not yet available for use but promising research is underway. Clinical trials with DH-AP may still be conducted with the commercially available glucagon used for severe hypoglycemia treatment but needs to be reconstituted every 24 h (62). Meanwhile, another pressing aspect is proving the safety profile of chronic glucagon use in its different formulations or analogs given its multisystemic effects in humans (63).

CONCLUSIONS

Technological advances have endowed individuals with T1D with important tools to help them better manage their blood glucose during exercise mainly allowing more secure conditions with reduced hypoglycemia risks. Some limitations to the different technologies have been detailed in this review and future research areas that need to be explored have been highlighted as well. The hope is that optimizing the use of these different technologies during exercise will encourage the majority of patients with T1D to regularly engage in physical activity.

AUTHOR CONTRIBUTIONS

ST, NT, and RR-L conceived the study design and content. ST and NT drafted the manuscript which was critically reviewed by RR-L.

ACKNOWLEDGMENTS

ST is supported by a fellowship grant from SFD (Société Francophone du Diabète) and FRM (Fondation de Recherche Médicale). NT is recipient of scholarship of CIHR (Canadian Institutes of Health Research) and FRSQ (Fonds de Recherche Santé Québec) scholarships. RR-L is holding the J-A DeSève diabetes research chair, a Diabetes Canada program grant (DI-5-17-5282-RR) and a NIH grant for artificial pancreas research that all supported this work.

REFERENCES

1. Chimen M, Kennedy A, Nirantharakumar K, Pang TT, Andrews R, Narendran P. What are the health benefits of physical activity in type 1 diabetes mellitus? A literature review. *Diabetologia* (2012) 55:542–51. doi: 10.1007/s00125-011-2403-2
2. Brazeau A-S, Rabasa-Lhoret R, Strychar I, Mircescu H. Barriers to physical activity among patients with type 1 diabetes. *Diabetes Care* (2008) 31:2108–9. doi: 10.2337/dc08-0720
3. Leroux C, Brazeau A-S, Gingras V, Desjardins K, Strychar I, Rabasa-Lhoret R. Lifestyle and cardiometabolic risk in adults with type 1 diabetes: a review. *Can J Diabetes* (2014) 38:62–9. doi: 10.1016/j.jcjd.2013.08.268
4. Younk LM, Mikeladze M, Tate D, Davis SN. Exercise-related hypoglycemia in diabetes mellitus. *Expert Rev Endocrinol Metab.* (2011) 6:93–108. doi: 10.1586/eem.10.78
5. Riddell MC, Gallen IW, Smart CE, Taplin CE, Adolfsson P, Lumb AN, et al. Exercise management in type 1 diabetes: a consensus statement. *Lancet Diabetes Endocrinol.* (2017) 5:377–90. doi: 10.1016/S2213-8587(17)30014-1
6. Riddell MC, Zaharieva DP, Yavelberg L, Cinar A, Jamnik VK. Exercise and the development of the artificial pancreas: one of the more difficult series of hurdles. *J Diabetes Sci Technol.* (2015) 9:1217–26. doi: 10.1177/1932296815609370
7. Taleb N, Rabasa-Lhoret R. Can somatostatin antagonism prevent hypoglycaemia during exercise in type 1 diabetes? *Diabetologia* (2016) 59:1632–5. doi: 10.1007/s00125-016-3978-4
8. Yardley J, Mollard R, MacIntosh A, MacMillan F, Wicklow B, Berard L, et al. Vigorous intensity exercise for glycemic control in patients with type 1 diabetes. *Can J Diabetes* (2013) 37:427–32. doi: 10.1016/j.jcjd.2013.08.269
9. Yardley JE, Colberg SR. Update on management of type 1 diabetes and type 2 diabetes in athletes. *Curr Sports Med Rep.* (2017) 16:38–44. doi: 10.1249/JSR.0000000000000327
10. Turner D, Luzio S, Gray BJ, Dunseath G, Rees ED, Kilduff LP, et al. Impact of single and multiple sets of resistance exercise in type 1 diabetes. *Scand J Med Sci Sports* (2015) 25:e99–109. doi: 10.1111/sms.12202
11. Koivisto VA, Sane T, Fyhrquist F, Pelkonen R. Fuel and fluid homeostasis during long-term exercise in healthy subjects and type I diabetic patients. *Diabetes Care* (1992) 15:1736–41.
12. American Diabetes Association. Physical activity/exercise and diabetes. *Diabetes Care* (2004) 27(Suppl. 1):S58–62. doi: 10.2337/dc06-9910
13. Kemmer FW. Prevention of hypoglycemia during exercise in type I diabetes. *Diabetes Care* (1992) 15:1732–5.
14. Grimm JJ, Ybarra J, Berné C, Muchnick S, Golay A. A new table for prevention of hypoglycaemia during physical activity in type 1 diabetic patients. *Diabetes Metab* (2004) 30:465–70.
15. Riddell MC, Bar-Or O, Ayub BV, Calvert RE, Heigenhauser GJ. Glucose ingestion matched with total carbohydrate utilization attenuates hypoglycemia during exercise in adolescents with IDDM. *Int J Sport Nutr.* (1999) 9:24–34.
16. Francescato MP, Geat M, Accardo A, Blokar M, Cattin L, Noacco C. Exercise and glycemic imbalances: a situation-specific estimate of glucose supplement. *Med Sci Sports Exerc.* (2011) 43:2–11. doi: 10.1249/MSS.0b013e3181e6d6a1
17. Mauvais-Jarvis F, Sobngwi E, Porcher R, Garnier JP, Vexiau P, Duvallet A, et al. Glucose response to intense aerobic exercise in type 1 diabetes: maintenance of near euglycemia despite a drastic decrease in insulin dose. *Diabetes Care* (2003) 26:1316–7. doi: 10.2337/diacare.26.4.1316
18. Rabasa-Lhoret R, Bourque J, Ducros F, Chiasson JL. Guidelines for premeal insulin dose reduction for postprandial exercise of different intensities and durations in type 1 diabetic subjects treated intensively with a basal-bolus insulin regimen (ultralente-lispro). *Diabetes Care* (2001) 24:625–30. doi: 10.2337/diacare.24.4.625
19. Lenhard MJ, Reeves GD. Continuous subcutaneous insulin infusion: a comprehensive review of insulin pump therapy. *Arch Intern Med.* (2001) 161:2293–300. doi: 10.1001/archinte.161.19.2293
20. Pickup J, Keen H. Continuous subcutaneous insulin infusion at 25 years: evidence base for the expanding use of insulin pump therapy in type 1 diabetes. *Diabetes Care* (2002) 25:593–8. doi: 10.2337/diacare.25.3.593
21. Thabit H, Hovorka R. Continuous subcutaneous insulin infusion therapy and multiple daily insulin injections in type 1 diabetes mellitus: a comparative overview and future horizons. *Expert Opin Drug Deliv.* (2016) 13:389–400. doi: 10.1517/17425247.2016.1115013
22. Misso ML, Egberts KJ, Page M, O'Connor D, Shaw J. Continuous subcutaneous insulin infusion (CSII) versus multiple insulin injections for type 1 diabetes mellitus. *Cochr Database Syst Rev.* (2010) 1:CD005103. doi: 10.1002/14651858.CD005103.pub2
23. Pickup JC. Insulin-pump therapy for type 1 diabetes mellitus. *N Engl J Med.* (2012) 366:1616–24. doi: 10.1056/NEJMct1113948
24. Reznik Y, Cohen O, Aronson R, Conget I, Runzis S, Castaneda J, et al. Insulin pump treatment compared with multiple daily injections for treatment of type 2 diabetes (OpT2mise): a randomised open-label controlled trial. *Lancet* (2014) 384:1265–72. doi: 10.1016/S0140-6736(14)61037-0
25. Campbell MD, Walker M, Trenell MI, Jakovljevic DG, Stevenson EJ, Bracken RM, et al. Large pre- and postexercise rapid-acting insulin reductions preserve glycemia and prevent early- but not late-onset hypoglycemia in patients with type 1 diabetes. *Diabetes Care* (2013) 36:2217–24. doi: 10.2337/dc12-2467
26. Franc S, Daoudi A, Pochat A, Petit M-H, Randazzo C, Petit C, et al. Insulin-based strategies to prevent hypoglycaemia during and after exercise in adult patients with type 1 diabetes on pump therapy: the DIABRASPORT randomized study. *Diabetes Obes Metab.* (2015) 17:1150–57. doi: 10.1111/dom.12552
27. Zaharieva D, Yavelberg L, Jamnik V, Cinar A, Turksoy K, Riddell MC. The effects of basal insulin suspension at the start of exercise on blood glucose levels during continuous versus circuit-based exercise in individuals with type 1 diabetes on continuous subcutaneous insulin infusion. *Diabetes Technol Ther.* (2017) 19:370–8. doi: 10.1089/dia.2017.0010
28. Admon G, Weinstein Y, Falk B, Weintrob N, Benzaquen H, Ofan R, et al. Exercise with and without an insulin pump among children and adolescents with type 1 diabetes mellitus. *Pediatrics* (2005) 116:e348–55. doi: 10.1542/peds.2004-2428
29. Diabetes Research in Children Network (DirecNet) Study Group, Tsalikian E, Kollman C, Tamborlane WB, Beck RW, Fiallo-Scharer R, et al. Prevention of hypoglycemia during exercise in children with type 1 diabetes by suspending basal insulin. *Diabetes Care* (2006) 29:2200–4. doi: 10.2337/dc06-0495
30. Heinemann L, Nosek L, Kapitza C, Schweitzer M-A, Krinelke L. Changes in basal insulin infusion rates with subcutaneous insulin infusion: time until a change in metabolic effect is induced in patients with type 1 diabetes. *Diabetes Care* (2009) 32:1437–9. doi: 10.2337/dc09-0595
31. Roy-Fleming A, Taleb N, Messier V, Suppère C, Cameli C, Elbekri S, et al. Timing of insulin basal rate reduction to reduce hypoglycemia during late post-prandial exercise in adults with type 1 diabetes using insulin pump therapy: a randomized crossover trial. *Diabetes Metab.* (2018). doi: 10.1016/j.diabet.2018.08.002. [Epub ahead of print].
32. McAuley SA, Horsburgh JC, Ward GM, Gerche AL, Gooley JL, Jenkins AJ, et al. Insulin pump basal adjustment for exercise in type 1 diabetes: a randomised crossover study. *Diabetologia* (2016) 59:1636–44. doi: 10.1007/s00125-016-3981-9
33. Desjardins K, Brazeau A-S, Strychar I, Rabasa-Lhoret R. Are bedtime nutritional strategies effective in preventing nocturnal hypoglycaemia in patients with type 1 diabetes? *Diabetes Obes Metab.* (2014) 16:577–87. doi: 10.1111/dom.12232
34. Taplin CE, Cobry E, Messer L, McFann K, Chase HP, Fiallo-Scharer R. Preventing post-exercise nocturnal hypoglycemia in children with type 1 diabetes. *J Pediatr.* (2010) 157:784–8.e1. doi: 10.1016/j.jpeds.2010.06.004
35. Aronson R, Brown RE, Li A, Riddell MC. Optimal insulin correction factor in post-high-intensity exercise hyperglycemia in adults with type 1 diabetes: the FIT study. *Diabetes Care* (2018). doi: 10.2337/dc18-1475. [Epub ahead of print].
36. Gandhi GY, Kovalaske M, Kudva Y, Walsh K, Elamin MB, Beers M, et al. Efficacy of continuous glucose monitoring in improving glycemic control and reducing hypoglycemia: a systematic review and meta-analysis of randomized trials. *J Diabetes Sci Technol.* (2011) 5:952–65. doi: 10.1177/193229681100500419
37. Tumminia A, Crimi S, Sciacca L, Buscema M, Frittitta L, Squatrito S, et al. Efficacy of real-time continuous glucose monitoring on glycaemic control and glucose variability in type 1 diabetic patients treated with either insulin pumps or multiple insulin injection therapy: a randomized controlled crossover trial. *Diabetes Metab Res Rev.* (2015) 31:61–8. doi: 10.1002/dmrr.2557

38. Reddy M, Jugnee N, El Laboudi A, Spanudakis E, Anantharaja S, Oliver N. A randomized controlled pilot study of continuous glucose monitoring and flash glucose monitoring in people with Type 1 diabetes and impaired awareness of hypoglycaemia. *Diabet Med.* (2018) 35:483–90. doi: 10.1111/dme.13561
39. Houlder SK, Yardley JE. Continuous glucose monitoring and exercise in type 1 diabetes: past, present and future. *Biosensors* (2018) 8:E73. doi: 10.3390/bios8030073
40. Riddell MC, Milliken J. Preventing exercise-induced hypoglycemia in type 1 diabetes using real-time continuous glucose monitoring and a new carbohydrate intake algorithm: an observational field study. *Diabetes Technol Ther.* (2011) 13:819–25. doi: 10.1089/dia.2011.0052
41. Breton MD, Patek SD, Lv D, Schertz E, Robic J, Pinnata J, et al. Continuous glucose monitoring and insulin informed advisory system with automated titration and dosing of insulin reduces glucose variability in type 1 diabetes mellitus. *Diabetes Technol Ther.* (2018) 20:531–40. doi: 10.1089/dia.2018.0079
42. Dyck RA, Kleinman NJ, Funk DR, Yeung RO, Senior P, Yardley JE. We can work (It) out together: type 1 diabetes boot camp for adult patients and providers improves exercise self-efficacy. *Can J Diabetes* (2018) 42:619–25. doi: 10.1016/j.jcjd.2018.02.006
43. Radermecker R-P, Fayolle C, Brun J-F, Bringer J, Renard E. Accuracy assessment of online glucose monitoring by a subcutaneous enzymatic glucose sensor during exercise in patients with type 1 diabetes treated by continuous subcutaneous insulin infusion. *Diabetes Metab.* (2013) 39:258–62. doi: 10.1016/j.diabet.2012.12.004
44. Yardley JE, Sigal RJ, Kenny GP, Riddell MC, Lovblom LE, Perkins BA. Point accuracy of interstitial continuous glucose monitoring during exercise in type 1 diabetes. *Diabetes Technol Ther.* (2013) 15:46–9. doi: 10.1089/dia.2012.0182
45. Taleb N, Emami A, Suppere C, Messier V, Legault L, Chiasson J-L, et al. Comparison of two continuous glucose monitoring systems, dexcom G4 platinum and medtronic paradigm veo enlite system, at rest and during exercise. *Diabetes Technol Ther.* (2016) 18:561–7. doi: 10.1089/dia.2015.0394
46. Bally L, Zueger T, Pasi N, Carlos C, Paganini D, Stettler C. Accuracy of continuous glucose monitoring during differing exercise conditions. *Diabetes Res Clin Pract.* (2016) 112:1–5. doi: 10.1016/j.diabres.2015.11.012
47. Moser O, Mader JK, Tschakert G, Mueller A, Groeschl W, Pieber TR, et al. Accuracy of continuous glucose monitoring (CGM) during continuous and high-intensity interval exercise in patients with type 1 diabetes mellitus. *Nutrients* (2016) 8:E489. doi: 10.3390/nu8080489
48. Kowalski A. Pathway to artificial pancreas systems revisited: moving downstream. *Diabetes Care* (2015) 38:1036–43. doi: 10.2337/dc15-0364
49. Šoupal J, PetruŽelková L, Flekač M, Pelcl T, Matoulek M, Danková M, et al. Comparison of different treatment modalities for type 1 diabetes, including sensor-augmented insulin regimens, in 52 weeks of follow-up: a COMISAIR study. *Diabetes Technol Ther.* (2016) 18:532–8. doi: 10.1089/dia.2016.0171
50. Bergenstal RM, Welsh JB, Shin JJ. Threshold insulin-pump interruption to reduce hypoglycemia. *N Engl J Med.* (2013) 369:1473–4. doi: 10.1056/NEJMc1310365
51. Thabit H, Hovorka R. Coming of age: the artificial pancreas for type 1 diabetes. *Diabetologia* (2016) 59:1795–805. doi: 10.1007/s00125-016-4022-4
52. Bekiari E, Kitsios K, Thabit H, Tauschmann M, Athanasiadou E, Karagiannis T, et al. Artificial pancreas treatment for outpatients with type 1 diabetes: systematic review and meta-analysis. *BMJ* (2018) 361:k1310. doi: 10.1136/bmj.k1310
53. Weisman A, Bai J-W, Cardinez M, Kramer CK, Perkins BA. Effect of artificial pancreas systems on glycaemic control in patients with type 1 diabetes: a systematic review and meta-analysis of outpatient randomised controlled trials. *Lancet Diabetes Endocrinol.* (2017) 5:501–12. doi: 10.1016/S2213-8587(17)30167-5
54. Dovc K, Macedoni M, Bratina N, Lepej D, Nimri R, Atlas E, et al. Closed-loop glucose control in young people with type 1 diabetes during and after unannounced physical activity: a randomised controlled crossover trial. *Diabetologia* (2017) 60:2157–67. doi: 10.1007/s00125-017-4395-z
55. Breton MD, Cherñavvsky DR, Forlenza GP, DeBoer MD, Robic J, Wadwa RP, et al. Closed-loop control during intense prolonged outdoor exercise in adolescents with type 1 diabetes: the artificial pancreas Ski study. *Diabetes Care* (2017) 40:1644–50. doi: 10.2337/dc17-0883
56. Patel NS, Van Name MA, Cengiz E, Carria LR, Tichy EM, Weyman K, et al. Mitigating reductions in glucose during exercise on closed-loop insulin delivery: the ex-snacks study. *Diabetes Technol Ther.* (2016) 18:794–9. doi: 10.1089/dia.2016.0311
57. Jacobs PG, El Youssef J, Reddy R, Resalat N, Branigan D, Condon J, et al. Randomized trial of a dual-hormone artificial pancreas with dosing adjustment during exercise compared with no adjustment and sensor-augmented pump therapy. *Diabetes Obes Metab.* (2016) 18:1110–9. doi: 10.1111/dom.12707
58. Taleb N, Emami A, Suppere C, Messier V, Legault L, Ladouceur M, et al. Efficacy of single-hormone and dual-hormone artificial pancreas during continuous and interval exercise in adult patients with type 1 diabetes: randomised controlled crossover trial. *Diabetologia* (2016) 59:2561–71. doi: 10.1007/s00125-016-4107-0
59. Breton MD, Brown SA, Karvetski CH, Kollar L, Topchyan KA, Anderson SM, et al. Adding heart rate signal to a control-to-range artificial pancreas system improves the protection against hypoglycemia during exercise in type 1 diabetes. *Diabetes Technol Ther.* (2014) 16:506–11. doi: 10.1089/dia.2013.0333
60. Jacobs PG, Resalat N, El Youssef J, Reddy R, Branigan D, Preiser N, et al. Incorporating an exercise detection, grading, and hormone dosing algorithm into the artificial pancreas using accelerometry and heart rate. *J Diabetes Sci Technol.* (2015) 9:1175–84. doi: 10.1177/1932296815609371
61. Castle JR, El Youssef J, Wilson LM, Reddy R, Resalat N, Branigan D, et al. Randomized outpatient trial of single- and dual-hormone closed-loop systems that adapt to exercise using wearable sensors. *Diabetes Care* (2018) 41:1471–7. doi: 10.2337/dc18-0228
62. Taleb N, Coriati A, Khazzaka C, Bayonne J, Messier V, Rabasa-Lhoret R. Stability of commercially available glucagon formulation for dual-hormone artificial pancreas clinical use. *Diabetes Technol Ther.* (2017) 19:589–94. doi: 10.1089/dia.2017.0204
63. Taleb N, Haidar A, Messier V, Gingras V, Legault L, Rabasa-Lhoret R. Glucagon in artificial pancreas systems: potential benefits and safety profile of future chronic use. *Diabetes Obes Metab.* (2017) 19:13–23. doi: 10.1111/dom.12789

14

Using the T Cell Receptor as a Biomarker in Type 1 Diabetes

Maki Nakayama [1,2,3*] *and Aaron W. Michels* [1,2,3,4]

[1] *Barbara Davis Center for Childhood Diabetes, University of Colorado School of Medicine, Aurora, CO, United States,* [2] *Department of Pediatrics, University of Colorado School of Medicine, Aurora, CO, United States,* [3] *Department of Immunology and Microbiology, University of Colorado School of Medicine, Aurora, CO, United States,* [4] *Department of Medicine, University of Colorado School of Medicine, Aurora, CO, United States*

Correspondence:
Maki Nakayama
maki.nakayama@cuanschutz.edu

T cell receptors (TCRs) are unique markers that define antigen specificity for a given T cell. With the evolution of sequencing and computational analysis technologies, TCRs are now prime candidates for the development of next-generation non-cell based T cell biomarkers, which provide a surrogate measure to assess the presence of antigen-specific T cells. Type 1 diabetes (T1D), the immune-mediated form of diabetes, is a prototypical organ specific autoimmune disease in which T cells play a pivotal role in targeting pancreatic insulin-producing beta cells. While the disease is now predictable by measuring autoantibodies in the peripheral blood directed to beta cell proteins, there is an urgent need to develop T cell markers that recapitulate T cell activity in the pancreas and can be a measure of disease activity. This review focuses on the potential and challenges of developing TCR biomarkers for T1D. We summarize current knowledge about TCR repertoires and clonotypes specific for T1D and discuss challenges that are unique for autoimmune diabetes. Ultimately, the integration of large TCR datasets produced from individuals with and without T1D along with computational 'big data' analysis will facilitate the development of TCRs as potentially powerful biomarkers in the development of T1D.

Keywords: T cells, TCR sequencing, autoimmunity, type 1 diabetes, HLA, MHC

INTRODUCTION

A T cell receptor (TCR) determines antigen specificity of T cells by interacting with a peptide-major histocompatibility complex (peptide-MHC), and signals received through the TCR along with the CD3 complex are the primary components that regulate function and fate of T cells. Individual T cells express unique TCRs, and therefore TCR sequences can be used as an identifier of T cells that are specific to particular antigens and involved in immune responses. In this review, we will focus on the potential use of TCR sequences as non-cell based T cell biomarkers for type 1 diabetes (T1D), a tissue-specific autoimmune disease targeting insulin-secreting pancreatic beta cells (1–3).

Several features of self-reactive T cells make it challenging to develop T cell biomarkers in diabetes (4). First, the frequency of autoreactive T cells is extremely low in the peripheral blood, estimated to be $1/10^5$ – $1/10^6$. Second, response to peptide-MHC by autoreactive T cells tends to be minimal compared to anti-cancer or anti-pathogen T cell responses (5, 6). Third, healthy individuals with T1D-risk MHC molecules can have autoreactive T cells that are quantitatively and functionally similar to those in T1D patients (7). TCR sequencing allows for the analysis of TCR clonotypes from tens of millions of T cells using nucleotide samples rather than living cell biospecimens and may overcome many of these challenges when appropriately utilized. Advantages provided by TCR biomarkers include (1) living T cells are not required for assays; (2) intra- and inter-assay variations due to cell conditions and operator performance are minimized; and (3) extremely infrequent and low-responding T cells are detectable by recently emerging high-throughput sequencing technologies. Here, we will review current knowledge about TCR repertoires and clonotypes specific for T1D and address the knowledge gaps to develop TCR biomarkers that can stratify individuals throughout the stages of T1D development.

TRI-MOLECULAR COMPLEX CONSISTING OF TCR, PEPTIDE, AND MHC MOLECULES

TCRs expressed by classical T cells are composed of alpha and beta chains, both of which are formed by somatic recombination of the variable (V) and joining (J) segment genes (and diversity [D] for beta chains). In humans, 45 TRAV and 52 TRAJ genes have been identified as functional V and J segment genes for alpha chains (8, 9). Likewise, there are 49 TRBV, 2 TRBD, and 13 TRBJ functional V, D, and J segment genes in the beta chain locus (10, 11). During maturation in the thymus, individual T cells undergo rearrangement of segment genes, resulting in one V, one D (for beta), and one J segment genes assembled adjacent to each other. Since additional nucleotides are often inserted or deleted between the segments, billions of junction sequences with hundreds of different V, D, J combinations are possibly assembled (12–14). Experimentally, each adult person is expected to have over 100 million TCR clonotypes uniquely expressed by hundreds of billions of individual T cells in the body (15–19). There are three regions, called complementarity determining regions (CDR), that directly interact with peptide-MHC complexes, thereby crucial to determine antigen specificity (20–22). Two CDR regions, CDR1 and CDR2, are included in the V segment, and the CDR3 region is formed at the junction between V, D (for beta), and J segments. Amino acid residues in the CDR3 regions closely interact with peptide, and thus are considered to be important to determine antigen specificity and are often used as a property of each TCR clonotype for TCR repertoire analysis.

MHC MOLECULES IN T1D

The major genetic determinant in susceptibility to most autoimmune diseases reside in the human MHC that contains the human leukocyte antigen (HLA) region. MHC molecules are heterodimers formed between alpha and beta chains that function to present peptides to TCRs on T cells. Class I molecules are on all nucleated cells and present antigens to CD8 T cells, while class II molecules are expressed by antigen presenting cells (e.g. B cells, dendritic cells, and macrophages) and present peptides to CD4 T cells. In T1D, specific HLA class I and II alleles are associated with increased risk (23, 24). Several HLA class I and II alleles confer risk for T1D and are associated with other autoimmune disorders (**Table 1**) (25, 26). DR is in close linkage disequilibrium with DQ such that the DR4-DQ8 and DR3-DQ2 haplotypes confer the greatest risk for T1D development. Both the alpha and beta chains of DQ molecules are polymorphic, and have the ability to form mixed molecules in cis and trans. As an example, the alpha chain of DQ2 can pair with the beta chain of DQ8 to form DQ8-trans (*DQA1*05:01-DQB1*03:02*) when both DQ2 and DQ8 are in the genotype. DQ8-trans has an odds ratio of disease development for T1D at 35 (35 times more likely to develop diabetes compared to those without these alleles), compared to odds ratios of ~11 and ~4 for DQ8 and DQ2, respectively (27, 28). Interestingly, HLA-DQ6 (*DQA1*01:02-DQB1*06:02*) provides dominant protection for T1D development with an odds ratio of only 0.03 (29, 30). The stark dichotomy of risk between DQ molecules highlights the important role of antigen presentation to TCRs in T1D.

TABLE 1 | Common HLA alleles associated with type 1 diabetes risk.

Name	Allele	Associated Autoimmune Diseases
HLA Class II		
DQ8	*DQA1*03:01-DQB1*03:02*	Celiac disease, Addison's disease
DQ2	*DQA1*05:01-DQB1*02:01*	Celiac disease, Addison's disease
	*DQA1*02:01-DQB1*02:02*	Celiac disease, Addison's disease
DQ8-trans	*DQA1*05:01-DQB1*03:02*	Celiac disease
DR4	*DRB1*04:01*	Rheumatoid Arthritis, Thyroid disease, Addison's disease, Alopecia Areata
	*DRB1*04:02*	Rheumatoid Arthritis (protective), Thyroid disease, Addison's disease
	*DRB1*04:04*	Rheumatoid Arthritis, Thyroid disease, Addison's disease
	*DRB1*04:05*	Rheumatoid Arthritis, Thyroid disease, Addison's disease
DR3	*DRB1*03:01*	Systemic Lupus Erythematous (SLE), Neuromyelitis Optica (NMO), Myasthenia Gravis, Thyroid disease, Addison's disease
HLA Class I		
A2	*A*02:01*	Vitiligo
A24	*A*24:02*	unknown
B39	*B*39:06*	unknown
B18	*B*18:01*	unknown
B7	*B*07:05*	unknown

DIVERSITY OF TCR REPERTOIRES

Adults have approximately 10^8-10^{10} unique TCR clonotypes (15, 17, 18, 31). With an assumption that the TCR repertoire size may represent a capacity for responding to diverse antigens, the TCR repertoire diversity in the blood has been examined to determine whether it is associated with immune conditions. For example, having diverse TCR repertoires is associated with desirable responses to immune therapies in cancer (32–34). In T1D, it has been reported that TCR repertoires in peripheral blood of T1D patients are less diverse compared with those without T1D (35). Thus, there may be trends of TCR repertoire sizes that are preferred by a certain immune condition. However, it should be noted that the diversity of TCR repertoires cannot specify a certain disease.

USE OF TCR CLONOTYPES AS SURROGATES TO QUANTIFY ANTIGEN-SPECIFIC T CELLS

TCR clonotypes determine antigen specificity, and therefore they can be utilized as a surrogate marker to evaluate the presence and prevalence of antigen-specific T cells in the blood. Frequencies of these antigen-specific TCR clonotypes can be quantified by high-throughput sequencing, which is expected to be more specific to individual diseases compared to surveying the broad TCR repertoire. Furthermore, once a panel of antigen-specific TCR clonotypes are determined, a single TCR sequencing assay allows for evaluating specificity to many antigens rather than needing to test specificity to each individual antigen. TCR sequencing has been done from different tissues in many disease states (36), including autoimmune disorders (37) and cancer (38–40). Remarkably, TCR sequencing has been shown to differentiate early-stage cancer patients from healthy individuals (41, 42). This strategy requires a list of TCR clonotypes beforehand that can be searched in blood samples, and such TCR clonotypes used as surrogate biomarkers need to satisfy three factors: (1) publicity (i.e. commonality and shared between individuals), (2) abundancy, and (3) disease specificity. Namely, T cells expressing the same or similar TCR clonotypes need to be commonly present in a number of people; frequency of such T cells in the blood of each person needs to be high enough for quantification; and presence or absence of such T cells needs to be associated with a disease state. In addition, with larger numbers of TCR clonotypes in a given panel, the more specific and sensitive an assay will become. Thus, identifying disease-specific TCR candidates is essential to establish a robust TCR sequencing assay that can discriminate a subset of individuals having a specific stage or feature of T1D such as those who have potential to respond to an interventional therapy.

There are several strategies to identify disease-specific TCR clonotypes. Since a significant portion of disease-specific TCRs are likely to recognize islet antigens, TCR clonotypes expressed by islet antigen-specific T cells are reasonable candidates for TCR biomarkers. Such T cell sources include peripheral blood T cells responding to islet antigen stimulation or enriched by staining with fluorescence-conjugated multimers consisting of an islet-derived peptide and a particular HLA molecule (43–45). Alternatively, TCR clonotypes identified in the target organ (i.e. pancreas or pancreatic islets) or draining lymph nodes may be also disease-specific. In any of these T cell sources, specificity (i.e. potential contamination of non-disease associated T cells) as well as sensitivity (i.e. missing a portion of antigen-specific T cells) needs to be carefully considered. For example, T cell samples enriched by antigen stimulation may contain only a few clonotypes that readily proliferate in response to the stimulation or could be non-specific T cells that proliferate due to "bystander effect." Likewise, T cells in the pancreas and pancreatic lymph nodes may not necessarily be islet-reactive or disease-specific (46). On the other hand, T cell populations enriched by multimer staining may contain only those having high affinity to bind peptide-MHC complexes, and TCRs weakly binding to peptide-MHC may be missed. This possibility is likely important for autoreactive TCRs since T cell responsiveness to self-antigens tends to be low compared to pathogen T cell responses. Nevertheless, identifying TCR clonotypes from samples enriched with antigen-specific T cells is indispensable to identify disease-specific TCR candidates. These TCR clonotypes should then be assessed for frequency in peripheral blood of individuals with different stages of T1D to determine the ultimate association with disease status. The next subsections will summarize features of TCR clonotypes specific to islet-specific autoantigens as well as those potentially associated with T1D pathogenesis.

Lessons From Islet-Specific TCRs in T1D Animal Models

Non-diabetic (NOD) mice spontaneously develop autoimmune diabetes and represent many features of human T1D including a T1D-susceptible MHC allele (I-A^{g7}), homologous to HLA-DQ8, the development of insulin autoantibodies prior to diabetes onset, and insulitis. A number of T cell clones reacting with islet tissues have been isolated from pancreatic islets and spleens of NOD mice in the past few decades and further characterized for antigen specificity as well as TCR clonotypes (47). In the 1990's, Santamaria and colleagues discovered that a large portion of CD8 T cells infiltrating NOD islets share an identical Valpha segment (i.e. TRAV16) along with a specific junction motif (i.e. MRD or MRE) (48), and subsequently identified a peptide derived from islet-specific glucose-6-phosphatase catalytic subunit-related protein (IGRP) as an epitope targeted by these CD8 T cells (49). Likewise, CD4 T cell clones as well as T-hybridoma cells that are reactive to insulin B-chain peptides have been established from NOD islets by a number of investigators using different methods (50–56). The majority of these T cells expresses TCRs containing specific Valpha and Jalpha segment motifs, TRAV5D-4 or TRAV10 along with TRAJ53 or TRAJ42. When mice are forced to have only T cells expressing TCRs containing TRAV5D-4, approximately one percent of CD4 T cells becomes specific to an insulin B chain 9-23 peptide (57), and the mice are susceptible to develop anti-insulin autoimmunity (58, 59).

Alanine scanning and crystal structure analyses identified several amino acid residues in the TRAV5D-4 and TRAV10 CDR1 and CDR2 regions that are crucial to interact with the insulin peptide-MHC complex (59, 60). Also, among insulin B chain-specific CD4 T cells, those particularly recognize an insulin B chain 12-20 peptide prefer to express TCR beta chains containing a negatively charged amino acid (i.e. aspartic acid [D] or glutamic acid [E]) in the junction region (56). This observation is consistent with a notion that the I-A^{g7} T1D-susceptible MHC class II molecule, which has a positively charged patch in the surface area near the p9 pocket due to the lack of a negatively charged amino acid residue at the beta 57 position, engage TCRs having a negatively charged residue when p9 of peptides is not negatively charged (the position 20 of insulin B chain is glycine). Thus, these studies provide a molecular elucidation of how TCR motif selection occurs by interaction with a particular peptide-MHC complex.

T1D-specific TCR repertoires in rat models have been extensively studied by the group of Mordes and Blankenhorn (61). Of note, diabetes-susceptible rat strains have a T1D risk MHC haplotype (RT1B/D^{u}), which lacks a negatively charged amino acid residue at the beta chain 57 position and is homologous to HLA-DQ8 (61). In addition to the HLA gene locus, *Iddm14*, which contains the TCR beta chain genes, is a T1D-susceptible locus (62). The group identified a TCR Vbeta allele, *Tcrb-V13S1A1*, that is shared among T1D-susceptible rat strains but not with T1D-resistant ones (63), and demonstrated that genetic elimination of this allele or depletion of T cells expressing TCRs containing Vbeta13a (product of the *Tcrb-V13S1A1* gene) abrogates diabetes development in T1D-susceptible rats (64–66). A series of these studies elegantly linked the genetic risk with a functional mechanism in which a particular TCR motif facilitates T1D development with a specific MHC molecule.

In sum, these animal studies demonstrate the presence of preferred TCR motifs in both germline-encoded and rearranged regions to recognize particular epitope sequences, which can be reasonably explained by molecular interaction between the TCR – peptide – MHC molecule. From a view of TCR biomarker development, TCR motifs shared by antigen-specific or disease-susceptible T cells can be utilized to enrich and classify TCR clonotypes that are distinctive of T1D.

TCR Repertoires in the Pancreas of Humans

Emerging sequencing technologies and increasing availability of human samples, in particular pancreas and peripheral immune tissues isolated from organ donors having T1D, facilitate identification of islet antigen-specific or T1D-associated T cells and TCR clonotypes (7, 67–74). In the 1990's, two groups in Spain and Japan separately analyzed TCR repertoires in the pancreas and demonstrated clonal expansion of T cells with particular Vgene segment usage in individual patients (75, 76). Importantly, the same group in Spain demonstrated that a clonally expanding TCR in islet and pancreas samples was detected in the blood of the same individual, indicating that islet-residing TCR clonotypes are detectable in peripheral blood samples (77). More recently, Brusko and colleagues further corroborated this concept by studying a larger number of individuals using a next generation sequencing technology that allows to analyze much higher numbers of T cells (72, 78). This high resolution analysis discovered that CD8 TCR clonotypes in the pancreas and draining lymph nodes are detected in peripheral blood more frequently than those expressed by CD4 T cells and provided important insights about the depth of TCR sequencing to achieve quantitative measurement.

Another important concept is to consider commonality of TCR repertoires in the pancreas across patients. We recently determined thousands of TCR clonotypes expressed by T cells in the islets of organ donors with and without T1D (73, 74). Our analysis indicated clonal expansion in the pancreas of individual donors regardless of the disease, but also found that the frequency of TCR clonotypes shared between donors is limited. This low frequency of shared TCR clonotypes may be due to diverse HLA restrictions present in different individuals. Another reason could be the fact that T cells in the islets may not be necessarily islet-specific. Indeed, multiple studies analyzing islet T cell specificity found that over half of T cell clones and lines derived from the islets did not respond to preproinsulin and other known islet epitopes (46, 70, 71, 73, 74). However, it should be noted that collecting TCR clonotypes from a larger number of donors significantly increases the number of shared clonotypes and such large TCR repertoire information allows for identifying common motifs even when not sharing entire TCR sequences, which will be essential to precisely cluster TCRs recognizing the same epitope (see below regarding TCR clustering). Thus, continuing efforts to accumulate TCR sequence information from the target organ along with epitope identification is crucial to establish a sufficient list of TCR clonotypes that can be used for disease-associated TCR biomarkers.

Islet Antigen-Specific TCR Clonotypes in Humans

TCRs expressed by islet-reactive T cells may be another optimal source that can be used as clonotypes for T1D biomarkers, especially if they circulate in the peripheral blood. Such clonotypes could come from T cell clones, T cell lines, hybridomas, and transductant cells that have been confirmed to respond to islet antigens, cell subsets enriched by multimer staining, and those activated or proliferated by antigen stimulation. TCR clonotypes for which reactivity to epitopes has been confirmed at a single cell level would be the most reliable source. Here we summarize islet antigen-specific TCR clonotypes that were isolated from individuals having T1D (**Table 2**). To date, over a hundred TCR alpha and beta paired sequences specific to common islet epitopes have been reported by a number of investigators, and it is notable that the majority of these TCRs were identified in the past several years (7, 45, 70, 73, 74, 79–99). However, hundreds of disease-associated TCR clonotypes are far too small to cover T1D patients having heterogeneous antigen specificity. With rapidly evolving sequencing technologies, future efforts to identify islet epitope-

TABLE 2 | T cell receptors specific to islet epitopes.

Clone/ Sequence ID	Epitope	Epitope sequence	HLA[#]	TRAV	TRAJ	CDR3a	TRBV	TRBJ	CDR3b	Source of T cells	Method to confirm reactivity	Reference
BRI4.13	GAD65:555-567	NFFRMVISNPAAT	DR4	TRAV19	TRAJ44	CALSENRGGTASKLTF	TRBV5-1	TRBJ1-1	CASSLVGGPSSEAFF	PBMC CD4	Clone/ Transgenic cells	(79–81)
BRI164	GAD65:555-567	NFFRMVISNPAAT	DR4	TRAV19	TRAJ56	CALSEEGGGANSKLTF	TRBV5-1	TRBJ1-6	CASSLAGGANSPLHF	PBMC CD4	Clone/ Transgenic cells	(80, 82)
T1D2-1&2	IGRP:305-324	QLYHFLQIPTHEEHLFYVLS	DR4	TRAV29	TRAJ40	CAATRTSGTYKYIF	TRBV6-6	TRBJ2-3	CASSPWGAGGTDTQYF	PBMC CD4	Clone/TCR transductant	(81)
T1D4-3&4	IGRP:305-324	KWCANPDWIHIDTTPFAGLV	DR4	TRAV2	TRAJ15	CAVEDLNQAGTALIF	TRBV5-1	TRBJ2-1	CASSLALGQGNQQFF	PBMC CD4	Clone/TCR transductant	(81)
23.G8	PPI:36-50	VEALYLVCGERGFFY	DR4	TRAV39	TRAJ56	CAWFTGANSKLTF	TRBV24-1	TRBJ2-2	CATGLAANTGELFF	Islet CD4	TCR transductant	(83)
SD52.c1	PPI:72-90	PGAGSLQPLALEGSLQKRG	DR4	TRAV4	TRAJ27	CLVGDSLNTNAGKSTF	TRBV27	TRBJ1-5	CASSWSSIGNQPQHF	PBMC CD4	Clone	(82, 84)
95.A9-1	PPI:87-101	QKRGIVEQCCTSICS	DR4.4	TRAV9-2	TRAJ18	CALRTDRGSTLGRLYF	TRBV11-2	TRBJ1-6	CASSLQSSYNSPLHF	Islet CD4	TCR transductant	(83)
Mi.1	Insulin A:1-15 (PPI: 90-104)	GIVEQCCTSICSLYQ	DR4	TRAV8-3	TRAJ44	CAVGALAGTASKLTF	TRBV29-1	TRBJ2-3	CSVEATRADTQYF	PLN CD4	Clone	(85)
Ba.14	Insulin A:1-15 (PPI: 90-104)	GIVEQCCTSICSLYQ	DR4	TRAV39	TRAJ33	CAVVNMDSNYQLIW	TRBV5-1	TRBJ2-3	CASSLATSGGGSDTQYF	PLN CD4	Clone	(85)
Ba.11	Insulin A:1-15 (PPI: 90-104)	GIVEQCCTSICSLYQ	DR4	TRAV22 TRAV26-2 ##	TRAJ52 TRAJ47	CADAGGTSYKLF CIPGSEEYGNKLVF	TRBV5-1	TRBJ2-3	CASSLATSGGGSDTQYF	PLN CD4	Clone	(85)
6.H11	PPI:94-108	QCCTSICSLYQLENY	DR4.2	TRAV26-1	TRAJ13	CIVRVYSGGYQKVTF	TRBV30	TRBJ2-3	CAWSARLAGGPRTQYF	Islet CD4	TCR transductant	(83)
SD32.5	PPI:94-110	QCCTSICSLYQLENYCN	DR4	TRAV26-1	TRAJ23	CIVRVSSAYYNQGGKLIF	TRBV27	TRBJ2-3	CASSPRANTDTQYF	PBMC CD4	Clone	(82, 84)
B3.3	Proinsulin:52-62 (PPI:76-86)	SLQPLALEGSL	DR4	TRAV17	TRAJ54	CATGPIQGAQKLVF	TRBV6-5	TRBJ1-1	CASSYAWGRATEAFF	PBMC CD4	Clone	(86)
K4.4/K6.4	Proinsulin:54-63 (PPI:78-87)	QPLALEGSLQ	DR4	TRAV10	TRAJ17	CVVSAKAAGNKLTF	TRBV7-8	TRBJ2-7	CASSLAGTDHYEQYF	PBMC CD4	Clone	(86)
23.F7	PPI:24-38	AFVNQHLCGSHLVEA	DR1	TRAV8-2	TRAJ29	CAVIASGNTPLVF	TRBV19	TRBJ2-3	CASKGPGTVIRADTQYF	Islet CD4	TCR transductant	(83)
55.B3	PPI:37-51	EALYLVCGERGFFYT	DR9	TRAV21	TRAJ29	CAVLPPTPLVF	TRBV18	TRBJ1-1	CASSYPGTGGARTEAFF	Islet CD4	TCR transductant	(83)
55.C10	PPI:58-72	AEDLQVGQVELGGGP	DR53	TRAV26-1	TRAJ26	CIVRSHGQNFVF	TRBV20-1	TRBJ2-7	CSARPGTRNYEQYF	Islet CD4	TCR transductant	(83)
Clone 5	Insulin B:9-23 (PPI: 33-47)	SHLVEALYLVCGERG	DQ8	TRAV21	TRAJ6	CAVKRTGGSYIPTF	TRBV11-2	TRBJ2-2	CASSSFWGSDTGELFF	PBMC CD4	Clone/TCR transductant	(82, 87, 88)
GSE.6H9	Insulin B:9-23 (PPI: 33-47)	SHLVEALYLVCGERG	DQ8, DQ8-trans	TRAV26-1	TRAJ40	CIVRVDSGTYKYIF	TRBV7-2	TRBJ2-1	CASSLTAGLASTYNEQFF	Islet CD4	TCR transductant	(73, 83)
GSE.20D11	Insulin B:9-23 (PPI: 33-47)	SHLVEALYLVCGERG	DQ8	TRAV12-3	TRAJ4	CAILSGGYNKLIF	TRBV2	TRBJ2-5	CASSAETQYF	Islet CD4	TCR transductant	(73, 83)
T1D#3 C8	Insulin B:11-23 (PPI: 35-47)[R22E]	LVEALYLVCGEEG	DQ8	TRAV17	TRAJ23	CATDAGYNQGGKLIF	TRBV5-1	TBBJ1-3	CASSAGNTIYF	PBMC CD4	Clone	(82, 89)

(Continued)

TABLE 2 | Continued

Clone/ Sequence ID	Epitope	Epitope sequence	HLA#	TRAV	TRAJ	CDR3a	TRBV	TRBJ	CDR3b	Source of T cells	Method to confirm reactivity	Reference
T1D#3 C10	Insulin B:11-23 (PPI: 35-47)^{R22E}	LVEALYLVCGEEG	DQ8	TRAV12-3	TRAJ26	CATAYGQNFVF	TRBV4-1	TRBJ2-2	CASSRGGGNTGELFF	PBMC CD4	Clone	(82, 89)
19.A4	PPI:55-69	RREAEDLQVGQVELG	DQ8	TRAV8-6	TRAJ32	CAVRETGATNKLIF	TRBV20-1	TRBJ2-7	CSARPQGFSSYEQYF	Islet CD4	TCR transductant	(83)
GSE.8E3	PPI:72-87 hEL:C-peptide (HIP11)	PGAGSLQPLALEGSLQ SLQPLALEAEDLQV	DQ8, DQ8-trans	TRAV2	TRAJ37	CAVDGSGNTGKLIF	TRBV4-1	TRBJ2-7	CASSQDLAGVREQYF	Islet CD4	TCR transductant	(73, 83)
6.G4	PPI:86-100	LQKRGIVEQCCTSIC	DQ8, DQ8-trans	TRAV26-1	TRAJ8	CIVRVRNTGFQKLVF	TRBV27	TRBJ1-1	CASSPGPGNTEAFF	Islet CD4	TCR transductant	(83)
56.B1	PPI:40-54	YLVCGERGFFYTPKT	DQ2	TRAV13-1	TRAJ40	CAVLSPSGTYKYIF	TRBV7-9	TRBJ1-4	CASSLMGNPHEKLFF	Islet CD4	TCR transductant	(83)
53.A4-1	PPI:72-87	PGAGSLQPLALEGSLQ	DQ2	TRAV39	TRAJ33	CAVDPMDSNYQLIW	TRBV29-1	TRBJ2-6	CSVGTDPSGANVLTF	Islet CD4	TCR transductant	(83)
23.G6	PPI:29-43	HLCGSHLVEALYLVC	DP4	TRAV9-2	TRAJ6	CALSISGGSYIPTF	TRBV5-1	TRBJ2-5	CASSFRQGEQETQYF	Islet CD4	TCR transductant	(83, 90)
A4.13	Proinsulin:41-51 (PPI:65-75)	QVELGGGPGAG	DQ8	TRAV6	TRAJ36	CALKYGANNLFF	TRBV18	TRBJ1-1	CASSPTTGGDEAFF	Islet CD4	Clone	(70)
A1.1	Proinsulin:50-59 (PPI:74-83)	AGSLQPLALE	DQ8	TRAV25	TRAJ16	CAGGFSDGQKLLF	TRBV20-1	TRBJ2-7	CSARTEAYEQYF	Islet CD4	Clone	(70)
A1.2	Proinsulin:50-58 (PPI:74-82)	AGSLQPLAL	DQ8	TRAV20	TRAJ58	CAVIETSGSRLTF	TRBV20-1	TRBJ2-3	CSARDQQRVDTQYF	Islet CD4	Clone	(70)
A2.4	Proinsulin:52-62 (PPI:76-86)	SLQPLALEGSL	DQ8-trans	TRAV19	TRAJ49	CALSRAGTGNQFYF	TRBV5-1	TRBJ2-4	CASSLGLRGENIQYF	Islet CD4	Clone	(70)
B3.1	Proinsulin:48-59 (PPI:72-83)	PGAGSLQPLALE	DQ8	TRAV12-1	TRAJ9	CVVKSTGGFKTIF	TRBV20-1	TRBJ2-5	CSAGGLAGASQETQYF	PBMC CD4	Clone	(86)
K3.2/K9.5	Proinsulin:54-62 (PPI:78-86)	QPLALEGSL	DQ2	TRAV3	TRAJ31	CAVRGDNNARLMF	TRBV7-2	TRBJ2-2	CASSPIIWGTGELFF	PBMC CD4	Clone	(86)
K6.2	Proinsulin:49-58 (PPI:73-82)	GAGSLQPLAL	DQ8-trans	TRAV8-2/8-4	TRAJ11	CAVTPKSGYSTLTF	TRBV20-1	TRBJ2-3	CSARDLAIPDTQYF	PBMC CD4	Clone	(86)
K9.6	Proinsulin:41-51 (PPI:65-75)	QVELGGGPGAG	DQ8	TRAV26-1	TRAJ54	CIVRVEIQGAQKLVF	TRBV3-2	TRBJ2-1	CASSSPGTEYNEQFF	PBMC CD4	Clone	(86)
D1.1/D1.4	Proinsulin:34-43 (PPI:58-67)	AEDLQVGQVE	DQ8	TRAV13-1	TRAJ38	CAARNAGNNRKLIW	TRBV4-2	TRBJ2-3	CASSFRGLGGGTDTQYF	PBMC CD4	Clone	(86)
T6.1	Proinsulin:52-63 (PPI:76-87)	SLQPLALEGSLQ	DQ2, DQ2-trans	Functional alpha not detected			TRBV9	TRBJ2-1	CASSVDPGVYNEQFF	PBMC CD4	Clone	(86)
T6.6	Proinsulin:56-62 (PPI:80-86)	LALEGSL	DQ2	TRAV35	TRAJ28	CAAALSGAGSYQLTF	TRBV19	TRBJ2-3	CASRLDPSTDTQYF	PBMC CD4	Clone	(86)
T17.1	Proinsulin:56-62 (PPI:80-86)	LALEGSL	DQ2, DQ2-trans	TRAV35	TRAJ28	CAAALSGAGSYQLTF	TRBV19	TRBJ2-3	CASRLDPSTDTQYF	PBMC CD4	Clone	(86)
H3.3/H6.4	Proinsulin:52-61 (PPI:76-85)	SLQPLALEGS	DQ8-trans	TRAV19	TRAJ57	CALSGRGSEKLVF	TRBV5-1	TRBJ2-7	CASSTRTGQGGNEQYF	PBMC CD4	Clone	(86)
H3.7/H7.4/ H8.5	Proinsulin:50-58 (PPI:74-82)	AGSLQPLAL	DQ8	TRAV12-1	TRAJ20	CVVNPTDDYKLSF	TRBV20-1	TRBJ2-3	CSARSLASGGPDTQYF	PBMC CD4	Clone	(86)

(Continued)

TABLE 2 | Continued

Clone/ Sequence ID	Epitope	Epitope sequence	HLA[#]	TRAV	TRAJ	CDR3a	TRBV	TRBJ	CDR3b	Source of T cells	Method to confirm reactivity	Reference
H11.5	Proinsulin:42-51 (PPI:66-75)	VELGGGPGAG	DQ8	TRAV26-1	TRAJ36	CIVRVVTGANNLFF	TRBV5-1	TRBJ2-5	CASSLERETQYF	PBMC CD4	Clone	(86)
E2.3	Proinsulin:54-62 (PPI:78-86)	QPLALEGSL	DQ2	TRAV30	TRAJ37	CGTEKPGSGNTGKLIF	TRBV20-1	TRBJ1-4	CSARDGARGEKLFF	PBMC CD4	Clone	(86)
E2.5	Proinsulin:35-46 (PPI:59-70)	EDLQVGQVELGG	DQ8	TRAV12-3	TRAJ5	CVISPPGRRALTF	TRBV5-4	TRBJ2-2	CASSSGTSAGTGELFF	PBMC CD4	Clone	(86)
A3.10	hEGGG : IAPP2 (HIP6)	GQVELGGGNAVEVLK	DQ8	TRAV38-1	TRAJ54	CAFFGQGAGKLVF	TRBV5-1	TRBJ2-3	CASSLSASGGATDTQYF	Islet CD4	Clone	(70, 91, 92)
A1.9	Proinsulin:42-50 (PPI:66-74) hEGGG : IAPP2 (HIP6)	VELGGGPGA GQVELGGGNAVEVLK	DQ8	TRAV20	TRAJ7	CAVQAGGNNRLAF	TRBV5-1	TRBJ1-2	CASSLERDGYTF	Islet CD4	Clone	(70, 92)
A6.15/A5.8	Proinsulin:42-50 (PPI:66-74) hEGGG : IAPP2 (HIP6)	VELGGGPGA GQVELGGGNAVEVLK	DQ8	TRAV26-1	TRAJ21	CIAIYNFNKFYF	TRBV5-1	TRBJ1-6	CASSLEASSYNSPLHF	Islet CD4	Clone	(70, 92)
A2.13	Proinsulin:42-50 (PPI:66-74) hEGGG : IAPP2 (HIP6)	VELGGGPGA GQVELGGGNAVEVLK	DQ8	TRAV26-1	TRAJ39	CIVSHNAGNMLTF	TRBV5-1	TRBJ2-5	CASSLERETQYF	Islet CD4	Clone	(70, 92)
A5.5	Proinsulin:42-50 (PPI:66-74) hEGGG : IAPP2 (HIP6)	VELGGGPGA GQVELGGGNAVEVLK	DQ8	TRAV26-1	TRAJ54	CIVRVEIQGAQKLVF	TRBV5-1	TRBJ2-5	CASSLGPGQRETQYF	Islet CD4	Clone	(70, 92)
A2.11	hEGGG : IAPP2 (HIP6)	GQVELGGGNAVEVLK	Not reported	TRAV38-1	TRAJ54	CAFMGAGAQKLVF	TRBV4-3	TRBJ2-3	CASSQILRGGPPDTQYF	Islet CD4	Clone	(70, 91)
HIP14-G10/D3	hEL : IAPP2 (HIP14)	SLQPLALNAVEVLK	DR	TRAV16 TRAV5 ##	TRAJ37 TRAJ40	CARSHGSGNTGKLIF CAESIASGTYKYIF	TRBV27	TRBJ2-5	CASSSGYGGETQYF	PBMC CD4	Clone	(93)
E2b	hEL:C-peptide (HIP11)	SLQPLALEAEDLQV	DQ2	TRAV8-4	TRAJ43	CAVGATNNNDMRF	TRBV5-4	TRBJ2-1	CASSPIGASGGNEQFF	PBMC CD4	Clone	(94)
ET650-2	Proinsulin:42-50 (PPI:66-74) hEGGG : IAPP2 (HIP6) HIPL11C	VELGGGPGA GQVELGGGNAVEVLK GQVELGGGNAVEVCK	DQ8	TRAV26-1	TRAJ39	CIVRVGYNAGNMLTF	TRBV20-1	TRBJ1-5	CSAIAGPNQPQHF	PBMC CD4	Clone	(92)
ET650-4	Proinsulin:42-50 (PPI:66-74) hEGGG : IAPP2 (HIP6) HIPL11C	VELGGGPGA GQVELGGGNAVEVLK GQVELGGGNAVEVCK	DQ8	TRAV26-1	TRAJ42	CIVRVAIEGSQGNLIF	TRBV5-1	TRBJ1-3	CASSLRRGDTIYF	PBMC CD4	Clone	(92)
ET650-5	hEGGG : IAPP2 (HIP6) HIPL11C	GQVELGGGNAVEVLK GQVELGGGNAVEVCK	DQ8	TRAV26-1	TRAJ9	CIVRLQSGGFKTIF	TRBV20-1	TRBJ1-2	CSAYSPGDRDFSNYGYTF	PBMC CD4	Clone	(92)
ET672-1	Proinsulin:42-50 (PPI:66-74) hEGGG : IAPP2 (HIP6) HIPL11C	VELGGGPGA GQVELGGGNAVEVLK GQVELGGGNAVEVCK	DQ8	TRAV12-2	TRAJ48	CAVNHGNEKLTF	TRBV18	TRBJ1-1	CASSPWEGRMDTEAFF	PBMC CD4	Clone	(92)
1E6	PPI:15-24	ALWGPDPAAA	A*02:01	TRAV12-3	TRAJ12	CAMRGDSSYKLIF	TRBV12-4	TRBJ2-4	CASSLWEKLAKNIQYF	PBMC CD8	Clone	(82, 95)
1D5/1D10/2B3/4C6/3E7	PPI:3-11	LWMRLLPLL	A*24:02	TRAV5	TRAJ37	CAEPSGNTGKLIF	TRBV7–9	TRBJ2-7	CASSLHHEQYF	PBMC CD8	Clone	(96)

(Continued)

TABLE 2 | Continued

Clone/ Sequence ID	Epitope	Epitope sequence	HLA[#]	TRAV	TRAJ	CDR3a	TRBV	TRBJ	CDR3b	Source of T cells	Method to confirm reactivity	Reference
Clone 7	IGRP:265-273	VLFGLGFAI	A*02:01	TRAV41	TRAJ48	CAVTSNFGNEKLTF	TRBV6-2/6-3	TRBJ2-7	CASSSRFVGEGLFRYGYEQYF	PBMC CD8	Clone/ Transgenic cells	(97, 98)
Clone 32	IGRP:265-273	VLFGLGFAI	A*02:01	TRAV12-1	TRAJ48	CVVNILSNFGNEKLTF	TRBV20-1	TRBJ2-1	CSASRQGWVNEQFF	PBMC CD8	Clone/ Transgenic cells	(97, 98)
Clone 16/17	IGRP:265-273	VLFGLGFAI	A*02:01	TRAV25	TRAJ53	CAGLGDSGGSNYKLTF	TRBV3-1	TRBJ2-4	CASSQDRWDVMSKNIQYF	PBMC CD8	Clone	(45)
Clone 22/27	IGRP:265-273	VLFGLGFAI	A*02:01	TRAV29/DV5	TRAJ53	CAASGGSNYKLTF	TRBV10-3	TRBJ1-2	CAISDRFMREGMTYGYTF	PBMC CD8	Clone	(45)
Clone#1	INS-DRiP:1-9	MLYQHLLPL	A*02:01	TRAV12-2	TRAJ34	CAVNKTDKLIF	TRBV6-1	TRBJ1-2	CASSVTGNGYTF	PBMC CD8	Clone	(99)
Clone#2	INS-DRiP:1-9	MLYQHLLPL	A*02:01	TRAV10	TRAJ8	CVVNMNTGFQKLVF	TRBV12-3/12-4	TRBJ2-2	CASSPPQGGNTGELFF	PBMC CD8	Clone	(99)
1.C1	INS-DRiP:1-9	MLYQHLLPL	A*02:01	TRAV12-1	TRAJ39	CGENNAGNMLTF	TRBV27	TRBJ2-5	CASSLQPPGTSTETQYF	Islet CD8	TCR transductant	(74)
96.A9	INS-DRiP:1-9	MLYQHLLPL	B*08:01	TRAV12-2	TRAJ39	CAVNVYNAGNMLTF	TRBV30	TRBJ1-1	CAWSVRGGSYMNTEAFF	Islet CD8	TCR transductant	(74)
D222D Clones 2	ZNT8:186-194	VAANIVLTV	A*02:01	TRAV17	TRAJ36	CAVTGANNLFF	TRBV19	TRBJ2-2	CASSIEGPTGELF	PBMC CD8	Clone	(7)
D010R clone 1E2	ZNT8:186-194	VAANIVLTV	A*02:01	TRAV35	TRAJ36	CAGTRNNLFF	TRBV19	TRBJ2-7	CASGGSSYEQYF	PBMC CD8	Clone	(7)
D010R clone 1D3	ZNT8:186-194	VAANIVLTV	A*02:01	TRAV25	TRAJ20	CAGGSNDYKLSF	TRBV6-1	TRBJ2-3	CASSSVGVDTQYF	PBMC CD8	Clone	(7)
D267T 33B8	ZNT8:186-194	VAANIVLTV	A*02:01	TRAV19	TRAJ23	CALSEATYNQGGKLIF	TRBV19	TRBJ1-3	CASSIFPNPGNTIYF	PBMC CD8	Clone	(7)
D349D 178B9	ZNT8:186-194	VAANIVLTV	A*02:01	TRAV14/DV4	TRAJ9	CAMREGLTGGFKTIF	TRBV11-2	TRBJ1-1	CASSPFLTGSNTEAFF	PBMC CD8	Clone	(7)
D351D 188D3	ZNT8:186-194	VAANIVLTV	A*02:01	TRAV19	TRAJ20	CALSPAETSDYKLSF	TRBV19	TRBJ1-1	CASTLTGFAEAFF	PBMC CD8	Clone	(7)
23.F9	PPI:1-11	MALWMRLLPLL	C*03:04	TRAV12-3	TRAJ48	CAMSALGNFGNEKLTF	TRBV19	TRBJ2-1	CASSIAGGNEQFF	Islet CD8	TCR transductant	(74)
19.A1	PPI:1-11	MALWMRLLPLL	C*03:04	TRAV8-4	TRAJ11	CAVSDQGSGYSTLTF	TRBV28	TRBJ1-5	CASSWTANQPQHF	Islet CD8	TCR transductant	(74)
20.E5	PPI:1-11	MALWMRLLPLL	C*03:04	TRAV14/DV4	TRAJ52	CAMSNAGGTSYGKLTF	TRBV28	TRBJ1-4	CASSLARYNEKLFF	Islet CD8	TCR transductant	(74)
20.F1	PPI:1-11	MALWMRLLPLL	C*03:04	TRAV14/DV4	TRAJ43	CAMRLHNNNDMRF	TRBV28	TRBJ1-5	CASIASRYNQPQHF	Islet CD8	TCR transductant	(74)
22.A10	PPI:1-11	MALWMRLLPLL	C*03:04	TRAV8-1	TRAJ13	CAVNAAGGYQKVTF	TRBV28	TRBJ2-1	CASIPDRYNEQFF	Islet CD8	TCR transductant	(74)
1.C8	PPI:1-11/2-12/2-10	MALWMRLLPLL ALWMRLLPLLA ALWMRLLPL	A*02:01	TRAV24	TRAJ58	CAFKRETSGSRLTF	TRBV13	TRBJ2-1	CASSTRLAGDEQFF	Islet CD8	TCR transductant	(74)
1.F3	PPI:2-12	ALWMRLLPLLA	A*02:01	TRAV39	TRAJ39	CAVENAGNMLTF	TRBV10-2	TRBJ2-1	CASWTVSYNEQFF	Islet CD8	TCR transductant	(74)

(Continued)

TABLE 2 | Continued

Clone/ Sequence ID	Epitope	Epitope sequence	HLA#	TRAV	TRAJ	CDR3a	TRBV	TRBJ	CDR3b	Source of T cells	Method to confirm reactivity	Reference
96.F5	PPI:3-11	LWMRLLPLL	A*02:01	TRAV8-6	TRAJ48	CAVSDISNFGNEKLTF	TRBV9	TRBJ2-3	CASSVVGLGTDTQYF	Islet CD8	TCR transductant	(74)
23.H5	PPI:3-13	LWMRLLPLLAL	A*02:01	TRAV38-2/DV8	TRAJ22	CAYRSPARQLTF	TRBV6-1	TRBJ2-7	CASSEGWGVPSYEQYF	Islet CD8	TCR transductant	(74)
1.B10-1	PPI:15-23	ALWGPDPAA	A*02:01	TRAV8-3	TRAJ33	CAVVADSNYQLIW	TRBV4-2/4-3	TRBJ2-2	CASSQTKGTGELFF	Islet CD8	TCR transductant	(74)
1.F1	PPI:15-24	ALWGPDPAAA	A*02:01	TRAV39	TRAJ41	CAVSNSGYALNF	TRBV29-1	TRBJ2-5	CSVFHRGETQYF	Islet CD8	TCR transductant	(74)
23.C12	PPI:15-24/15-25	ALWGPDPAAA ALWGPDPAAAF	A*02:01	TRAV41	TRAJ42	CAVSGGSQGNLIF	TRBV28	TRBJ1-2	CASSPPTGWGGYTF	Islet CD8	TCR transductant	(74)
93.D1	PPI:15-25	ALWGPDPAAAF	A*02:01	TRAV5	TRAJ8	CAVTKDTGFQKLVF	TRBV20-1	TRBJ2-1	CSARDHFGGSGYEQFF	Islet CD8	TCR transductant	(74)
10.C6-1	PPI:23-32	AAFVNQHLCG	C*12:03	TRAV19	TRAJ39	CALSGALNNAGNMLTF	TRBV27	TRBJ2-5	CASSLFGYRQETQYF	Islet CD8	TCR transductant	(74)
28.D3	PPI:31-41/34-41	CGSHLVEALYL HLVEALYL	A*02:01	TRAV26-2	TRAJ26	CILTDNYGQNFVF	TRBV27	TRBJ1-1	CASSLIGLNTEAFF	Islet CD8	TCR transductant	(74)
28.E6	PPI:46-54/47-54	RGFFYTPKT GFFYTPKT	A*29:02	TRAV19	TRAJ28	CALSEAGAGSYQLTF	TRBV2	TRBJ2-5	CASSPSGTSSQETQYF	Islet CD8	TCR transductant	(74)
20.G1	PPI:69-77/69-79	GGGPGAGSL GGGPGAGSLQP	C*03:04	TRAV1-2	TRAJ8	CAVRMNTGFQKLVF	TRBV9	TRBJ2-1	CASSVGMDPGLGYNEQFF	Islet CD8	TCR transductant	(74)
96.B4	PPI:91-99	IVEQCCTSI	C*05:01	TRAV12-2	TRAJ31	CAVNNARLMF	TRBV6-5	TRBJ2-1	CASRPTSGGYNEQFF	Islet CD8	TCR transductant	(74)
86.C1	PPI:91-100/92-100/ 92-102	IVEQCCTSIC VEQCCTSIC VEQCCTSICSL	B*41:02	TRAV19	TRAJ16	CALSEAGFSDGQKLLF	TRBV19	TRBJ2-1	CASSIQFSYNEQFF	Islet CD8	TCR transductant	(74)
84.D9	PPI:91-100/92-100/ 92-102	IVEQCCTSIC VEQCCTSIC VEQCCTSICSL	B*41:02	TRAV29/ DV5	TRAJ43	CAASNSNDMRF	TRBV7-9	TRBJ2-1	CASSLAQREQFF	Islet CD8	TCR transductant	(74)
28.E11	PPI:91-100	IVEQCCTSIC	B*18:01	TRAV12-2	TRAJ49	CAVSMNTGNQFYF	TRBV29-1	TRBJ2-1	CSVQVYNEQFF	Islet CD8	TCR transductant	(74)
1.E9-1	PPI:92-99	VEQCCTSI	B*50:01	TRAV12-2	TRAJ34	CAVNIRYNTDKLIF	TRBV6-2/6-3	TRBJ1-5	CASSSIQGSGSGQPQHF	Islet CD8	TCR transductant	(74)
86.G3-2	PPI:94-102	QCCTSICSL	B*35:01	TRAV8-6	TRAJ33	CAVSDGYQLIW	TRBV6-1	TRBJ2-7	CASSGREAPYEQYF	Islet CD8	TCR transductant	(74)
54.F1	PPI:96-103	CTSICSLY	A*01:01	TRAV3	TRAJ26	CAVPDNYGQNFVF	TRBV7-2	TRBJ2-2	CASSLVVELFF	Islet CD8	TCR transductant	(74)

#*HLA class II alleles: DR4 (DRB1*04:01); DR4.4 (DRB1*04:04); DR4.2 (DRB1*04:02); DR1 (DRB1*01:01); DR9 (DRB1*09:01); DR53 (DRB4*01:01); DQ8 (DQA1*03:01-DQB1*03:02); DQ8-trans (DQA1*05:01-DQB1*03:02); DQ2 (DQA1*05:01-DQB1*02:01/02:02), DQ2-trans (DQA1*03:01-DQB1*02:01); DP4 (DPA1*01:03-DPB1*04:01).*

##*Two in-frame alpha chains detected. Functional alpha not determined.*

specific TCR clonotypes is essential to develop TCR biomarkers for T1D. In addition to TCR clonotypes listed in **Table 2**, Bonifacio and colleagues reported hundreds of TCR sequences expressed by T cells that were stained with multimer composed of islet epitopes or those proliferated in response to islet antigens (44, 45). While it is necessary to carefully validate true reactivity to antigens, this type of analysis is an excellent resource to gain T1D-associated TCR clonotypes. Computational tools to decrease the "noise" (i.e. eliminating non-specific binding TCR clonotypes) may help to enrich truly antigen-specific clonotypes (100, 101). Further, these candidate TCR clonotypes could be validated for disease specificity using larger cohorts analyzed with whole blood TCR sequencing, and then clonotypes that were detected only in individuals having various stages of T1D could be assessed for functional reactivity (**Figures 1A–C**). Retro/lentiviral transduction systems, especially in a moderate to high throughput multiplex assay, will facilitate verifying reactivity to antigens (82, 98, 102, 103).

Identification of Disease-Specific TCR Clonotypes Using Big Data

Big data analysis, which seeks to classify TCR repertoires in a specific condition using a large number of TCR samples, is an emerging strategy to identify disease-associated TCR clonotypes. A major advantage of this approach is the capability to identify disease-associated TCR clonotypes without knowing antigen specificity, thereby allowing one to include TCRs that are potentially disease-associated but not islet-specific and also those having low affinity to antigens. Indeed, specificities of large proportions of T cells in the islets are unknown (46, 70–74). Virus infections such as enterovirus and coxsackie B virus (CVB) are suggested to be involved in T1D development (104–106), and TCRs specific to these viruses could be identified by big data analysis by comparing TCR repertoires of individuals having or not having different stages of T1D. Although it has been demonstrated in infectious diseases that big data analyses can identify pathogen-specific TCR clonotypes, it has not yet been successful at identifying T1D-associated TCR clonotypes using PBMC samples from individuals with or without different stages of T1D. This could be explained by several possibilities: (1) the frequency of T1D-associated T cells may be lower than that of pathogen-specific T cells; (2) antigens involved in T1D pathogenesis, especially those at different stages of T1D, may be more heterogeneous than those in infectious diseases; (3) autoreactive TCRs could be more private (i.e. not common between patients) than those of conventional T cells; and (4) sample sizes studied to date have not been large enough. However, having large TCR data sets produced by next generation sequencing will enable machine learning algorithms to cluster and classify TCR clonotypes. Using these newly developed techniques, even infrequent disease-specific TCRs having less publicity (i.e. commonality) between people may be identified from relatively small numbers of samples. Indeed, some computational TCR classifying methods are now capable of identifying cancer patients responding to immune checkpoint inhibitors (40), and also early stages of cancer can be differentiated from healthy individuals using this type of technique (107, 108). In the next section, we will discuss how to take advantages of the latest TCR clustering/classifying techniques for T1D TCR biomarkers.

Clustering and Classification of TCR Clonotypes

TCR clonotypes recognizing the same peptide-MHC complex often share similar motifs and features. For example, influenza-specific TCRs prefer to use TRAV38-1/TRAJ52/TRBV19/TRBJ1-2 (109–111), and melanoma (MART-1)-specific TCRs often contain an alpha chain with TRAV12-2 (112). Likewise, several features common for islet antigen-specific TCRs have been reported. We discovered that insulin B-chain-specific TCRs tend to use TRAV38-1/38-2 and other Valpha segments having similar motifs in the CDR1 and CDR2 regions (113). Also, it has been shown that a specific motif "SGGSNYKLTF" is contained in the CDR3 region of alpha chains specific to an IGRP peptide (45). More recently, crystal structure analysis of TCRs specific to a hybrid insulin peptide composed of proinsulin and islet amyloid polypeptide (IAPP) demonstrated that motifs in the TRBV5-1 segment commonly interact with amino acid residues in IAPP (92). Our work also indicates that T cell responses to hybrid insulin peptides precede clinical T1D onset (114), making these TCR clonotypes excellent candidates for biomarkers. Thus, autoreactive TCRs share commonalities and similarities, which provide clues to cluster TCRs and stratify those specific to a certain condition.

A number of algorithms to cluster or classify TCR clonotypes have been developed. Each algorithm has advantages and disadvantages as reviewed by others (115, 116), but in respect to TCR biomarker development for T1D, the algorithms can be divided to two groups. First, those that clusters TCRs by assessing similarities of TCR sequences with each other in datasets. Second, those that seek to classify TCRs by identifying similar to known antigen-specific or disease-specific TCR clonotypes. The former algorithms such as TCRdist (111), GLIPH/GLIPH2 (117, 118), ClusTCR (119), and GIANA (108) do not need information about T1D-specific epitopes and TCR sequences beforehand, and thus can be used to predict disease-specific TCR clonotypes that are specifically detected in T1D patients but not in non-diabetic subjects. On the other hand, machine learning-based algorithms that assess similarities to known antigen-specific TCR datasets to predict epitopes, such as DeepTCR (101), DeepCAT (107), TCRmatch (120), and TCRAI (100) need prior information about disease-specific TCR sequences. These algorithms show excellent performance when classifying TCRs specific to the same epitopes that were used to develop the machine learning algorithm but not for those having different specificities. Therefore, large sets of disease-specific TCR sequence information for machine training are necessary to achieve high specificity and sensitivity. Typically these types of algorithms show better performance to detect antigen-specific TCR clonotypes than the clustering-based algorithms, thereby being useful to validate TCR clonotypes once epitopes or disease-specificity are determined.

Alternatively, they can be also used to 'clean up' (i.e. eliminate non-specific TCR clonotypes) TCR datasets that are obtained from multimer-stained T cells or those activated by antigen stimulation (**Figure 1B**).

In any case, it is essential to prepare TCR datasets from a large number of individuals with and without T1D at multiple time points to elicit the best performance by machine learning and clustering algorithms. Typically, diverse datasets rather than large data but from a limited number of samples improve learning efficiency (100). In addition, it is also important to prepare accurate TCR clonotype information to differentiate T1D patients from healthy subjects. There are now several TCR databases available, which accumulate and curate information about TCR sequences along with target peptide-MHC complexes, such as VDJbase (121, 122), IEDB (123), VDJdb (124), iReceptor (125), and McPAS-TCR (126). While these are incredibly useful resources, a proportion of islet-specific clonotypes is still very small, accounting for only ~100 out of tens of thousands of clonotypes, the majority of which are specific to viruses and tumor antigens. Assuming that self-reactive TCR clonotypes are more heterogeneous and rarer compared to pathogen-specific ones, there is a need for higher numbers of clonotypes specific to T1D. Thus, identifying a large set of accurate disease-specific TCR clonotypes will be a key component to achieve successful big data analysis, which will ultimately lead us to establish TCR biomarkers in T1D (**Figure 1**).

PERSPECTIVE

It is still controversial whether T1D patients have distinct islet antigen-specific T cell subsets in the blood compared to healthy individuals. Even in the pancreas, non-diabetic organ donors have preproinsulin-specific T cells in the exocrine compartment, but such antigen-specific T cells accumulate into the islets over the course of T1D progression (127). In the islets, we recently demonstrated that only T1D donors have CD8 T cells highly reactive to preproinsulin (74). Mallone and colleagues also reported that pancreata of T1D donors have a higher number of zinc transporter-8-specific T cells than non-diabetic controls (7). Thus, multiple studies demonstrate that islets of T1D individuals have distinct T cell repertoires from those without diabetes. However, a number of studies indicate that healthy individuals have islet-antigen specific T cells in the blood (7, 113, 128–131), and depending on cell subsets examined, some studies including those looking into pathogenic T cells show that T1D patients have higher numbers of islet-specific T cells, whereas others do not detect differential islet-specific T cells in T1D patients. This controversy could be explained by either (1) detectable numbers of pathogenic T cells in the islets do not leak into the peripheral blood (**Figure 2A**); or (2) pathogenic T cells in the islets do indeed circulate, but because there are already a number of islet-specific (but not harmful) T cells in the circulation, the total numbers of islet-specific T cells (i.e. pathogenic T cells leaked from the islets plus non-pathogenic T cells) are not differentiated enough in the blood of T1D patients from healthy individuals (**Figure 2B**). Given evidence that a portion of T cell repertoires are shared between pancreas, pancreatic lymph nodes, and peripheral blood cells (72), and that TCR repertoires in the islets of T1D organ donors are clonally distinct from those of non-diabetic donors (74), if the latter hypothesis (**Figure 2B**) is correct, islet-derived TCR sequences will be a powerful marker to discriminate pathogenic from physiological T cells, thereby capable of stratifying individuals with active insulitis prior to clinical T1D onset.

To develop practical TCR biomarkers in T1D, a number of obstacles need to be overcome, some of which may be unique to autoimmune diseases. These challenges can be considered from the view of (1) publicity, (2) abundancy, and (3) disease-specificity.

1. Publicity

   It will be important to understand the frequencies of public *vs* private TCR clonotypes that are specific to the T1D disease state, and these likely fluctuate over time during T1D development. Given the genetic risk associated with HLA class II genes, heterogeneity provided by HLA diversity could be smaller than other diseases for TCR clonotypes expressed by CD4 T cells. However, autoreactive T cells, which often bind to peptide-MHC complexes with low affinity, may have a larger TCR repertoire than conventional anti-pathogen T cells, resulting in less commonality. Therefore, frequency of public T1D-specific TCR clonotypes may be low. Strategies that compare TCR repertoires in each individual such as pre and post treatment (40) do not need to consider publicity of clonotypes, and therefore may be more easily applicable to T1D immune intervention studies.

2. Abundancy

   Theoretically, 10^{15}-10^{16} diverse TCR clonotypes can be assembled (12–14); however, a practical TCR repertoire size is estimated to be about 10^{8}-10^{10} per person (15, 17, 18). This indicates that the frequency of target clonotypes is extremely low. However, there is evidence that identical clonotypes are persistently detected from the same individuals over time (44, 81, 93, 132). We believe quantitative resolution of TCRs will need to be increased. This could be achieved by enriching samples before sequencing (e.g. beads enrichment by antigen-specific multimers). Another very attractive approach is to target sequencing to TCRs containing a preferred Vgene segment of interest, thus greatly enhancing the depth of sequencing by analyzing clonotypes that can be obtained for a specific V allele. Blood sample volume needed to quantitatively evaluate frequency of disease-associated TCR clonotypes is another important consideration, which will need to be addressed given that the T1D disease process does begin in young children.

3. Disease-Specificity

   Identification of disease-specific TCR clonotypes is an essential component to develop robust T1D TCR biomarkers. A larger number of TCR clonotypes with higher specificity to the disease that are in place will allow for more sensitive and specific assays. Therefore, the key

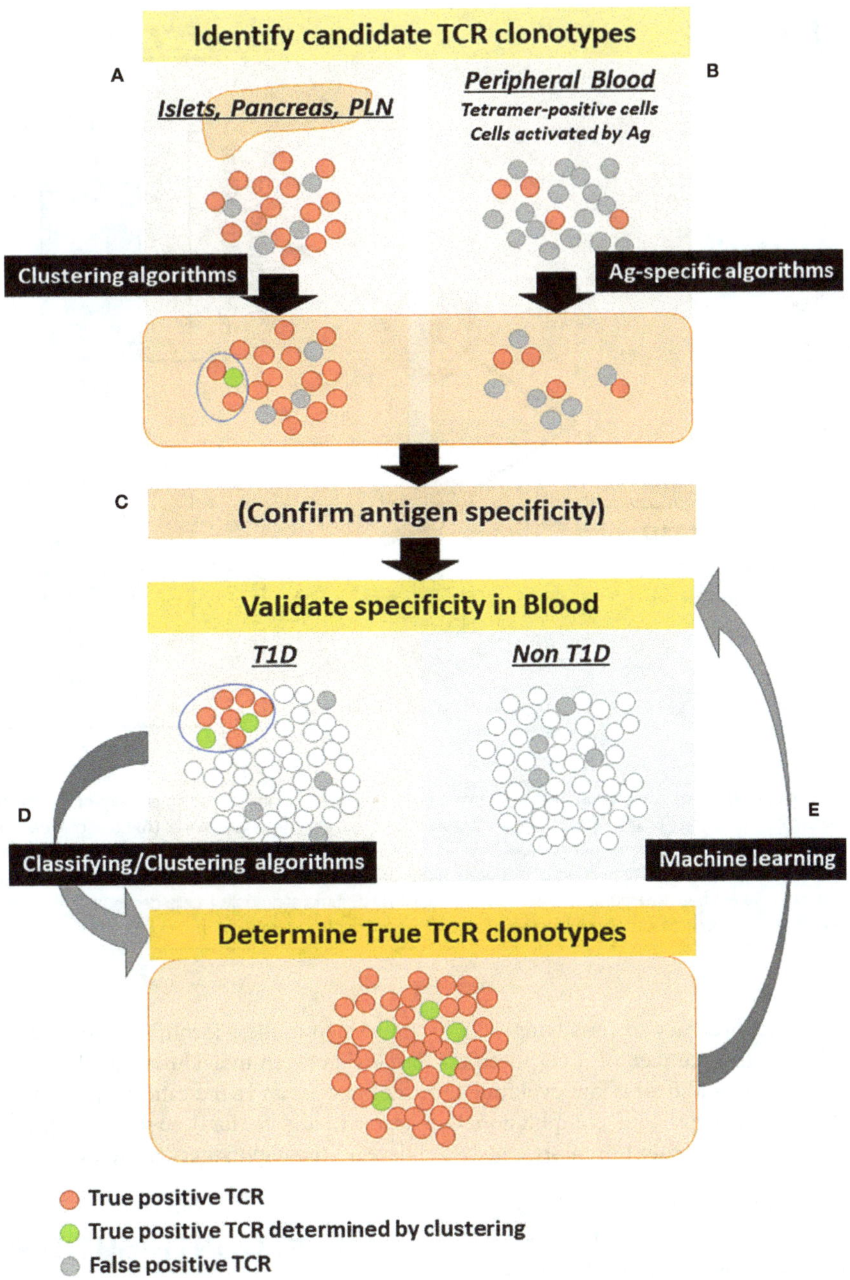

FIGURE 1 | Strategy to determine disease-specific TCR clonotypes. Red and gray circles represent true and false disease-specific TCR clonotypes, respectively. Green circles are true disease-specific clonotypes determined by clustering with known disease-specific TCR clonotypes. **(A)** TCRs detected in the islets, pancreata, and pancreatic lymph nodes, in particular those for which antigen specificity has been determined as well as those that are clustered with known disease-specific TCRs, can be the initial source for disease-specific TCR candidates. **(B)** TCRs detected from peripheral blood T cells enriched by antigen stimulation or peptide-MHC-conjugated multimers are also an initial source. Antigen-specific algorithms can enrich TCR clonotypes that are truly specific to antigens. **(C)** Candidate TCR clonotypes may be assessed for specificity to islet tissues, proteins, and peptides. **(D)** Using classifying algorithms, candidate TCR clonotypes are assessed for frequency in the blood of individuals with and without T1D to determine disease specificity. Simultaneously, clustering algorithms can select additional clonotypes that are clustered with known disease-specific TCR clonotypes. **(E)** TCR clonotypes selected by classifying and clustering algorithms are used for machine learning of antigen-specific algorithms to further determine true disease-specificity.

is how to select such truly disease-specific TCR clonotypes. As illustrated in **Figure 1**, both accumulation of actual TCR datasets produced from individuals with and without T1D and computational big data analysis will facilitate the development of biomarkers. While the majority of TCR big data analysis currently uses only CDR3-beta sequences, it has been demonstrated that inclusion of entire sequence information such as V and J segments, in particular CDR1

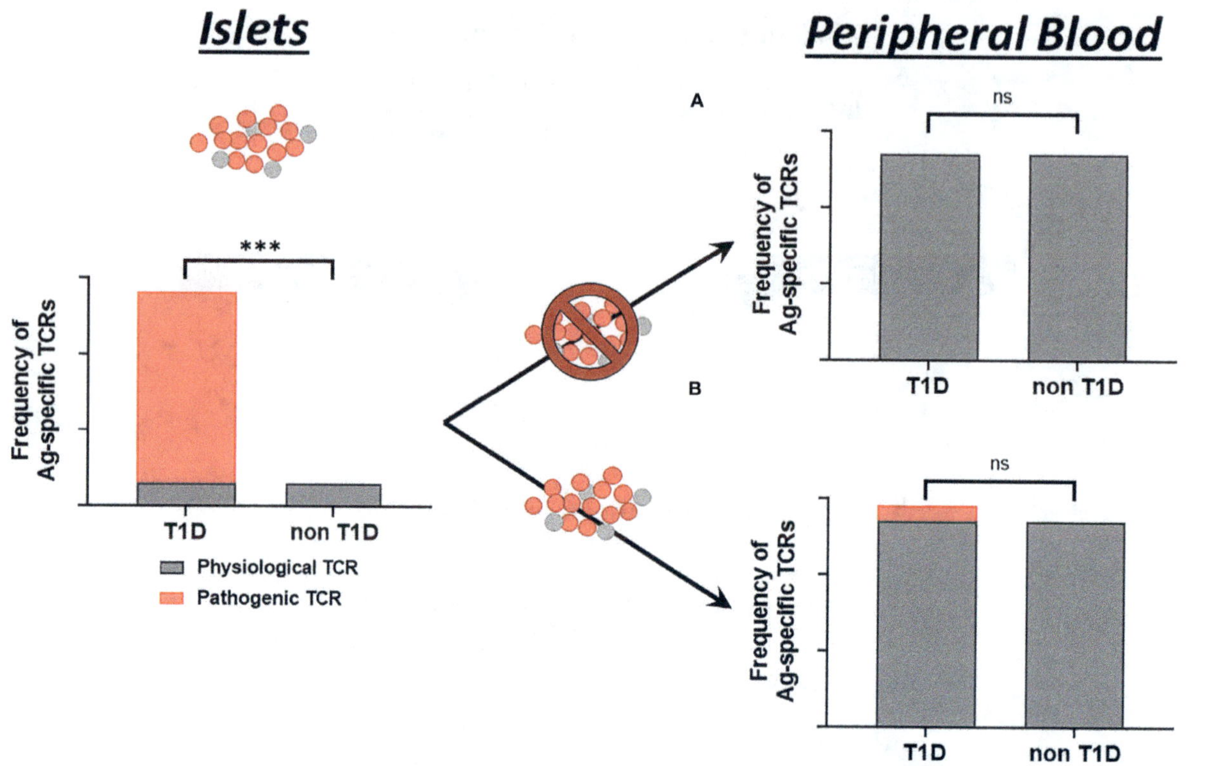

FIGURE 2 | Proposed models of islet-specific T cell detection in the blood. While pancreatic islets contain a certain amount of T cells regardless of disease status (gray bars), only islets of individuals with T1D contain T cells that are highly reactive to islet antigens (red bar). Model **(A)** Leak of T cells from the islets to peripheral blood is limited. T cell repertoires specific to islet antigens are not different between individuals with and without T1D. Model **(B)** There are substantial amounts of islet-specific but not disease-specific T cells in the blood regardless of disease status (gray bars). T cells in the islets do circulate in the blood (red bar), but the total numbers of islet-specific T cells are not different between individuals with and without T1D. Enumerating only T cells derived from the islets can identify individuals having T1D. TCR clonotypes are a distinct property to identify islet-derived T cells. *** significantly different. ns, not significant.

and CDR2 sequences, increases accuracy of classifying TCR clonotypes (100, 120). While the number of T1D-specific clonotypes that have been determined so far is low, evolutions in both TCR sequencing technologies and computational analysis strategies will dramatically impact this effort.

In conclusion, the antigen receptor on disease specific T cells holds promise for a non-cell based biomarker of not only the presence of T1D but disease activity as well. Efforts to define the TCR repertoire within the human pancreas of T1D and non-T1D organ donors is underway with a need to define the antigen specificity and HLA restriction of these identified clonotypes. Those clonotypes that are shared between individuals with T1D, frequent, and circulate from the pancreas and pancreatic lymph nodes to the peripheral blood are prime candidates for deep sequencing and clustering of TCRs using developed computational analyses.

AUTHOR CONTRIBUTIONS

MN and AM wrote and edited the manuscript. All authors contributed to the article and approved the submitted version.

REFERENCES

1. Atkinson MA, Eisenbarth GS, Michels AW. Type 1 Diabetes. *Lancet (London England)* (2014) 383:69–82. doi: 10.1016/S0140-6736(13)60591-7
2. Katsarou A, Gudbjörnsdottir S, Rawshani A, Dabelea D, Bonifacio E, Anderson BJ, et al. Type 1 Diabetes Mellitus. *Nat Rev Dis Primers* (2017) 3:17016. doi: 10.1038/nrdp.2017.16
3. Bluestone JA, Buckner JH, Herold KC. Immunotherapy: Building a Bridge to a Cure for Type 1 Diabetes. *Sci (New York NY)* (2021) 373:510–6. doi: 10.1126/science.abh1654
4. Ahmed S, Cerosaletti K, James E, Long SA, Mannering S, Speake C, et al. Standardizing T-Cell Biomarkers in Type 1 Diabetes: Challenges and Recent Advances. *Diabetes* (2019) 68:1366–79. doi: 10.2337/db19-0119
5. Cole DK, Pumphrey NJ, Boulter JM, Sami M, Bell JI, Gostick E, et al. Human TCR-Binding Affinity Is Governed by MHC Class Restriction. *J Immunol (Baltimore Md. 1950)* (2007) 178:5727–34. doi: 10.4049/jimmunol.178.9.5727
6. Unger WW, Velthuis J, Abreu JR, Laban S, Quinten E, Kester MG, et al. Discovery of Low-Affinity Preproinsulin Epitopes and Detection of Autoreactive CD8 T-Cells Using Combinatorial MHC Multimers. *J Autoimmun* (2011) 37:151–9. doi: 10.1016/j.jaut.2011.05.012

7. Culina S, Lalanne AI, Afonso G, Cerosaletti K, Pinto S, Sebastiani G, et al. Islet-Reactive CD8(+) T Cell Frequencies in the Pancreas, But Not in Blood, Distinguish Type 1 Diabetic Patients From Healthy Donors. *Sci Immunol* (2018) 3(20):eaao4013. doi: 10.1126/sciimmunol.aao4013
8. Scaviner D, Lefranc MP. The Human T Cell Receptor Alpha Variable (TRAV) Genes. *Exp Clin Immunogenetics* (2000) 17:83–96. doi: 10.1159/000019128
9. Scaviner D, Lefranc MP. The Human T Cell Receptor Alpha Joining (TRAJ) Genes. *Exp Clin Immunogenetics* (2000) 17:97–106. doi: 10.1159/000019129
10. Folch G, Lefranc MP. The Human T Cell Receptor Beta Variable (TRBV) Genes. *Exp Clin Immunogenetics* (2000) 17:42–54. doi: 10.1159/000019123
11. Folch G, Lefranc MP. The Human T Cell Receptor Beta Diversity (TRBD) and Beta Joining (TRBJ) Genes. *Exp Clin Immunogenetics* (2000) 17:107–14. doi: 10.1159/000019130
12. Davis MM, Bjorkman PJ. T-Cell Antigen Receptor Genes and T-Cell Recognition. *Nature* (1988) 334:395–402. doi: 10.1038/334395a0
13. Elhanati Y, Marcou Q, Mora T, Walczak AM. repgenHMM: A Dynamic Programming Tool to Infer the Rules of Immune Receptor Generation From Sequence Data. *Bioinf (Oxford England)* (2016) 32:1943–51. doi: 10.1093/bioinformatics/btw112
14. Zarnitsyna VI, Evavold BD, Schoettle LN, Blattman JN, Antia R. Estimating the Diversity, Completeness, and Cross-Reactivity of the T Cell Repertoire. *Front Immunol* (2013) 4:485. doi: 10.3389/fimmu.2013.00485
15. Robins HS, Campregher PV, Srivastava SK, Wacher A, Turtle CJ, Kahsai O, et al. Comprehensive Assessment of T-Cell Receptor Beta-Chain Diversity in Alphabeta T Cells. *Blood* (2009) 114:4099–107. doi: 10.1182/blood-2009-04-217604
16. Qi Q, Liu Y, Cheng Y, Glanville J, Zhang D, Lee JY, et al. Diversity and Clonal Selection in the Human T-Cell Repertoire. *Proc Natl Acad Sci USA* (2014) 111:13139–44. doi: 10.1073/pnas.1409155111
17. Farber DL, Yudanin NA, Restifo NP. Human Memory T Cells: Generation, Compartmentalization and Homeostasis. *Nat Rev Immunol* (2014) 14:24–35. doi: 10.1038/nri3567
18. Lythe G, Callard RE, Hoare RL, Molina-París C. How Many TCR Clonotypes Does a Body Maintain? *J Theor Biol* (2016) 389:214–24. doi: 10.1016/j.jtbi.2015.10.016
19. Kumar BV, Connors TJ, Farber DL, Development HTC. Localization, and Function Throughout Life. *Immunity* (2018) 48:202–13. doi: 10.1016/j.immuni.2018.01.007
20. Marrack P, Scott-Browne JP, Dai S, Gapin L, Kappler JW. Evolutionarily Conserved Amino Acids That Control TCR-MHC Interaction. *Annu Rev Immunol* (2008) 26:171–203. doi: 10.1146/annurev.immunol.26.021607.090421
21. Rossjohn J, Gras S, Miles JJ, Turner SJ, Godfrey DI, McCluskey J. T Cell Antigen Receptor Recognition of Antigen-Presenting Molecules. *Annu Rev Immunol* (2015) 33:169–200. doi: 10.1146/annurev-immunol-032414-112334
22. La Gruta NL, Gras S, Daley SR, Thomas PG, Rossjohn J. Understanding the Drivers of MHC Restriction of T Cell Receptors. *Nat Rev Immunol* (2018) 18:467–78. doi: 10.1038/s41577-018-0007-5
23. Concannon P, Rich SS, Nepom GT. Genetics of Type 1A Diabetes. *New Engl J Med* (2009) 360:1646–54. doi: 10.1056/NEJMra0808284
24. Robertson CC, Rich SS. Genetics of Type 1 Diabetes. *Curr Opin Genet Dev* (2018) 50:7–16. doi: 10.1016/j.gde.2018.01.006
25. Nejentsev S, Howson JM, Walker NM, Szeszko J, Field SF, Stevens HE, et al. Localization of Type 1 Diabetes Susceptibility to the MHC Class I Genes HLA-B and HLA-A. *Nature* (2007) 450:887–92. doi: 10.1038/nature06406
26. Noble JA, Valdes AM, Varney MD, Carlson JA, Moonsamy P, Fear AL, et al. And Genetic Susceptibility to Type 1 Diabetes: Results From the Type 1 Diabetes Genetics Consortium. *Diabetes* (2010) 59:2972–9. doi: 10.2337/db10-0699
27. Erlich H, Valdes AM, Noble J, Carlson JA, Varney M, Concannon P, et al. And Genotypes and Type 1 Diabetes Risk: Analysis of the Type 1 Diabetes Genetics Consortium Families. *Diabetes* (2008) 57:1084–92. doi: 10.2337/db07-1331
28. Hu X, Deutsch AJ, Lenz TL, Onengut-Gumuscu S, Han B, Chen WM, et al. Additive and Interaction Effects at Three Amino Acid Positions in HLA-DQ and HLA-DR Molecules Drive Type 1 Diabetes Risk. *Nat Genet* (2015) 47:898–905. doi: 10.1038/ng.3353
29. Pugliese A, Boulware D, Yu L, Babu S, Steck AK, Becker D, et al. HLA-DRB1*15:01-DQA1*01:02-DQB1*06:02 Haplotype Protects Autoantibody-Positive Relatives From Type 1 Diabetes Throughout the Stages of Disease Progression. *Diabetes* (2016) 65:1109–19. doi: 10.2337/db15-1105
30. Pecher SA, de Castro GB, Borrás MR. Anemophilus Fungi in the Brazilian-Colombian Border. *Rev da Sociedade Bras Medicina Trop* (1988) 21:63–6. doi: 10.1590/S0037-86821988000200006
31. Jenkins MK, Chu HH, McLachlan JB, Moon JJ. On the Composition of the Preimmune Repertoire of T Cells Specific for Peptide-Major Histocompatibility Complex Ligands. *Annu Rev Immunol* (2010) 28:275–94. doi: 10.1146/annurev-immunol-030409-101253
32. Snyder A, Nathanson T, Funt SA, Ahuja A, Buros Novik J, Hellmann MD, et al. Contribution of Systemic and Somatic Factors to Clinical Response and Resistance to PD-L1 Blockade in Urothelial Cancer: An Exploratory Multi-Omic Analysis. *PloS Med* (2017) 14:e1002309. doi: 10.1371/journal.pmed.1002309
33. Tumeh PC, Harview CL, Yearley JH, Shintaku IP, Taylor EJ, Robert L, et al. PD-1 Blockade Induces Responses by Inhibiting Adaptive Immune Resistance. *Nature* (2014) 515:568–71. doi: 10.1038/nature13954
34. Sheikh N, Cham J, Zhang L, DeVries T, Letarte S, Pufnock J, et al. Clonotypic Diversification of Intratumoral T Cells Following Sipuleucel-T Treatment in Prostate Cancer Subjects. *Cancer Res* (2016) 76:3711–8. doi: 10.1158/0008-5472.CAN-15-3173
35. Tong Y, Li Z, Zhang H, Xia L, Zhang M, Xu Y, et al. T Cell Repertoire Diversity Is Decreased in Type 1 Diabetes Patients. *Genomics Proteomics Bioinf* (2016) 14:338–48. doi: 10.1016/j.gpb.2016.10.003
36. Pai JA, Satpathy AT. High-Throughput and Single-Cell T Cell Receptor Sequencing Technologies. *Nat Methods* (2021) 18:881–92. doi: 10.1038/s41592-021-01201-8
37. Mitchell AM, Michels AW. T Cell Receptor Sequencing in Autoimmunity. *J Life Sci (Westlake Village Calif.)* (2020) 2:38–58. doi: 10.36069/jols/20201203
38. Li N, Yuan J, Tian W, Meng L, Liu Y. T-Cell Receptor Repertoire Analysis for the Diagnosis and Treatment of Solid Tumor: A Methodology and Clinical Applications. *Cancer Commun (London England)* (2020) 40:473–83. doi: 10.1002/cac2.12074
39. Joshi K, Milighetti M, Chain BM. Application of T Cell Receptor (TCR) Repertoire Analysis for the Advancement of Cancer Immunotherapy. *Curr Opin Immunol* (2021) 74:1–8. doi: 10.1016/j.coi.2021.07.006
40. Fairfax BP, Taylor CA, Watson RA, Nassiri I, Danielli S, Fang H, et al. Peripheral CD8(+) T Cell Characteristics Associated With Durable Responses to Immune Checkpoint Blockade in Patients With Metastatic Melanoma. *Nat Med* (2020) 26:193–9. doi: 10.1038/s41591-019-0734-6
41. Beausang JF, Wheeler AJ, Chan NH, Hanft VR, Dirbas FM, Jeffrey SS, et al. T Cell Receptor Sequencing of Early-Stage Breast Cancer Tumors Identifies Altered Clonal Structure of the T Cell Repertoire. *Proc Natl Acad Sci USA* (2017) 114:E10409–e10417. doi: 10.1073/pnas.1713863114
42. Zhang H, Liu L, Zhang J, Chen J, Ye J, Shukla S, et al. Investigation of Antigen-Specific T-Cell Receptor Clusters in Human Cancers. *Clin Cancer Res an Off J Am Assoc Cancer Res* (2020) 26:1359–71. doi: 10.1158/1078-0432.CCR-19-3249
43. Estorninho M, Gibson VB, Kronenberg-Versteeg D, Liu YF, Ni C, Cerosaletti K, et al. A Novel Approach to Tracking Antigen-Experienced CD4 T Cells Into Functional Compartments *via* Tandem Deep and Shallow TCR Clonotyping. *J Immunol (Baltimore Md. 1950)* (2013) 191:5430–40. doi: 10.4049/jimmunol.1300622
44. Eugster A, Lindner A, Catani M, Heninger AK, Dahl A, Klemroth S, et al. High Diversity in the TCR Repertoire of GAD65 Autoantigen-Specific Human CD4+ T Cells. *J Immunol (Baltimore Md. 1950)* (2015) 194:2531–8. doi: 10.4049/jimmunol.1403031
45. Fuchs YF, Eugster A, Dietz S, Sebelefsky C, Kühn D, Wilhelm C, et al. CD8(+) T Cells Specific for the Islet Autoantigen IGRP Are Restricted in Their T Cell Receptor Chain Usage. *Sci Rep* (2017) 7:44661. doi: 10.1038/srep44661
46. Rodriguez-Calvo T, Christoffersson G, Bender C, von Herrath MG, Mallone R, Kent SC, et al. Means, Motive, and Opportunity: Do Non-Islet-Reactive Infiltrating T Cells Contribute to Autoimmunity in Type 1 Diabetes? *Front Immunol* (2021) 12:683091. doi: 10.3389/fimmu.2021.683091

47. Haskins K. Pathogenic T-Cell Clones in Autoimmune Diabetes: More Lessons From the NOD Mouse. *Adv Immunol* (2005) 87:123–62. doi: 10.1016/S0065-2776(05)87004-X
48. Santamaria P, Utsugi T, Park BJ, Averill N, Kawazu S, Yoon JW. Beta-Cell-Cytotoxic CD8+ T Cells From Nonobese Diabetic Mice Use Highly Homologous T Cell Receptor Alpha-Chain CDR3 Sequences. *J Immunol (Baltimore Md. 1950)* (1995) 154:2494–503.
49. Lieberman SM, Evans AM, Han B, Takaki T, Vinnitskaya Y, Caldwell JA, et al. Identification of the Beta Cell Antigen Targeted by a Prevalent Population of Pathogenic CD8+ T Cells in Autoimmune Diabetes. *Proc Natl Acad Sci USA* (2003) 100:8384–8. doi: 10.1073/pnas.0932778100
50. Daniel D, Gill RG, Schloot N, Wegmann D. Epitope Specificity, Cytokine Production Profile and Diabetogenic Activity of Insulin-Specific T Cell Clones Isolated From NOD Mice. *Eur J Immunol* (1995) 25:1056–62. doi: 10.1002/eji.1830250430
51. Simone E, Daniel D, Schloot N, Gottlieb P, Babu S, Kawasaki E, et al. T Cell Receptor Restriction of Diabetogenic Autoimmune NOD T Cells. *Proc Natl Acad Sci USA* (1997) 94:2518–21. doi: 10.1073/pnas.94.6.2518
52. Abiru N, Wegmann D, Kawasaki E, Gottlieb P, Simone E, Eisenbarth GS. Dual Overlapping Peptides Recognized by Insulin Peptide B:9-23 T Cell Receptor AV13S3 T Cell Clones of the NOD Mouse. *J Autoimmun* (2000) 14:231–7. doi: 10.1006/jaut.2000.0369
53. Levisetti MG, Suri A, Petzold SJ, Unanue ER. The Insulin-Specific T Cells of Nonobese Diabetic Mice Recognize a Weak MHC-Binding Segment in More Than One Form. *J Immunol (Baltimore Md. 1950)* (2007) 178:6051–7. doi: 10.4049/jimmunol.178.10.6051
54. Mohan JF, Levisetti MG, Calderon B, Herzog JW, Petzold SJ, Unanue ER. Unique Autoreactive T Cells Recognize Insulin Peptides Generated Within the Islets of Langerhans in Autoimmune Diabetes. *Nat Immunol* (2010) 11:350–4. doi: 10.1038/ni.1850
55. Mohan JF, Calderon B, Anderson MS, Unanue ER. Pathogenic $CD4^+$ T Cells Recognizing an Unstable Peptide of Insulin Are Directly Recruited Into Islets Bypassing Local Lymph Nodes. *J Exp Med* (2013) 210:2403–14. doi: 10.1084/jem.20130582
56. Gioia L, Holt M, Costanzo A, Sharma S, Abe B, Kain L, et al. Position β57 of I-A(g7) Controls Early Anti-Insulin Responses in NOD Mice, Linking an MHC Susceptibility Allele to Type 1 Diabetes Onset. *Sci Immunol* (2019) 4 (38):eaaw6329. doi: 10.1126/sciimmunol.aaw6329
57. Zhang L, Jasinski JM, Kobayashi M, Davenport B, Johnson K, Davidson H, et al. Analysis of T Cell Receptor Beta Chains That Combine With Dominant Conserved TRAV5D-4*04 Anti-Insulin B:9-23 Alpha Chains. *J Autoimmun* (2009) 33:42–9. doi: 10.1016/j.jaut.2009.02.003
58. Kobayashi M, Jasinski J, Liu E, Li M, Miao D, Zhang L, et al. Conserved T Cell Receptor Alpha-Chain Induces Insulin Autoantibodies. *Proc Natl Acad Sci USA* (2008) 105:10090–4. doi: 10.1073/pnas.0801648105
59. Nakayama M, Castoe T, Sosinowski T, He X, Johnson K, Haskins K, et al. Germline TRAV5D-4 T-Cell Receptor Sequence Targets a Primary Insulin Peptide of NOD Mice. *Diabetes* (2012) 61:857–65. doi: 10.2337/db11-1113
60. Wang Y, Sosinowski T, Novikov A, Crawford F, White J, Jin N, et al. How C-Terminal Additions to Insulin B-Chain Fragments Create Superagonists for T Cells in Mouse and Human Type 1 Diabetes. *Sci Immunol* (2019) 4(34): eaav7517. doi: 10.1126/sciimmunol.aav7517
61. Mordes JP, Bortell R, Blankenhorn EP, Rossini AA, Greiner DL. Rat Models of Type 1 Diabetes: Genetics, Environment, and Autoimmunity. *ILAR J* (2004) 45:278–91. doi: 10.1093/ilar.45.3.278
62. Mordes JP, Cort L, Norowski E, Leif J, Fuller JM, Lernmark A, et al. Analysis of the Rat Iddm14 Diabetes Susceptibility Locus in Multiple Rat Strains: Identification of a Susceptibility Haplotype in the Tcrb-V Locus. *Mamm Genome Off J Int Mamm Genome Soc* (2009) 20:162–9. doi: 10.1007/s00335-009-9172-y
63. Stienekemeier M, Hofmann K, Gold R, Herrmann T. A Polymorphism of the Rat T-Cell Receptor Beta-Chain Variable Gene 13 (BV13S1) Correlates With the Frequency of BV13S1-Positive CD4 Cells. *Immunogenetics* (2000) 51:296–305. doi: 10.1007/s002510050623
64. Liu Z, Cort L, Eberwine R, Herrmann T, Leif JH, Greiner DL, et al. Prevention of Type 1 Diabetes in the Rat With an Allele-Specific Anti-T-Cell Receptor Antibody: Vβ13 as a Therapeutic Target and Biomarker. *Diabetes* (2012) 61:1160–8. doi: 10.2337/db11-0867
65. Bogdani M, Faxius L, Fex M, Ramelius A, Wernersson A, Mordes JP, et al. The Vbeta13 T Cell Receptor Monoclonal Antibody Reduces Hyaluronan and CD68+, CD3+, and CD8+ Cell Infiltrations to Delay Diabetes in Congenic BB DRLyp/Lyp Rats. *Front Endocrinol* (2021) 12:629242. doi: 10.3389/fendo.2021.629242
66. Mordes JP, Cort L, Liu Z, Eberwine R, Blankenhorn EP, Pierce BG, et al. Cell Receptor Genotype and Ubash3a Determine Susceptibility to Rat Autoimmune Diabetes. *Genes* (2021) 12(6):852. doi: 10.3390/genes12060852
67. Campbell-Thompson M, Wasserfall C, Kaddis J, Albanese-O'Neill A, Staeva T, Nierras C, et al. Network for Pancreatic Organ Donors With Diabetes (nPOD): Developing a Tissue Biobank for Type 1 Diabetes. *Diabetes/Metabolism Res Rev* (2012) 28:608–17. doi: 10.1002/dmrr.2316
68. Kaddis JS, Pugliese A, Atkinson MA. A Run on the Biobank: What Have We Learned About Type 1 Diabetes From the nPOD Tissue Repository? *Curr Opin Endocrinol Diabetes Obes* (2015) 22:290–5. doi: 10.1097/MED.0000000000000171
69. Coppieters KT, Dotta F, Amirian N, Campbell PD, Kay TW, Atkinson MA, et al. Demonstration of Islet-Autoreactive CD8 T Cells in Insulitic Lesions From Recent Onset and Long-Term Type 1 Diabetes Patients. *J Exp Med* (2012) 209:51–60. doi: 10.1084/jem.20111187
70. Pathiraja V, Kuehlich JP, Campbell PD, Krishnamurthy B, Loudovaris T, Coates PT, et al. Proinsulin-Specific, HLA-DQ8, and HLA-DQ8-Transdimer-Restricted CD4+ T Cells Infiltrate Islets in Type 1 Diabetes. *Diabetes* (2015) 64:172–82. doi: 10.2337/db14-0858
71. Babon JA, DeNicola ME, Blodgett DM, Crèvecoeur I, Buttrick TS, Maehr R, et al. Analysis of Self-Antigen Specificity of Islet-Infiltrating T Cells From Human Donors With Type 1 Diabetes. *Nat Med* (2016) 22:1482–7. doi: 10.1038/nm.4203
72. Seay HR, Yusko E, Rothweiler SJ, Zhang L, Posgai AL, Campbell-Thompson M, et al. Tissue Distribution and Clonal Diversity of the T and B Cell Repertoire in Type 1 Diabetes. *JCI Insight* (2016) 1:e88242. doi: 10.1172/jci.insight.88242
73. Michels AW, Landry LG, McDaniel KA, Yu L, Campbell-Thompson M, Kwok WW, et al. Islet-Derived CD4 T Cells Targeting Proinsulin in Human Autoimmune Diabetes. *Diabetes* (2017) 66:722–34. doi: 10.2337/db16-1025
74. Anderson AM, Landry LG, Alkanani AA, Pyle L, Powers AC, Atkinson MA, et al. Human Islet T Cells Are Highly Reactive to Preproinsulin in Type 1 Diabetes. *Proc Natl Acad Sci USA* (2021) 118(41):e2107208118. doi: 10.1073/pnas.2107208118
75. Somoza N, Vargas F, Roura-Mir C, Vives-Pi M, Fernández-Figueras MT, Ariza A, et al. Pancreas in Recent Onset Insulin-Dependent Diabetes Mellitus. Changes in HLA, Adhesion Molecules and Autoantigens, Restricted T Cell Receptor V Beta Usage, and Cytokine Profile. *J Immunol (Baltimore Md. 1950)* (1994) 153:1360–77.
76. Yamagata K, Nakajima H, Tomita K, Itoh N, Miyagawa J, Hamaguchi T, et al. Dominant TCR Alpha-Chain Clonotypes and Interferon-Gamma Are Expressed in the Pancreas of Patients With Recent-Onset Insulin-Dependent Diabetes Mellitus. *Diabetes Res Clin Pract* (1996) 34:37–46. doi: 10.1016/S0168-8227(96)01328-9
77. Codina-Busqueta E, Scholz E, Muñoz-Torres PM, Roura-Mir C, Costa M, Xufré C, et al. TCR Bias of *In Vivo* Expanded T Cells in Pancreatic Islets and Spleen at the Onset in Human Type 1 Diabetes. *J Immunol (Baltimore Md. 1950)* (2011) 186:3787–97. doi: 10.4049/jimmunol.1002423
78. Jacobsen LM, Posgai A, Seay HR, Haller MJ, Brusko TM. T Cell Receptor Profiling in Type 1 Diabetes. *Curr Diabetes Rep* (2017) 17:118. doi: 10.1007/s11892-017-0946-4
79. Reijonen H, Mallone R, Heninger AK, Laughlin EM, Kochik SA, Falk B, et al. GAD65-Specific CD4+ T-Cells With High Antigen Avidity Are Prevalent in Peripheral Blood of Patients With Type 1 Diabetes. *Diabetes* (2004) 53:1987–94. doi: 10.2337/diabetes.53.8.1987
80. Gebe JA, Yue BB, Unrath KA, Falk BA, Nepom GT. Restricted Autoantigen Recognition Associated With Deletional and Adaptive Regulatory Mechanisms. *J Immunol (Baltimore Md. 1950)* (2009) 183:59–65. doi: 10.4049/jimmunol.0804046
81. Cerosaletti K, Barahmand-Pour-Whitman F, Yang J, DeBerg HA, Dufort MJ, Murray SA, et al. Single-Cell RNA Sequencing Reveals Expanded Clones

of Islet Antigen-Reactive CD4(+) T Cells in Peripheral Blood of Subjects With Type 1 Diabetes. *J Immunol (Baltimore Md. 1950)* (2017) 199:323–35. doi: 10.4049/jimmunol.1700172
82. Yeh WI, Seay HR, Newby B, Posgai AL, Moniz FB, Michels A, et al. Avidity and Bystander Suppressive Capacity of Human Regulatory T Cells Expressing *De Novo* Autoreactive T-Cell Receptors in Type 1 Diabetes. *Front Immunol* (2017) 8:1313. doi: 10.3389/fimmu.2017.01313
83. Landry LG, Anderson AM, Russ HA, Yu L, Kent SC, Atkinson MA, et al. Proinsulin-Reactive CD4 T Cells in the Islets of Type 1 Diabetes Organ Donors. *Front Endocrinol* (2021) 12:622647. doi: 10.3389/fendo.2021.622647
84. Endl J, Rosinger S, Schwarz B, Friedrich SO, Rothe G, Karges W, et al. Coexpression of CD25 and OX40 (CD134) Receptors Delineates Autoreactive T-Cells in Type 1 Diabetes. *Diabetes* (2006) 55:50–60. doi: 10.2337/diabetes.55.01.06.db05-0387
85. Kent SC, Chen Y, Bregoli L, Clemmings SM, Kenyon NS, Ricordi C, et al. Expanded T Cells From Pancreatic Lymph Nodes of Type 1 Diabetic Subjects Recognize an Insulin Epitope. *Nature* (2005) 435:224–8. doi: 10.1038/nature03625
86. So M, Elso CM, Tresoldi E, Pakusch M, Pathiraja V, Wentworth JM, et al. Proinsulin C-Peptide Is an Autoantigen in People With Type 1 Diabetes. *Proc Natl Acad Sci USA* (2018) 115:10732–7. doi: 10.1073/pnas.1809208115
87. Eerligh P, van Lummel M, Zaldumbide A, Moustakas AK, Duinkerken G, Bondinas G, et al. Functional Consequences of HLA-DQ8 Homozygosity Versus Heterozygosity for Islet Autoimmunity in Type 1 Diabetes. *Genes Immun* (2011) 12:415–27. doi: 10.1038/gene.2011.24
88. Tan S, Li Y, Xia J, Jin CH, Hu Z, Duinkerken G, et al. Type 1 Diabetes Induction in Humanized Mice. *Proc Natl Acad Sci USA* (2017) 114:10954–9. doi: 10.1073/pnas.1710415114
89. Yang J, Chow IT, Sosinowski T, Torres-Chinn N, Greenbaum CJ, James EA, et al. Autoreactive T Cells Specific for Insulin B:11-23 Recognize a Low-Affinity Peptide Register in Human Subjects With Autoimmune Diabetes. *Proc Natl Acad Sci USA* (2014) 111:14840–5. doi: 10.1073/pnas.1416864111
90. Williams T, Krovi HS, Landry LG, Crawford F, Jin N, Hohenstein A, et al. Development of T Cell Lines Sensitive to Antigen Stimulation. *J Immunol Methods* (2018) 462:65–73. doi: 10.1016/j.jim.2018.08.011
91. Delong T, Wiles TA, Baker RL, Bradley B, Barbour G, Reisdorph R, et al. Pathogenic CD4 T Cells in Type 1 Diabetes Recognize Epitopes Formed by Peptide Fusion. *Sci (New York NY)* (2016) 351:711–4. doi: 10.1126/science.aad2791
92. Tran MT, Faridi P, Lim JJ, Ting YT, Onwukwe G, Bhattacharjee P, et al. T Cell Receptor Recognition of Hybrid Insulin Peptides Bound to HLA-Dq8. *Nat Commun* (2021) 12:5110. doi: 10.1038/s41467-021-25404-x
93. Baker RL, Rihanek M, Hohenstein AC, Nakayama M, Michels A, Gottlieb PA, et al. Hybrid Insulin Peptides Are Autoantigens in Type 1 Diabetes. *Diabetes* (2019) 68:1830–40. doi: 10.2337/db19-0128
94. Wiles TA, Hohenstein A, Landry LG, Dang M, Powell R, Guyer P, et al. Characterization of Human CD4 T Cells Specific for a C-Peptide/C-Peptide Hybrid Insulin Peptide. *Front Immunol* (2021) 12:668680. doi: 10.3389/fimmu.2021.668680
95. Skowera A, Ellis RJ, Varela-Calviño R, Arif S, Huang GC, Van-Krinks C, et al. CTLs Are Targeted to Kill Beta Cells in Patients With Type 1 Diabetes Through Recognition of a Glucose-Regulated Preproinsulin Epitope. *J Clin Invest* (2008) 118:3390–402. doi: 10.1172/JCI35449
96. Kronenberg D, Knight RR, Estorninho M, Ellis RJ, Kester MG, de Ru A, et al. Circulating Preproinsulin Signal Peptide-Specific CD8 T Cells Restricted by the Susceptibility Molecule HLA-A24 Are Expanded at Onset of Type 1 Diabetes and Kill β-Cells. *Diabetes* (2012) 61:1752–9. doi: 10.2337/db11-1520
97. Unger WW, Pearson T, Abreu JR, Laban S, van der Slik AR, der Kracht SM, et al. Islet-Specific CTL Cloned From a Type 1 Diabetes Patient Cause Beta-Cell Destruction After Engraftment Into HLA-A2 Transgenic NOD/scid/IL2RG Null Mice. *PloS One* (2012) 7:e49213. doi: 10.1371/journal.pone.0049213
98. Babad J, Mukherjee G, Follenzi A, Ali R, Roep BO, Shultz LD, et al. Generation of β Cell-Specific Human Cytotoxic T Cells by Lentiviral Transduction and Their Survival in Immunodeficient Human Leucocyte Antigen-Transgenic Mice. *Clin Exp Immunol* (2015) 179:398–413. doi: 10.1111/cei.12465
99. Kracht MJ, van Lummel M, Nikolic T, Joosten AM, Laban S, van der Slik AR, et al. Autoimmunity Against a Defective Ribosomal Insulin Gene Product in Type 1 Diabetes. *Nat Med* (2017) 23:501–7. doi: 10.1038/nm.4289
100. Zhang W, Hawkins PG, He J, Gupta NT, Liu J, Choonoo G, et al. A Framework for Highly Multiplexed Dextramer Mapping and Prediction of T Cell Receptor Sequences to Antigen Specificity. *Sci Adv* (2021) 7(20): eabf5835. doi: 10.1126/sciadv.abf5835
101. Sidhom JW, Larman HB, Pardoll DM, Baras AS. DeepTCR Is a Deep Learning Framework for Revealing Sequence Concepts Within T-Cell Repertoires. *Nat Commun* (2021) 12:1605. doi: 10.1038/s41467-021-21879-w
102. Mann SE, Zhou Z, Landry LG, Anderson AM, Alkanani AK, Fischer J, et al. Multiplex T Cell Stimulation Assay Utilizing a T Cell Activation Reporter-Based Detection System. *Front Immunol* (2020) 11:633. doi: 10.3389/fimmu.2020.00633
103. Landry LG, Mann SE, Anderson AM, Nakayama M. Multiplex T-Cell Stimulation Assay Utilizing a T-Cell Activation Reporter-Based Detection System. *Bio-Protocol* (2021) 11:e3883. doi: 10.21769/BioProtoc.3883
104. Stene LC, Oikarinen S, Hyöty H, Barriga KJ, Norris JM, Klingensmith G, et al. Enterovirus Infection and Progression From Islet Autoimmunity to Type 1 Diabetes: The Diabetes and Autoimmunity Study in the Young (DAISY). *Diabetes* (2010) 59:3174–80. doi: 10.2337/db10-0866
105. Beyerlein A, Wehweck F, Ziegler AG, Pflueger M. Respiratory Infections in Early Life and the Development of Islet Autoimmunity in Children at Increased Type 1 Diabetes Risk: Evidence From the BABYDIET Study. *JAMA Pediatr* (2013) 167:800–7. doi: 10.1001/jamapediatrics.2013.158
106. Ashton MP, Eugster A, Walther D, Daehling N, Riethausen S, Kuehn D, et al. Incomplete Immune Response to Coxsackie B Viruses Associates With Early Autoimmunity Against Insulin. *Sci Rep* (2016) 6:32899. doi: 10.1038/srep32899
107. Beshnova D, Ye J, Onabolu O, Moon B, Zheng W, Fu YX, et al. *De Novo* Prediction of Cancer-Associated T Cell Receptors for Noninvasive Cancer Detection. *Sci Trans Med* (2020) 12(557):eaaz3738. doi: 10.1126/scitranslmed.aaz3738
108. Zhang H, Zhan X, Li B. GIANA Allows Computationally-Efficient TCR Clustering and Multi-Disease Repertoire Classification by Isometric Transformation. *Nat Commun* (2021) 12:4699. doi: 10.1038/s41467-021-25006-7
109. Ishizuka J, Stewart-Jones GB, van der Merwe A, Bell JI, McMichael AJ, Jones EY. The Structural Dynamics and Energetics of an Immunodominant T Cell Receptor Are Programmed by Its Vbeta Domain. *Immunity* (2008) 28:171–82. doi: 10.1016/j.immuni.2007.12.018
110. Song I, Gil A, Mishra R, Ghersi D, Selin LK, Stern LJ. Broad TCR Repertoire and Diverse Structural Solutions for Recognition of an Immunodominant CD8(+) T Cell Epitope. *Nat Struct Mol Biol* (2017) 24:395–406. doi: 10.1038/nsmb.3383
111. Dash P, Fiore-Gartland AJ, Hertz T, Wang GC, Sharma S, Souquette A, et al. Quantifiable Predictive Features Define Epitope-Specific T Cell Receptor Repertoires. *Nature* (2017) 547:89–93. doi: 10.1038/nature22383
112. Cole DK, Yuan F, Rizkallah PJ, Miles JJ, Gostick E, Price DA, et al. Germ Line-Governed Recognition of a Cancer Epitope by an Immunodominant Human T-Cell Receptor. *J Biol Chem* (2009) 284:27281–9. doi: 10.1074/jbc.M109.022509
113. Nakayama M, McDaniel K, Fitzgerald-Miller L, Kiekhaefer C, Snell-Bergeon JK, Davidson HW, et al. Regulatory vs. Inflammatory Cytokine T-Cell Responses to Mutated Insulin Peptides in Healthy and Type 1 Diabetic Subjects. *Proc Natl Acad Sci USA* (2015) 112:4429–34. doi: 10.1073/pnas.1502967112
114. Mitchell AM, Alkanani AA, McDaniel KA, Pyle L, Waugh K, Steck AK, et al. T-Cell Responses to Hybrid Insulin Peptides Prior to Type 1 Diabetes Development. *Proc Natl Acad Sci USA* (2021) 118(6):e2019129118. doi: 10.1073/pnas.2019129118
115. Lee CH, Salio M, Napolitani G, Ogg G, Simmons A, Koohy H. Predicting Cross-Reactivity and Antigen Specificity of T Cell Receptors. *Front Immunol* (2020) 11:565096. doi: 10.3389/fimmu.2020.565096
116. Vujovic M, Degn KF, Marin FI, Schaap-Johansen AL, Chain B, Andresen TL, et al. T Cell Receptor Sequence Clustering and Antigen Specificity. *Comput Struct Biotechnol J* (2020) 18:2166–73. doi: 10.1016/j.csbj.2020.06.041

117. Glanville J, Huang H, Nau A, Hatton O, Wagar LE, Rubelt F, et al. Identifying Specificity Groups in the T Cell Receptor Repertoire. *Nature* (2017) 547:94–8. doi: 10.1038/nature22976
118. Huang H, Wang C, Rubelt F, Scriba TJ, Davis MM. Analyzing the Mycobacterium Tuberculosis Immune Response by T-Cell Receptor Clustering With GLIPH2 and Genome-Wide Antigen Screening. *Nat Biotechnol* (2020) 38:1194–202. doi: 10.1038/s41587-020-0505-4
119. Valkiers S, Van Houcke M, Laukens K, Meysman P. ClusTCR: A Python Interface for Rapid Clustering of Large Sets of CDR3 Sequences With Unknown Antigen Specificity. *Bioinf (Oxford England)* (2021) btab446. doi: 10.1101/2021.02.22.432291
120. Chronister WD, Crinklaw A, Mahajan S, Vita R, Koşaloğlu-Yalçın Z, Yan Z, et al. TCRMatch: Predicting T-Cell Receptor Specificity Based on Sequence Similarity to Previously Characterized Receptors. *Front Immunol* (2021) 12:640725. doi: 10.3389/fimmu.2021.640725
121. Shugay M, Bagaev DV, Zvyagin IV, Vroomans RM, Crawford JC, Dolton G, et al. VDJdb: A Curated Database of T-Cell Receptor Sequences With Known Antigen Specificity. *Nucleic Acids Res* (2018) 46:D419–d427. doi: 10.1093/nar/gkx760
122. Omer A, Shemesh O, Peres A, Polak P, Shepherd AJ, Watson CT, et al. VDJbase: An Adaptive Immune Receptor Genotype and Haplotype Database. *Nucleic Acids Res* (2020) 48:D1051–6. doi: 10.1093/nar/gkz872
123. Vita R, Mahajan S, Overton JA, Dhanda SK, Martini S, Cantrell JR, et al. The Immune Epitope Database (IEDB): 2018 Update. *Nucleic Acids Res* (2019) 47:D339–d343. doi: 10.1093/nar/gky1006
124. Bagaev DV, Vroomans RMA, Samir J, Stervbo U, Rius C, Dolton G, et al. VDJdb in 2019: Database Extension, New Analysis Infrastructure and a T-Cell Receptor Motif Compendium. *Nucleic Acids Res* (2020) 48:D1057–d1062. doi: 10.1093/nar/gkz874
125. Corrie BD, Marthandan N, Zimonja B, Jaglale J, Zhou Y, Barr E, et al. Ireceptor: A Platform for Querying and Analyzing Antibody/B-Cell and T-Cell Receptor Repertoire Data Across Federated Repositories. *Immunol Rev* (2018) 284:24–41. doi: 10.1111/imr.12666
126. Tickotsky N, Sagiv T, Prilusky J, Shifrut E, Friedman N. McPAS-TCR: A Manually Curated Catalogue of Pathology-Associated T Cell Receptor Sequences. *Bioinf (Oxford England)* (2017) 33:2924–9. doi: 10.1093/bioinformatics/btx286
127. Bender C, Rodriguez-Calvo T, Amirian N, Coppieters KT, von Herrath MG. The Healthy Exocrine Pancreas Contains Preproinsulin-Specific CD8 T Cells That Attack Islets in Type 1 Diabetes. *Sci Adv* (2020) 6(42):eabc5586. doi: 10.1126/sciadv.abc5586
128. Lindley S, Dayan CM, Bishop A, Roep BO, Peakman M, Tree TI. Defective Suppressor Function in CD4(+)CD25(+) T-Cells From Patients With Type 1 Diabetes. *Diabetes* (2005) 54:92–9. doi: 10.2337/diabetes.54.1.92
129. Tree TI, Lawson J, Edwards H, Skowera A, Arif S, Roep BO, et al. Naturally Arising Human CD4 T-Cells That Recognize Islet Autoantigens and Secrete Interleukin-10 Regulate Proinflammatory T-Cell Responses *via* Linked Suppression. *Diabetes* (2010) 59:1451–60. doi: 10.2337/db09-0503
130. Chadt A, Immisch A, de Wendt C, Springer C, Zhou Z, Stermann T, et al. "Deletion of Both Rab-GTPase–Activating Proteins TBC1D1 and TBC1D4 in Mice Eliminates Insulin- and AICAR-Stimulated Glucose Transport [Corrected]. *Diabetes* (2015) 64:746–59. doi: 10.2337/db14-0368
131. Skowera A, Ladell K, McLaren JE, Dolton G, Matthews KK, Gostick E, et al. β-Cell-Specific CD8 T Cell Phenotype in Type 1 Diabetes Reflects Chronic Autoantigen Exposure. *Diabetes* (2015) 64:916–25. doi: 10.2337/db14-0332
132. Risnes LF, Christophersen A, Dahal-Koirala S, Neumann RS, Sandve GK, Sarna VK, et al. Disease-Driving CD4+ T Cell Clonotypes Persist for Decades in Celiac Disease. *J Clin Invest* (2018) 128:2642–50. doi: 10.1172/JCI98819

15

Tolerance to Proinsulin-1 Reduces Autoimmune Diabetes in NOD Mice

Gaurang Jhala[1,2], Claudia Selck[1†], Jonathan Chee[3,4], Chun-Ting J. Kwong[1], Evan G. Pappas[1], Helen E. Thomas[1,2], Thomas W.H. Kay[1,2‡] and Balasubramanian Krishnamurthy[1,2‡]*

[1] St. Vincent's Institute, Fitzroy, VIC, Australia, [2] Department of Medicine, The University of Melbourne, St Vincent's Hospital, Fitzroy, VIC, Australia, [3] National Centre for Asbestos Related Diseases, Institute of Respiratory Health, University of Western Australia, Perth, WA, Australia, [4] School of Biomedical Sciences, University of Western Australia, Perth, WA, Australia

***Correspondence:**
Thomas W.H. Kay
tkay@svi.edu.au

†Present address:
Imperial College London, United Kingdom

‡These authors have contributed equally to this work and share senior authorship

T-cell responses to insulin and its precursor proinsulin are central to islet autoimmunity in humans and non-obese diabetic (NOD) mice that spontaneously develop autoimmune diabetes. Mice have two proinsulin genes proinsulin -1 and 2 that are differentially expressed, with predominant proinsulin-2 expression in the thymus and proinsulin-1 in islet beta-cells. In contrast to proinsulin-2, proinsulin-1 knockout NOD mice are protected from autoimmune diabetes. This indicates that proinsulin-1 epitopes in beta-cells maybe preferentially targeted by autoreactive T cells. To study the contribution of proinsulin-1 reactive T cells in autoimmune diabetes, we generated transgenic NOD mice with tetracycline-regulated expression of proinsulin-1 in antigen presenting cells (TIP-1 mice) with an aim to induce immune tolerance. TIP-1 mice displayed a significantly reduced incidence of spontaneous diabetes, which was associated with reduced severity of insulitis and insulin autoantibody development. Antigen experienced proinsulin specific T cells were significantly reduced in in TIP-1 mice indicating immune tolerance. Moreover, T cells from TIP-1 mice expressing proinsulin-1 transferred diabetes at a significantly reduced frequency. However, proinsulin-1 expression in APCs had minimal impact on the immune responses to the downstream antigen islet-specific glucose-6-phosphatase catalytic subunit-related protein (IGRP) and did not prevent diabetes in NOD 8.3 mice with a pre-existing repertoire of IGRP reactive T cells. Thus, boosting immune tolerance to proinsulin-1 partially prevents islet-autoimmunity. This study further extends the previously established role of proinsulin-1 epitopes in autoimmune diabetes in NOD mice.

Keywords: type 1 diabetes, proinsulin-1, CD4+ T cells, immune tolerance, NOD mice

INTRODUCTION

Recognition of proinsulin by the immune system is a major determinant in the pathogenesis of autoimmune diabetes in both humans and non-obese diabetic (NOD) mice (1, 2). A polymorphic variable number of tandem repeats (VNTR) located in the promoter region of the insulin locus controls the transcription level of the *Ins* gene and is strongly associated with susceptibility to type 1 diabetes (T1D) in humans (3–5). Mice do not have a VNTR upstream of the insulin locus; however, they have two Insulin genes, *Ins1* and *Ins2* encoding proteins that are highly homologous with 92% identity at the amino acid level. Proinsulin 1 and 2 proteins have identical A chains but differ by two amino acids in the B chain, three amino acids in the connecting peptide (C-peptide) and six amino acids in the leader peptide (6). The two proinsulin isoforms are differentially expressed with proinsulin 1 (PIns1) predominantly expressed in the pancreatic beta-cells and proinsulin 2 (PIns2) being the predominant isoform detected in the thymus (7–9).

Immune responses to native insulin peptides, in particular the B chain amino acids 9-23 (Ins B:9-23), are essential for autoimmune diabetes in NOD mice (10, 11). The two proinsulin isoforms differ by a single amino acid in the B: 9-23 region (PIns1: B9 proline, PIns2: B9 serine) and strong cross-reactivity of T cells for the Ins B: 9-23 epitope in both proinsulin molecules has also been reported (12). Despite the high degree of homology in the B:9-23 epitope and cross-reactivity of T cells for the Ins B: 9-23 epitope, a divergent immune response was observed when NOD mice were immunized with either Ins1 B:9-23 or Ins2 B:9-23 peptides, with Ins2 peptide conferring protection from diabetes onset, whereas Ins1 peptide did not prevent disease (13, 14). Further differences in cellular and humoral immune responses to both proinsulin isoforms have been highlighted by individual gene knockouts. NOD mice lacking *Ins2* gene develop accelerated diabetes, ascribed to loss of central tolerance to insulin peptides; however, development of insulin autoantibodies (IAA) in *Ins2 -/-* mice suggests that immune responses against PIns1 epitopes are intact (15). In contrast, genetic deletion of *Ins1* or replacement of murine *Ins1* with human insulin gene (*INS*) in NOD mice provides significant protection from diabetes (16, 17). Protection from diabetes in NOD mice lacking *Ins1* is likely due to the absence of cognate antigen in the target tissue, indicating that PIns1 peptides may be primarily targeted by insulin reactive T cells. Immunogenic epitopes in the PIns1 molecule have been reported (18), and T cells recognizing PIns1 amino acids 47-64 in the C-peptide region induce diabetes in NOD.SCID recipients (19). Thus, epitopes in PIns1 molecule may contribute to islet autoimmunity.

In contrast to NOD mice, non-autoimmune strains lacking *Ins2* globally (20), or in medullary thymic epithelial cells (mTECs) did not develop pathological islet destruction however, when C57Bl/6 mice lacking Ins2 in mTECs were crossed to *Ins1* knockout mice, the progeny developed spontaneous autoimmune diabetes within 3 weeks after birth (21). These studies suggest that thymic expression of PIns1 may add to the effect of PIns2 in eliminating insulin-specific autoreactive T cells. Constitutive or temporal expression of PIns2 in APCs induces recessive tolerance to PIns2 as it provides lasting protection from autoimmune diabetes in NOD mice (22). These mice were also thought to be tolerant to PIns1 epitopes because of cross-reactivity of the T cells to the conserved Ins B: 9-23 epitope. However, the role of PIns1 specific immune responses in pathogenesis of islet autoimmunity in NOD mice remains unclear, given the differential immune response observed upon immunization with Ins1 B:9-23 or Ins2 B:9-23 peptide. To resolve this, we investigated the impact of induced PIns1 expression in APCs on the development of antigen-specific T cells as well as insulitis and diabetes in NOD mice.

MATERIALS AND METHODS

TetO-Ins1 Mice

To generate the TetO-Ins1 construct, a 411 bp cDNA fragment spanning the coding region of murine PIns1 was amplified by PCR using NOD pancreatic islet cDNA as a template and cloned into HindIII and EcoRV sites of the pTRE-tight plasmid (Clontech). A 1100 bp transgene cassette comprising of the TetO-minimal CMV promoter, followed by the PIns1 gene and a polyA signal was excised between Xho I sites and purified for injection into fertilized NOD/Lt ova using standard techniques. Founders and transgene positive offspring were screened by PCR using primers spanning the PIns1 gene (5'-TTAAGATATCTTCATTCATTATAGAACTC -3') and the tetO-CMV promoter (5'-TCAGTGATAGAGAACGTATGTCG -3').

Other Mice

NOD/Lt mice were bred and housed at the bioresources center St. Vincent's Hospital, Fitzroy. The NOD-IEα-tTA mice that drive the expression of tetracycline transactivator (tTA) under the control of MHC class II IEα promoter have been previously described (23) and were obtained from Prof. C. Benoist and Prof. D. Mathis (Dept of Pathology, Harvard Medical School, Boston, Massachusetts, USA). Generation of NOD8.3 mice, which express the TCRαβ rearrangements of the H-2Kd-restricted, β cell-reactive, CD8+ T cell clone NY8.3, was previously described in detail (24). TIP-1/8.3 mice were generated by crossing NOD-IEα-tTA-TetO-Ins1double transgenic TIP-1 mice with TCR transgenic NOD8.3 mice. All mice were bred, maintained and used under specific pathogen free conditions at St Vincent's Institute (Melbourne, Australia). All experimental procedures followed the guidelines approved by the institutional animal ethics committee.

Doxycycline Treatment

Untreated TIP-1 mice constitutively express proinsulin-1 in antigen presenting cells (APCs). To turn-off proinsulin-1 expression, doxycycline hyclate (Dox) (Sigma-Aldrich) was administered *via* drinking water at concentration of 2mg/ml. Water bottles were changed thrice weekly.

RT-PCR

For total RNA extraction, whole spleen and thymus were harvested in cold Phosphate Buffered Saline (PBS). Tissue homogenates were prepared in RNA lysis buffer RA1 (Macherey-Nagel) from a 15mg slice of tissue using a tissue homogenizer. RNA was isolated using Nucleospin RNA II-isolate kits (Macherey-Nagel), and first strand cDNA was generated from 500ng RNA using High Capacity cDNA Reverse Transcription kits (Applied Biosystem) according to the manufacturers' instructions. cDNA was diluted (1:20) and Real-time PCR analysis was performed using Rotor-Gene-RG-3000 cycler (Corbett Research, Sydney, Australia). Taqman gene expression primers murine insulin 1 (*Ins1*; Mm01950294_s1), murine β-actin (*Actb*; Mm00607939_s1) and murine Glyceraldehyde 3-phosphate dehydrogenase (*Gapdh*; Mm99999915_g1) were purchased from Applied Biosystems. To determine relative expression, Ct values of Insulin were subtracted from Ct values of reference genes for each sample and the difference (dCt) was plotted to determine the abundance of the gene of interest.

Histology and Immunohistochemistry

For immunohistochemistry, pancreata were snap-frozen in optimal cutting temperature compound (OCT Compound; Sakura Finetek, Torrance, CA) and stored at −80°C. For histological analysis 5-µm frozen sections of pancreas were prepared from three levels (200 µm apart), acetone fixed, stained with guinea pig anti-insulin followed by horseradish peroxidase–conjugated anti–guinea pig Ig (Dako Cytomation, Carpenteria, CA) and counterstained with hematoxylin. Insulitis was graded using the following scale: 0 = no infiltrate, 1 = peri-islet infiltrate, 2 = extensive (>50%) peri-islet infiltrate, 3 = intraislet infiltrate, and 4 = extensive intraislet infiltrate (>80%) or total β-cell loss. The percentage of islets with each grade per pancreas was calculated by addition of the grades for the three sections. Individual insulitis scoring for each mouse was performed as previously described (22).

Incidence of Diabetes and Insulitis

Diabetes onset was monitored by weekly measurement of urine glucose levels using Diastix (Bayer Diagnostics). Blood glucose levels were measured in mice with glycosuria using Advantage II Glucose strips (Roche). Animals displaying two consecutive blood glucose measurements of ≥ 15mmol/L were considered diabetic. For adoptive transfer of diabetes, 2 $x10^7$ splenocytes from 13-17 week old pre-diabetic TIP-1 mice or control NOD mice were transferred (i.v.) into 9-12week old NOD Rag-/- recipients and diabetes development was monitored as above.

Flow Cytometry

Antibodies used were anti-CD4 (RM4-5) conjugated to PerCpCy5.5, anti-CD3 (145-2C11) conjugated to FITC or anti-CD3 (500 A2) V500, anti-CD44 (1M7) conjugated to AlexaFlour700 (all BD Biosciences), anti-CD11c (N418), anti-B220 (RA3-6B2), anti-CD11b (M1/70), anti-F4/80 (BM8) conjugated to eFlour450 and anti-FoxP3 (FJK-16S) conjugated to APC (all eBiosciences), anti-CD8a (5H10) conjugated to Pacific Orange (Invitrogen) or anti-CD8a (53-6.7) conjugated to PE-Cy7, anti-CD62L (MEL-14) conjugated to APC-Cy7 (BD Biosciences). FoxP3 was stained intracellularly using FoxP3/Transcription Factor Fixation/Permeabilization kit (eBiosciences). Data were collected on an LSR Fortessa flow-cytometer (BD) and analyzed using FlowJo (Treestar) software.

Tetramer and Magnetic Bead-Based Enrichment

The tetramer and magnetic bead-based enrichment method was previously described (25). I-Ag7 tetramers were obtained from NIH tetramer core facility (Emory University, Georgia, USA), Kd-tetramers were obtained from ImmunoID (Parkville, Victoria, Australia). To enrich insulin-specific CD4+ T cells single cell suspensions from peripheral lymphoid organs (PLO), (pooled spleen and non-draining lymph nodes), were stained with phycoerythrin (PE)-conjugated I-Ag7-$INSB_{10-23}$ (HLVERLYLVCGGEG) tetramer for 1 hour at room temperature. The Ins B_{10-23} peptide in the I-Ag7-$INSB_{10-23}$ tetramer has been mutated (Glutamic acid to Glycine (E-G) at position 20 and Arginine to Glycine (R-G) at position 21) to improve its binding to the I-Ag7 molecule, which allows for better detection of insulin-specific CD4+ T cells (26). Insulin-specific CD8+ T cells were enriched from pooled PLO by staining the cell suspensions with APC-conjugated H-2Kd- $INSB_{15-23}$ (LYLVCGGEG) tetramer for 1 hour on ice. Hen Egg Lysozyme I-Ag7-HEL (AMKRHGLDNYRGYSL) tetramer or H-2Kd-TUM (KYQAVTTTL) were used as controls. Cells were then washed and stained with anti-PE or anti-APC microbeads (Miltenyi Biotec) followed by magnetic separation using an AutoMACSpro (Miltenyi Biotec) according to manufacturer's instructions. $IGRP_{206-214}$ specific CD8+ T cells (H2-Kd, VYLKTNVFL) were stained and enriched as previously described (27). The separated fractions were stained and analyzed by flow cytometry. Gating strategy for tetramer enrichment was as follows: single cells were gated on forward and side scatter, and dead cells excluded using propidium iodide. From the live cell population, CD11c-CD11b-B220-F4/80-CD3+ cells were gated as the T cell population for analysis. Further selection of CD4+ T cells or CD8+ T cells was followed by analysis of the insulin or IGRP tetramer positive population respectively.

Insulin Autoantibody (IAA) Assay

A non-competitive IAA assay was performed in a 96 well ELISA format as previously described (28, 29). Briefly, an ELISA plate (Costar) was coated with or without human insulin (10 µg/ml, Actrapid, Novo Nordisk) overnight at 4°C. Wells were blocked with PBS containing 2% BSA for 2 hours and room-temperature and then probed with sera from 12-15 weeks old TIP mice, NOD or C57BL/6 mice (1:10 dilution) for 2 hours. Wells were washed 4 times and a biotinylated anti-mouse IgG1 (AbCam, 1:10000 dilution) antibody was added for 30 minutes. After washing, horse-radish-peroxidase conjugated streptavidin (BioLegend) was added for 15 minutes. The plate was washed five times, TMB substrate solution (BioLegend) was added and absorbance was measured at 450 nm using a Polarstar (BMG labtech) microplate reader. Each sample was run in duplicate and absorbance (450 nm) of test sample without plate bound insulin was subtracted from absorbance of test sample with plate bound insulin to calculate the actual absorbance value for each sample.

Statistical Analysis

Statistical analysis was performed using GraphPad Prism 8 Software (GraphPad, San Diego, CA, USA). Pooled data are shown as dot-plots with individual mice and the mean ± SEM. Data were tested for normal distribution using D'Agostino-Pearson omnibus normality test or Shapiro-Wilks test. Comparisons between two groups were performed using two-tailed unpaired student *t*-tests. Multiple comparisons were performed using One-way ANOVA with Sidak's post-hoc test. Survival curves were compared using Log-Rank (Mantel-Cox) test. Statistical significance was defined as $P < 0.05$.

RESULTS

Conditional Expression of Proinsulin-1 in NOD Mice

To test whether inducing immune tolerance to proinsulin-1 (PIns1) influenced autoimmune diabetes we generated transgenic NOD mice to facilitate conditional expression of PIns1 in the antigen presenting cells (APCs). Reporter NOD mice expressing PIns1 under the control of the tetracycline-responsive CMV promoter (TetO-Ins1 mice) were bred with previously described driver NOD mice expressing TetR-VP16 tetracycline transactivator protein (tTA) under the control of IEα-MHC-II promoter referred to as TA-NOD mice (23). Bi-transgenic progeny referred to as TIP-1 (Tet Inducible PIns1) mice (**Figure 1A**) express Pins1 in the APCs, which can be turned-off upon doxycycline (Dox) treatment. Analysis of PIns1 expression in TIP-1 mice revealed that PIns1 transgene was expressed in the thymus and spleen as measured by RT-PCR (**Figure 1B**). After one week of Dox treatment, PIns1 expression dropped to baseline levels (**Figure S1**). Thus, PIns1 expression in TIP-1 mice was conditional, and tightly regulated.

TIP-1 Mice Have Reduced Insulitis and Insulin Autoantibody Expression

We recently reported that constitutive or temporal expression of PIns2 (PIns2) in the APCs limited to the perinatal period prevented insulitis and diabetes in NOD mice (22). To test whether PIns1 expression in the APCs influenced the progression of islet autoimmunity, we examined the immune infiltrate (insulitis) in the pancreata of TIP-1 mice expressing PIns1 continuously. At 12-14 weeks of age, insulitis was significantly reduced in TIP-1 mice expressing PIns1 compared to age matched NOD mice or TIP-1 mice fed dox to suppress PIns1 expression (**Figures 2A–C**). Analysis of pancreas histology from TIP-1 mice at 20-25 weeks of age revealed that approximately 50% of the islets examined were free of insulitis, whereas more than 80% of the islets examined from non-transgenic littermates were infiltrated (**Figures 2D, E** and **Table S1**), indicating that PIns1 expression in the APCs decreased but did not completely abolish development of insulitis, which progressed over time. Production of insulin autoantibodies (IAA) indicates spontaneous anti-insulin autoimmunity and IAA are frequently detected prior to diabetes onset in both humans and NOD mice (30, 31). We examined whether induced PIns1 expression in TIP-1 mice influenced B cell mediated humoral responses against insulin by measuring IAA in TIP-1 mice. IAA was significantly reduced in 12-15 weeks old TIP-1 mice as compared to age matched non-transgenic NOD mice (**Figure 2F**). Previously described PIns2 tolerant NOD-PI mice that are protected from diabetes and non-autoimmune prone C57BL/6 mice were used to set the baseline. Collectively, these results indicate that immune tolerance to PIns1 influenced progression of insulitis and reduced the development of IAA.

PIns1 Overexpression Partially Suppresses Spontaneous Diabetes in NOD Mice

Reduced insulitis and IAA suggest that diabetes development may be altered in TIP-1 mice. A cohort of female TIP-1 mice expressing PIns1 continuously and control NOD mice were observed for incidence of spontaneous diabetes. TIP-1 mice developed diabetes but at a significantly reduced incidence compared to non-transgenic control NOD mice. By 300 days of age 40% of TIP-1 mice and 65% of the control mice developed diabetes (**Figure 3A**). In addition, we investigated whether PIns1 expression in TIP-1 mice influenced the pathogenic potential of effector T cells. Splenocytes from 15-18 weeks old TIP-1 mice with ongoing expression of PIns1 and age matched control NOD mice were transferred into NOD.Rag1 -/- recipients. All recipient mice receiving control splenocytes developed diabetes between 50-70 days post-transfer, whereas only 2 out of 6 (33%) animals that received splenocytes from TIP-1 mice developed diabetes 70-90 days post-transfer (**Figure 3B**). Taken together these results suggest that overexpression of PIns1 in APCs is able to partially dampen immune responses against insulin and reduce diabetes incidence in NOD mice.

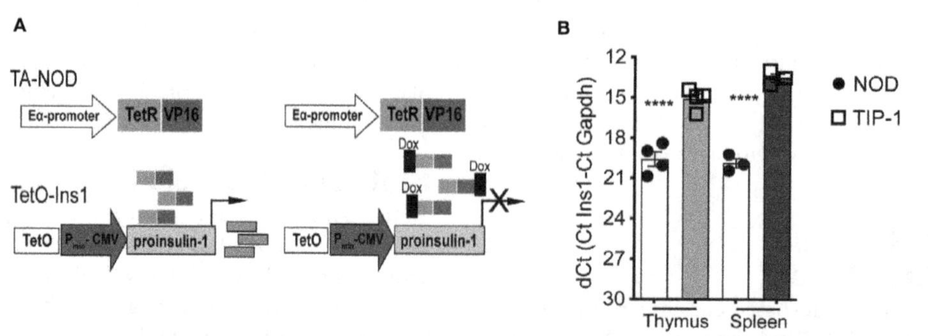

FIGURE 1 | Conditional proinsulin 1 expression in TIP-1 mice **(A)** Scheme of generation of tetracycline regulated NOD.IEα-tTA (TA-NOD) and tetO-Ins1 dual transgenic mice referred to herein as TIP-1 mice. TA-NOD mice were crossed with tetO-Ins1 mice. Bi-transgenic animals constitutively express PIns1 in APCs **(B)** Quantitative RT-PCR was performed using Taqman probes for *Ins1* and *Gapdh* in thymic and splenic lysates of WT-NOD mice TIP-1 mice. Data represent dCT values (Mean ± SEM) from 2-3 independent experiments run in duplicate for each probe. ****P < 0.0001. Data compared using One-way ANOVA with Sidak's multiple comparisons test.

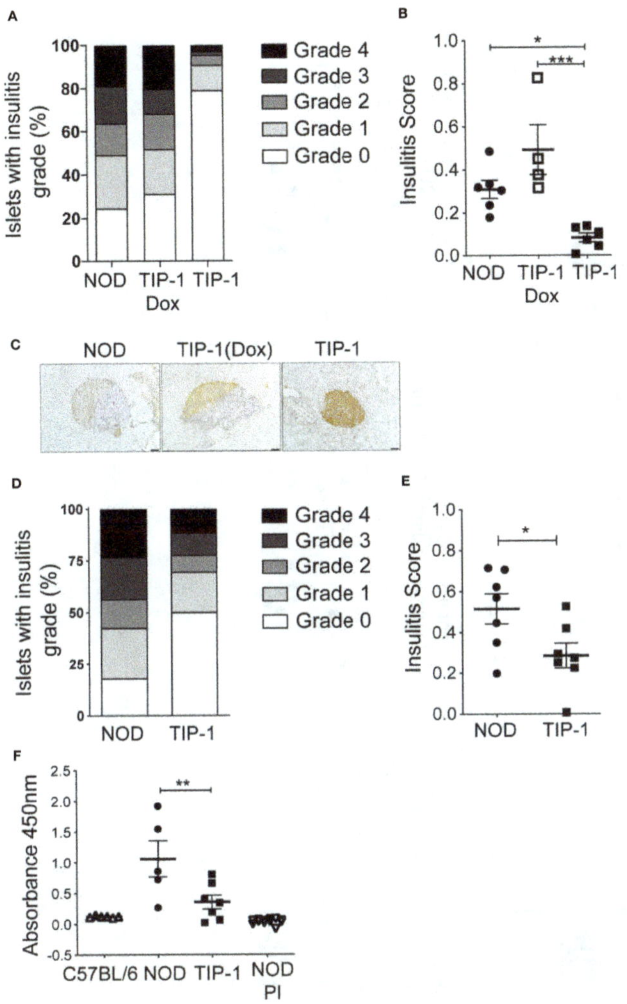

FIGURE 2 | Insulitis and insulin autoantibodies (IAA) in TIP-1 mice **(A, B)** Histological grading and individual insulitis scores in NOD mice, Doxycycline treated and untreated TIP-1 mice at 12-14 weeks of age. **(C)** Representative images of islet histology from 12-14 week old NOD, TIP-1 and Dox treated TIP-1 mice, 200x magnification, scale bar 50 μm. **(D, E)** Histological grading and individual insulitis scores at 20-25 weeks of age in NOD mice and TIP-1 mice (n=4-7, > 60 islets scored per mouse). **(F)** Sera from 12-16 weeks old C57BL/6 mice, NOD mice, TIP-1 and NOD-PI mice were tested for the presence of insulin autoantibodies (IAA) by ELISA assay. Absorbance values at 450nm are plotted. Each symbol in the scatter plot represents data from individual animals. Data plotted as Mean ± SEM, $^{***}P < 0.001$, $^{**}P < 0.01$, $^{*}P < 0.05$. Data compared using One-way ANOVA with Sidak's multiple comparisons test **(B, F)** and 2-tailed unpaired t-test **(E)**.

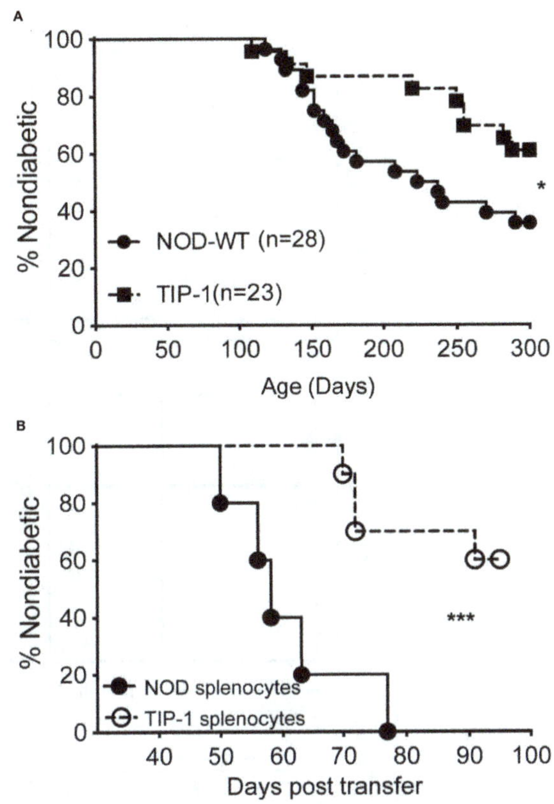

FIGURE 3 | Spontaneous diabetes incidence in TIP-1 mice **(A)** Incidence of spontaneous diabetes in female TIP-1 mice and non-transgenic littermates until 300 days of age. Numbers in parentheses indicate the number of mice analyzed. **(B)** Incidence of diabetes following transfer of splenocytes (2 x 10^7 cells/recipient) from 13-17 weeks old non-diabetic TIP-1 mice or NOD mice into 8-9 weeks old NOD.Rag1$^{-/-}$ recipients (n > 5 each). $^{*}P < 0.05$; $^{***}P < 0.0001$. Survival curves were compared using log-rank (Mantel-Cox) test.

Proinsulin-Specific Tolerance in TIP-1 Mice

The partial protection from insulitis and diabetes in TIP-1 mice expressing PIns1 in the APCs could be due to immune tolerance to PIns1 epitopes. To demonstrate tolerance to PIns1, we enumerated the frequency of Insulin B $_{9-23}$ reactive CD4+ T cells and Insulin B $_{15-23}$ reactive CD8+ T cells in the peripheral lymphoid organs (PLO) (pooled spleen and non-draining lymph nodes) of 20-25 weeks old non-diabetic TIP-1 mice and age matched control mice using respective I-A (g^7) and K^d tetramers. There was a significant reduction in the absolute number of insulin B:$_{9-23}$ specific CD4+ T cells binding to insulin B:$_{10-23}$/I-A (g^7) tetramer (26) and the antigen-experienced CD44^{hi} subset of insulin B:$_{9-23}$ specific CD4+ T cells in TIP-1 mice (**Figures 4A–D**). The absolute number of CD8+T cells recognizing insulin B:$_{15-23}$ epitope (32) as well as the number of antigen-experienced CD44^{hi} subset of insulin B:$_{15-23}$ specific CD8+ T cells were comparable in both TIP-1 mice and controls (**Figures 4E–H**). While the significant reduction of insulin-specific CD4+ and CD8+ T cells in TIP-1 is suggestive of deletional tolerance, it is possible that transgenic antigen expression in APCs may induce regulatory T cells (Tregs) that confer dominant tolerance and prevent diabetes in TIP-1 mice. We examined the expression of Foxp3 on insulin B:$_{9-23}$ specific CD4+ T cells in PLO of TIP-1 mice and non-transgenic controls and did not observe any significant differences (**Figure S2A, B**), In addition we examined the frequency of Foxp3+ CD4+ Tregs in the thymus and pancreatic lymph node (PLN). The proportion of Tregs was similar in both TIP-1 and control mice (**Figure S2C, D**).Taken together our data indicate that ectopic PIns1 expression induces deletion of cognate CD4+

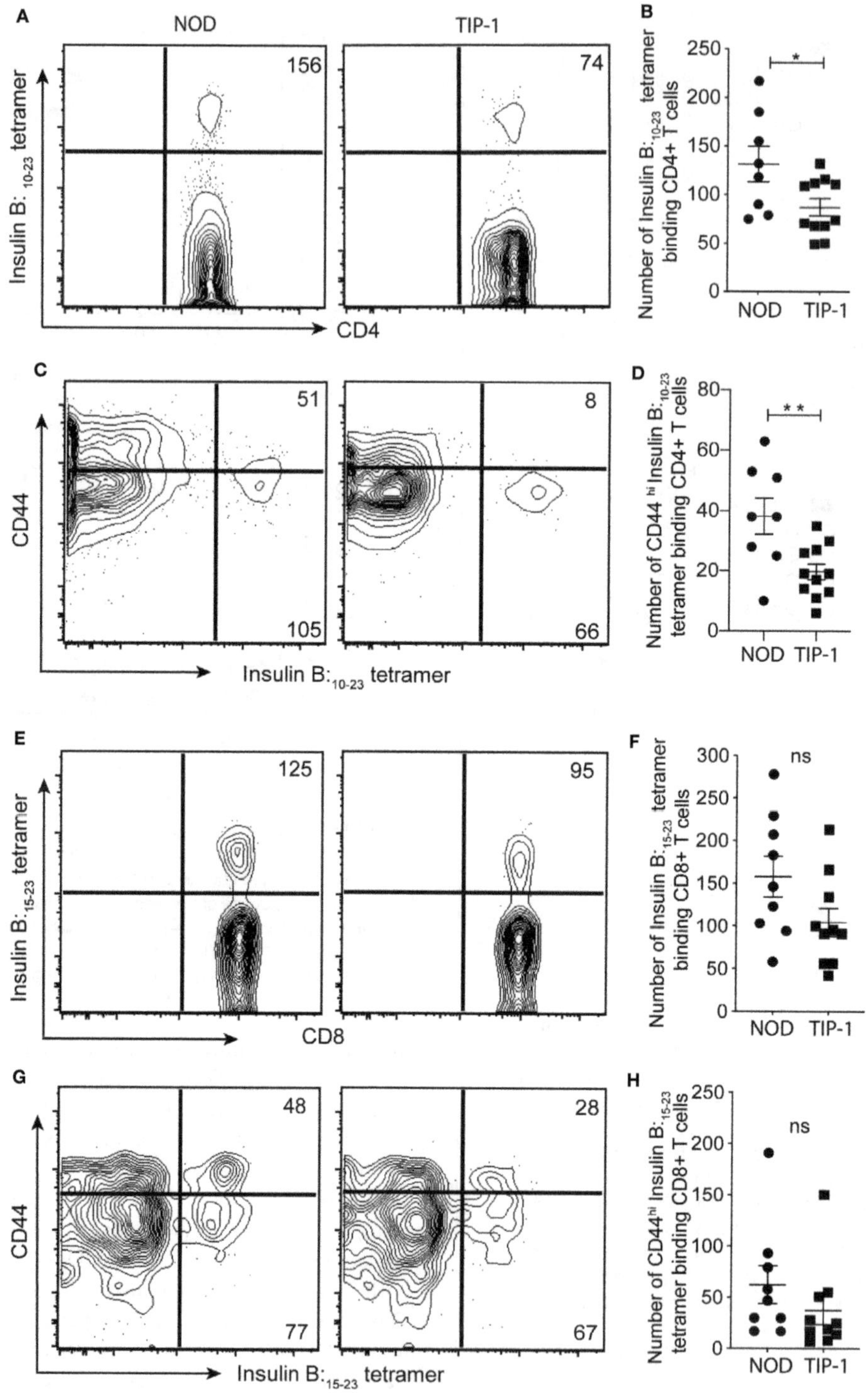

FIGURE 4 | Immune tolerance to insulin specific T cells in TIP-1 mice Insulin B:$_{10\text{-}23}$-specific CD4+ T cells or Insulin B:$_{15\text{-}23}$-specific CD8+ T cells were stained with respective tetramers and enriched from pooled peripheral lymphoid organs (PLO) of 20-25 weeks old TIP-1 mice and NOD mice using magnetic beads and enumerated by flow-cytometry. Representative FACS plots **(A, C, E, G)** and enumeration of insulin tetramer+ CD4+ T **(B)** cells, insulin tetramer+ CD8+ T cells **(F)**, CD44^{hi} Insulin tetramer + CD4+ T cells **(D)** and CD44^{hi} Insulin tetramer + CD8+ T cells **(H)** in TIP-1 and NOD mice. Values in the FACS plots indicate absolute number of tetramer binding cells. Each symbol in the scatter plots (Mean ± SEM) represents data from an individual mouse. **P < 0.01, *P < 0.05, ns= not significant. Data compared using 2-tailed unpaired t-test.

T cells, but does not induce antigen specific Tregs. The few remaining insulin reactive CD4+T cells could not be activated by the expressed antigen, whereas the low-affinity insulin B:$_{15-23}$ reactive CD8+ T cells (33) are not influenced by transgenic PIns1 expression.

Downstream Responses to IGRP Are Delayed in TIP-1 Mice

Previous work from our group has demonstrated that autoreactive responses to islet-specific glucose-6-phosphatase catalytic subunit-related protein (IGRP) are dependent upon immune response to PIns2 (1). To investigate if tolerance to PIns1 influenced the immune response to IGRP we examined the frequency of pathogenic IGRP $_{206-214}$ reactive CD8+ T cells in TIP-1 mice. The number of IGRP $_{206-214}$ specific CD8+ T cells was significantly reduced in 12-14 weeks old TIP-1 mice expressing PIns1 as compared to age matched controls. However, the frequency of IGRP $_{206-214}$ specific CD8+ T cells in TIP-1 mice expressing PIns1 did not differ from age-matched controls at 20-25 weeks of age (**Figures 5A, B**). This indicates that tolerance to PIns1 delays but does not prevent the spreading of immune responses to downstream antigen IGRP.

Immune Response to Proinsulin-1 Is Not Required for Diabetes in NOD 8.3 Mice

Autoreactivity to PIns2 is required for diabetes development in NOD 8.3 mice that have a pre-existing repertoire of IGRP specific T cells (34). Since we observed reduced frequency of IGRP reactive CD8+ T cells in 12-14 weeks old TIP-1 mice, we wished to know if immune responses to PIns1 were necessary for diabetes development in NOD 8.3 mice. TIP-1 mice were crossed with NOD 8.3 mice to generate offspring that were TIP-1/NOD8.3 double transgenic or NOD 8.3 transgenic alone. TIP-1/8.3 mice developed diabetes with significantly delayed kinetics (median survival 97 days) compared to NOD8.3 mice (median survival 70 days) but all mice eventually developed disease (**Figure 5C**). The frequency of insulin specific T cells is very low even in NOD mice and with a skewed T cell repertoire in NOD 8.3 transgenic mice it is not possible to detect any insulin specific T cells. We were unable to detect insulin-specific T cells

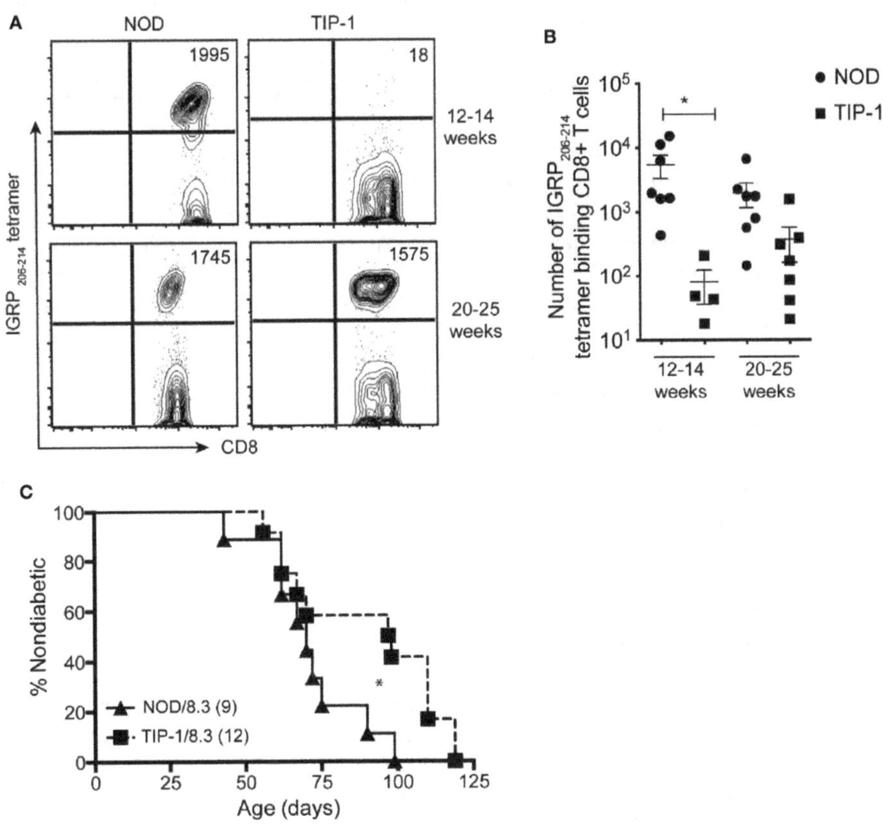

FIGURE 5 | Enumeration of IGRP specific CD8+ T cells in TIP-1 mice IGRP $_{206-214}$-specific CD8+ T cells were stained with Kd- IGRP tetramer and enriched from pooled peripheral lymphoid organs (PLO) of 12-14 weeks and 20-25 weeks old NOD mice and TIP-1 mice. Representative FACS plots **(A)** and quantification **(B)** of absolute number of IGRP $_{206-214}$ tetramer + CD8+ T cells at indicated ages. Values in the FACS plots indicate absolute number of tetramer binding cells. Each symbol in the scatter plots (Mean ± SEM) represents data from an individual mouse. *P<0.05, data in **(B)** compared using one-way ANOVA with Sidak's multiple comparisons test. **(C)** Incidence of spontaneous diabetes in female TIP-1/8.3 mice and NOD 8.3 littermates. Numbers in parentheses indicate the number of mice analyzed. *P < 0.05. Survival curves were compared using log-rank (Mantel-Cox) test.

in TIP-1/8.3 mice (data not shown). Therefore, tolerance to PIns1 significantly delays but does not prevent diabetes development in NOD 8.3 mice.

DISCUSSION

In this study we generated transgenic NOD mice to induce PIns1 expression in the APCs and examined the impact of antigen specific tolerance on autoimmune diabetes. The main findings of this study are 1) TIP-1 mice expressing PIns1 in the APCs show significantly reduced incidence of diabetes, which is associated with reduced insulitis and insulin autoantibody (IAA) expression. 2) Proinsulin specific CD4+ T cells are detectable in TIP-1 mice at a reduced frequency and are not activated. 3) Immune responses to downstream antigen IGRP are delayed but not absent in TIP-1 mice.

Given the high degree of homology between proinsulin 1 and 2 proteins, especially in the immunodominant insulin B chain epitope Ins B:$_{9\text{-}23}$ we expected to achieve robust protection from diabetes onset in TIP-1 mice, similar to previously described proinsulin-2 tolerant NOD mice (35); however, the partial protection from insulitis and diabetes observed in TIP-1 mice points to the existence of distinct pathogenic peptide epitopes in the PIns2 protein that can precipitate autoimmunity in NOD mice. A previous study characterizing immunogenic epitopes in NOD mice reported existence of multiple epitopes on both PIns1 and PIns2 molecules recognized by CD4+T cells (18). Importantly, epitopes outside of the highly homologous Ins B:$_{9\text{-}23}$ peptide were identified in the leader and A chain sequences of PIns2 molecule. Thus, it is likely that PIns2 reactive T-cells recognizing these unique epitopes may induce islet destruction and subsequent diabetes onset in TIP-1 mice.

Our data complement the previous observations that reported detection of PIns1 reactive T cells (18, 19) in NOD mice. While the previous studies did not directly demonstrate the role of PIns1-reactive T cells in spontaneous disease, the significant reduction in diabetes incidence in TIP-1 mice suggests that PIns1 specific T cells participate in autoimmune destruction of beta cells. On the other hand, development of IAA and diabetes in TIP-1 mice may be related to ongoing immune responses to PIns2 epitopes.

A drawback of our study is that we have analyzed a single transgenic founder line expressing PIns1 in the APCs. Varying levels of transgenic insulin expression in the thymus may influence the diabetes progression in NOD mice. PIns2 levels were 7-fold higher in the spleen (~140 pmol/L) as compared to thymus (~20pmol/L) in the partially protected Pins2 tolerant mice previously described by Jaeckel et al. (12), whereas in the recently described TIP mice with robust protection from autoimmune diabetes upon conditional PIns2 expression in APCs, the level of thymic Pins2 expression (100pmol/L) was 5-fold more compared to peripheral tissues(20pmol/L) (22). TIP-1 mice may have relatively reduced transgenic expression of PIns1 in the thymic APCs as compared to transgenic PIns2 expression in the previously described TIP mice, thus imparting incomplete protection from autoimmune diabetes. Chentoufi and Polychronakos previously reported that Ins2 is expressed at a level more than 3-fold higher than Ins1 in the thymus of NOD mice (9). In TIP-1 mice analyzed here, induction of PIns1 results in approximately 5-fold higher expression as compared to non-transgenic NOD mice or uninduced TIP-1 mice. Moreover, protection from insulitis in TIP-1 mice is associated with the expression of PIns1 transgene, as TIP-1 mice fed doxycycline to suppress PIns1 expression develop islet infiltration comparable to non-transgenic controls indicating that ectopic PIns1 expression in APCs influences anti-islet immunity.

Does the reduction in the incidence of spontaneous diabetes in TIP-1 mice correlate with deletion of PIns1 specific T cells? Insulin B:$_{10\text{-}23}$ and Insulin B:$_{15\text{-}23}$ specific tetramers used in our study are likely to detect both PIns1 and 2 reactive CD4+ and CD8 +T cells, due to the invariant nature of the Insulin B:$_{9\text{-}23}$ peptide between the two isoforms. Immune responses to Insulin B:$_{9\text{-}23}$ epitope are required for both priming and effector phase of islet autoimmunity in NOD mice. Moreover, Insulin B:$_{9\text{-}23}$ primed CD4+ T cells are able to induce islet autoimmunity evidenced by IAA production (36). The significant reduction in absolute number of Insulin B:$_{9\text{-}23}$ tetramer binding CD4+T cells, and the antigen-experienced subset of tetramer binding CD4+ T cells, coupled with reduced IAA production in TIP-1 mice is suggestive of antigen-specific tolerance. While Tregs are an important tolerance mechanism, we did not find any evidence to suggest that the partial protection from diabetes in TIP-1mice is due to antigen-specific Tregs. We are currently unable to conclude whether central or peripheral tolerance mechanisms regulate the insulin specific T cells in TIP-1 mice; however, future studies with ectopic antigen expression induced after the exit of antigen-specific T cells from the thymus may resolve this question.

Autoimmunity to insulin determines immune responses to other downstream antigens such as IGRP (1). IGRP $_{206\text{-}214}$ reactive CD8+ T cells were reduced in TIP-1 mice at 12-14 weeks; but ongoing tolerance to PIns1 did not prevent development of diabetes onset in TIP-1/8.3 mice. The precursor frequency of IGRP reactive CD8+ T cells is low in NOD mice (27), and the residual immune response to PIns2 in TIP-1 mice may be reduced as compared to control mice. The reduced CD4+ T cell help possibly accounts for the delayed expansion of IGRP specific T cells seen in TIP-1 mice. However, the residual immune response to PIns2 in TIP-1/8.3 mice with a pre-existing repertoire of IGRP specific T cells may be sufficient to help IGRP specific CD8+ T cells to mediate beta-cell destruction.

In summary, we find that immune tolerance to PIns1, whilst partly protective, is not sufficient to prevent spontaneous diabetes in NOD mice. Our data clarifies the role of PIns1 in the pathogenesis of autoimmune diabetes in NOD mice and extends the previously established role of PIns1 in autoimmune diabetes. The experimental model we have presented here, with its conditional gene-expression system, has the potential to delineate whether antigen-specific interventions can induce immune tolerance after islet autoimmunity is well established. Understanding this is important for development of strategies to induce antigen-specific tolerance clinically in people with stage 1 or 2 type 1 diabetes (37).

AUTHOR CONTRIBUTIONS

GJ performed experiments, analyzed data, and wrote the manuscript. CS, JC, C-TK, and EP performed experiments and analyzed data. HT, BK, and TK designed the study, analyzed data, and wrote the manuscript. BK and TK supervised the study. All authors contributed to the article and approved the submitted version.

ACKNOWLEDGMENTS

We thank S. Fynch, T. Catterall, I. Voelcker, V. Moshovakis, E. Tonkin, H. Barlow, and A. Cornelisz (St Vincent's Institute) for excellent technical support and animal husbandry.

REFERENCES

1. Krishnamurthy B, Dudek NL, McKenzie MD, Purcell AW, Brooks AG, Gellert S, et al. Responses against islet antigens in NOD mice are prevented by tolerance to proinsulin but not IGRP. *J Clin Invest* (2006) 116(12):3258–65. doi: 10.1172/JCI29602
2. Mannering SI, Pathiraja V, Kay TW. The case for an autoimmune aetiology of type 1 diabetes. *Clin Exp Immunol* (2016) 183(1):8–15. doi: 10.1111/cei.12699
3. Lucassen AM, Julier C, Beressi J-P, Boitard C, Froguel P, Lathrop M, et al. Susceptibility to insulin dependent diabetes mellitus maps to a 4.1 kb segment of DNA spanning the insulin gene and associated VNTR. *Nat Genet* (1993) 4 (3):305–10. doi: 10.1038/ng0793-305
4. Pugliese A, Zeller M, Fernandez A Jr., Zalcberg LJ, Bartlett RJ, Ricordi C, et al. The insulin gene is transcribed in the human thymus and transcription levels correlated with allelic variation at the INS VNTR-IDDM2 susceptibility locus for type 1 diabetes. *Nat Genet* (1997) 15(3):293–7. doi: 10.1038/ng0397-293
5. Vafiadis P, Bennett ST, Todd JA, Nadeau J, Grabs R, Goodyer CG, et al. Insulin expression in human thymus is modulated by INS VNTR alleles at the IDDM2 locus. *Nat Genet* (1997) 15(3):289–92. doi: 10.1038/ng0397-289
6. Wentworth BM, Schaefer IM, Villa-Komaroff L, Chirgwin JM. Characterization of the two nonallelic genes encoding mouse preproinsulin. *J Mol Evol* (1986) 23(4):305–12. doi: 10.1007/BF02100639
7. Deltour L, Leduque P, Blume N, Madsen O, Dubois P, Jami J, et al. Differential expression of the two nonallelic proinsulin genes in the developing mouse embryo. *Proc Natl Acad Sci U S A* (1993) 90(2):527–31. doi: 10.1073/pnas.90.2.527
8. Heath VL, Moore NC, Parnell SM, Mason DW. Intrathymic expression of genes involved in organ specific autoimmune disease. *J Autoimmun* (1998) 11 (4):309–18. doi: 10.1006/jaut.1998.0210
9. Chentoufi AA, Polychronakos C. Insulin expression levels in the thymus modulate insulin-specific autoreactive T-cell tolerance: the mechanism by which the IDDM2 locus may predispose to diabetes. *Diabetes* (2002) 51 (5):1383–90. doi: 10.2337/diabetes.51.5.1383
10. Wegmann DR, Norbury-Glaser M, Daniel D. Insulin-specific T cells are a predominant component of islet infiltrates in pre-diabetic NOD mice. *Eur J Immunol* (1994) 24(8):1853–7. doi: 10.1002/eji.1830240820
11. Nakayama M, Abiru N, Moriyama H, Babya N, Liu E, Miao D, et al. Prime role for an insulin epitope in the development of type 1 diabetes in NOD mice. *Nature* (2005) 435(7039):220–3. doi: 10.1038/nature03523
12. Jaeckel E, Lipes MA, von Boehmer H. Recessive tolerance to preproinsulin 2 reduces but does not abolish type 1 diabetes. *Nat Immunol* (2004) 5 (10):1028–35. doi: 10.1038/ni1120
13. Daniel D, Wegmann DR. Protection of nonobese diabetic mice from diabetes by intranasal or subcutaneous administration of insulin peptide B-(9-23). *Proc Natl Acad Sci U S A* (1996) 93(2):956–60. doi: 10.1073/pnas.93.2.956
14. Devendra D, Paronen J, Moriyama H, Miao D, Eisenbarth GS, Liu E, et al. Differential immune response to B:9-23 insulin 1 and insulin 2 peptides in animal models of type 1 diabetes. *J Autoimmun* (2004) 23(1):17–26. doi: 10.1016/j.jaut.2004.03.008
15. Thebault-Baumont K, Dubois-Laforge D, Krief P, Briand J-P, Halbout P, Vallon-Geoffroy K, et al. Acceleration of type 1 diabetes mellitus in proinsulin 2-deficient NOD mice. *J Clin Invest* (2003) 111(6):851–7. doi: 10.1172/JCI16584
16. Moriyama H, Abiru N, Paronen J, Sikora K, Liu E, Miao D, et al. Evidence for a primary islet autoantigen (preproinsulin 1) for insulitis and diabetes in the nonobese diabetic mouse. *Proc Natl Acad Sci U S A* (2003) 100(18):10376–81. doi: 10.1073/pnas.1834450100
17. Elso CM, Scott NA, Mariana L, Masterman EI, Sutherland APR, Thomas HE, et al. Replacing murine insulin 1 with human insulin protects NOD mice from diabetes. *PLoS One* (2019) 14(12):e0225021. doi: 10.1371/journal.pone.0225021
18. Halbout P, Briand J-P, Becourt C, Muller S, Boitard C. T cell response to preproinsulin I and II in the nonobese diabetic mouse. *J Immunol* (2002) 169 (5):2436–43. doi: 10.4049/jimmunol.169.5.2436
19. Levisetti MG, Lewis DM, Suri A, Unanue ER. Weak proinsulin peptide-major histocompatibility complexes are targeted in autoimmune diabetes in mice. *Diabetes* (2008) 57(7):1852–60. doi: 10.2337/db08-0068
20. Faideau B, Lotton C, Lucas B, Tardivel I, Elliott JF, Boitard C, et al. Tolerance to proinsulin-2 is due to radioresistant thymic cells. *J Immunol* (2006) 177 (1):53–60. doi: 10.4049/jimmunol.177.1.53
21. Fan Y, Rudert WA, Grupillo M, He J, Sisino G, Trucco M. Thymus-specific deletion of insulin induces autoimmune diabetes. *EMBO J* (2009) 28 (18):2812–24. doi: 10.1038/emboj.2009.212
22. Jhala G, Chee J, Trivedi PM, Selck C, Gurzov EN, Graham KL, et al. Perinatal tolerance to proinsulin is sufficient to prevent autoimmune diabetes. *JCI Insight* (2016) 1(10):e86065. doi: 10.1172/jci.insight.86065
23. Guerau-de-Arellano M, Martinic M, Benoist C, Mathis D. Neonatal tolerance revisited: a perinatal window for Aire control of autoimmunity. *J Exp Med* (2009) 206(6):1245–52. doi: 10.1084/jem.20090300
24. Verdaguer J, Schmidt D, Amrani A, Anderson B, Averill N, Santamaria P, et al. Spontaneous autoimmune diabetes in monoclonal T cell nonobese diabetic mice. *J Exp Med* (1997) 186(10):1663–76. doi: 10.1084/jem.186.10.1663
25. Moon JJ, Chu HH, Hataye J, Pagan AJ, Pepper M, McLachlan JB, et al. Tracking epitope-specific T cells. *Nat Protoc* (2009) 4(4):565–81. doi: 10.1038/nprot.2009.9
26. Crawford F, Stadinski B, Jin N, Michels A, Nakayama M, Pratt P, et al. Specificity and detection of insulin-reactive CD4+ T cells in type 1 diabetes in the nonobese diabetic (NOD) mouse. *Proc Natl Acad Sci U S A* (2011) 108 (40):16729–34. doi: 10.1073/pnas.1113954108
27. Chee J, Ko H-J, Skowera A, Jhala G, Catterall T, Graham KL, et al. Effector-memory T cells develop in islets and report islet pathology in type 1 diabetes. *J Immunol* (2014) 192(2):572–80. doi: 10.4049/jimmunol.1302100
28. Babaya N, Liu E, Miao D, Li M, Yu L, Eisenbarth GS, et al. Murine high specificity/sensitivity competitive europium insulin autoantibody assay. *Diabetes Technol Ther* (2009) 11(4):227–33. doi: 10.1089/dia.2008.0072
29. Daniel C, Weigmann B, Bronson R, von Boehmer H. Prevention of type 1 diabetes in mice by tolerogenic vaccination with a strong agonist insulin mimetope. *J Exp Med* (2011) 208(7):1501–10. doi: 10.1084/jem.20110574
30. Yu L, Robles DT, Abiru N, Kaur P, Rewers M, Kelemen GS. Early expression of antiinsulin autoantibodies of humans and the NOD mouse: evidence for early determination of subsequent diabetes. *Proc Natl Acad Sci U S A* (2000) 97(4):1701–6. doi: 10.1073/pnas.040556697
31. Ziegler AG, Rewers M, Simell O, Simell T, Lempainen J, Steck A, et al. Seroconversion to multiple islet autoantibodies and risk of progression to diabetes in children. *JAMA* (2013) 309(23):2473–9. doi: 10.1001/jama.2013.6285
32. Wong FS, Karttunen J, Dumont C, Wen L, Visintin I, Pilip IM, et al. Identification of an MHC class I-restricted autoantigen in type 1 diabetes

by screening an organ-specific cDNA library. *Nat Med* (1999) 5(9):1026–31. doi: 10.1038/12465

33. Wong FS, Siew LK, Scott G, Thomas IJ, Chapman S, Viret C, et al. Activation of insulin-reactive CD8 T-cells for development of autoimmune diabetes. *Diabetes* (2009) 58(5):1156–64. doi: 10.2337/db08-0800
34. Krishnamurthy B, Mariana L, Gellert SA, Colman PG, Harrison LC, Lew AM, et al. Autoimmunity to both proinsulin and IGRP is required for diabetes in nonobese diabetic 8.3 TCR transgenic mice. *J Immunol* (2008) 180 (7):4458–64. doi: 10.4049/jimmunol.180.7.4458
35. French MB, Allison J, Cram DS, Thomas HE, Dempsey-Collier M, Silva A, et al. Transgenic expression of mouse proinsulin II prevents diabetes in nonobese diabetic mice. *Diabetes* (1997) 46(1):34–9. doi: 10.2337/diabetes.46.1.34
36. Nakayama M, Beilke JN, Jasinski JM, Kobayashi M, Miao D, Li M, et al. Priming and effector dependence on insulin B:9-23 peptide in NOD islet autoimmunity. *J Clin Invest* (2007) 117(7):1835–43. doi: 10.1172/JCI31368
37. Insel RA, Dunne JL, Atkinson MA, Chiang JL, Dabelea D, Gottlieb PA, et al. Staging presymptomatic type 1 diabetes: a scientific statement of JDRF, the Endocrine Society, and the American Diabetes Association. *Diabetes Care* (2015) 38(10):1964–74. doi: 10.2337/dc15-1419

16

Identification of Sorafenib as a Treatment for Type 1 Diabetes

Qin Zeng[1,2†], Jianfeng Song[1,2†], Dandan Wang[1,2], Xiaoxiao Sun[1,2], Yalun Xiao[1,2], Haowei Zhang[1,2], Yang Xiao[1,2], Zhiguang Zhou[1,2] and Tuo Deng[1,2,3*]*

[1] National Clinical Research Center for Metabolic Diseases, and Department of Metabolism and Endocrinology, The Second Xiangya Hospital of Central South University, Changsha, China, [2] Key Laboratory of Diabetes Immunology, Ministry of Education, and Metabolic Syndrome Research Center, The Second Xiangya Hospital of Central South University, Changsha, China, [3] Clinical Immunology Center, The Second Xiangya Hospital of Central South University, Changsha, China

***Correspondence:**
Tuo Deng
dengtuo@csu.edu.cn
Zhiguang Zhou
zhouzhiguang@csu.edu.cn

[†]These authors have contributed equally to this work

Th1 cell activation is considered a key mediator of the pathogenesis of type 1 diabetes. Targeting IL-12-induced Th1 cell differentiation seems to be an effective way to block the development of type 1 diabetes. However, given the critical function of Th1 in the immune system, the potential side effects hinder the application of anti-Th1 therapy in the treatment of type 1 diabetes. To identify safe anti-Th1 treatment(s), we screened the FDA-approved tyrosine kinase inhibitor (TKI) drug library using an IL-12-induced Th1 differentiation cell model. We found that among the TKIs with little effect on T cell viability, sorafenib is the top contender for the inhibition of Th1 differentiation. Treatment of NOD mice with sorafenib significantly impeded the development of type 1 diabetes and ameliorated insulitis, which coincided with a specifically decreased accumulation of Th1 cell population in the pancreas but not in peripheral immune organs. Mechanistically, sorafenib indirectly inhibited janus kinase 2 (JAK2) activity and blocked IL-12-induced phosphorylations of JAK2 and signal transducer and activator of transcription 4 (STAT4). Since sorafenib is classified as an FDA-approved drug, it serves as a preliminary lead point for additional experimentation and may be a promising therapy for type 1 diabetes in humans.

Keywords: type 1 diabetes, Th1, sorafenib, IL-12, NOD mice

INTRODUCTION

Type 1 diabetes is an immune-mediated disease characterized by the impairment of insulin-producing pancreatic beta cells. Since the destruction of beta cells in type 1 diabetes is mainly mediated by pathogenic autoreactive T cells, targeting autoreactive T cells shows promise in treating type 1 diabetes. T cell-based immunotherapies, such as an anti-CD3 monoclonal antibody, CTLA4-Ig fusion protein and low-dose anti-thymocyte globulin, have emerged for the treatment of type 1 diabetes (1). These immunotherapies indeed have shown some benefits in human clinical trials, but

Abbreviations: APCs, antigen-presenting cells; Cy, Cyclophosphamide; I-A2, insulinoma-associated antigen 2; JAK2, janus kinase 2; LADA, latent autoimmune diabetes in adults; MLN, mesenteric lymph node; PBMCs, Peripheral blood mononuclear cells; PDGFR, platelet derived growth factor receptor; PLNs, pancreatic lymph nodes; PPI, preproinsulin; STAT4, signal transducer and activator of transcription 4; TKI, tyrosine kinase inhibitor; Tregs, regulatory T cells; TYK2, tyrosine kinase 2; VEGFR, vascular endothelial growth factor receptor; ZnT8, zinc transporter 8; Cy, cyclophosphamide; MLN, mesenteric lymph node; PMBC, peripheral blood mononuclear cells.

their systemic immunosuppressive effects and transient efficiency limit the success of application. In the face of an increasing type 1 diabetes population, it is urgent to development more effective and safer T cell-based immunotherapies.

In the early stage of type 1 diabetes, antigen-presenting cells (APCs) present autoantigens such as preproinsulin (PPI), insulinoma-associated antigen 2 (I-A2), GAD, and zinc transporter (ZnT8) to $CD4^+$ T cells (2). Meanwhile, APCs secrete IL-12 to trigger the differentiation of naïve $CD4^+$ T cells into Th1 cells. The Th1 cells produce inflammatory cytokines including IFN-γ and IL-2 to activate $CD8^+$ cytotoxic T lymphocytes and macrophages (3), and cooperate with them to attack pancreatic beta cells. Transfer of pathogenic Th1 cells into neonatal NOD mice initiated the onset of type 1 diabetes (4), while the depletion of Th1 cells by disrupting Tbet, a key transcription factor for Th1 cell polarization, effectively blocked insulitis and type 1 diabetes in NOD mice (5). Therefore, Th1 cell population is a critical mediator of type 1 diabetes pathogenesis. IL-12 is a key cytokine for the induction of Th1 cell differentiation, and IL-12-induced signal transducer and activator of transcription 4 (STAT4) activation is a paramount signaling pathway for Th1 cell differentiation (6). In NOD mice, daily administration of IL-12 increased type 1 diabetes incidence (7), while addition of an IL-12 antagonist decreased type 1 diabetes incidence (8, 9). In addition, disruption of STAT4 activation prevented the development of type 1 diabetes in NOD mice completely (10). In humans, *IL-12b* was identified as a susceptible type 1 diabetes gene (11). These studies suggest that IL-12 played an essential role, inducing Th1 cell differentiation in pathogenesis of type 1 diabetes. Therefore, targeting the IL-12/STAT4 axis to suppress Th1 cell may be an effective strategy for the treatment of type 1 diabetes.

Tyrosine kinases possess a catalytic subunit that transfers a phosphate group from ATP to one or more tyrosine residues in a protein, leading to conformational changes, affecting protein function. They are important mediators of the signaling transduction, regulating cellular activity such as cell division, differentiation, apoptosis, and metabolism, in response to external and internal stimuli (12, 13). Due to multiple functions of tyrosine kinases in a variety of biological processes, tyrosine kinase inhibitors (TKIs) have been developed for the treatment of many diseases, including cancer, autoimmune and inflammatory diseases, degenerative disease and infectious disease (14, 15). Up until now, 39 TKIs have been approved by FDA, and more are being tested in clinical trials (16). IL-12/STAT4 pathway is directly mediated by a tyrosine kinase, janus kinase 2 (JAK2) (17, 18), and may be indirectly regulated by tyrosine kinase 2 (TYK2) or other tyrosine kinases (19, 20). To identify new and safe Th1 cell differentiation inhibitors that can be used to treat type 1 diabetes, we screened the FDA-approved TKI drug sub-library in an *in-vitro* cell culture model of IL-12-induced Th1 cell differentiation. We found that sorafenib, a TKI mainly targeting Raf for the treatment of renal and liver cancers, strongly blocked IL-12-induced Th1 cell differentiation by inhibiting the phosphorylations of JAK2 and STAT4. Treatment with sorafenib in NOD mice inhibited Th1 cell accumulation in the pancreas, and prevented insulitis and diabetes. These results suggest that sorafenib may be a potential treatment for type 1 diabetes.

MATERIAL AND METHODS

Experimental Animals

Female NOD mice were purchased from the Model Animal Research Center of Nanjing University (Nanjing, China), 017581-B6.129S4-*Ifng*$^{tm3.1Lky}$/J (GREAT) mice were purchased from the Jackson Laboratory (Bar Harbor, ME, USA), C57BL/6J mice were purchased from Slac Laboratory Animal Inc (Shanghai, China). All mice were housed in a specific-pathogen-free animal facility at Central South University (Changsha, China). 12-week-old female NOD mice were monitored for blood glucose twice per week and considered diabetic after two consecutive blood glucose readings were >250 mg/dl. All animal experiments were performed in accordance with the guidelines from the Department of Laboratory Animal Science, Central South University.

Drugs and Treatments

Sorafenib tosylate (Nexavar) tablets were purchased from Byer (Leverkusen, Germany) and suspended in 1% sodium carboxymethyl cellulose for *in vivo* use. Eight-week-old female NOD mice were treated with 10 mg/kg body weight of sorafenib or vehicle once daily by oral gavage. Administration time varies by experiment. Cyclophosphamide (Cy, Sigma-Aldrich, St. Louis, MO) was diluted to 35 mg/ml with 0.9% sodium chloride solution before i.p. for the treatment of 12-week-old mice (300 mg/kg) to induce the onset of diabetes in female NOD mice. For the therapeutic treatment, diabetic female NOD mice were treated with 10 or 50 mg/kg body weight of sorafenib or vehicle once daily by oral gavage for three weeks.

Histological Analysis of Insulitis

Pancreatic tissues from vehicle-treated or sorafenib-treated mice were fixed with 4% paraformaldehyde, embedded in paraffin, and 5-μm-thick sections were stained with hematoxylin and eosin. Insulitis scores were calculated by using the following scale: 0 = no infiltrate, 1 = peri-insulitis, 2 = moderate insulitis (<50%), 3 = severe insulitis (>50%).

Isolation of Lymphocytes From Tissues and Intracellular Staining

The pancreas was dissected from vehicle and sorafenib-treated mice, and digested in 1.5 mg/ml collagenase IV (Worthington Biochemical, Lakewood, NJ) for 45 min at 37°C. Pancreatic lymph nodes (PLNs) and spleens were mechanically disrupted. Cells were filtered through a 70 μm filter to get single cell suspension. Lymphocytes from tissues were stimulated for 6 h with phorbol myristate acetate (50 ng/ml) and ionomycin (5 μM) in the presence of brefeldin A and monensin (Biolegend, San Diego, CA, USA). Cells were collected to stain with antibodies, and then fixed and permeabilized in cytofix/cytoperm buffer (BD Biosciences, San Jose, CA).

Mouse T Cell Isolation and Th1 Differentiation

Naive $CD4^+$ T cells from the spleens of 6-8 weeks old male GREAT mice were prepared using magnetic bead cell sorting (Miltenyi Biotec, Bergisch-Gladbach, Germany). The purity of $CD4^+CD44^{low}CD62L^{high}$ T cell subset was validated by flow cytometry. These naïve $CD4^+$ T cells were stimulated with 5 μg/ml pre-coated anti-CD3ϵ antibody (Biolegend) and 1 μg/ml soluble anti-CD28 antibody (Biolegend) in culture medium containing 10 ng/ml IL-12 (Peprotech, Cranbury, NJ, USA), 10 ng/ml IL-2 (Peprotech) and 10 μg/ml anti–IL-4 antibody (BD Biosciences) for 3 days. The culture medium was RPMI 1640 medium (plus 50 μM β-mercaptoethanol) supplemented with 10% FBS, 1% GlutaMax, and 1% Pen/Strep (Gibco, Shanghai, China). 1×10^5 naive $CD4^+$ T cells were cultured in 96-well plates with 100 μl culture medium per well.

Human T Cell Isolation and Th1 Differentiation

Healthy volunteers were recruited from the medical students at the Second Xiangya Hospital and written informed consent was obtained. Human study was approved by the Ethics Committee of the Second Xiangya Hospital of Central South University. Peripheral blood mononuclear cells (PBMCs) from the peripheral blood of healthy volunteers were separated by Histopaque (Sigma-Aldrich, St. Louis, MO). Naive $CD4^+$ T cells from PBMC were isolated by negative selection using Miltenyi beads according to the manufacturer's instructions. The purity of $CD4^+CD45RA^+CD45RO^-$ T cell subset was validated by flow cytometry. The purified naïve $CD4^+$ T cells were stimulated with 5 μg/ml pre-coated anti-CD3ϵ antibody (Biolegend) and 2 μg/ml soluble anti-CD28 antibody (Biolegend) in culture medium containing 10 ng/ml IL-12 (Peprotech, Cranbury, NJ, USA), 10 ng/ml IL-2 (Peprotech) and 10 μg/ml anti–IL-4 antibody (eBioscience) for 5 days. The culture medium was RPMI 1640 medium supplemented with 10% FBS, 1% GlutaMax, and 1% Pen/Strep (Gibco, Shanghai, China). 1×10^5 naive $CD4^+$ T cells were cultured in 96-well plates with 100 μl culture medium per well. The culture medium was refreshed on day 3.

Drug Screen

The FDA-approved TKI drug library was purchased from Selleck Chemicals (Houston, TX, USA), and was dissolved in DMSO or water to get a 10 mM concentration for screening. Naive $CD4^+$ T cells were prepared from the spleens of 8-week-old male GREAT mice, 1×10^5 Th0 cells/well were plated into 96-well plates and cultured for 72 h. Th0 cells were cultured with Th1 differentiation medium containing 10 μM of individual FDA-approved TKI drug, and the IFN-γ–expressing Th1 cells were defined by detection of YFP expression.

Cell Viability Assay

Cell viability of Th0 cells was performed using standard trypan blue exclusion method and ATP chemiluminescence assay. After isolation of naïve $CD4^+$ T cells (Th0) cells, 5×10^4 Th0 cells/well were plated into 96-well plates and cultured for 48 h. Viable cells were assessed by trypan blue staining. Similarly, 1×10^3 Th0 cells/well were plated into opaque 96-well plates and cultured for 48 h, and then detected by using the CellTiter-Lumi™ luminescent cell viability assay kit (Beyotime, Beijing, China), the absorbance of 570 nm was measured using a microplate reader (Enspire Multimode Plate Reader, Perkin Elmer).

E. coli-Infection Mouse Model

Eight weeks old male C57BL/6J mice were treated with 10 mg/kg body weight of sorafenib or vehicle once daily by oral gavage. Two days after sorafenib treatment, C57BL/6J mice were injected intraperitoneally with 0.2 ml of suspensions of *E. coli* (ATCC 8739) at 10^7 CFU. Bacteria were harvested by centrifugation at 4000 rpm for 15 min and washed twice in PBS, and then diluted in PBS to obtain the desired concentration for infection experiments. To determine injection success, bacteria in peritoneal lavage fluid from the infected mice were collected at 24 hours after infection, and cultured overnight at 37°C on Luria-Bertani Agar plates.

In-Vitro Kinase Assay

Enzyme activity was measured using mobility shift assay in duplicate in 384-well plates. Dilution series of ten different concentrations were diluted in DMSO. Sorafenib was diluted to 50X of the final desired highest inhibitor concentration in DMSO, 10 μl of the compound was mixed with 90 μl of 1x kinase buffer to each well of the 96-well plate for shaking 10 min, then the mixture was transferred to a 384-well plate in duplicates. After assay plate preparation, enzyme solution and carboxyfluorescein-labeled peptide and ATP were added into the assay plate in turn. Luminescence signal was measured on Caliper (Perkin Elmer).

Real-Time Quantitative PCR

Total RNA was extracted from the pancreas using the Trizol reagent (Invitrogen, Life Technologies, NY) following manufacturer's instructions. cDNA was synthesized using the cDNA Synthesis Kit (Thermo-Fisher Scientific, MA) and primers (Sangon Biotech Shanghai, China). RT-qPCR was performed using the FastStart Universal Master mix (Roche, Germany) in an ABI ViiA 7 Real-Time Polymerase Chain Reaction System. Relative gene expression levels were normalized to housing-keeping gene beta-actin. The following primers were used: mouse Tbet (Tbx21; forward: 5'-TTCAACCAGCACCAGACAG-3', reverse: 5'-AGACCACATCC ACAAACATCC-3'), mouse IFN-γ (Ifng; forward: 5'-CTTTGGACCCTCTGACTTGAG-3', reverse: 5'-TCTTCCA CATCTATGCCACTTG-3'), mouse IL-1β (forward: 5'-TGAA ATGCCACCTTTTGACAG-3', reverse: 5'-CACGGGAAAGA CACAGGTAG-3'), mouse IL-6 (forward: 5'-TGGAAATGAG AAAAGAGTTGTGC-3', reverse: 5'-CTCTGAAGGACTC

TGGCTTTG-3'), mouse TNF-α (forward: 5'-CTTCTG TCTACTGAACTTCGGG-3', reverse: 5'-TGTCTTTGAGA TCCATGCCG-3'), mouse Bcl6 (forward: 5'-CCATACAAAT GTGATCGCTGC-3', reverse: 5'- GTAGGGCTTTTCT CCAGAGTG-3'), mouse Rorc (forward: 5'-GCACCAACCT CTTTTCACG-3', reverse: 5'-ACGACTTCCATTGCTCCTG-3'), mouse Foxp3 (forward: 5'-ACCCAGGAAAGACAGCAAC-3', reverse: 5'-CTTCTCCTTTTCCAGCTCCAG-3'), mouse Gata3 (forward: 5'-CTTATCAAGCCCAAGCGAAG-3', reverse: 5'-TCGATTTGCTAGACATCTTCCG-3'), mouse IL-21 (forward: 5'-ATCATTGACCTCGTGGCC-3', reverse: 5'-CTTCGG GTCCTATGTGTTCTAG-3'), mouse Stat4 (forward: 5'-CTGGGAGTAAAGGAAACGAGG-3', reverse: 5'-GCTG GTCTCTAGGTTAATGGTG-3'), mouse Jak2 (forward: 5'-TGAGGCCACCAGTAAAAGACA-3', reverse: 5'-TTTTG CCAGACAAGAGTGATG-3'), mouse beta-actin (forward: 5'-ACCGTGAAAAGATGACCCAG-3', reverse: 5'-GAGCA TAGCCCTCGTAGATG-3').

In-Vitro Phosphorylation Assay

The purified naive CD4$^+$ T cells were cultured in RPMI 1640 with 10% FBS and 1% Pen/Strep. 2×10^6 Th0 cells/well were pre-treated with gradient concentrations of sorafenib for 3 h and then stimulated with 10 ng/ml IL-12 for 5 min to induce the phosphorylations of JAK2 and STAT4. Finally, cell extracts were collected for western blots analysis.

Western Blots Analysis

Total protein was extracted using RIPA buffer containing a cocktail of proteinase and phosphatase inhibitors (Sigma-Aldrich). Protein concentration was measured using BCA kit (Thermo Scientific, Pierce) and 30 μg/lane of total protein was loaded onto 10% polyacrylamide gels. The membranes were first incubated with following anti-phosphotyrosine antibodies at 4°C overnight: anti-pJAK2 (Cell Signaling Technology, Cat#3771, dilute 1:1000) and anti-pSTAT4 (Santa Cruz, Cat#sc-28296, dilute 1:100). The membranes were subsequently stripped using a solution containing 100 mM β-mercaptoethanol, 2% SDS, and 62.5 mM Tris-HCl (pH 7.6) at 50°C for 30 min, and re-incubated with anti-JAK2 (Cell Signaling Technology, Cat#3230, dilute 1:1000) or anti-STAT4 (Cell Signaling Technology, Cat#2653, dilute 1:1000) antibodies at 4°C overnight.

Flow Cytometry

Cells were stained with fluorochrome-conjugated mAbs and analyzed on CYTEK northern lights NL-3000 or BD FACS Canto II. For surface markers detection, cells were incubated with FcR blocking antibody (Biolegend, Cat#101302 and 422302) for 15 min at room temperature, and stained with antibodies against surface markers for 30 min at 4°C in the dark. Stained cells were washed in PBS and then incubated with 7-AAD viability staining solution (Biolegend, Cat#420404) for 5 min at room temperature. For intracellular staining, cells were incubated with Zombie NIR (Biolegend, Cat#423106) for 15 min at room temperature, and then blocked with CD16/32 antibody and stained with fluorochrome-labeled mAbs against cell-surface antigens for 30 min at 4°C. Cells subsequently were fixed and permeabilized with foxp3/transcription factor staining buffer set (eBioscience, 00-5523-00) or cytofix/cytoperm buffer, and stained with fluorochrome-conjugated antibodies for an additional 30 minutes at 4°C in the dark. The following mAbs were used: CD45 (Biolegend, Cat#103108, 103132 and BD, Cat#562420), CD3e (Biolegend, Cat#100330, 100306, 100216), CD4 (Biolegend, Cat#100406, 100408, 100414, 980804 and eBioscience, Cat#11-0049-41), CD8a (Biolegend, Cat#100721), IFN-γ (Biolegend, Cat#505810, 505832 and 502512), IL-4 (Biolegend, Cat# 504123), IL-17A (Biolegend, Cat#506903), CD25 (Biolegend, Cat#102012 and eBioscience, Cat#56-0251-80), Foxp3 (Biolegend, Cat#126403 and eBioscience, Cat#17-57773-82), CD62L (Biolegend, Cat#104427), CD44 (Biolegend, Cat#103012), CD45RA (Biolegend, Cat#983002) and CD45RO (Biolegend, Cat#304230). Data were analyzed using FlowJo software.

Statistical Analysis

Data are presented as means ± SEM. Statistical analysis was performed using SPSS Version 19.0 software (Chicago, IL, USA). Diabetes incidence was compared using log-rank test. Insulitis was analyzed with χ^2 test. The other group differences were analyzed with 2-tailed Student's t test.

RESULTS

Sorafenib Inhibits IL-12-Induced Th1 Cell Differentiation

To identify new inhibitors of Th1 cell differentiation, we utilized the 'GREAT' (IFN-γ reporter with endogenous polyA transcript) mice model (21), which allows analysis of IFN-γ–expressing cells through the detection of YFP expression. We screened a mini compound library including all TKI drugs approved by FDA between 2001 and 2019 (**Supplementary Figures 1A–C**). To exclude the TKIs with significant cytotoxicity to T cells, we assessed the toxic effects of TKIs on T cells first. We found that 10 TKIs have minimal cytotoxic effects on T cells at a concentration of 10 μM. Among them, sorafenib, an oral multikinase inhibitor with antitumor properties, was identified as the most potent inhibitor of IL-12-induced Th1 cell differentiation. As shown in **Figures 1A, B**, sorafenib inhibited IL-12-induced Th1 cell differentiation in a dose-dependent manner. The gating strategy and purity of sorted mouse naïve CD4$^+$ T cells were shown in **Supplementary Figures 2A, B**. To confirm that the inhibitory effect of sorafenib on Th1 cell differentiation was not due to cytotoxicity, we treated naïve CD4$^+$ T (Th0) cells with different doses of sorafenib for 2 days and examined the viability of naïve CD4$^+$ T cells by performing an ATP chemiluminescence assay. We found that the number of viable cells did not differ by the treatment of 10 μM of sorafenib (**Figure 1C**), which strongly inhibited IL-12-induced Th1 cell differentiation. However, sorafenib was not able to inhibit IFN-γ production in Th1 cells at non-toxic doses (**Supplementary**

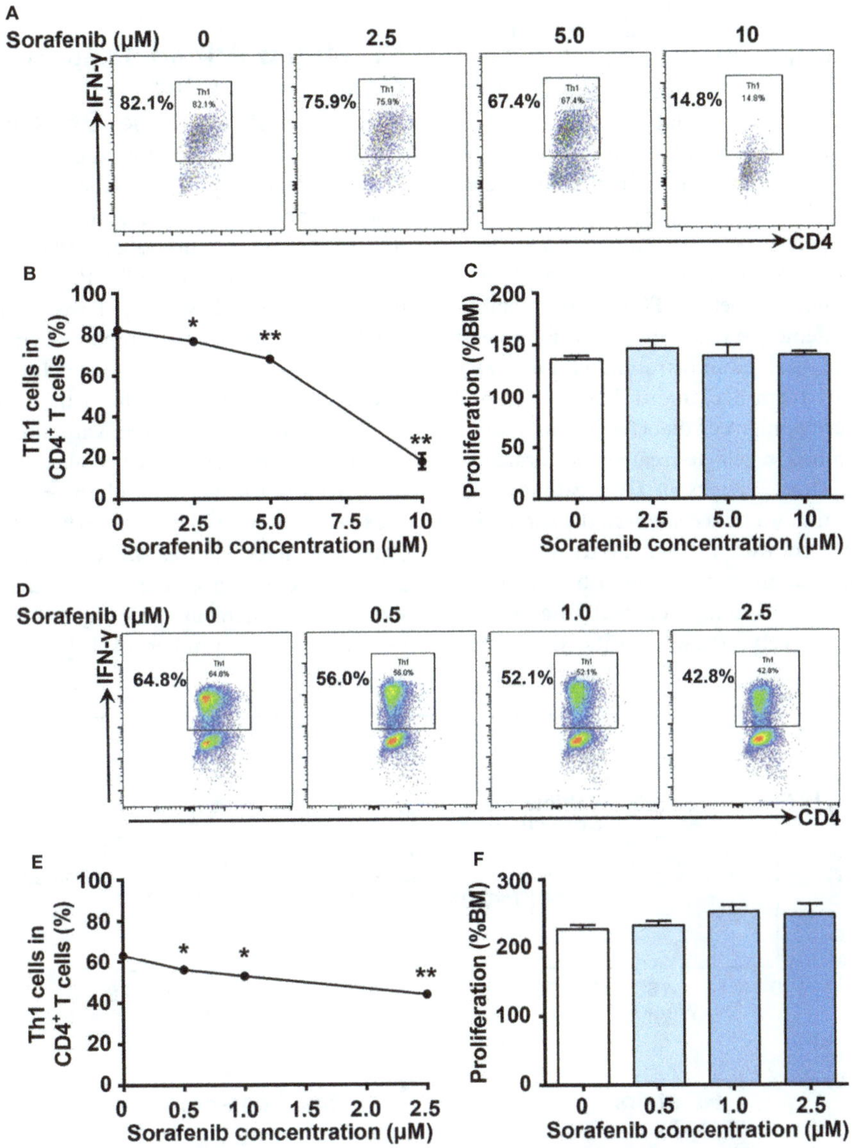

FIGURE 1 | Sorafenib inhibits IL-12-induced Th1 cell differentiation in a dose-dependent manner in both mice and humans. **(A, B)** Flow cytometry analysis of Th1 cells in mouse naïve splenic CD4$^+$ T cells stimulated with IL-12 in medium containing different concentrations of sorafenib as indicated. **(C)** CellTiter-Lumi assay to assess viable cells in the naïve splenic Th0 cells cultured in medium containing different concentrations of sorafenib as indicated. **(D, E)** Flow cytometry analysis of Th1 cells in human naïve PBMC CD4$^+$ T cells stimulated with IL-12 in medium containing different concentrations of sorafenib as indicated. **(F)** CellTiter-Lumi assay to assess viable cells in the naïve PBMC Th0 cells cultured in medium containing different concentrations of sorafenib as indicated. BM, blank medium. Data are representative of 3 independent experiments. Data represent means ± s.e.m; $^*P < 0.05$ or $^{**}P < 0.01$ versus 0 μM by t-test.

Figures 3A, B). To determine whether sorafenib inhibits Th1 cell differentiation in humans, naïve CD4$^+$ T cells were isolated from PBMC of healthy donors by cell sorting and subsequently were differentiated into Th1 cells by IL-12 stimulation. The gating strategy and purity of sorted naïve CD4$^+$ T cells were shown in **Supplementary Figures 2C, D**. As shown in **Figures 1D–F**, sorafenib effectively inhibited IL-12-induced Th1 cell differentiation in human T cells without altering their viability. Collectively, our results indicate that sorafenib is a strong inhibitor of Th1 differentiation.

Sorafenib Administration Prevents Development of Type 1 Diabetes

Type 1 diabetes is characterized by the activation of pathogenic autoreactive Th1 cells in the pancreas (3). To investigate whether sorafenib inhibits the development of type 1 diabetes, sorafenib was administered to NOD mice, a widely used type 1 diabetes mice model, once daily by oral gavage at a dose of 10 mg/kg body weight. Oral administration was initiated at 8 weeks of age and continued to 20 weeks of age. During the development of natural diabetes, vehicle-treated mice had a higher incidence (32%) than sorafenib-treated mice (19%) at 17 weeks of age, and the gap between two groups grew over time. By 32 weeks of age, the endpoint of this experiment, 43% of the mice treated with sorafenib were diabetic, as opposed to 74% of the vehicle-treated mice (**Figure 2A**). Next, we assessed the effects of sorafenib on cyclophosphamide (Cy)-induced type 1 diabetes. Cy treatment leads to a rapid onset of type 1 diabetes both in human and NOD mice through suppression of regulatory T cells (Tregs) (22–25). Our data showed that more than half of the vehicle-treated mice developed diabetes within 6 weeks after Cy injection, in contrast, only 24% of the sorafenib-treated mice developed diabetes during the same period (**Figure 2B**). Notably, the protective effects of sorafenib persisted and lasted for at least 5 weeks after cessation of oral administration (**Figure 2B**), suggesting that the short-term treatment had prolonged beneficial effects on the development of diabetes in this setting. Pancreatic islets were examined in vehicle-treated and sorafenib-treated prediabetic mice. After 2 weeks of Cy treatment, the mononuclear cell accumulation was less evident in the sorafenib-treated group when compared with the vehicle-treated group (**Figure 2C**), and mice treated with sorafenib showed a significantly lower insulitis score compared with the control mice (**Figure 2D**). Collectively, these results show that sorafenib impedes the development of type 1 diabetes and alleviates insulitis in NOD mice.

Sorafenib Administration Diminishes Th1 Cells Accumulation in Pancreas but Not in Peripheral Immune Organs in NOD Mice

T cells play an important role in the development of type 1 diabetes (2). Our data (**Figure 1**) has shown sorafenib inhibits Th1 cell differentiation *in vitro*. To examine the effects of sorafenib on T cells *in vivo*, 8-week-old prediabetic NOD mice were treated with a therapeutic dose of sorafenib (10 mg/kg/day) for 6 weeks. These mice were injected with Cy 4 weeks after the beginning of the sorafenib treatment to promote accumulation of Th1 cells in pancreas. At the end of the sorafenib treatment, the T cells in the spleen, PLN and pancreas from the vehicle-treated or sorafenib-treated mice were analyzed with flow cytometry. Preventative treatment of sorafenib did not alter the $CD4^+$ and $CD8^+$ T cell ratio (data not shown) in spleen or PLNs, nor the $CD4^+$ T cell subsets such as Th1, Th2, Th17 cell and Tregs populations (**Supplementary Figures 4A–C**). These data have indicated that prophylactic administration of sorafenib does not modify T cell subsets in peripheral immune organs. However, in the pancreas, the percentage and number of IFN-γ-producing Th1 cell were

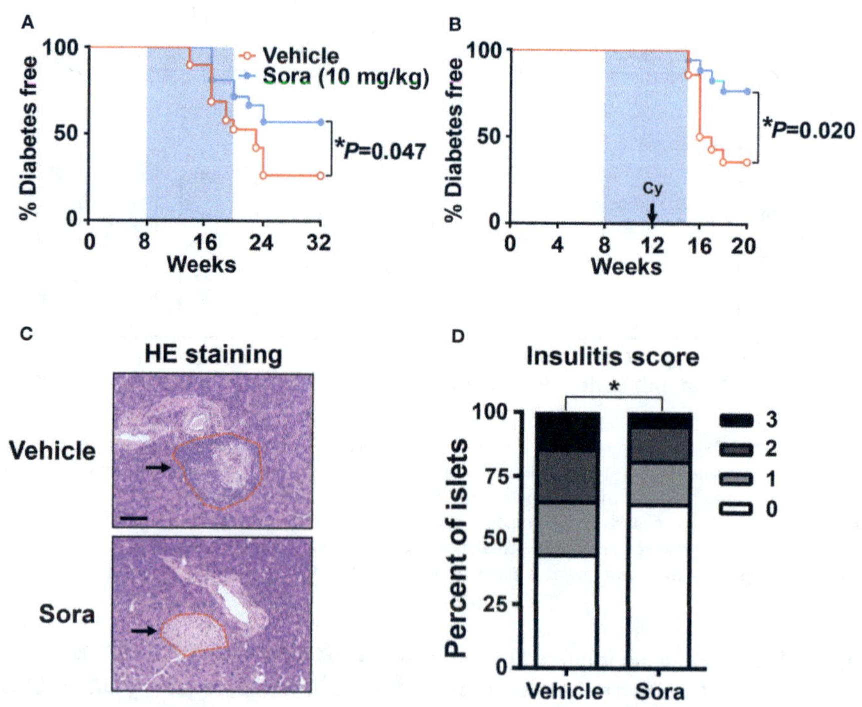

FIGURE 2 | Sorafenib prevents the development of autoimmune diabetes in NOD mice. **(A)** Diabetes incidence of female NOD mice having been treated (gavage) daily with vehicle (n = 19) or sorafenib (10 mg/kg, n = 21) for 12 weeks (blue shaded area). **(B)** Diabetes incidence of female NOD mice having been treated daily with vehicle (n = 14) or sorafenib (10 mg/kg, n = 17) for 7 weeks. Cyclophosphamide (Cy, 300 mg/kg) was injected i.p., 4 weeks after beginning of sorafenib treatment. Statistical significance: $^*P < 0.05$ versus vehicle by long-rank test. **(C)** Representative images of HE staining for pancreatic sections from 14-week-old prediabetic NOD mice having been treated daily with sorafenib (10 mg/kg) or vehicle for 6 weeks, Cy (300 mg/kg) was injected i.p., 4 weeks after beginning of sorafenib treatment, the arrows point to the islet in pancreas. (scale bar indicates 100 μm). **(D)** Insulitis scores from 14-week-old prediabetic NOD mice, data are combined from two independent experiments. $^*P < 0.05$, χ^2 test.

dramatically reduced by sorafenib administration, while the percentage and number of other CD4$^+$ T cell subsets (Th2, Th17 and Treg cells) and CD8$^+$ T cell subsets (Tc1 and Tc2 cells) were unchanged (**Figures 3A–F**). In addition, the mRNA levels of Th1 cell marker genes (*Tbet*) and proinflammatory cytokines (*IFN-γ, IL-1β, TNF-α*) were notably decreased in pancreas of sorafenib-treated mice when compared with vehicle-treated mice, but the mRNA levels of marker genes for Th2 (*Gata3*), Th17 (*Rorc*), Treg (*Foxp3*), and Tfh (*Bcl6*) cells and cytokine (*IL-21*) regulating Th1/Th17 cell differentiation were not different between the two groups (**Figure 3G**). To determine whether the inhibitory effect of sorafenib on Th1 differentiation is specific in pancreas, we investigated the effects of sorafenib on Th1 activation in mesenteric lymph node (MLN) and spleen of *E. coli*-infected

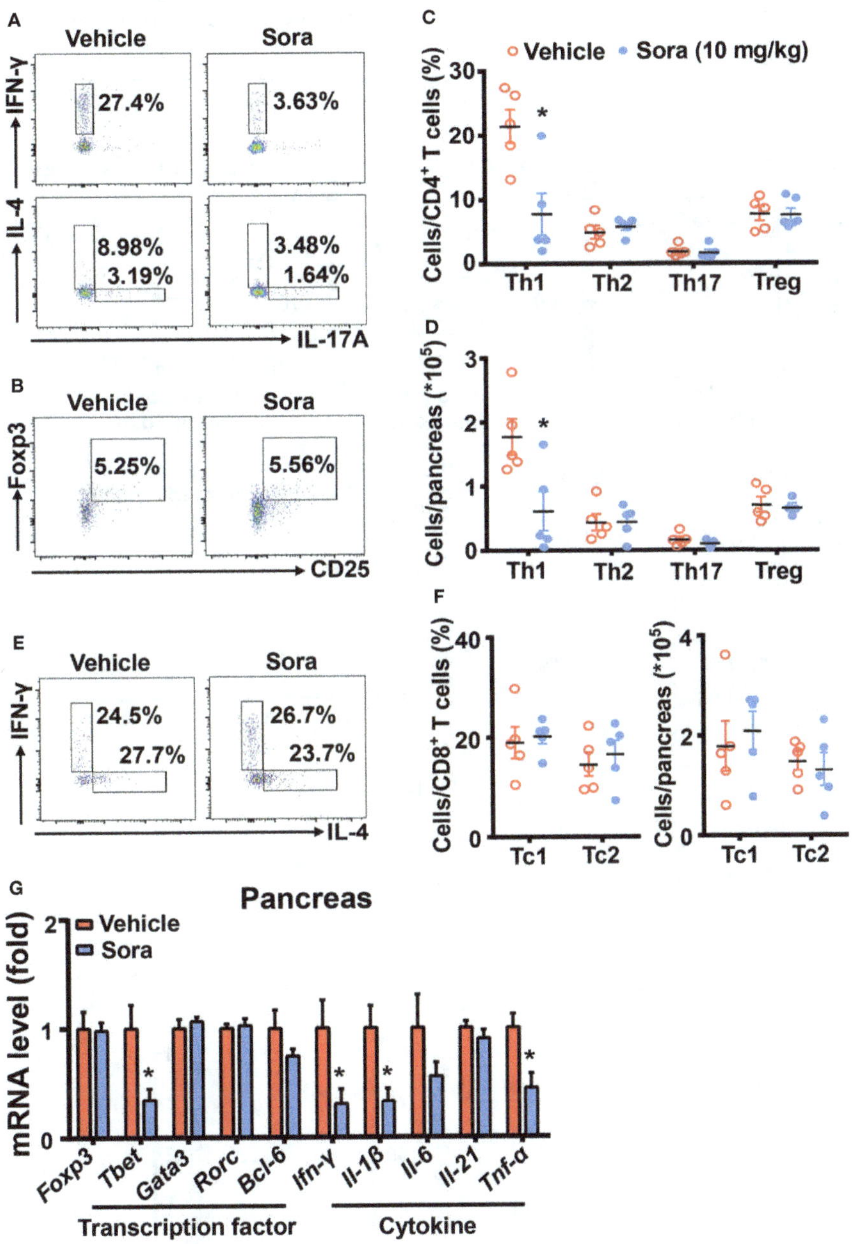

FIGURE 3 | Sorafenib decreases inflammatory Th1 cells in the pancreas of prediabetic NOD mice. Flow cytometry analysis of the frequency and number **(A–D)** of Th1, Th2, Th17 cells and Tregs in pancreas from vehicle-treated or sorafenib-treated prediabetic NOD mice. Flow cytometry analysis of the frequency and number **(E, F)** of Tc1 and Tc2 cells in pancreas from vehicle-treated or sorafenib-treated prediabetic NOD mice. **(G)** RT-PCR analysis of transcription factors (Foxp3, Tbet, Gata3, Rorc and Bcl-6) and cytokines (Ifn-γ, Il-1β, Il-6, Il-21 and Tnf-α) in pancreas from vehicle-treated or sorafenib-treated prediabetic NOD mice. Sora, sorafenib. Data represent means ± s.e.m. and data were pooled from 2 or more independent experiments. n = 5-7 mice per group in each experiment. Statistical significance: *$P < 0.05$ versus vehicle by t-test.

C57BL/6J mice, an animal model of Th1 activation (26). The flow data showed that sorafenib effectively inhibited *E. coli*-induced Th1 cell activation in both MLN and spleen (**Supplementary Figures 5A–C**). Thus, it is likely that sorafenib, as an inhibitor of Th1 cell differentiation, induces Th1 deficiency and immunosuppression in the tissues accumulated with Th1 cells.

Sorafenib Reverses Autoimmune Diabetes in NOD Mice

In addition to defining its prevention role, we also tested whether sorafenib can reverse type 1 diabetes in NOD mice. Once diagnosed with diabetes, the mice were divided into three groups, including vehicle, low dose (10 mg/kg/day) and high dose (50 mg/kg/day) sorafenib groups. A low dose of sorafenib (10 mg/kg/day) did not reduce hyperglycemia in NOD mice with diabetes (data not shown). However, a high dose of sorafenib (50 mg/kg/day) significantly ameliorated hyperglycemia in diabetic NOD mice after one to three weeks of treatment (**Figures 4A–C**). The flow data showed that sorafenib did not alter the $CD4^+$ T cell subsets such as Th1, Th2, Th17 cell and Tregs populations in the peripheral immune organs, PLN and spleen (**Supplementary Figures 6A–C**). In the pancreas, the frequency and number of

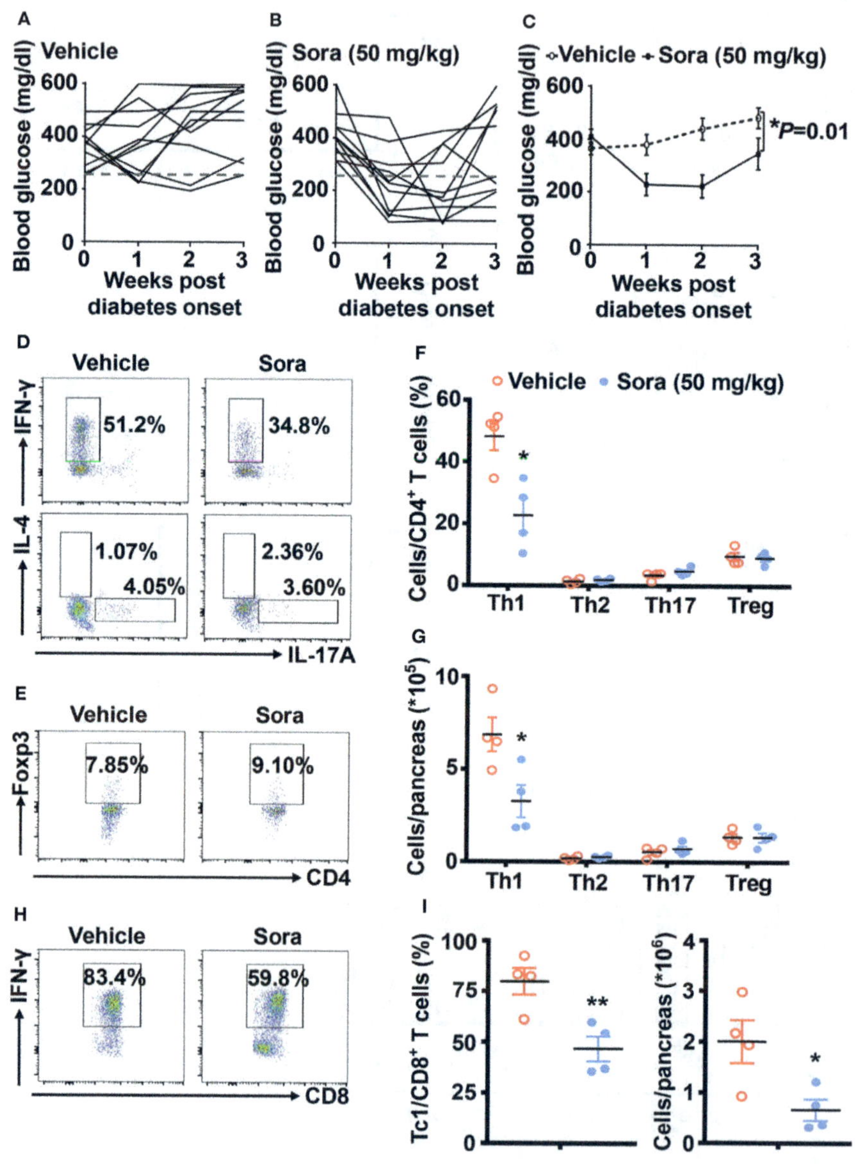

FIGURE 4 | Sorafenib reverses autoimmune diabetes in NOD mice. The trend of blood glucose **(A–C)** from vehicle-treated (n = 11) and sorafenib-treated (50 mg/kg, n = 10) new-onset diabetic NOD mice (diagnosed by two consecutive readings of blood glucose>250 mg/dl). Flow cytometry analysis of the frequency and number **(D–G)** of Th1, Th2, Th17 cells and Tregs in pancreas from vehicle-treated or sorafenib-treated diabetic NOD mice. Flow cytometry analysis of the frequency and number **(H, I)** of Tc1 cells in pancreas from vehicle-treated or sorafenib-treated diabetic NOD mice. Sora, sorafenib. Data represent means ± s.e.m. N = 4 mice per group in each experiment. Statistical significance: $^*P < 0.05$, $^{**}P < 0.01$ versus vehicle by t-test.

Th2, Th17 and Treg cells were also unchanged, but Th1 and Tc1 cells were significantly decreased in the group of sorafenib-treated diabetic NOD mice (**Figures 4D–I**). These results suggest that sorafenib may create a less-inflammatory environment in pancreas of diabetic NOD mice, which leads to the functional recovery of islet beta cells and eventually the remission of autoimmune diabetes.

Sorafenib Indirectly Inhibits the Activation of JAK2/STAT4 Pathway in IL-12-Induced Th1 Cell Differentiation

STAT4 is a transcription factor that mediates IL-12 induced Th1 cell differentiation (6). Disruption of STAT4 activation in NOD mice reduced Th1 type cytokine production and prevented the development of spontaneous type 1 diabetes (10). STAT4 protein is phosphorylated and activated by JAK2 (17, 18). To test whether JAK2 and STAT4 are involved in the inhibitory effects of sorafenib on Th1 cell differentiation, we measured the effects of sorafenib on JAK2 and STAT4 activity in IL-12 pretreated naive $CD4^+$ T cells. As shown in **Figures 5A–F**, sorafenib had no effects on protein and mRNA levels of JAK2 and STAT4 at the concentration of 1-5 μM, but it strongly inhibited IL-12-induced phosphorylations of JAK2 and STAT4. Notably, the dose of sorafenib that inhibited JAK2 activation matched the dose that inhibited Th1 cell differentiation. Moreover, in order to determine whether sorafenib directly affects JAK2, we tested the effect of sorafenib on JAK2 protein. The results from *in-vitro* kinase assay showed that sorafenib had almost no inhibitory effects on JAK2 activity at a concentration from 1 μM to 10 μM (**Figure 5G**), indicating an indirect inhibitory effect of sorafenib on JAK2. Thus, these results suggested that sorafenib suppresses IL-12-induced Th1 cell differentiation by indirectly inhibiting JAK2/STAT4 axis activation.

DISCUSSION

To date, insulin therapy is still the standard treatment for type 1 diabetes. In most cases, blood glucose was well controlled by precise insulin administration, but hypoglycemia and complications are inevitable in some patients (27–29). With the unremitting efforts of researchers, islet or stem cell transplantation is explored as an emerging treatment for type 1 diabetes patients (30, 31). However, long-term immune rejection and islet autoantigen-specific T cells destroy the newly transplanted islet or stem cells, leading to failure of transplantation (32). Currently, a comprehensive cure for type 1 diabetes is not available. Since type 1 diabetes is basically an autoimmune disease, many have high expectations for controlling the excessive immune response in pancreas as a means for curing type 1 diabetes. Type 1 diabetes is mainly mediated by pathogenic autoreactive T cells, among which Th1 cells play a key role in the pathogenesis of type 1 diabetes (4, 5). Utilizing an *in-vitro* cell culture model, we found that sorafenib can effectively block IL-12-induced Th1 cell differentiation in a dose-dependent manner without affecting the viability of T cell in both mice and humans. This finding suggests that sorafenib may be able to fight type 1 diabetes, which is characterized by the over-expansion of Th1 cells in pancreas. Indeed, sorafenib administration prevented and reversed autoimmune type 1 diabetes in NOD mice by decreasing Th1 cells accumulation and expression of inflammatory cytokines in pancreas. Thus, sorafenib may have the potential to protect against type 1 diabetes by improving the immuno-environment in the pancreas.

The NOD mouse model is the most popular animal model of type 1 diabetes. However, it has some limitations for treatment assessment. In NOD mice, about 60%-80% female and 20%-30% male mice spontaneously develop type 1 diabetes, while the sexual discrepancy is not existed in human (33). The insulitis in diabetic NOD mice was more severe than that in patients with type 1 diabetes (34, 35). High numbers of $CD4^+$ T cells and B cells predominate in NOD mice, while relatively small numbers of $CD8^+$ T cells and macrophages were observed in patients with type 1 diabetes (36, 37). In addition, multiple susceptibility loci for type 1 diabetes, such as *Idd*3 and *Idd*5 loci, which have been found in human, are not directly shown to be dysregulated in NOD mice (33), highlighting the difference in the pathogenesis of type 1 diabetes between humans and NOD mice. Despite its limitations, the NOD mouse model is currently the sole animal model to test therapies for autoimmune diabetes *in vivo*.

Importantly, scattered clinical reports have provided evidence that sorafenib can affect blood glucose in malignancy patients. Sorafenib was reported to significantly reduce blood glucose in a patient with advanced diabetic hepatocellular carcinoma (38). In addition, a previous retrospective study showed that sorafenib can markedly reduce blood glucose levels in both diabetic and nondiabetic patients with cancers (39). These clinical studies suggest that sorafenib may have the ability to affect blood glucose in humans. Further studies are warranted to explore the therapeutic effect of sorafenib in patients with type 1 diabetes.

Since type 1 diabetes is an immune-mediated disease, the targeting of immune pathways is a continued focus on either preventing or reversing type 1 diabetes. Currently, there are no approved successful immunotherapies for type 1 diabetes, and past failures were mainly due to the various side effects from systemic immunosuppression (1). Given the comprehensive function of Th1 cells in the immune system, the potential side effects hinder the application of anti-Th1 therapy in the treatment of type 1 diabetes. Although sorafenib was identified as an inhibitor of Th1 differentiation, we believe it is quite a safe option for the treatment of type 1 diabetes. First, sorafenib has been approved by FDA for the treatment of multiple cancers for more than 15 years and has shown limited side effects (40, 41). Second, the dose of sorafenib (10 mg/kg/day for prevention and 50 mg/kg/day for remission) used in NOD mice to treat type 1 diabetes is lower or equal to the generally effective dose for the treatment of cancer (30-50 mg/kg/day) in animal models (42, 43), suggesting that the dose used to treat diabetes may be lower than the current clinical dose for cancer, which also means lower side effects. Third, our *in vivo* data showed that in NOD mice sorafenib decreased Th1 cells and inhibited inflammation

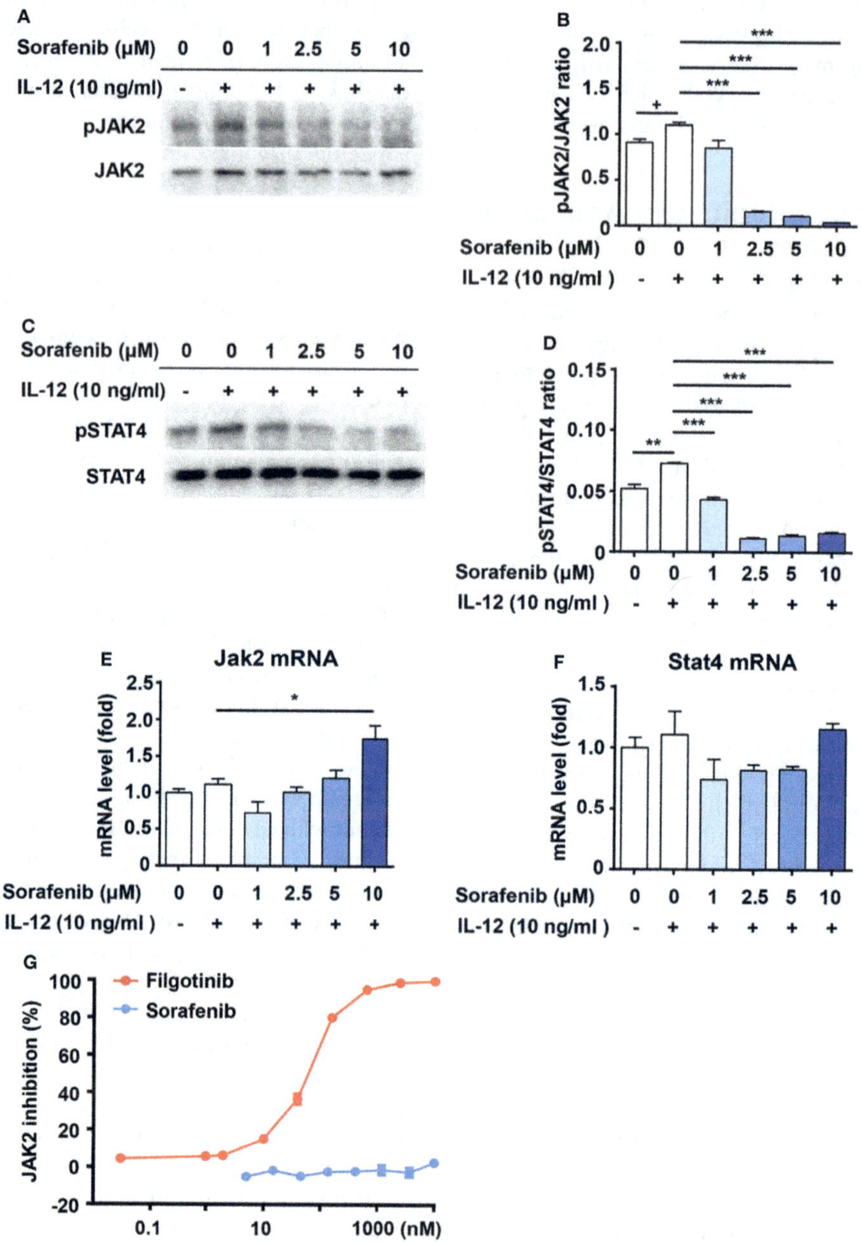

FIGURE 5 | Sorafenib indirectly inhibits phosphorylations of JAK2 and STAT4. Immunoblots and quantitation of pJAK2 **(A, B)** and pSTAT4 **(C, D)** in naive $CD4^{+}$ T cells, which were stimulated with IL-12 in medium containing different concentration sorafenib as indicated. Quantitation of phosphorylated JAK2 and STAT4 normalized to total JAK2 and STAT4. RT-PCR analysis of JAK2 and STAT4 in naive $CD4^{+}$ T cells, which were stimulated with IL-12 in medium containing different concentration sorafenib **(E, F)** as indicated. **(G)** The inhibition ratio of filgotinib and sorafenib on JAK2 activity. Data are representative of 3 independent experiments. Data represent means ± s.e.m. Statistical significance: $^{+}P < 0.1$, $^{*}P < 0.05$, $^{**}P < 0.01$ or $^{***}P < 0.001$. T-test used for statistical analysis.

specifically in the pancreas, but not in peripheral immune organs (**Figures 3A–C** and **Supplementary Figures 4A, B**), suggesting that sorafenib may not have significant effects on systemic immunity in certain condition. Notably, sorafenib repressed Th1 activation in spleens and MLNs of bacteria-infected mice. Since Th1 cells play a critical role in fighting bacterial infection, sorafenib may not be suitable to be used in patients with infectious diseases.

To date, the treatment of type 1 diabetes is still in a dilemma. Successful interventions at any stage of type 1 diabetes will be a breakthrough. Our study found that a low dose of sorafenib (10 mg/kg/day) has the ability to prevent (**Figures 2A, B**) but cannot reverse type 1 diabetes in NOD mice. However, high dose of sorafenib (50 mg/kg/day) treatment induces the remission of established type 1 diabetes (**Figures 4A–C**) in NOD mice, which may due to the suppression of Th1 and Tc1 cells in pancreas.

This result indicates a therapeutic effect of sorafenib on autoimmune diabetes. We think sorafenib can be applied to treat type 1 diabetes, particularly under certain conditions. Sorafenib may be used for the treatment of latent autoimmune diabetes in adults (LADA), a subtype of type 1 diabetes which is characterized by a slower progression to insulin dependence. Patients with LADA were enriched with a subclass of GAD65 IgG1 autoantibodies, reflecting a dominant Th1 cell response to GAD65 in the pancreas (44). Moreover, compared with classic type 1 diabetes, LADA has a less functional deterioration of beta cells and a slower decline of C-peptide serum level (45). GAD autoantibody has been reported as a predictor of insulin requirement in LADA patients. The higher GAD autoantibody titers indicated the higher risk of early insulin dependence (46). Therefore, sorafenib may be particularly suitable for the treatment of LADA patients with higher GAD autoantibody titers. Another possible application area for sorafenib is the honeymoon phase of type 1 diabetes, a remission period where insulin usage can be sharply reduced or even withdrawn during the treatment of type 1 diabetes (47). Although the underlying mechanisms of honeymoon phase of type 1 diabetes are unclear, some clinical studies have indicated that the lower level of serum IFN-γ was associated with the remission of type 1 diabetes (48–50), suggesting that the sorafenib may be used to maintain and extend the honeymoon phase by reducing the accumulation of IFN-γ producing Th1 cells in the pancreas. These possible clinical applications of sorafenib are warranted to be explored in future studies.

Recent studies investigated the role of JAK-STAT signaling pathway in the pathogenesis of type 1 diabetes. The JAK1/JAK2 inhibitor AZD1480 reversed autoimmune diabetes in newly diagnosed mice by blocking the $CD8^+$ T cell-mediated damage of beta cells (51). A case report showed that JAK1/JAK2 inhibitor ruxolitinib normalized blood-glucose levels and discontinued exogenous insulin in a patient with type 1 diabetes caused by STAT1 gain-of-function (52). A recent review summarized the roles of STAT (STAT1, STAT3 and STAT5b) monogenic mutations in type 1 diabetes. These mutations are associated with an increased susceptibility to type 1 diabetes due to the perturbation of Th17/Treg equilibrium (53). These findings suggest that JAK/STAT inhibitor is a potential therapy for type 1 diabetes. IL-12/JAK2/STAT4 signaling has been defined as an essential way for Th1 cell differentiation (17, 18). In our study, we found that sorafenib significantly suppressed IL-12-induced activations of JAK2 and STAT4 in a dose-dependent manner (**Figures 5A–D**), suggesting that sorafenib is a new JAK2 inhibitor. To further explore whether sorafenib directly affects JAK2, we examined the effect of sorafenib on JAK2 activity in an *in-vitro* kinase assay. The classic JAK2 inhibitor, filgotinib, almost completely inhibited JAK2 activity at concentrations as low as 0.6 μM (**Figure 5G**), indicating that the assay system worked very well. In this *in-vitro* kinase assay, sorafenib had little inhibitory effects on JAK2 activity at a concentration of 10 μM. However, this concentration of sorafenib was sufficient to inhibit the IL-12-induced phosphorylation of JAK2 in T cells. (**Figures 5A, B**). This result suggested that sorafenib cannot directly target JAK2, and may indirectly inhibit IL-12-induced JAK2 activation by targeting an unknown factor. Sorafenib is a multiple kinase inhibitor and directly targets Raf and several receptor tyrosine kinases, including vascular endothelial growth factor receptor (VEGFR), platelet derived growth factor receptor (PDGFR), FLT-3, c-Kit, p38 and RET (40). Although we cannot exclude the possibility that the known sorafenib targets mediate its inhibitory effects on JAK2 activation, it is more likely that sorafenib suppresses the IL-12-induced JAK2 activation through its unidentified target. Further studies are warranted to identify the new target of sorafenib.

CONCLUSION

In summary, we identified sorafenib as an inhibitor of Th1 differentiation and an indirect inhibitor of JAK2 and found that sorafenib prevents and reverses type 1 diabetes in NOD mice by decreasing the accumulation of Th1 cells and the expression of inflammatory cytokines in pancreas. Our findings emphasize the importance of Th1 cells in the pathogenesis of type 1 diabetes and suggest that sorafenib may prove to be an important new therapy for clinical treatment in type 1 diabetes.

AUTHOR CONTRIBUTIONS

QZ and JS contributed to the study design, acquisition of data, analysis and interpretation of results, as well as drafting and revision of the manuscript. DW, XS, YLX, and HZ contributed to the acquisition of the data and revision of the manuscript. YX and ZZ contributed to the design of study, analysis of results and revision of the manuscript. TD contributed to the conception and design of the study, analysis of results and the revision of the manuscript. All authors gave their approval for the final manuscript to be published.

ACKNOWLEDGMENTS

We are grateful to Wanyu Hu, Xiyan Liao, Wufuer ■ Aini, Yujin Ding, Hui Zhou and Zhixia Li for their technical supports in our project.

SUPPLEMENTARY MATERIAL

Supplementary Figure 1 | The effects of 34 FDA-approved TKIs on IL-12-induced Th1 cell differentiation. **(A)** Cell counts using trypan blue exclusion to assess viable cells and **(B, C)** flow cytometry analysis of Th1 cells in naïve splenic CD4+ T cells stimulated with IL-12 in medium containing 10 μM of individual FDA-approved TKI as indicated. Data represent means ± s.e.m; *P < 0.05 or **P < 0.01 versus vehicle by t-test.

Supplementary Figure 2 | Gating strategy for flow cytometry analysis of T cells. **(A)** Gating of naïve CD4+ T cells in mouse splenocyte (upper panel); the purity of sorted naïve CD4+ T cells (down panel). **(B)** Gating of Th1 cells in mouse CD4+ T cells. **(C)** Gating of naïve CD4+ T cells in human PBMC (upper panel); the purity of sorted naïve CD4+ T cells (down panel). **(D)** Gating of Th1 cells in human CD4+ T cells. PBMC, peripheral blood mononuclear cells.

Supplementary Figure 3 | Sorafenib does not alter IFN-γ expression in Th1 cell. **(A, B)** Flow cytometry analysis of IFN-γ + Th1 cells treated with different concentrations of sorafenib (μM) as indicated.

Supplementary Figure 4 | Sorafenib does not alter T cell subsets in peripheral immune tissues of prediabetic NOD mice. Flow cytometry analysis of the frequency of Th1, Th2, and Th17 cells in PLN **(A)** and splenic **(B)** CD4+ T cells from vehicle-treated or sorafenib-treated NOD mice. **(C)** Flow cytometry analysis of the frequency of Tregs in PLN and splenic CD4+ T cells, respectively. Sora, sorafenib; PLN, pancreatic lymph nodes. Data represent means ± s.e.m. and data were pooled from 2 or more independent experiments. n = 5-7 mice per group in each experiment.

Supplementary Figure 5 | Sorafenib decreases activate Th1 cells in MLN and spleen of E. coli-infected mice. **(A)** Image of E coli on Luria-Bertani Agar plates from vehicle-treated or sorafenib-treated C57BL/6J mice injected with PBS or E.coli (1*107 CFU). Flow cytometry analysis of the frequency of Th1 cells in MLN **(B)** and splenic **(C)** CD4+ T cells from the three groups mice as indicated. Sora, sorafenib; MLN, mesenteric lymph node. Data represent means ± s.e.m.. n = 4 mice per group in this experiment. Statistical significance: *P <0.05 or **P <0.01 versus vehicle by t-test.

Supplementary Figure 6 | Sorafenib does not alter T-cell subsets in peripheral immune tissues of diabetic NOD mice. Flow cytometry analysis of the frequency of Th1, Th2, and Th17 cells in PLN **(A)** and splenic **(B)** $CD4^+$ T cells from vehicle-treated or sorafenib-treated diabetic NOD mice. **(C)** Flow cytometry analysis of the frequency of Tregs in PLN and splenic $CD4^+$ T cells, respectively. Sora, sorafenib; PLN, pancreatic lymph nodes. Data represent means ± s.e.m. n = 4 mice per group in each experiment.

REFERENCES

1. Warshauer JT, Bluestone JA, Anderson MS. New Frontiers in the Treatment of Type 1 Diabetes. *Cell Metab* (2020) 31(1):46–61. doi: 10.1016/j.cmet.2019.11.017
2. Todd JA. Etiology of Type 1 Diabetes. *Immunity* (2010) 32(4):457–67. doi: 10.1016/j.immuni.2010.04.001
3. Adorini L. Interleukin 12 and Autoimmune Diabetes. *Nat Genet* (2001) 27 (2):131–2. doi: 10.1038/84732
4. Katz JD, Benoist C, Mathis D. T Helper Cell Subsets in Insulin-Dependent Diabetes. *Science* (1995) 268(5214):1185–8. doi: 10.1126/science.7761837
5. Esensten JH, Lee MR, Glimcher LH, Bluestone JA. T-Bet-Deficient NOD Mice Are Protected From Diabetes Due to Defects in Both T Cell and Innate Immune System Function. *J Immunol* (2009) 183(1):75–82. doi: 10.4049/jimmunol.0804154
6. Murphy KM, Ouyang W, Farrar JD, Yang J, Ranganath S, Asnagli H, et al. Signaling and Transcription in T Helper Development. *Annu Rev Immunol* (2000) 18:451–94. doi: 10.1146/annurev.immunol.18.1.451
7. Trembleau S, Penna G, Bosi E, Mortara A, Gately MK, Adorini L. Interleukin 12 Administration Induces T Helper Type 1 Cells and Accelerates Autoimmune Diabetes in NOD Mice. *J Exp Med* (1995) 181(2):817–21. doi: 10.1084/jem.181.2.817
8. Rothe H, O'Hara C.OMMAJr RM, Martin S, Kolb H. Suppression of Cyclophosphamide Induced Diabetes Development and Pancreatic Th1 Reactivity in NOD Mice Treated With the Interleukin (IL)-12 Antagonist IL-12(P40)2. *Diabetologia* (1997) 40(6):641–6. doi: 10.1007/s001250050728
9. Nitta Y, Kawamoto S, Tashiro F, Aihara H, Yoshimoto T, Nariuchi H, et al. IL-12 Plays a Pathologic Role at the Inflammatory Loci in the Development of Diabetes in NOD Mice. *J Autoimmun* (2001) 16(2):97–104. doi: 10.1006/jaut.2000.0469
10. Yang Z, Chen M, Ellett JD, Fialkow LB, Carter JD, McDuffie M, et al. Autoimmune Diabetes Is Blocked in Stat4-Deficient Mice. *J Autoimmun* (2004) 22(3):191–200. doi: 10.1016/j.jaut.2003.08.006
11. Morahan G, Huang D, Ymer SI, Cancilla MR, Stephen K, Dabadghao P, et al. Linkage Disequilibrium of a Type 1 Diabetes Susceptibility Locus With a Regulatory IL12B Allele. *Nat Genet* (2001) 27(2):218–21. doi: 10.1038/84872
12. Hubbard SR, Till JH. Protein Tyrosine Kinase Structure and Function. *Annu Rev Biochem* (2000) 69:373–98. doi: 10.1146/annurev.biochem.69.1.373
13. Manning G, Whyte DB, Martinez R, Hunter T, Sudarsanam S. The Protein Kinase Complement of the Human Genome. *Science* (2002) 298(5600):1912–34. doi: 10.1126/science.1075762
14. Ferguson FM, Gray NS. Kinase Inhibitors: The Road Ahead. *Nat Rev Drug Discovery* (2018) 17(5):353–77. doi: 10.1038/nrd.2018.21
15. Levitzki A. Protein Kinase Inhibitors as a Therapeutic Modality. *Acc Chem Res* (2003) 36(6):462–9. doi: 10.1021/ar0201207
16. Roskoski RJR. Properties of FDA-Approved Small Molecule Protein Kinase Inhibitors: A 2020 Update. *Pharmacol Res* (2020) 152:104609. doi: 10.1016/j.phrs.2019.104609
17. Watford WT, Hissong BD, Bream JH, et al. Signaling by IL-12 and IL-23 and the Immunoregulatory Roles of STAT4. *Immunol Rev* (2004) 202:139–56. doi: 10.1111/j.0105-2896.2004.00211.x
18. Zundler S, Neurath MF. Interleukin-12: Functional Activities and Implications for Disease. *Cytokine Growth Factor Rev* (2015) 26(5):559–68. doi: 10.1016/j.cytogfr.2015.07.003
19. Karaghiosoff M, Neubauer H, Lassnig C, Kovarik P, Schindler H, Pircher H, et al. Partial Impairment of Cytokine Responses in Tyk2-Deficient Mice. *Immunity* (2000) 13(4):549–60. doi: 10.1016/S1074-7613(00)00054-6
20. Pignata C, Sanghera JS, Cossette L, Pelech SL, Ritz J. Interleukin-12 Induces Tyrosine Phosphorylation and Activation of 44-Kd Mitogen-Activated Protein Kinase in Human T Cells. *Blood* (1994) 83(1):184–90. doi: 10.1016/S1074-7613(00)00054-6
21. Reinhardt RL, Liang HE, Locksley RM. Cytokine-Secreting Follicular T Cells Shape the Antibody Repertoire. *Nat Immunol* (2009) 10(4):385–93. doi: 10.1038/ni.1715
22. Harada M, Makino S. Promotion of Spontaneous Diabetes in Non-Obese Diabetes-Prone Mice by Cyclophosphamide. *Diabetologia* (1984) 27(6):604–6. doi: 10.1007/BF00276978
23. Atlan-Gepner C, Bouabdallah R, Valero R, Coso D, Vialettes B. A Cyclophosphamide-Induced Autoimmune Diabetes. *Lancet* (1998) 352 (9125):373–4. doi: 10.1016/S0140-6736(05)60474-6
24. Brode S, Raine T, Zaccone P, Cooke A. Cyclophosphamide-Induced Type-1 Diabetes in the NOD Mouse Is Associated With a Reduction of CD4+CD25+Foxp3+ Regulatory T Cells. *J Immunol* (2006) 177(10):6603–12. doi: 10.4049/jimmunol.177.10.6603
25. Louvet C, Szot GL, Lang J, Lee MR, Martinier N, Bollag G, et al. Tyrosine Kinase Inhibitors Reverse Type 1 Diabetes in Nonobese Diabetic Mice. *Proc Natl Acad Sci USA* (2008) 105(48):18895–900. doi: 10.1073/pnas.0810246105
26. Nagayama M, Yano T, Atarashi K, Tanoue T, Sekiya M, Kobayashi Y, et al. TH1 Cell-Inducing Escherichia Coli Strain Identified From the Small Intestinal Mucosa of Patients With Crohn's Disease. *Gut Microbes* (2020) 12(1):1788898. doi: 10.1080/19490976.2020.1788898
27. Action to Control Cardiovascular Risk in Diabetes Study, G, Gerstein HC, Miller ME, Byington RP, Goff DC Jr, Bigger JT, et al. Effects of Intensive Glucose Lowering in Type 2 Diabetes. *N Engl J Med* (2008) 358(24):2545–59. doi: 10.1056/NEJMoa0802743
28. Group AC, Patel A, MacMahon S, Chalmers J, Neal B, Billot L, et al. Intensive Blood Glucose Control and Vascular Outcomes in Patients With Type 2 Diabetes. *N Engl J Med* (2008) 358(24):2560–72. doi: 10.1056/NEJMoa0802987

29. Duckworth W, Abraira C, Moritz T, Reda D, Emanuele N, Reaven PD, et al. Glucose Control and Vascular Complications in Veterans With Type 2 Diabetes. *N Engl J Med* (2009) 360(2):129–39. doi: 10.1056/NEJMoa0808431
30. Shapiro AM, Lakey JR, Ryan EA, Korbutt GS, Toth E, Warnock GL, et al. Islet Transplantation in Seven Patients With Type 1 Diabetes Mellitus Using a Glucocorticoid-Free Immunosuppressive Regimen. *N Engl J Med* (2000) 343 (4):230–8. doi: 10.1056/NEJM200007273430401
31. Voltarelli JC, Couri CE, Stracieri AB, Oliveira MC, Moraes DA, Pieroni F, et al. Autologous Nonmyeloablative Hematopoietic Stem Cell Transplantation in Newly Diagnosed Type 1 Diabetes Mellitus. *JAMA* (2007) 297(14):1568–76. doi: 10.1001/jama.297.14.1568
32. Sneddon JB, Tang Q, Stock P, Bluestone JA, Roy S, Desaiet T, et al. Stem Cell Therapies for Treating Diabetes: Progress and Remaining Challenges. *Cell Stem Cell* (2018) 22(6):810–23. doi: 10.1016/j.stem.2018.05.016
33. Anderson MS, Bluestone JA. The NOD Mouse: A Model of Immune Dysregulation. *Annu Rev Immumnol* (2005) 23:447–85. doi: 10.1146/annurev.immunol.23.021704.115643
34. Sherry NA, Kushner JA, Glandt M, Kitamura T, Brillantes AB, Herold KC, et al. Effects of Autoimmunity and Immune Therapy on Beta-Cell Turnover in Type 1 Diabetes. *Diabetes* (2006) 55(12):3238–45. doi: 10.2337/db05-1034
35. Coppieters KT, Dotta F, Amirian N, Campbell PD, Kay TW, Atkinson MA, et al. Demonstration of Islet-Autoreactive CD8 T Cells in Insulitic Lesions From Recent Onset and Long-Term Type 1 Diabetes Patients. *J Exp Med* (2012) 209(1):51–60. doi: 10.1084/jem.20111187
36. Willcox A, Richardson SJ, Bone AJ, Foulis AK, Morgan NG. Analysis of Islet Inflammation in Human Type 1 Diabetes. *Clin Exp Immunol* (2009) 155 (2):173–81. doi: 10.1111/j.1365-2249.2008.03860.x
37. Reed JC, Herold KC. Thinking Bedside at the Bench: The NOD Mouse Model of T1DM. *Nat Rev Endocrinol* (2015) 11(5):308–14. doi: 10.1038/nrendo.2014.236
38. Holstein A, Kovacs P, Beil W. Severe Hypoglycemia Due to Possible Interaction Between Glibenclamide and Sorafenib in a Patient With Hepatocellular Carcinoma. *Curr Drug Saf* (2013) 8(2):148–52. doi: 10.2174/15748863113089990027
39. Agostino NM, Chinchilli VM, Lynch CJ, Koszyk-Szewczyk A, Gingrich R, Sivik J, et al. Effect of the Tyrosine Kinase Inhibitors (Sunitinib, Sorafenib, Dasatinib, and Imatinib) on Blood Glucose Levels in Diabetic and Nondiabetic Patients in General Clinical Practice. *J Oncol Pharm Pract* (2011) 17(3):197–202. doi: 10.1177/1078155210378913
40. Wilhelm S, Carter C, Lynch M, Lowinger T, Dumas J, Smith RA, et al. Discovery and Development of Sorafenib: A Multikinase Inhibitor for Treating Cancer. *Nat Rev Drug Discov* (2006) 5(10):835–44. doi: 10.1038/nrd2130
41. Jean GW, Mani RM, Jaffry A, Khan SA. Toxic Effects of Sorafenib in Patients With Differentiated Thyroid Carcinoma Compared With Other Cancers. *JAMA Oncol* (2016) 2(4):529–34. doi: 10.1001/jamaoncol.2015.5927
42. Horwitz E, Stein I, Andreozzi M, Nemeth J, Shoham A, Pappo O, et al. Human and Mouse VEGFA-Amplified Hepatocellular Carcinomas Are Highly Sensitive to Sorafenib Treatment. *Cancer Discovery* (2014) 4(6):730–43. doi: 10.1158/2159-8290.CD-13-0782
43. Wang C, Vegna S, Jin H, Benedict B, Lieftink C, Ramirez C, et al. Inducing and Exploiting Vulnerabilities for the Treatment of Liver Cancer. *Nature* (2019) 574(7777):268–72. doi: 10.1038/s41586-019-1607-3
44. Hillman M, Torn C, Thorgeirsson H, Landin-Olsson M. Igg4-Subclass of Glutamic Acid Decarboxylase Antibody Is More Frequent in Latent Autoimmune Diabetes in Adults Than in Type 1 Diabetes. *Diabetologia* (2004) 47(11):1984–9. doi: 10.1007/s00125-004-1558-5
45. Hernandez M, Mollo A, Marsal JR, Esquerda A, Capel I, Puig-Domingo M, et al. Insulin Secretion in Patients With Latent Autoimmune Diabetes (LADA): Half Way Between Type 1 and Type 2 Diabetes: Action LADA 9. *BMC Endocr Disord* (2015) 15:1. doi: 10.1186/1472-6823-15-1
46. Zampetti S, Campagna G, Tiberti C, Songini M, Arpi ML, Simone GD, et al. High GADA Titer Increases the Risk of Insulin Requirement in LADA Patients: A 7-Year Follow-Up (NIRAD Study 7). *Eur J Endocrinol* (2014) 171:697–704. doi: 10.1530/EJE-14-0342
47. van Belle TL, Coppieters KT, von Herrath MG. Type 1 Diabetes: Etiology, Immunology, and Therapeutic Strategies. *Physiol Rev* (2011) 91(1):79–118. doi: 10.1152/physrev.00003.2010
48. Alizadeh BZ, Hanifi-Moghaddam P, Eerligh P, Slik AR, Kolb H, Kharagjitsingh AV, et al. Association of Interferon-Gamma and Interleukin 10 Genotypes and Serum Levels With Partial Clinical Remission in Type 1 Diabetes. *Clin Exp Immunol* (2006) 145(3):480–4. doi: 10.1111/j.1365-2249.2006.03172.x
49. Karges B, Durinovic-Bello I, Heinze E, Debatin KM, Boehm B, Karges W. Immunological Mechanisms Associated With Long-Term Remission of Human Type 1 Diabetes. *Diabetes Metab Res Rev* (2006) 22(3):184–9. doi: 10.1002/dmrr.600
50. Schloot NC, Hanifi-Moghaddam P, Aabenhus-Andersen N, Alizadeh BZ, Saha MT, Knip M, et al. Association of Immune Mediators at Diagnosis of Type 1 Diabetes With Later Clinical Remission. *Diabetes Med* (2007) 24 (5):512–20. doi: 10.1111/j.1464-5491.2007.02096.x
51. Trivedi PM, Graham KL, Scott NA, Jenkins MR, Majaw S, Sutherland RM, et al. Repurposed JAK1/JAK2 Inhibitor Reverses Established Autoimmune Insulitis in NOD Mice. *Diabetes* (2017) 66(6):1650–60. doi: 10.2337/db16-1250
52. Chaimowitz NS, Ebenezer SJ, Hanson IC, Anderson M, Forbes LR. STAT1 Gain of Function, Type 1 Diabetes, and Reversal With JAK Inhibition. *N Engl J Med* (2020) 383(15):1494–6. doi: 10.1056/NEJMc2022226
53. Fabbri M, Frixou M, Degano M, Fousteri G. Type 1 Diabetes in STAT Protein Family Mutations: Regulating the Th17/Treg Equilibrium and Beyond. *Diabetes* (2019) 68(2):258–65. doi: 10.2337/db18-0627

17

Fruitarian Diet and Blood Glucose Control in Type 1 Diabetes

Claudia Vetrani[†], *Lutgarda Bozzetto*[†], *Giuseppe Della Pepa, Angela Albarosa Rivellese and Giovanni Annuzzi*[*]

Department of Clinical Medicine and Surgery, Federico II University, Naples, Italy

***Correspondence:**
Giovanni Annuzzi
annuzzi@unina.it

[†]*These authors have contributed equally to this work and share first authorship*

Diet is a key determinant of blood glucose control in individuals with type 1 diabetes. Although dietary education is part of their clinical follow-up, many patients show a propensity to self-treatment, adopting dietary changes, often extreme, that do not consider the overall impact on health. Here, we describe the case of a patient with type 1 diabetes who switched to a fruitarian diet because of ideological beliefs. A 25-year-old man with type 1 diabetes on an insulin pump and continuous glucose monitoring on optimal blood glucose control (HbA1c 6.5%, 48 mmol/mol; glucose time-in-range 70–180 mg/dl, TIR, 90%; coefficient of variation, CV, 36%) switched to a fruitarian diet because of ideological beliefs. After 3 months on this diet, blood glucose control was still optimal (TIR 88%, CV 33%), while plasma triglycerides and liver enzymes were above normal values. After 3 more months, blood glucose control had worsened (TIR 72%, CV 37%), plasma triglyceride and liver enzymes were within normal values, and hyperkalemia was detected. In this case report, a strict fruitarian diet was associated with early negative changes in some biochemical parameters, also in presence of optimal blood glucose control. Dietary counseling remains essential in the follow-up of patients with type 1 diabetes to ensure personalized medical nutrition therapy and monitor dietary changes that may affect health but with no major impact on blood glucose control.

Keywords: type 1 diabetes, eating habits, fruitarian diet, glucose control, insulin pump, continuous glucose monitoring

INTRODUCTION

Diet is a key determinant of blood glucose control in individuals with type 1 diabetes (1). Over the years, many dietary patterns have been proposed to address high glucose variability. A plant-based diet (2) and a low-carbohydrate diet (3) are becoming popular among individuals with diabetes mainly aiming at limiting hyperglycemia. According to international nutritional guidelines (1, 4), there is no ideal distribution of calories among carbohydrates, proteins, and fats for individuals with diabetes. Therefore, in clinical practice, each patient is advised to improve overall diet quality, considering his/her eating habits, food preferences, as much as possible, and metabolic targets. However, many patients show a propensity to self-treatment, adopting dietary changes, often extreme, that do not consider the overall impact on health. Here, we describe the case of a type 1 diabetes patient who switched to a fruitarian diet because of ideological beliefs. He used social media to increase his knowledge and obtain a meal plan.

CASE PRESENTATION

A 25-year-old man was diagnosed with type 1 diabetes at the age of 9. He is on an insulin pump and wears a sensor for continuous glucose monitoring (CGM).

TABLE 1 | Anthropometric, blood glucose control, and biochemical parameters.

	August 2020	November 2020	January 2021	April 2021
BMI (kg/m^2)	24.8	24.2	24.2	24.3
HbA1c (%)	6.5	-	6.2	6.6
HbA1c (mmol/mol)	48	-	44	49
Time in range (% blood glucose 70–180 mg/dl)	90	89	88	72
Time above range (% blood glucose >180 mg/dl)	8	9	10	26
Time below range (% blood glucose <70 mg/dl)	2	2	2	2
Mean glucose (mg/dl)	127 ± 46	127 ± 42	131 ± 44	153 ± 57
Coefficient of variation (%)	36	33	33	37
Total cholesterol (mg/dl)	142	-	125	151
LDL-cholesterol (mg/dl)	71	-	47	70
Triglyceride (mg/dl)	105	-	165	136
AST (U/l)	28	-	37	29
ALT (U/l)	22	-	45	28
GGT (U/l)	15	-	30	24

HbA1c, glycated hemoglobin; AST, aspartate transaminase; ALT, alanine transaminase; GGT, γ-glutamyl transferase.

At a follow-up out-patient visit in August 2020, his body mass index (BMI) was 24.8 kg/m^2 and his biochemical parameters were unremarkable (**Table 1**). Total daily insulin doses were 24.8 ± 3.1 IU (44% bolus and 56% basal infusion). He had an optimal blood glucose control, as shown by an HbA1c level of 6.5% (48 mmol/mol) and the glucose metrics derived by CGM (5) that also showed high daily glucose variability (coefficient of variation, CV, 36%) (**Table 1**). A diabetologist discussed the CGM profile (**Figure 1A**) with the patient and did not suggest changes in insulin therapy. Dietary habits, as evaluated by a 7-day food record, mainly showed a low intake of carbohydrates and a high intake of total fats and saturated fatty acids (**Table 2**). In accordance with the Standards of Medical Care by the American Diabetes Association (1), a dietitian advised him to reduce the intake of saturated fatty acids and increase carbohydrates from low glycemic index foods.

In November 2020, he joined an educational group to reinforce carbohydrate counting in accordance with our standard diabetes care for patients on an insulin pump. On this occasion, he told the dietitian that he had become a fruitarian in October 2020, experiencing, in his opinion, an improvement in blood glucose control. A 7-day food record confirmed that, according to the fruitarian diet, he had increased carbohydrates, mostly sugars and fructose, and fiber intake, while reducing the intake of proteins and fats (**Table 2**). CGM metrics confirmed an optimal blood glucose control (**Table 1**). Seven-day mean daily glucose variability was slightly lower (CV 33%), and the CGM profile was smoother than the previous one (**Figure 1B**). Total insulin doses were unchanged (24.8 ± 3.1 IU) with a shift to a

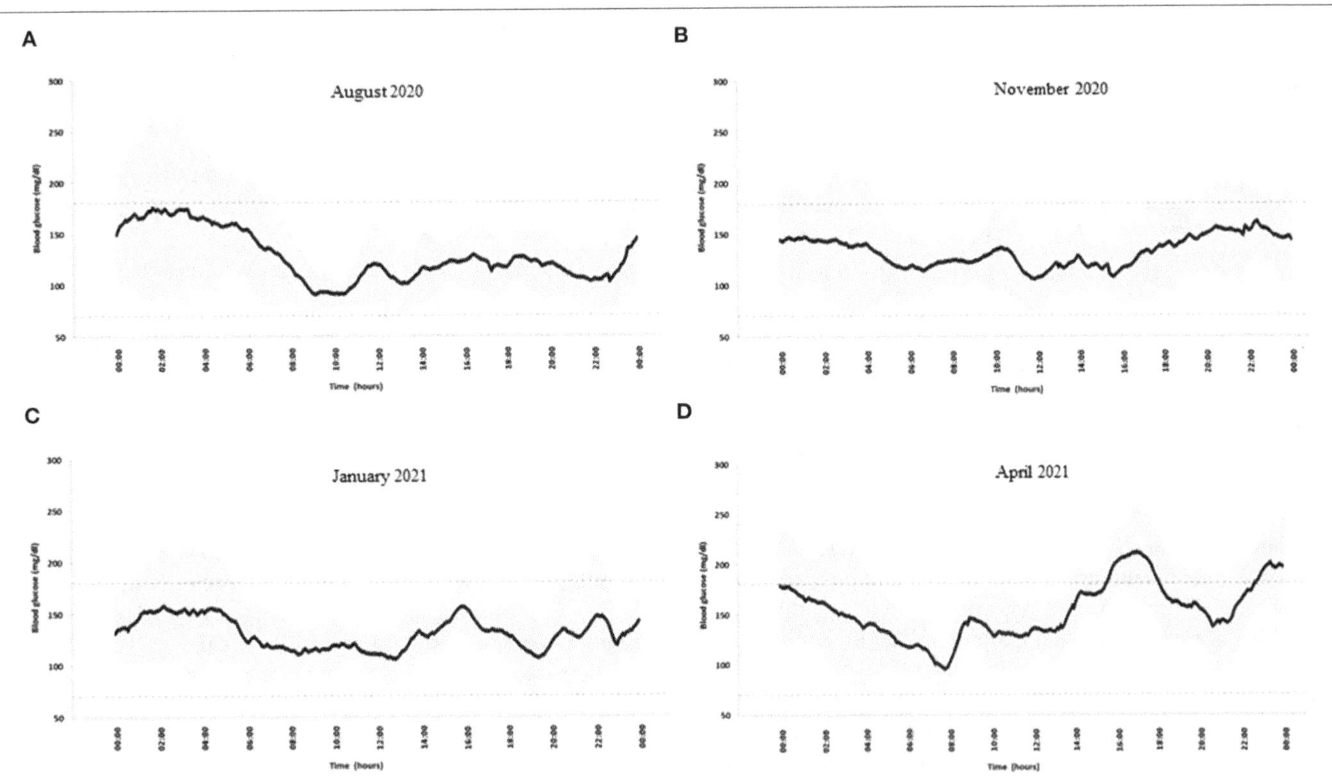

FIGURE 1 | Blood glucose profile in **(A)** August 2020, **(B)** November2020, **(C)** January 2021, and **(D)** April 2021. Black line: mean blood glucose concentrations; gray shadows: glucose variability expressed as SD. Dotted lines indicate blood glucose time in the range 70–180 mg/dl.

TABLE 2 | Mean daily energy intake and dietary composition obtained through 7-day food records during follow-up.

	August 2020	November 2020	April 2021	Absolute change November *vs.* August	Absolute change April *vs.* August
Energy (kcal)	1,977	2,030	1,980	+53	+3
Protein (g)	113.4	34.0	46.0	−79	−67
(% TEI)	24.1	7.0	9.8	−17	−14
-Animal (g)	76.8	0	0	−77	−77
(% TEI)	67.7	0	0	−68	−68
-Plant (g)	35.2	34.0	42.4	−1	+7
(% TEI)	31.0	6.7	8.6	−24	−22
Carbohydrate (g)	167.4	412.0	433.8	+245	+266
(% TEI)	33.4	79.4	86.4	+46	+53
-Starch (g)	115.3	18.0	24.0	−97	−91
(% TEI)	23.3	3.5	4.8	−20	−19
-Sugar (g)	32.6	392.5	398.7	+360	+366
(% TEI)	6.5	95.3	91.9	+89	+85
-Fructose (g)	1.59	125.3	64.5	+124	+63
Fat (g)	88.9	29.3	8.5	−60	−80
(% TEI)	42.6	13.6	4.1	−29	−39
-SFA (g)	19.5	3.8	1.8	−16	−18
-MUFA (g)	52.5	21.5	1.0	−31	−52
-PUFA (g)	12.5	2.7	2.5	−10	−10
Cholesterol (mg)	248.0	0	0	−248	−248
Fiber (g)	29.5	42.0	49.2	+13	+20
Glycemic index (%)	66.2	49.8	47.1	−16	−19
Glycemic load	98.1	155.2	156.1	+57	+58
Sodium (mg)	1,738	67.2	93.0	−1,671	−1,645
Potassium (g)	3.59	6.92	9.62	+3.3	+6.03
Calcium (mg)	738.8	269.3	420.5	−470	−318
Phosphorus (mg)	1,617	524.4	1,038	−1,093	−579
Iron (mg)	32.2	10.3	19.5	−22	−13
Vitamin C (mg)	124.6	275.8	875	+151	+750
Vitamin E (mg)	15.8	9.95	5.64	−6	−10
Vitamin D (μg)	6.98	0	0	−7	−7
Vitamin B12 (μg)	76.4	0	0	−76	−76

MUFAs, monounsaturated fatty acids; PUFAs, polyunsaturated fatty acids; SFAs, saturated fatty acids; TEI, total energy intake.

relatively higher proportion of pre-prandial insulin (66% bolus and 34% basal). He reported no changes in body weight and physical activity.

In January 2021, after 3 months on the fruitarian diet, biochemical laboratory analyses showed a 50% increase in plasma triglyceride and doubling of liver enzymes. A liver ultrasound examination showed no signs of steatosis. As compared to November 2020, no changes in glucose variability, CGM metrics and profile, total insulin doses, body weight, and physical activity were observed (**Table 1** and **Figure 1C**). Against the advice of health care providers, the patient chose to continue the fruitarian diet.

At the follow-up visit in April, blood glucose control was adequate according to CGM metrics, although glucose time-above-range had increased compared to the previous period (**Table 1**). Daily glucose variability had increased (37%), as also evidenced by the CGM profile (**Figure 1D**). Basal/bolus proportion was similar to that in August 2020 (47% bolus and 53% basal). As compared to November 2020, he had reintroduced raw protein-rich vegetables (artichokes, mushrooms, carrots, and zucchini) with no major changes in the mean dietary composition, except for reduced intake of fructose and monounsaturated fatty acids (**Table 2**). However, he reported occasional episodes of uncontrolled behavior, when he was consuming different foods, mainly pizza and bread, in considerable amounts. He did not report changes in body weight and physical activity. Plasma triglyceride and liver enzymes concentrations were within normal ranges (**Table 1**). An increased plasma potassium concentration was detected (6 mmol/L).

Healthcare providers cautioned the patient on the harmful effects of this diet on his long-term health (i.e., increased glucose variability, liver abnormalities, and hyperkaliemia).

The patient was provided a dietary plan to switch to a more balanced diet, suggesting to increase the intake of plant proteins and fats by favoring the consumption of legumes, sprouted grains, and extra-virgin olive oil (6). Moreover, the patient was asked to reduce the amount of K-rich foods (i.e., banana, dates) and total fruits to standard servings (400–500 g/day), preferring whole fruits over juices because of their higher fiber content and lower glycemic index (7). Nevertheless, the patient expressed his will to continue the fruitarian diet mainly because of its environmental and social implications.

Therefore, healthcare providers planned a strict follow-up to monitor circulating liver enzymes and electrolyte concentrations, liver fat content, and potential vitamin and mineral deficiencies.

DISCUSSION

The fruitarian diet is based on fruits, nuts, and seeds. Vegetables that are classified botanically as fruits (i.e., avocado and tomatoes) are included, while other vegetables, namely, grains and beans, and animal products are excluded (6). Concerns about the fruitarian diet have focused mainly on its high fructose content. Indeed, high fructose intake may increase triglyceride concentrations by promoting hepatic lipogenesis, and several epidemiological studies have suggested an association between average daily fructose intake and liver steatosis (8, 9). Evidence from randomized controlled clinical trials is not conclusive, although some studies reported increased liver fat accumulation after fructose consumption in healthy individuals (10) or people with type 2 diabetes (11). To the best of our knowledge, no studies evaluating the effect of fructose consumption on liver fat in individuals with type 1 diabetes are currently available.

Other potential major flaws related to the fruitarian diet refer to poor diet quality and nutritional deficiencies, particularly in terms of protein, omega-3 fatty acids (EPA and DHA), and micronutrients (i.e., vitamin B12, iron, and zinc) (6).

This case report shows that a short-term fruitarian diet increases plasma triglyceride and liver enzymes concentrations, particularly in the first 3 months, with no significant effects on liver fat accumulation evident on ultrasound evaluation. Unlike processed and refined foods with simple sugars, fruits contain several bioactive compounds with antioxidant activity (vitamins, minerals, fiber, polyphenols, and other phytochemicals). These compounds might reduce oxidative stress and inflammation that are major contributors to liver steatosis.

Plasma triglyceride and liver enzymes tended to reduce after 6 months. This might be related to lower adherence to the strict fruitarian diet, as also stated by the patient.

As for blood glucose control, it has been shown that fructose is a slow digestible carbohydrate that induces a lower postprandial blood glucose response than glucose in individuals with type 1 diabetes (12, 13). This could explain the reduction in glucose variability in the first 3 months of the fruitarian diet. Of note, the patient experienced more user-friendliness and feasibility in tracking the grams of carbohydrate since he had gone fruitarian. Indeed, his habitual meal plan (**Supplementary Table 1**) does not contain mixed meals that could require advanced knowledge of foodstuff composition to adjust insulin doses to compensate for delayed postprandial glycemic excursions (1). Therefore, optimal carbohydrate counting may have contributed to the achievement of optimal glycemic control with reduced glucose variability.

On the other hand, as stated by the patient, the fruitarian diet is highly restrictive (i.e., limited food options, difficulty in attending social events), and it affected his meal regularity, resulting in occasional loss of control with high consumption of highly gratifying comfort foods. This may have contributed to his worsened blood glucose control in the last period, in addition to the reported high intake of orange juice (**Supplementary Table 1**) that has recently been demonstrated to negatively affect blood glucose control in a cohort of individuals with type 1 diabetes (14).

Another reason of concern was the increased plasma potassium (K) concentration observed after 6 months on the fruitarian diet that is in line with the fact that daily dietary K intake reported by the patient was three-fold higher than the recommended one (3.9 g/day). Previous studies have shown increased circulating K concentrations with no changes in renal function after short-term oral K supplementation (15).

To the best of our knowledge, there is no evidence on short- or long-term effects of the fruitarian diet in patients with type 1 diabetes. Nevertheless, according to the evidence existing on high-glycemic index and sugars, we would at present strongly discourage the use of the fruitarian diet for patients with diabetes. Further experimental clinical research is required on the usefulness and safety of extreme plant-based diets.

In conclusion, this case emphasizes the importance of close dietary counseling in the follow-up of patients with type 1 diabetes to ensure personalized medical nutrition therapy, in accordance with the current guidelines. This may allow for the correction of early alterations, not recognizable based only on blood glucose control, before incurring harmful consequences. In the era of social media, patients are exposed to fashionable dietary trends and ready-to-use information that might endanger their health. At the present state of knowledge, the fruitarian diet is not recommended for patients with diabetes.

AUTHOR CONTRIBUTIONS

CV and LB wrote the report and analyzed the data. GD collected the data and contributed to commentary. AR and GA provided relevant intellectual contributions to the development of the report. GA is the guarantor of this study and as such, had full access to all the patient data and takes responsibility for the integrity and accuracy of the case presentation. All authors revised the manuscript and gave final approval of the version to be submitted for publication.

ACKNOWLEDGMENTS

The authors would like to thank the patient who accepted the collection and sharing of his data.

SUPPLEMENTARY MATERIAL

Supplementary Table 1 | Examples of the daily menu as reported in the 7-day food records.

REFERENCES

1. American Diabetes Association. Lifestyle management: standards of medical care in diabetes. *Diabetes Care.* (2019) 42(Suppl. 1):S46–60. doi: 10.2337/dc19-S005
2. Salas-Salvadó J, Becerra-Tomás N, Papandreou C, Bulló M. Dietary patterns emphasizing the consumption of plant foods in the management of type 2 diabetes: a narrative review. *Adv Nutr.* (2019) 10:S320–31. doi: 10.1093/advances/nmy102
3. Bolla AM, Caretto A, Laurenzi A, Scavini M, Piemonti L. Low-carb and ketogenic diets in type 1 and type 2 diabetes. *Nutrients.*(2019) 11:962. doi: 10.3390/nu11050962
4. Cosentino F, Grant PJ, Aboyans V, Bailey CJ, Ceriello A, Delgado V, et al. 2019 ESC Guidelines on diabetes, pre-diabetes, and cardiovascular diseases developed in collaboration with the EASD. *Eur Heart J.* (2020) 41:255–323. doi: 10.1093/eurheartj/ehz486
5. Battelino T, Danne T, Bergenstal RM, Amiel SA, Beck R, Biester T, et al. Clinical target for continuous glucose monitoring data interpretation: recommendations from the international consensus on time in range. *Diabetes Care.* (2019) 42:1593–603. doi: 10.2337/dci19-0028
6. Melina V, Craig W, Levin S. Position of the academy of nutrition and dietetics: vegetarian diets. *J AcadNutr Diet.* (2016) 116:1970–80. doi: 10.1016/j.jand.2016.09.025
7. Locke A, Schneiderhan J, Zick SM. Diets for health: goals and guidelines. *Am Fam Physician.* (2018) 97:721–8.
8. Ter Horst KW, Serlie MJ. Fructose consumption, lipogenesis, and non-alcoholic fatty liver disease. *Nutrients.* (2017) 9:981. doi: 10.3390/nu9090981
9. Della Pepa G, Vetrani C, Lombardi G, Bozzetto L, Annuzzi G, Rivellese AA. Isocaloric dietary changes and non-alcoholic fatty liver disease in high cardiometabolic risk individuals. *Nutrients.* (2017) 9:1065. doi: 10.3390/nu9101065
10. Schwarz JM, Noworolski SM, Wen MJ, Dyachenko A, Prior JL, Weinberg ME, et al. Effect of a high-fructose weight-maintaining diet on lipogenesis and liver fat. *J Clin Endocrinol Metab.* (2015) 100:2434–42. doi: 10.1210/jc.2014-3678
11. Taskinen MR, Söderlund S, Bogl LH, Hakkarainen A, Matikainen N, Pietiläinen KH, et al. Adverse effects of fructose on cardiometabolic risk factors and hepatic lipid metabolism in subjects with abdominal obesity. *J InternMed.* (2017) 282:187–201. doi: 10.1111/joim.12632
12. Souto DL, Lima ÉDS, Dantas JR, Zajdenverg L, Rodacki M, Rosado EL. Postprandial metabolic effects of fructose and glucose in type 1 diabetes patients: a pilot randomized crossover clinical trial. *Arch Endocrinol Metab.* (2019) 63:376–84. doi: 10.20945/2359-3997000000148
13. Dos Santos Lima É, Souto DL, Rodacki M, Pereira JRD, Zajdenverg L, Rosado EL. Metabolic and appetite effects of fructose and glucose in subjects with type 1 diabetes: a randomized crossover clinical trial. *Curr Diabetes Rev.* (2021) 17:e113020188536. doi: 10.2174/1573399816666201201092334
14. Basu A, Alman AC, Snell-Bergeon JK. Associations of dietary patterns and nutrients with glycated hemoglobin in participants with and without type 1 diabetes. *Nutrients.* (2021) 13:1035. doi: 10.3390/nu13031035
15. Cappuccio FP, Buchanan LA, Ji C, Siani A, Miller MA. Systematic review and meta-analysis of randomised controlled trials on the effects of potassium supplements on serum potassium and creatinine. *BMJ Open.*(2016) 6:e011716. doi: 10.1136/bmjopen-2016-011716

18

Soluble CD137 Ameliorates Acute Type 1 Diabetes by Inducing T Cell Anergy

Arata Itoh[1], *Lorenzo Ortiz*[1], *Kritika Kachapati*[1], *Yuehong Wu*[1], *David Adams*[1], *Kyle Bednar*[1], *Shibabrata Mukherjee*[2], *Claire Chougnet*[2], *Robert S. Mittler*[3,4], *Yi-Guang Chen*[5], *Laurence Dolan*[6] *and William M. Ridgway*[1*†]

[1] Division of Immunology, Allergy and Rheumatology, University of Cincinnati College of Medicine, Cincinnati, OH, United States, [2] Division of Immunobiology, Cincinnati Children's Hospital Medical Center, Cincinnati, OH, United States, [3] Department of Surgery, Emory University, Atlanta, GA, United States, [4] Emory Vaccine Center, Atlanta, GA, United States, [5] Department of Pediatrics, Medical College of Wisconsin, Milwaukee, WI, United States, [6] Division of Endocrinology, Cincinnati Children's Hospital Medical Center, Cincinnati, OH, United States

***Correspondence:**
William M. Ridgway
ridgwawm@ucmail.uc.edu

We show here that soluble CD137 (sCD137), the alternately spliced gene product of *Tnfsfr9*, effectively treats acute type 1 diabetes (T1D) in nonobese diabetic (NOD) mice. sCD137 significantly delayed development of end-stage disease, preserved insulin+ islet beta cells, and prevented progression to end-stage T1D in some mice. We demonstrate that sCD137 induces CD4+ T cell anergy, suppressing antigen-specific T cell proliferation and IL-2/IFN-γ secretion. Exogenous IL-2 reversed the sCD137 anergy effect. sCD137 greatly reduces inflammatory cytokine production by CD8 effector memory T cells, critical mediators of beta cell damage. We demonstrate that human T1D patients have decreased serum sCD137 compared to age-matched controls (as do NOD mice compared to NOD congenic mice expressing a protective *Tnfsfr9* allele), that human sCD137 is secreted by regulatory T cells (Tregs; as in mice), and that human sCD137 induces T cell suppression in human T cells. These findings provide a rationale for further investigation of sCD137 as a treatment for T1D and other T cell–mediated autoimmune diseases.

Keywords: type 1 diabetes, autoimmunity, T cells, T cell anergy, soluble CD137

INTRODUCTION

Type 1 diabetes (T1D) is a complex autoimmune disease resulting from specific immunological destruction of pancreatic insulin-producing beta cells, leading to hyperglycemia, and ketoacidosis (1, 2). Nonobese diabetic (NOD) mice are a well-established animal model of T1D that reflects many of the same features as human T1D (3, 4). NOD mice spontaneously develop T1D (typically ~80% of females spontaneously develop T1D by 30 weeks in many colonies), mediated by autoreactive CD4 and CD8 T cells recognizing many of the same autoantigens found in the human disease. NOD mice also demonstrate genetic control of T1D with key contributions from genes that are implicated in human disease, including MHC class II genes (3). CD4 and CD8 T cells, in combination with environmental factors and genetic background, play an essential role in beta cell destruction in both NOD mice and humans (5, 6). In NOD mice, dysregulation of both effector and regulatory T cells (Tregs) is well-described (7).

Wicker et al. originally established that the B10 chromosome 4 genetic region *Idd9.3*, which includes the candidate gene *Tnfsfr9* (expressing CD137, also known as 4-1bb), protects from T1D in NOD *Idd9.3* congenic mice (8). We published that treatment with an agonistic CD137 antibody prevented T1D in NOD mice, at least partly by targeting and increasing the numbers of the CD4+CD25+CD137+ Treg subset (9). We then showed that the protective B10 *Idd9.3* allele was associated with increased numbers of CD4+CD25+CD137+ Tregs, which were functionally superior to CD25+ Tregs (10). We further showed that CD137+ Tregs produce an alternately spliced, soluble form of CD137, "sCD137," and that NOD mice had a decreased serum level of sCD137 compared to protected NOD *Idd9.3* congenic mice (10, 11). We produced recombinant mouse sCD137, demonstrated that it formed a homo-dimer, and showed that sCD137 directly suppresses effector CD4+CD25− and CD8 T cell proliferation in an APC-independent but CD137 ligand (CD137L)–dependent manner (11, 12). Finally, "restoring" serum levels by administration of recombinant sCD137 into NOD mice significantly prevented autoimmune diabetes compared with control treatment (11).

Although these results showed a suppressive effect of sCD137 on T cells, the mechanism of this effect was unclear. In addition, "prevention" of T1D (especially in NOD mice) is much different (and much easier to accomplish) than therapeutic efficacy in acute disease. Finally, we had not yet demonstrated any relevance of this work to human T1D. We address these issues in the current manuscript and show that (1) recombinant sCD137 acts by inducing antigen-specific T cell anergy; (2) sCD137 can ameliorate acute T1D; and (3) human T1D patients show a deficit of serum sCD137 similar to that seen in NOD mice, human Tregs are the main immune cell source of sCD137 just as in mice, and human sCD137 suppresses human T cell proliferation. These results support further exploration of sCD137 as a novel treatment approach in human T1D and other T cell–mediated autoimmune diseases.

MATERIALS AND METHODS

Mice

NOD and NOD BDC2.5 transgenic mice were bred and maintained under specific pathogen-free conditions, and all procedures involving mice were conducted in accordance with the institutional animal care guidelines at the University of Cincinnati College of Medicine Laboratory Animal Medical Services.

Purification of sCD137

Recombinant *Mus musculus* sCD137 was purified as previously described (9). Briefly, HEK293 cells were stably transduced with a lentiviral vector, LeGO-iG2-sCD137, expressing recombinant mouse sCD137 cDNA from the construct's SFFV promoter. Secreted sCD137 protein was purified from the culture supernatants using anti-CD137 antibody (clone: 3H3) affinity chromatography. After elution from the column, purified protein was dialyzed against 2 × 4 L of 1×TBS, then 2 × 4 L of 1×PBS, and then concentrated using Amicon Ultra-15 Ultracel 10 K centrifugal filters. The amount of purified sCD137 was determined by spectrophotometry and its specificity tested by binding to *M. musculus* CD137L-Myc-DDK protein expressed on the surface of HEK293 cells. SDS-PAGE and western blotting were used to confirm the dimeric state of active protein, as previously described (9). Prior to injection into mice, concentrated protein was thawed and diluted in sterile vehicle (1×PBS).

In vivo Treatment of Diabetic NOD Mice With sCD137

Prediabetic female NOD mice were randomly assigned to either control or sCD137 treatment groups. These mice were assessed for diabetes onset using urine glucose paper testing (Tes-Tape, Nasco) and their glucose levels quantified with a standard one-step blood glucose meter. After onset of polyuria, and when two consecutive blood glucose measurements were between 200 and 250 mg/dl (group 1) or 250 and 300 mg/dl (group 2), mice were treated with sCD137 (120 μg/mice) intraperitoneally injected at day 0. At day 4 and after day 7, if their repeat BG was still 200 or 250 mg/dl, treatment with the same dose of sCD137 was continued weekly until they reached "end-stage diabetes," defined as BG>500 mg/dl, or reached the study end point (10 weeks). Mice were excluded from the study (1) if they never developed T1D or (2) if their initial BG was not in the pre-specified range. The age of onset of diabetes in the female NOD mice in group 1 (initial BG 200–250) in the sCD137 and control groups was 24 ± 1 and 22 ± 3 weeks old of age, respectively ($p = 0.4763$). In group 2 (initial BG 250–300 mg/dl), the age of onset of the treatment and control groups was 24 ± 3 and 27 ± 2 weeks of age, respectively ($p = 0.2797$). For controls, group 1 used untreated NOD mice; this group of mice was also used as the control for another concurrent study, which has already been published (13). For group 2, control mice were treated with PBS i.p. at the same time points described above. At the end points, the pancreas was harvested and fixed in formalin for processing by the CCHMC Department of Anatomic Pathology. Pancreatic insulitis on H&E-stained slides was blindly scored as previously described (11, 13) (0: no visible infiltration; 1: peri-insulitis with a cell depth <5; 2: peri-insulitis with a cell depth >5; 3: insulitis with <50% islet infiltration; 4: insulitis with more than 50% islet infiltration; 5: islet scar). For quantification of islet immunofluorescence, insulin was stained with Insulin guinea pig primary antibody (Roche, cat. # 760-2655), and glucagon was stained with Glucagon rabbit primary antibody (Roche, cat. # 760-2644) overnight at 4°C, followed by staining using Texas-Red conjugated anti–guinea pig IgG and FITC-conjugated anti-rabbit IgG antibodies as secondary antibodies. Then, the nucleus was stained with DAPI (Vecta-shield with DAPI, Vector, cat. # H-1500) at the CCHMC Pathology Core. We imaged sCD137-treated mice that had not progressed to end-stage T1D and five randomly chosen control mice that reached end-stage diabetes. One pancreatic section per animal was stained with immunofluorescence. Whole slide digital images were created using a Leica Aperio AT2 digital slide scanner. Digital dual-immunofluorescence histology slides were analyzed using Photomerge (Adobe Photoshop) and Aperio ImageScope software (Leica Biosystems), used to count insulin and glucagon positive-staining regions per section.

Antigen-Specific T Cell Proliferation Assay

CD4+CD25− effector T cells were magnetically isolated from 6- to 10-week-old female BDC2.5 transgenic female mice using the CD4+ T cell isolation kit followed by removal of CD25+ cells with the CD25+ microbeads kit (Myltenyi Biotec). Fifty thousand cells were co-cultured with antigen-presenting cells plus 10 nM of BDC2.5:insulin hybrid peptide [sequence: DLQTLALWSRMD (14)], in the presence or absence of 60 μg/ml of sCD137 for 4 days on a 96-well flat-bottom plate in triplicated manner. Cells were resuspended in 0.2 mL of T cell culture media (TCM), composed of RPMI-1640 media (Lonza) supplemented with 10% heat-inactivated FBS (GE Lifescience), 10 mM of HEPES (Gibco), 2 mM of L-glutamine (Gibco), 100 U/ml of penicillin/streptomycin (Gibco), 100 nM of sodium pyruvate (Gibco), non-essential amino acids (Gibco), and 150 μM of β-mercaptoethanol (Sigma). In some wells, 25 U/ml of recombinant mouse IL-2 (Invitrogen) was added at the start or 24 h after starting cell culture. In the last 18 h of cell culture, 1 μCi of [3H] thymidine was added to each well. Cells were harvested and counted using a β-scintillation counter.

Flow Cytometry for Cell-Surface and Intracellular Phosphorylated Proteins

CD4+CD25− or CD8 T cells (0.5×10^5) were negatively isolated with either a CD4 T cell isolation kit and CD25 microbeads (Miltenyi Biotec) or a CD8 T cell isolation kit (Miltenyi Biotec), respectively. Cells were resuspended in 0.2 mL of TCM and stimulated with CD3/28 dynabeads (cell-to-bead ratio 1:1) in the presence of sCD137 or rapamycin (10 nM at final concentration) for 24 h on a 96-well round-bottom plate. Harvested cells were stained with eFluor 450–conjugated rat anti-mouse CD4 (clone: GK1.5, Thermo Fisher Scientific), PE-conjugated rat anti-mouse CD71 (clone: RI7217, BioLegend), and Alexa647-conjugated rat anti-mouse CD98 (clone: RL388, BioLegend) followed by staining of the dead cell population with Fixable Viability Dye eFluor 780 (Thermo Fisher Scientific). In another cell culture, harvested cells were fixed in 0.8% formaldehyde (Sigma-Aldrich) PBS solution for 15 min at room temperature and then permeabilized using ice-cold 99.9% HPLC-grade methanol (Fisher Scientific) for 30 min on ice. To exclude dead cells, Fixable Viability Dye eFluor 780 (eBioscience) was added between the cell fixation and permeabilization steps. Intracellular phosphorylated proteins were then stained with Alexa-Fluor-488–conjugated anti-phospho-S6 ribosomal protein (S235/S236) (clone: D57.2.2E, Cell Signaling Technology) and APC-conjugated anti-phospho AKT (S473) (clone: SDRNR, eBioscience) for 30 min at 4°C. Cell-surface and intracellular phosphorylated protein were analyzed on LSRFortessa (Becton Dickenson).

Cytokine Secretion From Mouse T Cell Subsets Stimulated *in vitro*

Splenic CD4 or CD8 T cells from prediabetic NOD mice were purified using either CD4 or CD8 microbeads (Miltenyi Biotecs) or FACS-sorted using a FACSAria II (Becton Dickinson) into CD62L^{high}CD44^{low} (naïve), CD62L^{high}CD44^{high} (central memory, CM), or CD62L^{low}CD44^{high} (effector memory, EM) CD4 or CD8 T cell subsets using PE-conjugated rat anti-mouse CD62L (clone: MEL-14, BD Biosciences), Alexa-Fluor-700–conjugated rat anti-mouse CD44 (clone: IM7, BD Biosciences), FITC-conjugated rat anti-mouse CD4 (clone: GK1.5, BioLegend), and APC-conjugated rat anti-mouse CD3e (clone: 17A2, BioLegend) for CD4 T cell subset sorting, or BD Horizon V500-conjugated rat anti-mouse CD8 (clone: 53-6.7, BD Biosciences) and FITC-conjugated hamster anti-mouse TCRβ (clone: H57-597, BD Biosciences) for CD8 T cell subset sorting; 1×10^5 cells of each sorted cell subset were resuspended in 0.2 mL of TCM as described above and stimulated with 25,000 beads/well of CD3/CD28 dynabeads (Invitrogen) for 24 h in the presence or absence of recombinant sCD137 on a 96-well round-bottom plate. In some experiments, 1×10^5 cells of magnetically purified CD4 or CD8 T cells were stimulated with 25,000 CD3/28 dynabeads for a total of 72 h, and sCD137 was added at indicated time points. IL-2 and IFN-ɤ protein concentrations in collected supernatants were measured by ELISA using IL-2 ELISA ready-set-Go! (eBioscience) and IFN-ɤ ELISA ready-set-Go! (eBioscience), respectively, following the manufacturer's instruction.

Cell Cycle Analysis

Splenic CD4+ T cells were magnetically purified and stimulated as described above, with or without sCD137 for 48 h. The percentages of harvested CD4 T cells in G0/G1, S, or G2/M phase were analyzed using FITC BrdU Flow kit (BD Biosciences), following the manufacturer's protocol. Briefly, 10 μM (final concentration) of BrdU was added 45 min before harvesting, fixing, and permeabilizing cells. Cells were incubated for 1 h in the presence of 300 μg/mL of DNase-PBS solution at 37°C and stained with anti-BrdU FITC antibody and 7-AAD. The percentage of cells in each cell cycle phase was then evaluated on FACSCalibur (BD Biosciences).

Gene Expression Analysis

CD44-positive or -negative (naïve) CD4 or CD8 T cells were purified using CD4 or CD8 naïve T cell isolation kit (Miltenyi Biotec). Fifty thousand CD44-positive or CD44-negative (naïve) cells resuspended in 0.2 ml/well of TCM were stimulated with 50,000 CD3/28 beads and harvested at the indicated times in 96-well round-bottom plate. Messenger RNA was extracted from harvested cells using RNeasy Plus Mini Kits (QIAGEN). cDNA was synthesized by PrimeScript RT Master Mix (Takara, Inc.), and semi-quantitative PCR was performed using SYBR® FAST qPCR Master mix and other KAPA reagents (KAPA Biosystems, Inc.). All qRT-PCR experiments were performed in duplicate on a StepOnePlus Real-time PCR system (Applied Biosystems). *Tnfsf9* (CD137L) gene expression data were normalized to *Gapdh* expression. Mm_Gapdh_3_SG and Mm_Tnfsf9_1_SG

QuantiTect Primer Assay (Qiagen) for *gapdh* and *Tnfsf9* gene expression, respectively, were used as primers.

Induction and Restimulation of Differentiated Th1 Cells *in vitro*

Splenic CD4 T cells (1×10^6) isolated from 10-week-old prediabetic female NOD mice were stimulated with plate-bound anti-CD3 antibody (3 μg/ml, clone: 145-2C11, BD Biosciences, USA) and soluble anti-CD28 antibody (3 μg/ml, clone: 37.51, BD Biosciences) in the presence of recombinant mouse IL-12 (10 ng/mL, TONBO Biosciences), recombinant mouse IL-2 (5 ng/mL, Invitrogen, USA), and anti-IL-4 antibody (10 μg/ml, clone: 11B11, BD Biosciences, USA) in 12-well culture plates. After 5 days, cells were harvested and washed, and 1×10^6 differentiated Th1 cells were treated with plate-bound anti-CD3 antibody (1 μg/ml) and soluble anti-CD28 antibody (1 μg/ml) in the presence or absence of recombinant sCD137 (240 μg/mL) for 24 h. In some wells, recombinant mouse IL-2 (25 U/ml) was added. After 24 h, cells were washed and rested in fresh TCM without IL-2 for 48 h; 0.5×10^5 rested living cells were restimulated with plate-bound anti-CD3 antibody (0.5 μg/ml) and soluble anti-CD28 antibody (0.5 μg/ml) for 24 h. Supernatant was collected, and IL-2 concentration was measured by ELISA.

Production of CD137L-Expressing Cells Lines and Testing for Specific sCD137 Binding

(1) Construction of CD137L-expressing cell lines. TrueORF cDNA expression clones for C-terminal Myc- and DDK (Flag)-tagged *M. musculus* TNFSF9 were obtained (cat. # MR220933, Origen). Circular plasmid DNA was isolated and restricted with ApaLI (NEB) to linearize the vector DNA. Linearized DNA was then transfected into HEK293 cells using Lipofectamine 2000 and stable integrants selected for using 400–500 μg/ml of Geneticin (G418). After isolation and expansion of individual cell clones, high mouse CD137L-Myc-DDK expressers were stained with rat anti-mouse CD137L antibody (clone: TKS-1, BioLegend) or Rat IgG2a isotype control antibody (clone: RTK2758, BioLegend), followed by biotinylated mouse anti-Rat IgG2a antibody (clone: RG7/1.30, BD Biosciences) and streptavidin PE (BioLegend), identified using BD FACSCanto (BD Biosciences).

(2) Confirmation of specific binding of sCD137 to CD137L. HEK-mCD137L or control HEK293 cells (2×10^6) were preincubated with 1 ug/sample of anti-CD137L Ab (TKS-1) or the same volume of PBS for 30 min at 4°C. After washing cells to remove excess CD137L antibody, cells were incubated with titrated doses of sCD137 for 30 min at 4°C. Then cells were stained with biotinylated rat anti-mouse CD137 antibodies (clone: 17B5, BioLegend) followed by streptavidin PE (BioLegend). The level of bound CD137 was analyzed using FACSCanto (BD Bioscience).

Analysis of Human PBMC and Serum Samples for sCD137

Unused residual peripheral blood samples collected for routine clinical labs from pediatric T1D patients and age-matched unrelated controls (all patients between ages 2 and 18 years) were de-identified by clinical lab staff at Cincinnati Children's Hospital. The diabetic patients were equally split between new-onset and established patients; mean duration of disease in established patients was 6.7 years. Notably, however, all diabetic patients were admitted for acute T1D disease flares. Serum/plasma was tested for human sCD137 level by ELISA using the Human 4-1BB/TNFRSF9 DuoSet ELISA kit (R&D Systems, Minneapolis, MN), following the manufacturer's instructions.

Peripheral blood mononuclear cells from healthy donors were separated by centrifugation through Ficoll-Hypaque (GE, Fairfield, CT). Resting CD4+ T cells were purified by negative selection using a CD4+ T cell isolation kit (Miltenyi Biotec, Auburn, CA), following the manufacturer's instructions. To isolate CD4 T cell subsets, purified CD4+ T cells were stained with FITC-conjugated mouse anti-human CD8 (clone: RPA-T8, eBioscience), PE-conjugated anti-human CD25 (clone: REA945, Mitenyi Biotec), and APC-conjugated mouse anti-human CD127 (eBioRDR5, eBioscience), and sorted using a FACSAria (BD Biosciences). The subsets were defined as follows: Tregs (CD8–$CD25^{hi}CD127^{lo}$ cells), double positive T cells (Tdps, CD8–$CD25^{hi}CD127^{hi}$), and conventional T cells (Tconvs, CD8–$CD25^{lo}CD127^{hi}$). Purity of the sorted populations was >90%, as determined by post-sorting analysis of FOXP3 expression. Fifty thousand Treg, Tdp, and Tconv cells were separately cultured on a 96-well round-bottom cell culture plate with human recombinant IL-2 at indicated doses. In some wells, 50,000 CD3/28 beads were added. Cells were cultured for 72 h, and supernatant was collected. Human sCD137 protein concentration was measured by ELISA using the Human 4-1BB/TNFRSF9 DuoSet ELISA kit (R&D Systems, Minneapolis, MN) following the manufacturer's instructions.

Cell Proliferation Assay of Human CD4 T Cells With Human sCD137

Human CD4 T cells were sorted from human PBMCs by the method described above and stained with anti-human CD8-FITC (clone: RPA-T8, eBioscience), anti-human CD25-APC (clone: REA945, Miltenyi Biotec), and anti-human CD127-PE-Cy7 (R34.34, Beckman Coulter), and sorted using an SH800S cell sorter (Sony biotechnology). Tconv cells were labeled with carboxyfluorescein succinimidyl ester (CFSE, Invitrogen) at 0.5 μM final concentration. Fifty thousand CFSE-labeled Tconv cells were cultured on a 96-well flat-bottom cell culture plates with 50,000 human CD3/28 dynabeads (Thermo Fisher Scientific) in the presence or absence of 40 μg/ml of human 4-1BB Fc chimera protein (R&D Systems) for 72 h. CFSE dilution of harvested cells was analyzed on FACSCanto (BD Biosciences).

Data Analysis

All data acquired in flow cytometry were analyzed using FlowJo software version 10 (FlowJo, LLC). All statistical analysis was performed using GraphPad Prism version 6 for Windows (GraphPad software). Significance testing was done using either the unpaired *t*-test or Mann–Whitney tests for sample comparisons, ANOVA and *post hoc* analysis in continuing

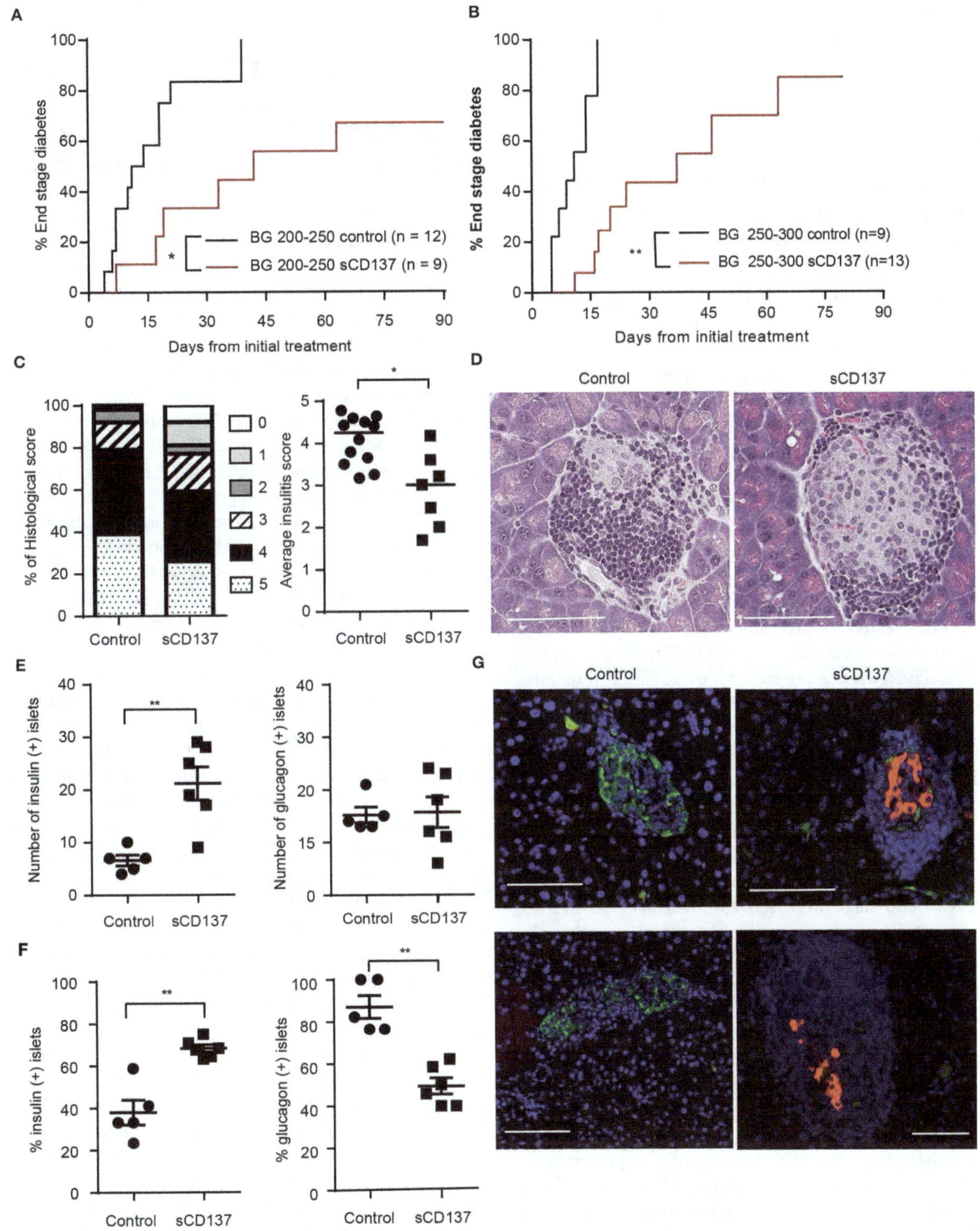

FIGURE 1 | Soluble CD137 (sCD137) ameliorates acute type 1 diabetes (T1D) in nonobese diabetic (NOD) mice. **(A,B)** Survival curves of acutely diabetic mice treated with sCD137 vs. controls. Female NOD mice were monitored until they became diabetic [blood glucose of **(A)** 200–250 mg/dl or **(B)** 250–300 mg/dl], and were then treated with sCD137 vs. untreated **(A)** or treated with PBS **(B)** (see methods). *$p < 0.05$, **$p < 0.01$, Mantel–Cox log-rank test. **(C)** Insulitis severity (see methods) in sCD137-treated mice ($n = 7$) that did not progress to end-stage T1D and control mice ($n = 12$) with end-stage diabetes. *$p < 0.05$, Mann–Whitney *U*-test. **(D)** Representative H&E-stained islets from each group. **(E–G)** The pancreatic islet was stained for insulin (red), glucagon (green), and nucleus (blue) and imaged by dual immunofluorescence in sCD137-treated mice ($n = 6$) compared to PBS-treated, end-stage diabetic mice ($n = 5$). The number **(E)** and percentages **(F)** of insulin- (**E,F**, left) and glucagon- (**E,F**, right) positive islets per section are shown. **$p < 0.01$, Mann–Whitney *U*-test **(E)** and unpaired *t*-test **(F)**. **(G)** Representative islets from two independent sCD137- vs. PBS-treated mice showing insulin preservation in sCD137-treated mice. White bars = 100 μm.

parametric data, and the log-rank test for survival curve analysis. Results in bar graphs are expressed as the mean ± standard error of the mean. *P*-values <0.05 were considered statistically significant.

RESULTS

sCD137 Treatment Ameliorates New-Onset Diabetes in NOD Mice and Can Preserve Insulin-Expressing Islet Beta Cells

Halting acute T1D remains an unachieved goal, and new therapeutic approaches are needed. Although we previously published that we can prevent T1D in NOD mice using sCD137 (11), this is not a good indicator of the ability of sCD137 to treat an acute autoimmune disease. Many agents that have "prevented" T1D in NOD, such as LPS, failed to reverse the acute disease (15). Therefore, we tested the effect of sCD137 on acute T1D. In the first treatment group, we started treatment with sCD137 in NOD mice with initial blood glucose between 200 and 250 mg/dl and showed a delay in progression to end-stage (BG >500 mg/dl) diabetes; in addition, three mice did not progress to end-stage disease (**Figure 1A**). In the second treatment group, we chose the more challenging criteria of initial BG between 250 and 300 mg/dl. PBS-treated control mice showed a more rapid progression to end-stage disease; the sCD137-treated mice had significantly delayed disease progression overall, and four mice did not progress to end-stage disease (**Figure 1B**). The individual blood glucose measurements at each time point are shown in **Supplemental Figure 1A**; clearly, all sCD137-treated mice (curves shown in red) are shifted to the right compared to the control mice (black curves). A direct ameliorative effect of sCD137 is shown by comparing the effects of sCD137 to PBS or no treatment on the next blood glucose measurement. As shown in **Supplemental Figure 1B**, in the seven mice that did not progress to end-stage T1D, sCD137 treatment on average reduced the next BG measurement by 22.1 mg/dl, a statistically significant difference compared to a mean blood glucose increase of 73.2 mg/dl in all the control mice (**Supplemental Figure 1B**). The mean ending BG level was >500 mg/dl in all control mice, compared with a mean of 213.9 mg/dl in the seven mice that did not progress (whose mean initial BG prior to treatment was 232.9 mg/dl). Histologically, successfully treated mice had a significantly decreased insulitis score, with decreased numbers of severely affected islets (**Figures 1C,D**). Beta cell immunohistochemistry demonstrated significant preservation of insulin+ beta cells, and an increase of insulin-positive islets as a percentage of all islets, in successfully treated mice (**Figures 1E–G**). The number of glucagon-positive islets was not statistically different between the two groups, but the percentage of glucagon-positive islets decreased in the sCD137-treated mice (**Figures 1E–G**, see discussion). Overall, treatment of new-onset diabetic NOD mice with sCD137 significantly delayed development of end-stage diabetes (blood glucose >500 mg/dl) compared with controls, and several mice did not progress to end-stage disease while being treated. These data indicate that sCD137 has a therapeutic potential in acute, new-onset autoimmune diabetes.

sCD137 Induces T Cell Anergy; Exogenous IL-2 Prevents and Reverses sCD137 Suppressive Effect on Antigen-Specific T Cell Proliferation and Cytokine Production

We previously showed that sCD137 can suppress both CD4+ (11) and CD8+ (12) T cell proliferation and that the suppressive effect of recombinant sCD137 could be blocked by an anti-CD137L antibody (TKS-1), but this did not directly show ligand specificity (11). We constructed a CD137L-expressing cell line (in a human cell line that does not express mouse CD137L) and showed that it expressed high levels of recombinant CD137L (**Supplemental Figure 2A**). Next, using a previously published approach (16), we showed that sCD137 specifically bound the recombinant CD137L (**Supplemental Figure 2B**) and that this binding could be blocked with the TKS-1 anti-CD137L antibody (**Supplemental Figure 2C**). These results confirmed the specificity of our sCD137 reagent.

The mechanism of the T cell suppressive effect was unclear, so we tested whether sCD137-treated T cells showed an anergic phenotype in antigen-specific CD4+ T cell proliferation assays, using T cells from NOD BDC2.5 congenic mice. Exogenous IL-2 added at the start of the T cell culture prevented sCD137-mediated antigen-specific T cell proliferation (**Figure 2A**). To meet the criteria for T cell anergy, however, the established, suppressed T cell phenotype must be reversible by IL-2. We tested the effect of adding IL-2 after induction of suppression and showed that IL-2 added 24 h after cell culture reversed the antigen-specific sCD137 suppressive effect on BDC 2.5 CD4+ transgenic T cells (**Figure 2B**). Consistent with **Figures 2A,B**, sCD137 suppressed the S phase of the cell cycle (**Figure 2C**). Cytokine secretion including IL-2 (**Figure 2D**) from CD3/28-stimulated CD4 and IFN-γ (**Figure 2E**) from CD3/28-stimulated CD4 and CD8 T cells was also suppressed by sCD137 (**Figure 2E**). To test whether the cytokine reduction induced by sCD137 was a reversible functional component of T cell anergy, we differentiated CD4 T cells into Th1 cells *in vitro*, restimulated them using CD3/28 plus/minus sCD137 and/or IL-2, washed them, and then rested them for 48 h in fresh TCM without IL-2 prior to restimulation. The reactivated Th1 cells that had been treated with sCD137 produced less IL-2 after restimulation, and this suppression of cytokine production was reversed by IL-2 treatment prior to restimulation (see methods) (**Figure 2F**). This result indicated that sCD137 treatment induces an anergic phenotype in T cells through its direct effect on T cells and that sCD137 could suppress antigen-experienced, cytokine differentiated cells and activated memory T cells, suggesting the ability to ameliorate ongoing autoimmunity against beta cells.

sCD137 Downregulates T Cells via the mTORC1 Signaling Pathway

Little is known about the CD137L pathway signaling in T cells, but in antigen-presenting cells, existing data suggest that membrane CD137/CD137L interaction acts via downstream Akt

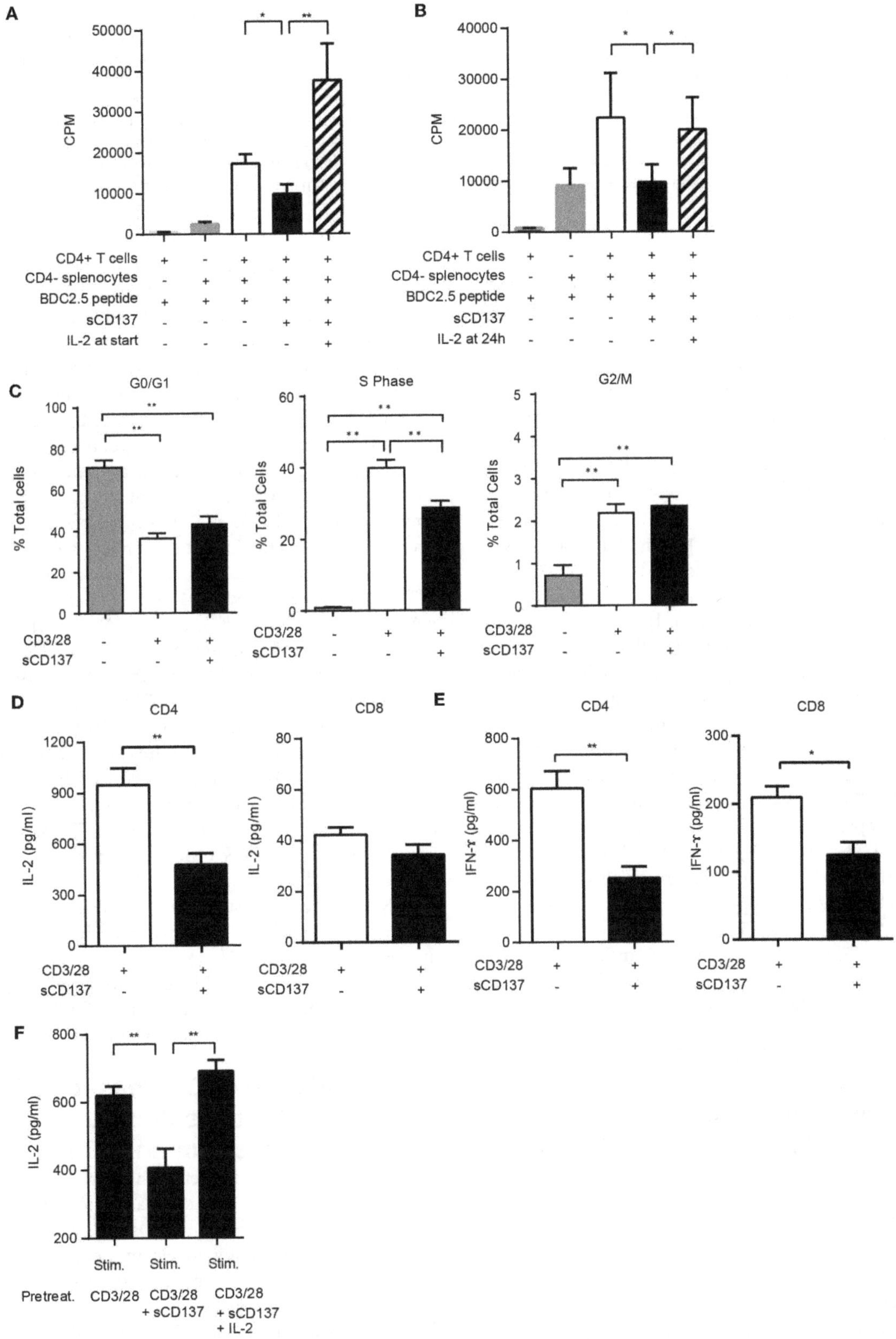

FIGURE 2 | sCD137 induces T cell anergy: IL-2 prevents and reverses sCD137 suppressive effect on antigen-specific T cell activation. **(A,B)** CD4+CD25– T cells and CD4-negative splenic antigen-presenting cells purified from non-diabetic NOD BDC2.5 transgenic mice were co-cultured with BDC2.5 peptide in the presence or

(Continued)

FIGURE 2 | absence of sCD137. In some wells, 25 U/ml of recombinant mouse IL-2 was added at the start **(A)** or 24 h **(B)** after starting cell culture. Cell proliferation was counted on a β-scintillation counter. Data expressed as mean/SEM from $n = 3$ **(A)** and $n = 5$ **(B)** independent samples in three independent experiments. $^{*}p < 0.05$, $^{**}p < 0.01$, unpaired *t*-test. **(C)** Magnetically isolated CD4 T cells were cultured with CD3/CD28 beads and sCD137 for 48 h, and cell cycle phases were analyzed by flow cytometry. Data expressed as mean/SEM, $n = 4$ mice. $^{*}p < 0.05$, $^{**}p < 0.01$, Mann–Whitney *U*-test. **(D,E)** MACS-bead-purified splenic NOD CD4+CD25− or CD8 T cells were stimulated with CD3/28 in the presence/absence of sCD137 for 24 h. After 24 h, supernatant was collected, and IL-2 **(D)** and IFN-ɤ **(E)** concentration was measured by ELISA. Data expressed as mean/SEM from three biologically independent experimental samples. **(F)** Differentiated Th1 cells (1×10^6) were stimulated for 24 h with CD3/28 beads, in the presence and absence of sCD137, with or without IL-2. Cells were then washed and rested in fresh cell culture media without IL-2 for 48 h, and then 0.5×10^5 rested living cells were restimulated for 24 h with plate-bound aCD3Ab (0.5 μg/ml) and soluble CD28 Ab (0.5 μg/ml). IL-2 in supernatant was measured by ELISA. Data expressed as mean and standard errors of mean from three independent experiments. $^{**}p < 0.01$, unpaired *t*-test.

and mTOR pathways (17). Therefore, we hypothesized that sCD137 caused decreased CD4/CD8 T cell proliferation via the AKT and/or mTOR pathways. In mammalian cells, mTOR forms two enzyme complexes, mTOR complex 1 (mTORC1), and mTOR complex 2 (mTORC2). We evaluated sCD137's effect on the mTOR pathway in T cells using phosphorylated S6 ribosomal protein at S235/236 as a marker of mTORC1 activity and phosphorylation of AKT at S473 as a maker of mTORC2 activity.

Phospho-flow cytometry showed that sCD137 significantly reduced p-S6 MFI in both CD4+ and CD8+ T cells (**Figure 3A**), while p-AKT (S473) expression did not change significantly (**Figure 3B**). The percentage of p-S6+ cells, but not p-AKT+ cells, was also significantly decreased in the sCD137-treated group (not shown). CD71 is a transferrin transporter that plays a crucial role in DNA synthesis in lymphocytes (18, 19), and CD98 is an amino acid transporter that is essential for cell expansion (20); both are regulated by mTORC1 activity in T cells (21, 22). sCD137 treatment significantly reduced CD71 and CD98 MFI in both CD4 and CD8 T cells, with a greater overall reduction in CD8 cells (**Figures 3C,D**). We compared these effects to the known mTORC1 inhibitor, rapamycin; sCD137 suppressed the expression of these molecules comparably to rapamycin in CD8 cells, with somewhat less suppression in CD4 cells (**Figures 3C,D**). We also directly compared sCD137 cytokine suppression of IFN-γ and IL-2 to rapamycin; both agents suppressed these cytokines with similar efficacy (**Supplemental Figure 3**). These results indicated that sCD137/CD137L interaction reduced mTORC1 activity, resulting in downregulation of T cell metabolic transporter expression and anergy induction.

sCD137 Acts on T Cells Early in the Cell Cycle, Related to Kinetics of CD137L Upregulation; Differential Effects of sCD137 on T Cell Memory Subsets

The studies in **Figure 3** showed a larger effect of sCD137 on CD8 T cell p-S6, CD71, and CD98 downregulation compared to CD4 cells. To understand this, we looked at the kinetics of CD137L expression on CD4 and CD8 T cell subsets. CD137L protein is difficult to detect on the T cell surface due to formation of cis-complexes with CD137 (23, 24) and possible limitations of the available antibodies (24), so we assessed *Tnfsf9* (encoding CD137L) gene expression using real-time PCR. *Tnfsf9* expression peaked 4 h after stimulation (**Figure 4A**), and *Tnfsf9* expression was significantly higher in CD44+ (activated/memory) T cells. CD8 memory/activated cells showed a significantly greater upregulation of *Tnfsf9* than CD4 cells after stimulation *in vitro* (**Figure 4A**). The early upregulation of CD137L suggested that sCD137 would act early after T cell activation but might be less effective later. To test this, we added sCD137 to CD4 and CD8 T cell cultures at different time points after CD3/CD28 stimulation and measured the cytokine production total 72 h post-CD3/28 stimulation. As in **Figure 2**, sCD137 added at the start of cell cultures significantly reduced IFN-ɤ (**Figure 4B**) concentration, but sCD137 added at either 24 or 48 h did not suppress CD4 or CD8 T cell cytokine production. These data confirmed that sCD137 mainly suppresses CD4 T cell cytokine production within the first 24 h after activation.

This result led us to study the functional effects of sCD137 in FACS-sorted CD4 and CD8 cell subsets. We sorted naïve ($CD62L^{high}CD44^{low}$), CM ($CD62L^{high}CD44^{high}$), and EM ($CD62L^{low}CD44^{high}$) subsets from splenic CD4 or CD8 T cells, stimulated with CD3/CD28 beads for 24 h, and assayed IL-2/IFN-ɤ expression. sCD137 reduced CD4 IL-2 concentration in all three subsets (**Figure 5A**, left panel). In CD8 subsets, only EM cells produced substantial amounts of IL-2 (**Figure 5A**, middle panel), and sCD137 significantly reduced IL-2 in EM CD8 cells (**Figure 5A**, right panel). In contrast, CD4 and CD8 EM T cells were the major source of IFN-ɤ, and sCD137 exerted most of its suppression of IFN-ɤ production in this subset (**Figure 5B**, right and middle panel, respectively). Overall, the vast majority of IFN-γ reduction resulted from sCD137 action on the CD8 EM subset (**Figure 5B**, right panel). These data indicate that upregulation of CD137L in memory cells predisposes these cells, and especially CD8 EM cells, to suppression by sCD137, resulting in significant downregulation of inflammatory cytokine expression, which plays a major role in T1D.

Human sCD137 Is Decreased in Type 1 Diabetic Patients, Is Secreted From Tregs, and Suppresses Human T Cells

Finally, we investigated whether human T1D patients showed decreased serum sCD137 compared to controls, analogous to NOD vs. disease-resistant NOD *Idd9.3* mice (10). Serum sCD137 was significantly lower in pediatric type 1 diabetic patients admitted with acute disease exacerbations compared to age-matched non-diabetic donors (**Figure 6A**). Next, we determined whether human Tregs were the primary source of sCD137, as we found in mice (10). $CD4+CD25^{high}CD127^{low}$ Tregs FACS-sorted from peripheral blood mononuclear cells secreted human sCD137, but $CD4+CD25^{low}CD127^{high}$ Tconvs, and $CD4+CD25^{high}CD127^{high}$ (Tdp) cells did not (**Figure 6B**).

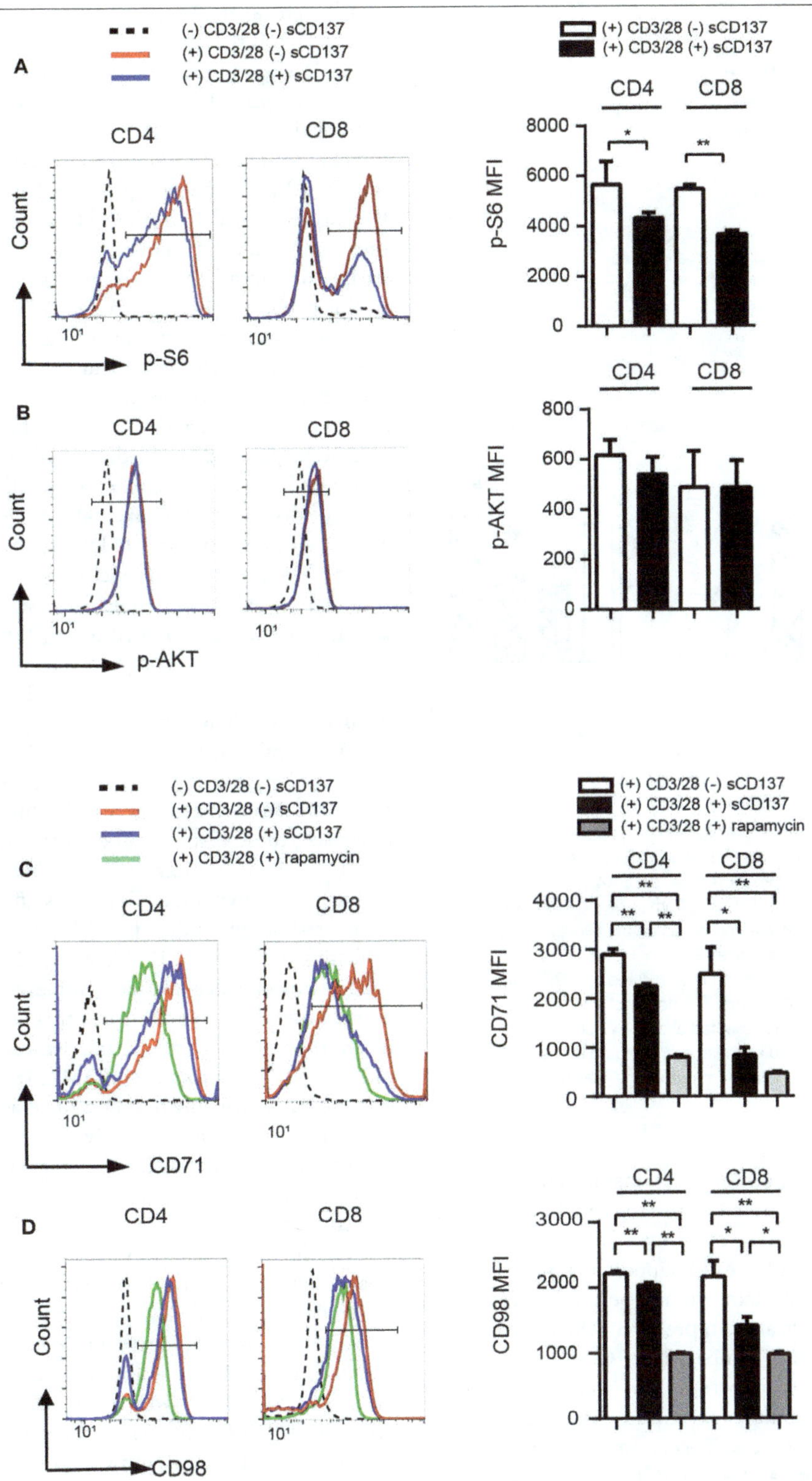

FIGURE 3 | sCD137-mediated suppression associated with reduced mTORC1 pathway activation; no effect on Akt pathway. NOD CD4+CD25− or CD8 T cells were stimulated with CD3/28 beads in the presence of sCD137 or rapamycin for 24 h. After 24 h culture, cells were harvested, and intracellular or cell-surface proteins were stained and analyzed as described in the *Materials and Methods* section. One representative histogram of intracellular p-S6 **(A)**, p-AKT **(B)**, cell-surface CD71 **(C)**, and CD98 **(D)** expression in CD4+CD25− and CD8+ cells is shown. Geometric MFI (far right) of the indicated populations is shown as mean/SEM from three to four biologically independent experimental samples. $^{*}p < 0.05$, $^{**}p < 0.01$, unpaired t-test.

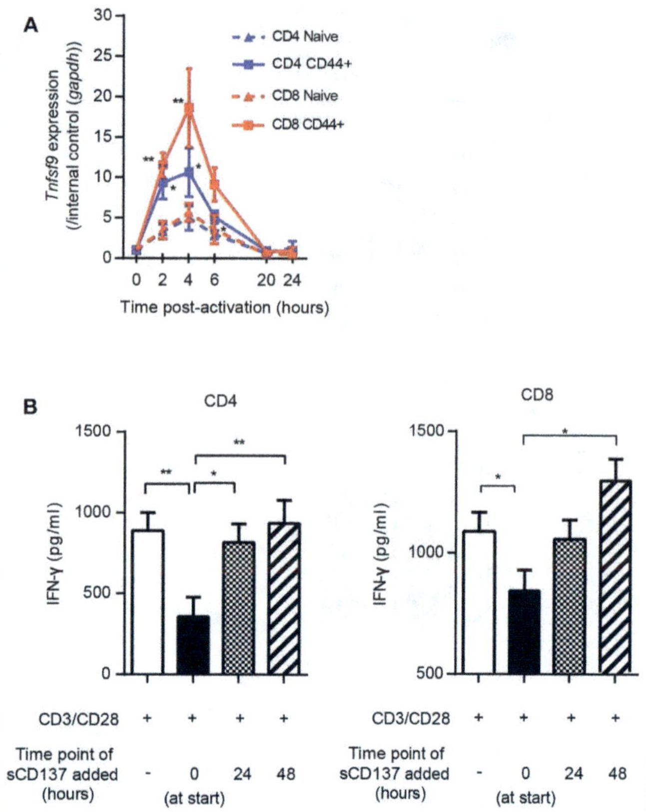

FIGURE 4 | Kinetics of CD137L upregulation; sCD137 suppresses T cell cytokine production only when administered within 24 h of T cell activation. **(A)** The kinetic profile of *Tnfsf9* gene expression in naïve (CD44–) and memory (CD44+) T cells stimulated with CD3/28 beads from three independent experiments. RT-PCR data were normalized based on the expression in each subset at 0 h (baseline). *$p < 0.05$ vs. naïve CD4, **$p < 0.05$ vs. naïve CD8, ANOVA. **(B)** NOD CD4+ or CD8+ T cells were stimulated with CD3/CD28 dynabeads and cultured with sCD137 added at indicated time points. After a total of 72 h culture, supernatant was collected and IFN-γ concentration measured by ELISA. Data expressed as mean and standard errors of mean from three biologically independent experiments and analyzed by ANOVA. *$p < 0.05$, **$p < 0.01$.

These data support the hypothesis that insufficient levels of anti-inflammatory sCD137 secreted from Tregs might contribute to the progression/exacerbation of human T1D. Finally, we tested whether human sCD137 could suppress human T cells. Using a human Fc-CD137 protein, human peripheral CD4 cell proliferation showed significant suppression when stimulated in the presence of sCD137 compared to CD3/CD28 alone (**Figure 6C**), very similar to our results in mice (11). These results suggest that the biology of sCD137 production and its biological effects to suppress T cells are very similar in humans compared to mice and support further investigation of sCD137 as a therapeutic agent in T cell–mediated human autoimmune disease.

DISCUSSION

T1D remains an incurable disease, despite much elucidation of its immunopathological basis in the last five decades. T cells are clearly central to the pathogenesis of the disease, yet antigen-specific T cell therapy has failed in over 20 human clinical trials (15). Clearly, ongoing investigation of T1D immunopathogenesis and development of new therapeutic approaches (including synergistic combination therapies) are both needed. We have focused on a genetically linked immune pathway in NOD mice: the *Tnfsf9* gene (encoding CD137) is most likely the causative B10 protective allele in the *Idd9.3* region and encodes a critical immune regulatory molecule that functions both on the cell surface and in an alternatively spliced, secreted form (sCD137). In this paper, we present strong evidence that sCD137 induces T cell anergy, sufficiently robust to ameliorate acute T1D. Disease amelioration shown here included a significant delay in disease progression, lack of progression to end-stage disease in some sCD137-treated mice (but in none of the controls), preservation of insulin-positive islets, decreased overall islet inflammation, and significant evidence of a therapeutic effect of sCD137 during flares of disease (**Supplemental Figure 1B**). In addition, we saw evidence of insulin-mediated paracrine suppression of glucagon in the islets (see below). Nonetheless, many sCD137-treated mice still progressed to end-stage disease, and evidence of disease activity continued in treated mice—this is clearly not a “cure” of T1D. This is perhaps an expected result, since sCD137 exclusively targets the immune pathogenesis of T1D, and there is no obvious means by which it can enhance beta cell regeneration. Hence, sCD137 would likely need to be used as a “combination” therapy in T1D, the need for which is increasingly appreciated in the field (25). Nonetheless, as a powerful new immunotherapeutic approach, these results support further investigation of sCD137 as a T cell directed therapy that could treat human T1D.

Little is known about CD137L signaling in T cells, compared to at least some studies in APCs. Partly this is a result of the difficulty in studying CD137L expression at the protein level; it is hard to detect, since it often complexes in *cis* with CD137 and is endocytosed (24). We overcame that issue by expressing CD137L in a non-expressing cell line and demonstrated specific binding of our recombinant protein to CD137L (**Supplemental Figure 2**). T cell anergy is probably best described as clonal unresponsiveness reversible by IL-2, as originally described by Schwartz (26), and our results meet that definition (**Figure 2B**). The mechanisms of anergy induction are complex and still incompletely understood; moreover, there are many forms of T cell unresponsiveness and several different anergy models (27). We show that CD4+ T cells treated with sCD137 have decreased p-S6, which is a downstream molecule in the mTORC1 pathway, while no effect is seen on pAKT, which is a downstream target in the mTORC2 pathway (**Figure 3B**) (28). In addition, we see decreased expression of CD71 and CD98, which are mTORC1-dependent proteins involved in DNA synthesis and cell proliferation. These results identify the mTORC1 pathway as a crucial aspect of sCD137-mediated unresponsiveness. Notably, we did not demonstrate antigen-specific CD8 T cell anergy, which should be done in future studies. We show that sCD137 has comparable effects on the expression of CD71 and CD98 (mTORC1 markers) as the mTORC1 specific immunomodulator rapamycin; especially in CD8 cells. This raises the interesting question as to whether sCD137 could function as an endogenous rapamycin equivalent. This comparison and hypothesis, however, will have to be

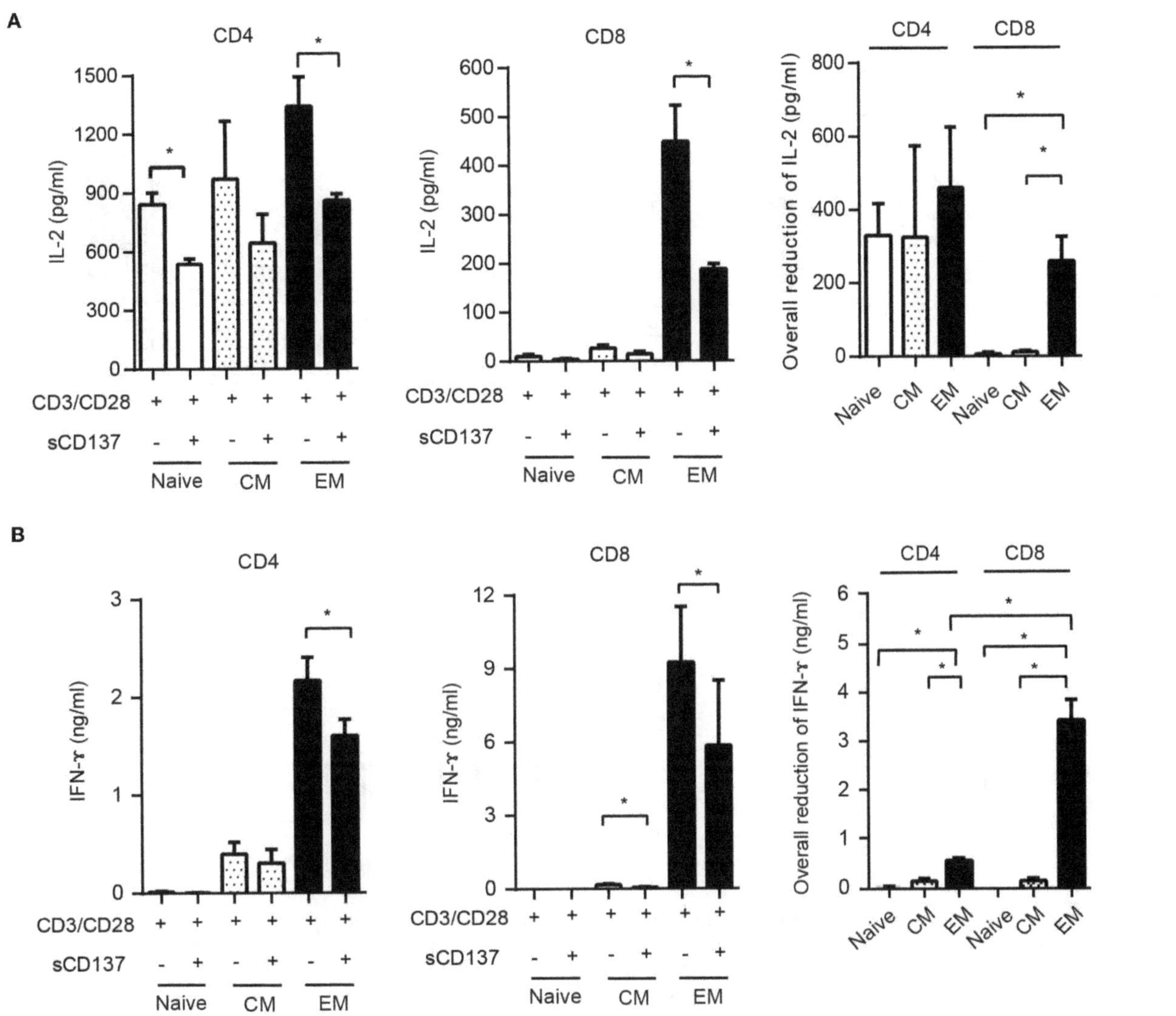

FIGURE 5 | Differential effect of sCD137 on cytokine production; CD8 effector memory T cells have the greatest reduction in cytokine expression. **(A,B)** Naïve (CD62L^{high}CD44^{low}), central memory (CD62L^{high}CD44^{high}), and effector memory (CD62L^{low}CD44^{high}) subsets were sorted from NOD CD4 or CD8 T cells and cultured with CD3/CD28 beads and sCD137 for 24 h. IL-2 **(A)** and IFN-γ **(B)** concentrations were measured by ELISA. Overall reduction of IL-2 or IFN-γ was calculated by subtraction of total cytokine in the sCD137-treated group from the cytokine level in the CD3/28 group in each individual experiment ($n = 3$ experiments). $^*p < 0.05$, $^{**}p < 0.01$, unpaired *t*-test. CM, central memory subset; EM, effector memory subset.

explored in future studies, which could also be extended to include *in vivo* effects of sCD137 on circulating and islet-infiltrating T cells.

We show that the EM CD8 T cell subset has the most marked reduction of IFN-γ production by sCD137 (**Figure 5B**); in addition, CD8 T cells show significantly more sCD137-mediated downregulation of p-S6, CD71, and CD98 in the mTORC1 pathway than CD4 cells (**Figures 3C,D**). A large amount of literature has documented the importance of CD8 T cells in T1D pathogenesis over the last three decades (29–31). The current consensus is that CD8 T cells are the ultimate mediator of beta cell destruction (32), most likely via perforin and Fas mediated pathways (33, 34). Of particular note is the critical role of EM CD8 T cells in the final phase of beta cell destruction; T EM CD8 cells are now well-recognized as a prime target for emergent T1D therapies (35, 36). Most strikingly, Herold et al. have recently used a T cell library approach to show that activated, memory CD8 T cells expressing IFN-γ are critical cell types in T1D patients that can now be tracked *in vivo* (37). These findings highlight the importance of our finding that sCD137 primarily targets EM CD8 T cells to dramatically lower IFN-γ, and support further investigation of this approach as a treatment for human T1D.

A central issue is understanding how sCD137 functions to suppress T cell activation. Membrane CD137 can induce activation signals in T cells, while the sCD137 form induces anergy. It has recently been demonstrated that the affinity of TNF/TNFR binding is largely determined by the number of

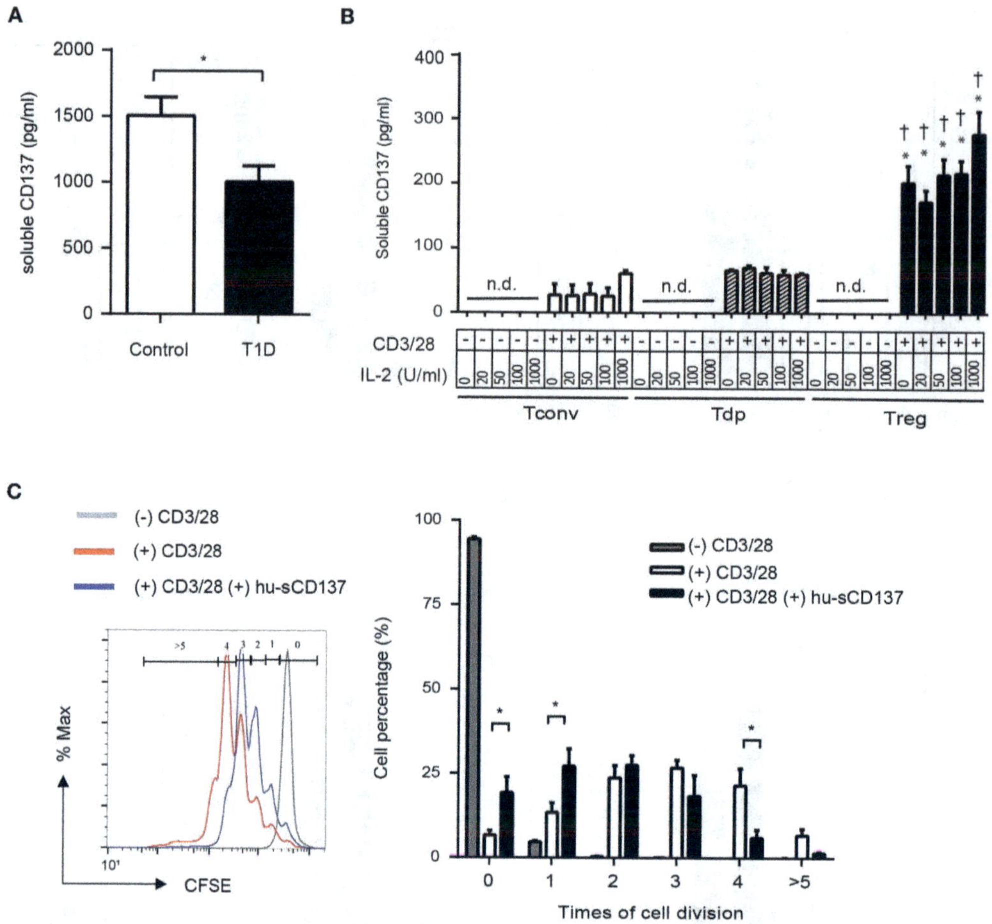

FIGURE 6 | Human T1D patients have decreased serum sCD137 levels, and sCD137 is secreted from human regulatory T cells. Human sCD137 suppresses human T cell proliferation. **(A)** sCD137 concentration in serum from pediatric type 1 diabetic patients ($n = 11$) or age-matched controls without T1D ($n = 10$) (all subjects were ages 2–18 years) was measured by ELISA. $^{*}p = 0.03$, unpaired *t*-test. **(B)** Human CD4+CD25^{low}CD127^{high} conventional T cells (Tconvs), CD4+CD25^{high}CD127^{high} double positive T cells (Tdps), and CD4+CD25^{high}CD127^{low} regulatory T cells (Tregs) from healthy donors were stimulated as indicated for 72 h. Supernatant was collected and human sCD137 concentration measured by ELISA. Data were expressed as mean/SEM from four subjects. $^{*}p < 0.01$ vs. Tconv in each dose of IL-2, $^{\dagger}p < 0.01$ vs. Tdp in each dose of IL-2, unpaired *t*-test. n.d., not detected. **(C)** carboxyfluorescein succinimidyl ester (CFSE)–labeled human CD4+ Tconv cells were stimulated with CD3/28 dynabeads in the presence or absence of hu-sCD137 for 3 days. CFSE dilution was analyzed on FACSCanto. One representative histogram (left panel) of CFSE is shown. Percentages of cells with the indicated number of cell divisions (gated as shown in the histogram) are shown in the right bar graph. Data expressed as average/SEM of $n = 5$ independent samples $^{*}p < 0.01$, unpaired *t*-test.

oligomers in the complex (38). As a result, two key observations may explain the difference between membrane and sCD137 signaling. First, we demonstrated previously that sCD137 exists as a dimer, not as a trimer as was previously reported (11). The interaction of a dimer with its ligand decreases the number of stimulating protein subunits (compared to a trimer) and may also completely change the geometry of receptor–ligand complex formation. Second, Croft et al. have recently reported that CD137L also exists as a dimer, not as a trimer as previously reported (39). This finding may completely change our understanding of CD137/CD137L biology and hence the differential effects of membrane vs. soluble forms of CD137.

We note some additional effects of sCD137 that go beyond its effects on T cell biology. First, in **Figures 1E–G**, we made the initially puzzling observations that while the number of glucagon+ islets in the sCD137-treated mice did not decrease, the percentage did: in other words, the increased number of insulin+ islets in treated mice didn't raise the percentage of glucagon+ islets. Inspection of individual islets confirmed (**Figure 1G**) that many insulin+ islets in the treated mice showed suppression of glucagon. This finding highlights an increasing awareness of the role of hyperglucagon production in acute T1D (40, 41). Physiologically, insulin suppresses glucagon secretion from alpha cells in the islets in a paracrine manner. Insulin preservation in the treated islets, therefore, likely has a secondary effect of intra-islet glucagon suppression, reflected in a decrease in glucagon+ insulin+ islets. Overall, both insulin preservation and glucagon suppression might contribute to amelioration of T1D, as suggested by a number of papers published in recent years (40, 41). We would predict that this is not an effect specific to sCD137 treatment, however, but to our knowledge, this has not been well-studied in acute T1D in NOD and should be explored in more depth in future studies.

In addition to the effect on T cells and on local glucagon production, it is possible that sCD137 has effects on other cell types and pathways beyond T cells and anergy. Recently, the role of IDO1 on pancreatic beta cells has been described, as well as a loss of indoleamine dioxygenase in T1D (42, 43). These results highlight possible regulatory roles of APCs and other immune cells; clearly, several APCs express CD137L and could be affected by sCD137 treatment, which has not been explored here. Furthermore, just as on the one hand, checkpoint inhibitors can precipitate acute T1D (44), harnessing immune checkpoints to induce T cell exhaustion is another therapeutic approach (45). Although we show that sCD137 specifically targets CD8 T cells and CD8 memory subsets, we do not show whether it induces immune exhaustion in these cells, which should be explored in future studies.

A major question that must be addressed is the use of the NOD mouse as a model of T1D and its relevance to human T1D. The major strengths of the NOD model of T1D include (1) development of spontaneous autoimmune diabetes, (2) an MHC class II molecule structurally similar to the human T1D disposing MHC class II, and (3) autoreactive T cells and autoantibodies directed at autoantigens shared between humans and mice (46, 47). In addition, multiple non-MHC susceptibility genes are shared between mouse and human, heavily weighted toward immune pathways and immune regulation (48). A major difference, however, is that T1D is easy to prevent in mice, whereas prevention trials have failed in human T1D to date. The existing literature is highly biased toward prevention trials in NOD, compared to the much more difficult task of reversing or ameliorating acute disease. Already in 2005, a review of the NOD literature showed 443 "prevention" studies but only 23 reversal studies (49); currently, ~1,000 prevention studies have been done in NOD compared to an estimated 40 or 50 reversal studies. Clearly, the main clinical issue in T1D is reversal of acute disease, which is entirely different from, and more difficult than, prevention. In fact, most of the published agents that "prevent" T1D in NOD have no effect on the acute disease (15). Prevention studies do show *in vivo* biological effects and can be useful to identify pathways in disease; however, we believe that reversal studies have been underutilized in NOD. A strength of the current study is that it demonstrates that sCD137 is active in acute autoimmunity. We do not show efficacy in all mice. This is likely explained by heterogeneity in the immune state of acutely diabetic NOD, which has been noted recently in the literature but is mechanistically unexplained (50). More studies should be performed on the immunobiology of acute T1D in NOD mice to understand the variable efficacy of therapies utilized at this stage. In addition, further dosing studies with sCD137 in acute disease need to be performed to ensure that our dosing regimens are maximized.

A final issue is the relevance of NOD studies for human T1D, a question emphasized by the failure of most agents that were successful in NOD mice to show efficacy in human studies. Given this, it is critical to extend any mouse results into human T1D patients and identify how closely the biology in the mouse reflects human immunobiology. We previously showed that protected NOD. *Idd9.3* congenic mice had higher serum levels of sCD137 compared to NOD mice (10); clearly, a deficit in an immunosuppressive/regulatory molecule could enhance autoimmune progression/severity. Here we tested pediatric T1D patients vs. controls and found that human T1D patients had decreased sCD137. Of great interest is that all the T1D patients tested in this study were admitted for T1D disease flares. As shown in **Supplemental Figure 1**, sCD137 can treat disease flares; this favors the potential use of this agent in acute T1D. A key unanswered question here, however, is whether sCD137 levels drop during human T1D disease flares—to answer this, more studies are needed using serum samples from T1D patients with stable, well-controlled disease. It is possible, for example, that loss of immunoregulation, reflected in a drop of serum/tissue sCD137, could contribute to disease exacerbations. These issues and the behavior of sCD137 serum levels need to be examined in larger populations; nonetheless, our results support a role for treatment with sCD137 in human T1D. In addition, we had previously shown that murine Tregs are the major source of sCD137, and here we confirm that this is also the case in humans: T effectors produce minimal sCD137, and Tregs are the major cellular source. Finally, we show that the functional effects of human sCD137 on human T cells are highly similar to those in mice; human sCD137 suppresses human T cells, which is an essential result to support further investigation of this approach for human autoimmunity. These experiments support further investigation into whether CD137L-mediated suppression can be a novel treatment pathway for human T1D and other autoimmune diseases.

AUTHOR CONTRIBUTIONS

AI, KK, DA, KB, CC, RM, Y-GC, and WR conceived and planned the experiments. AI, LO, KK, YW, DA, KB, and SM performed the experiments. CC and LD obtained and contributed human samples. AI and WR analyzed the data and wrote the manuscript with support from DA and SM. CC, Y-GC, and WR supervised the project.

SUPPLEMENTARY MATERIAL

Supplemental Figure 1 | Soluble CD137 treats acute T1D and induces treatment-related drops in serum blood glucose. **(A)** All individual blood glucose measurements from all the treated and control mice in **Figures 1A,B**. Control mice from **Figures 1A,B** are shown by black symbols/lines while sCD137 treated mice from **Figures 1A,B** are shown by red symbols/lines. **(B)** sCD137 reduces next blood glucose measurement compared to PBS/no treatment. All control BG measurements from **Figures 1A,B** were analyzed for the change in blood glucose at the next measurement (whether the mice received PBS or were untreated). All the sCD137 treatments of seven sCD137 treated mice that did not progress to end stage T1D were assessed for effect on next treatment. There were $n = 107$

events in the control group and $n = 64$ in the sCD137 treated group. **$p < 0.0001$, Mann-Whitney *U*-test.

Supplemental Figure 2 | Soluble CD137 specifically binds to CD137 ligand; binding is blocked by anti-CD137L antibody. **(A)** Mouse CD137L expression on HEK293 cell line overexpressing mouse CD137 ligand (HEK-mCD137L) vs. control HEK293 cells. 2×10^6 HEK-mCD137L or HEK293 cells were stained with anti-CD137L or isotype control Ab, followed with anti-Rat IgG2a biotin and streptavidin PE. Mouse CD137L expression was quantified by flow cytometry. One representative histogram of four independent experiments is shown. **(B,C)** sCD137 binding assay using HEK-mCD137L and recombinant sCD137. 2×10^6 HEK-mCD137L or control HEK293 cells were preincubated with 1 µg/sample of anti-CD137L Ab or PBS, then incubated with titrated doses of sCD137 for 30 min at 4°C. Cell bound mouse sCD137 **(B,C)** was analyzed by flow (see methods). One representative histogram of two independent experiments is shown.

Supplemental Figure 3 | Rapamycin and sCD137 comparably reduce cytokine expression in T cells. Splenic CD4+ T cells were magnetically isolated as above and stimulated with CD3/CD28 beads either alone, with sCD137, or with rapamycin. After 24 h, IL-2 (left panel) and IFN-γ (right panel) concentrations in the supernatant were measured by ELISA. Data expressed as mean/SEM from three biologically independent experimental samples. *$p < 0.05$, **$p < 0.01$, unpaired *t*-test.

REFERENCES

1. Bach JF. Insulin-dependent diabetes mellitus as an autoimmune disease. *Endocr Rev.* (1994) 15:516–42. doi: 10.1210/edrv-15-4-516
2. Atkinson MA, Eisenbarth GS, Michels AW. Type 1 diabetes. *Lancet.* (2014) 383:69–82. doi: 10.1016/S0140-6736(13)60591-7
3. Ridgway WM. Dissecting genetic control of autoimmunity in NOD congenic mice. *Immunol Res.* (2006) 36:189–95. doi: 10.1385/IR:36:1:189
4. Aoki CA, Borchers AT, Ridgway WM, Keen CL, Ansari AA, Gershwin ME. NOD mice and autoimmunity. *Autoimmun Rev.* (2005) 4:373–9. doi: 10.1016/j.autrev.2005.02.002
5. Yoon JW, Jun HS. Cellular and molecular pathogenic mechanisms of insulin-dependent diabetes mellitus. *Ann N Y Acad Sci.* (2001) 928:200–11. doi: 10.1111/j.1749-6632.2001.tb05650.x
6. Altobelli E, Petrocelli R, Verrotti A, Chiarelli F, Marziliano C. Genetic and environmental factors affect the onset of type 1 diabetes mellitus. *Pediatr Diabetes.* (2016) 17:559–66. doi: 10.1111/pedi.12345
7. D'Alise AM, Auyeung V, Feuerer M, Nishio J, Fontenot J, Benoist C, et al. The defect in T-cell regulation in NOD mice is an effect on the T-cell effectors. *Proc Natl Acad Sci USA.* (2008) 105:19857–62. doi: 10.1073/pnas.0810713105
8. Cannons JL, Chamberlain G, Howson J, Smink LJ, Todd JA, Peterson LB, et al. Genetic and functional association of the immune signaling molecule 4-1BB (CD137/TNFRSF9) with type 1 diabetes. *J Autoimmun.* (2005) 25:13–20. doi: 10.1016/j.jaut.2005.04.007
9. Irie J, Wu Y, Kachapati K, Mittler RS, Ridgway WM. Modulating protective and pathogenic CD4+ subsets via CD137 in type 1 diabetes. *Diabetes.* (2007) 56:186–96. doi: 10.2337/db06-0793
10. Kachapati K, Adams DE, Wu Y, Steward CA, Rainbow DB, Wicker LS, et al. The B10 Idd9.3 locus mediates accumulation of functionally superior CD137(+) regulatory T cells in the nonobese diabetic type 1 diabetes model. *J Immunol.* (2012) 189:5001–15. doi: 10.4049/jimmunol.1101013
11. Kachapati K, Bednar KJ, Adams DE, Wu Y, Mittler RS, Jordan MB, et al. Recombinant soluble CD137 prevents type one diabetes in nonobese diabetic mice. *J Autoimmun.* (2013) 47:94–103. doi: 10.1016/j.jaut.2013.09.002
12. Forsberg MH, Ciecko AE, Bednar KJ, Itoh A, Kachapati K, Ridgway WM, et al. CD137 plays both pathogenic and protective roles in type 1 diabetes development in NOD mice. *J Immunol.* (2017) 198:3857–68. doi: 10.4049/jimmunol.1601851
13. Bednar KJ, Tsukamoto H, Kachapati K, Ohta S, Wu Y, Katz JD, et al. Reversal of new-onset type 1 diabetes with an agonistic TLR4/MD-2 monoclonal antibody. *Diabetes.* (2015) 64:3614–26. doi: 10.2337/db14-1868
14. Delong T, Wiles TA, Baker RL, Bradley B, Barbour G, Reisdorph R, et al. Pathogenic CD4 T cells in type 1 diabetes recognize epitopes formed by peptide fusion. *Science.* (2016) 351:711–4. doi: 10.1126/science.aad2791
15. Itoh A, Ridgway WM. Targeting innate immunity to downmodulate adaptive immunity and reverse type 1 diabetes. *Immunotargets Ther.* (2017) 6:31–8. doi: 10.2147/ITT.S117264
16. Labiano S, Palazon A, Bolanos E, Azpilikueta A, Sanchez-Paulete AR, Morales-Kastresana A, et al. Hypoxia-induced soluble CD137 in malignant cells blocks CD137L-costimulation as an immune escape mechanism. *Oncoimmunology.* (2016) 5:e1062967. doi: 10.1080/2162402X.2015.1062967
17. Kim DK, Lee SC, Lee HW. CD137 ligand-mediated reverse signals increase cell viability and cytokine expression in murine myeloid cells: involvement of mTOR/p70S6 kinase and Akt. *Eur J Immunol.* (2009) 39:2617–28. doi: 10.1002/eji.200939292
18. Thorson JA, Smith KM, Gomez F, Naumann PW, Kemp JD. Role of iron in T cell activation: TH1 clones differ from TH2 clones in their sensitivity to inhibition of DNA synthesis caused by IgG Mabs against the transferrin receptor and the iron chelator deferoxamine. *Cell Immunol.* (1991) 134:126–37. doi: 10.1016/0008-8749(91)90336-A
19. Lo B. The requirement of iron transport for lymphocyte function. *Nat Genet.* (2016) 48:10–1. doi: 10.1038/ng.3478
20. Ablack JN, Metz PJ, Chang JT, Cantor JM, Ginsberg MH. Ubiquitylation of CD98 limits cell proliferation and clonal expansion. *J Cell Sci.* (2015) 128:4273–8. doi: 10.1242/jcs.178129
21. Johnson MO, Siska PJ, Contreras DC, Rathmell JC. Nutrients and the microenvironment to feed a T cell army. *Semin Immunol.* (2016) 28:505–13. doi: 10.1016/j.smim.2016.09.003
22. Sinclair LV, Rolf J, Emslie E, Shi YB, Taylor PM, Cantrell DA. Control of amino-acid transport by antigen receptors coordinates the metabolic reprogramming essential for T cell differentiation. *Nat Immunol.* (2013) 14:500–8. doi: 10.1038/ni.2556
23. Eun SY, Lee SW, Xu Y, Croft M. 4-1BB ligand signaling to T cells limits T cell activation. *J Immunol.* (2015) 194:134–41. doi: 10.4049/jimmunol.1401383
24. Mbanwi AN, Lin GHY, Wang KC, Watts TH. Constitutive interaction between 4-1BB and 4-1BBL on murine LPS-activated bone marrow dendritic cells masks detection of 4-1BBL by TKS-1 but not 19H3 antibody. *J Immunol Methods.* (2017) 450:81–9. doi: 10.1016/j.jim.2017.08.001
25. Boettler T, von Herrath M. Immunotherapy of type 1 diabetes–how to rationally prioritize combination therapies in T1D. *Int Immunopharmacol.* (2010) 10:1491–5. doi: 10.1016/j.intimp.2010.07.008
26. Beverly B, Kang SM, Lenardo MJ, Schwartz RH. Reversal of *in vitro* T cell clonal anergy by IL-2 stimulation. *Int Immunol.* (1992) 4:661–71. doi: 10.1093/intimm/4.6.661
27. Choi S, Schwartz RH. Molecular mechanisms for adaptive tolerance and other T cell anergy models. *Semin Immunol.* (2007) 19:140–52. doi: 10.1016/j.smim.2007.02.005
28. Waickman AT, Powell JD. mTOR, metabolism, and the regulation of T-cell differentiation and function. *Immunol Rev.* (2012) 249:43–58. doi: 10.1111/j.1600-065X.2012.01152.x
29. Graser RT, DiLorenzo TP, Wang F, Christianson GJ, Chapman HD, Roopenian DC, et al. Identification of a CD8 T cell that can independently mediate autoimmune diabetes development in the complete absence of CD4 T cell helper functions. *J Immunol.* (2000) 164:3913–8. doi: 10.4049/jimmunol.164.7.3913

30. Verdaguer J, Schmidt D, Amrani A, Anderson B, Averill N, Santamaria P. Spontaneous autoimmune diabetes in monoclonal T cell nonobese diabetic mice. *J Exp Med.* (1997) 186:1663–76. doi: 10.1084/jem.186.10.1663
31. Verdaguer J, Yoon JW, Anderson B, Averill N, Utsugi T, Park BJ, et al. Acceleration of spontaneous diabetes in TCR-beta-transgenic nonobese diabetic mice by beta-cell cytotoxic CD8+ T cells expressing identical endogenous TCR-alpha chains. *J Immunol.* (1996) 157:4726–35.
32. Presa M, Racine JJ, Dwyer JR, Lamont DJ, Ratiu JJ, Sarsani VK, et al. A Hypermorphic Nfkbid allele contributes to impaired thymic deletion of autoreactive diabetogenic CD8(+) T cells in NOD mice. *J Immunol.* (2018) 201:1907–17. doi: 10.4049/jimmunol.1800465
33. Knight RR, Kronenberg D, Zhao M, Huang GC, Eichmann M, Bulek A, et al. Human beta-cell killing by autoreactive preproinsulin-specific CD8 T cells is predominantly granule-mediated with the potency dependent upon T-cell receptor avidity. *Diabetes.* (2013) 62:205–13. doi: 10.2337/db12-0315
34. Varanasi V, Avanesyan L, Schumann DM, Chervonsky AV. Cytotoxic mechanisms employed by mouse T cells to destroy pancreatic beta-cells. *Diabetes.* (2012) 61:2862–70. doi: 10.2337/db11-1784
35. Ehlers MR, Rigby MR. Targeting memory T cells in type 1 diabetes. *Curr Diab Rep.* (2015) 15:84. doi: 10.1007/s11892-015-0659-5
36. Chee J, Ko HJ, Skowera A, Jhala G, Catterall T, Graham KL, et al. Effector-memory T cells develop in islets and report islet pathology in type 1 diabetes. *J Immunol.* (2014) 192:572–80. doi: 10.4049/jimmunol.1302100
37. Ogura H, Preston-Hurlburt P, Perdigoto AL, Amodio M, Krishnaswamy S, Clark P, et al. Identification and analysis of islet antigen-specific CD8(+) T cells with T cell libraries. *J Immunol.* (2018) 201:1662–70. doi: 10.4049/jimmunol.1800267
38. Lang I, Fullsack S, Wyzgol A, Fick A, Trebing J, Arana JA, et al. Binding studies of TNF receptor superfamily (TNFRSF) receptors on intact cells. *J Biol Chem.* (2016) 291:5022–37. doi: 10.1074/jbc.M115.683946
39. Bitra A, Doukov T, Wang J, Picarda G, Benedict CA, Croft M, et al. Crystal structure of murine 4-1BB and its interaction with 4-1BBL support a role for galectin-9 in 4-1BB signaling. *J Biol Chem.* (2018) 293:1317–29. doi: 10.1074/jbc.M117.814905
40. Unger RH, Cherrington AD. Glucagonocentric restructuring of diabetes: a pathophysiologic and therapeutic makeover. *J Clin Invest.* (2012) 122:4–12. doi: 10.1172/JCI60016
41. Bansal P, Wang Q. Insulin as a physiological modulator of glucagon secretion. *Am J Physiol Endocrinol Metab.* (2008) 295:E751–61. doi: 10.1152/ajpendo.90295.2008
42. Orabona C, Mondanelli G, Pallotta MT, Carvalho A, Albini E, Fallarino F, et al. Deficiency of immunoregulatory indoleamine 2,3-dioxygenase 1in juvenile diabetes. *JCI Insight.* (2018) 3:96244. doi: 10.1172/jci.insight.96244
43. Anquetil F, Mondanelli G, Gonzalez N, Rodriguez Calvo T, Zapardiel Gonzalo J, Krogvold L, et al. Loss of IDO1 expression from human pancreatic beta-cells precedes their destruction during the development of type 1 diabetes. *Diabetes.* (2018) 67:1858–66. doi: 10.2337/db17-1281
44. Mellati M, Eaton KD, Brooks-Worrell BM, Hagopian WA, Martins R, Palmer JP, et al. Anti-PD-1 and Anti-PDL-1 monoclonal antibodies causing type 1 diabetes. *Diabetes Care.* (2015) 38:e137–8. doi: 10.2337/dc15-0889
45. Linsley PS, Long SA. Enforcing the checkpoints: harnessing T-cell exhaustion for therapy of T1D. *Curr Opin Endocrinol Diabetes Obes.* (2019) 26:213–8. doi: 10.1097/MED.0000000000000488
46. Anderson MS, Bluestone JA. The NOD mouse: a model of immune dysregulation. *Annu Rev Immunol.* (2005) 23:447–85. doi: 10.1146/annurev.immunol.23.021704.115643
47. Chen YG, Mathews CE, Driver JP. The role of NOD mice in type 1 diabetes research: lessons from the past and recommendations for the future. *Front Endocrinol.* (2018) 9:51. doi: 10.3389/fendo.2018.00051
48. Bluestone JA, Herold K, Eisenbarth G. Genetics, pathogenesis and clinical interventions in type 1 diabetes. *Nature.* (2010) 464:1293–300. doi: 10.1038/nature08933
49. Shoda LK, Young DL, Ramanujan S, Whiting CC, Atkinson MA, Bluestone JA, et al. A comprehensive review of interventions in the NOD mouse and implications for translation. *Immunity.* (2005) 23:115–26. doi: 10.1016/j.immuni.2005.08.002
50. Mathews CE, Xue S, Posgai A, Lightfoot YL, Li X, Lin A, et al. Acute versus progressive onset of diabetes in NOD mice: potential implications for therapeutic interventions in type 1 diabetes. *Diabetes.* (2015) 64:3885–90. doi: 10.2337/db15-0449

19

Antigen-Specific Regulatory T Cells and Low Dose of IL-2 in Treatment of Type 1 Diabetes

*Minh N. Pham[1,2], Matthias G. von Herrath[1] and Jose Luis Vela[1]**

[1] *Novo Nordisk Research Center, Seattle, WA, USA,* [2] *Pacific Northwest Diabetes Research Institute, Seattle, WA, USA*

Correspondence:
Jose Luis Vela
jvl@novonordisk.com

Regulatory T cells (Tregs) play an important role in preventing effector T-cell (Teff) targeting of self-antigens that can lead to tissue destruction in autoimmune settings, including type 1 diabetes (T1D). Autoimmunity is caused in part by an imbalance between Teff and Tregs. Early attempts to treat with immunosuppressive agents have led to serious side effects, thus requiring a more targeted approach. Low-dose IL-2 (LD IL-2) can provide immunoregulation with few side effects by preferentially acting on Tregs to drive tolerance. The concept of LD IL-2 as a therapeutic approach is supported by data in mouse models where autoimmunity is cured and further strengthened by success in human clinical studies in hepatitis C virus-induced vasculitis, chronic graft-versus-host disease, and Alopecia areata. Treatment will require identification of a safe therapeutic window, which is a difficult task given that patients are reported to have deficient or defective IL-2 production or signaling and have experienced mild activation of NK cells and eosinophils with LD IL-2 therapy. In T1D, an LD IL-2 clinical trial concluded that Tregs can be safely expanded in humans; however, the study was not designed to address efficacy. Antigen-specific therapies have also aimed at regulation of the autoimmune response but have been filled with disappointment despite an extensive list of diverse islet antigens tested in humans. This approach could be enhanced through the addition of LD IL-2 to the antigenic treatment regimen to improve the frequency and function of antigen-specific Tregs, without global immunosuppression. Here, we will discuss the use of LD IL-2 and islet antigen to enhance antigen-specific Tregs in T1D and focus on what is known about their immunological impact, their safety, and potential efficacy, and need for better methods to identify therapeutic effectiveness.

Keywords: low-dose interleukin-2, antigen-specific therapy, type 1 diabetes, regulatory T-cell, immune biomarker

INTRODUCTION

Since the discovery of the 15.5 kDa protein Interleukin-2 (IL-2) numerous preclinical, clinical, and mechanistic studies have provided basic insights into its role in immunity (1–3). In 1998, Proleukin® (Aldesleukin, human recombinant IL-2) was approved by the FDA for use at a sustained high dose in patients with metastatic renal cell carcinoma (MRCC) or metastatic melanoma (MM) (4, 5). The high doses and repeated administration were based on the protein's short half-life (6). However, only a subset of treated patients exhibited improved outcome and the high-dose (HD) IL-2 treatment came with severe side effects (7, 8). Despite its long history, it is not understood why some patients respond to the therapy while most do not (7, 8). Subsequently, IL-2 has been pursued in different indications, using low doses which resulted in minimal side effects (8, 9). Studies have reported success of low-dose (LD) human recombinant IL-2 (LD IL-2) therapy in animal models of autoimmune pathology (10–14). In this context, the advantageous function of IL-2 appears to be expansion of antigen-specific regulatory T cells (Tregs) curing a number of autoimmune conditions in mice (10–14). This potential is further strengthened by success in human clinical studies in hepatitis C virus (HCV) induced vasculitis, chronic graft-versus-host disease (GVHD), T1D, systemic lupus erythematosus (SLE), and Alopecia areata (15–21).

Antigen-specific therapies in T1D aimed at regulation of the autoimmune response by tolerance induction have been filled with disappointments despite an extensive number of human trials. These trials tested primarily three autoantigens: insulin, glutamic acid decarboxylase (GAD), and heat shock protein 60 (Hsp60), either intact or components thereof (22–25). The combination of LD IL-2 together with an antigen-based therapy specific to a target organ or tissue may be a means to provide strong immunomodulation without general immunosuppression. The effect would likely involve the enhancement of antigen-specific Tregs in both their number and activity. The major question remains whether a proper dosing strategy for LD IL-2 as an induction agent can be identified that will include both an acceptable safety profile and measure of efficacy. A further consideration is how to best identify and predict efficacy of LD IL-2 therapy either with or without an antigen therapy. A dosing strategy for an antigen-based therapy is also required and the diversity of patients and the manifestation of disease must also be better understood. Currently, the common study end-points in intervention trials for T1D with LD IL-2 administration are clinical remission defined by preservation of C-peptide, decreased level of HbA1c, decreased insulin requirement, normal blood glucose, absence or reduced adverse events including vascular leak syndrome (VLS), serious infections, and allergic reactions, increased counts of eosinophils and neutrophils, and expansion of Tregs (15, 16). T1D is a complex autoimmune disease that presents in younger children in a faster, more aggressive onset, and progression. Intervention trials are mostly initiated at a later stage of disease development, when β-cell loss is well established and the intervention therapy is less likely to improve disease outcome or progression (26). Being able to conclude confidently that LD IL-2 administration is efficacious and safe for patients with T1D, we need reliable and robust immune biomarkers and assays that (1) will help to stratify the study population and (2) predict at which stage of disease progression the administration of LD IL-2 alone or in combination with an antigen-specific therapy will be efficacious in curing or preventing T1D.

IL-2 AND IL-2 RECEPTOR

IL-2 was the first cloned interleukin in 1983, and it is arguably the most investigated interleukin with a wide role in regulation of the immune system (27, 28). Initially, IL-2 was described as a T-cell growth factor with production mainly driven by antigen-activated $CD4^+$ T cells following the engagement of the T-cell receptor (TCR) and costimulation through CD28 (1, 28, 29). IL-2 is also produced, at a lower level, by activated $CD8^+$ T cells, dendritic cells, natural killer (NK) cells, and NKT cells (28, 30). After its secretion, IL-2 binds to its high affinity IL-2 receptor (IL-2R) consisting of three individual subunits IL-2Rα (CD25), IL-2Rβ (CD122), and IL-2Rγ (CD132) (31). IL-2 has low binding affinity to IL-2Rα and intermediate affinity to the dimeric complex IL-2Rβ/γ (31). Analysis of the crystal structure of this quaternary complex showed that IL-2 binds first to IL-2Rα and then to the two subunits IL-2Rβ and IL-2Rγ (32–34). Naïve $CD4^+$ T cells and immature and mature B-cells express almost none of the three subunits of IL-2R on their surface (28). Naïve $CD8^+$ T cells, memory $CD4^+$ and $CD8^+$ T cells, NK, and NKT cells show low expression of the IL-2Rβ and IL-2Rγ subunits (28). Cells that express higher levels of the dimeric complex IL-2Rβ/γ are more sensitive to HD IL-2 administration resulting in severe effects including VLS (28). On the cell surface of Tregs, high expression of the tri-complex IL-2Rα/β/γ can be detected and contributes to higher sensitivity of these cells to LD IL-2 (28). Independently of the existence of IL-2Rα, both IL-2Rβ and IL-2Rγ can induce fully competent IL-2 signaling resulting in activation of phosphoinositol 3-kinase (PI 3-K)/AKT, Ras-MAP kinase, and JAK-STAT pathways for mediating cell growth, survival, death, and differentiation (2, 28, 32, 35).

The IL-2 signal plays a major role in the homeostasis and activation of $CD4^+CD25^+Foxp3^+$ Tregs (31). The quaternary complex consisting of IL-2 and IL-2Rα/β/γ induces the phosphorylation of STAT5, resulting in increased expression of CD25 and Foxp3 on Tregs and activation of their suppressive activity (28, 36). *In vivo* as well as *in vitro* experiments have elucidated the roles of IL-2 and IL-2R in the homeostasis and activation of Tregs (1, 37–39) (**Figure 1**). Deficiency in signaling through IL-2, IL-2Rα, or IL-2Rβ, or STAT5 results in lethal autoimmunity, dysregulation and decline of Treg production, and uncontrolled Teff activity (37–40) leading to an imbalance between Tregs and Teff cells (**Figure 1**). Patients with autoimmune disease including SLE, T1D, or rheumatoid arthritis have defective expression and regulation of IL-2 and IL-2R resulting in dysregulated Treg function and impaired downstream signaling (41–45). Data from genome-wide association studies have shown that the IL-2 locus Idd3 in non-obese diabetic (NOD) mice and 4q27 in humans are risk factors for susceptibility to development of T1D (40, 46). Boosting with exogenous IL-2 in IL-2-deficient mice led to restoration of the impaired Treg population and also prevented disease development (10–12, 14, 47). It is unclear if clinical trials have seen a similar successful remission rate with the application of IL-2 in patients with a potential risk for the IL-2-, IL-2R-, or Treg-deficiency since these were not tested (15–21). In the case of IL-2R deficiency, there would likely be no therapeutic effect with LD IL-2.

MOVING FROM HD IL-2 IN CANCER TO LD IL-2 FOR AUTOIMMUNE DISEASES

Proleukin® was considered an attractive immunotherapy for patients with MRCC or MM. The first trial to use HD IL-2

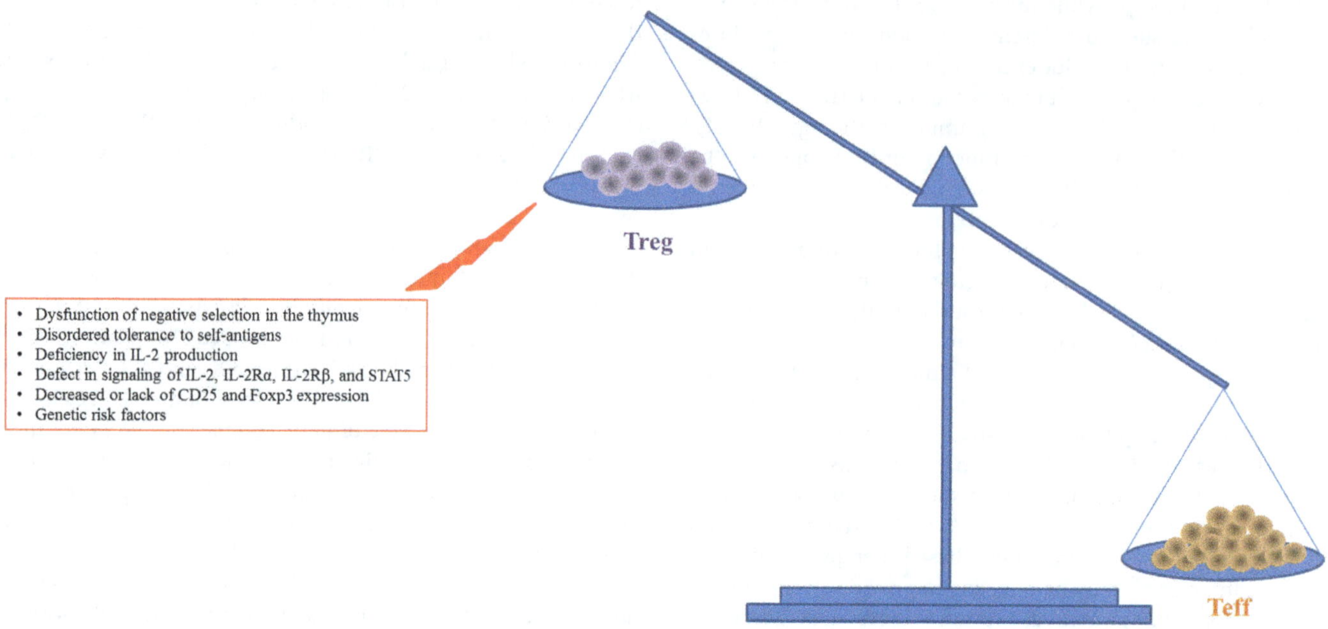

FIGURE 1 | Increased expansion and activity of Teff cells with reduced Treg number and function in autoimmune diseases like T1D are shown. This figure simplifies a complex situation in autoimmune disease. There is a balance required for tolerance to be maintained while allowing for efficient response to pathogen or other challenges. The main insight to this balance comes from lack of Foxp3 in humans and mice where the lack of Tregs leads to unchecked destruction and death by Teff cells.

was reported in 1985 by Rosenberg et al. (48). Seven percent of patients showed complete clinical remission from MM and MRCC with 13% showing partial regression after administration with HD IL-2 (7). The most life-threatening adverse effect with HD IL-2 is VLS. This acute toxicity is mediated primarily by neutrophils and eosinophils leading to higher expression of reactive oxygen, proteases, and proinflammatory cytokines (49). Modified versions of IL-2 and IL-2 complexes are currently under development with the goal to extend the half-life of IL-2, reduce the dose of IL-2, and fine-tune the activity of IL-2 on specific target cells with the aim of reducing or eliminating severe side effects (50, 51). The vision is for an engineered "superkine" IL-2 that will only activate Tregs without activating Teff, NK cells, or eosinophils (50, 51). This is a promising direction that needs to be strongly pursued, but FDA-approved Proleukin® is available now. Previous studies have shown that the administration of HD IL-2 can expand the population of Tregs in cancer patients. Subsequently, a lower dose of Proleukin® was tested in patients with autoimmune disease aiming to restore the defect in Tregs (17). The first clinical trial reporting successful induction of Tregs, safety, and clinical efficacy with LD IL-2 involved patients with HCV (17). In a preclinical study, Churlaud et al. revealed that long-term administration of LD IL-2 to NOD mice neither induced systemic toxicity nor impaired the immune response (52). Nevertheless, LD IL-2 is linked to increased eosinophil and neutrophil numbers in clinical trials (15, 20, 53). Further dosing studies are required to identify the optimal dose that provides efficacy and safety in humans while limiting these side effects. This is a complex issue, given patient heterogeneity and differences in IL-2 signaling among individuals (50, 51).

EFFECTIVE TREATMENT OF AUTOIMMUNE DISEASE IN MURINE MODELS WITH LD IL-2

In a study by Grinberg-Bleyer et al., the administration of LD IL-2 (25,000 IU) for five consecutive days resulted in remission of disease and normal blood glucose in 60% of treated NOD mice (10). The LD IL-2 induced a 1.5-fold increase in the number of Tregs in the pancreas of prediabetic mice as well as increased expression of CD25, Foxp3, CTLA-4, ICOS, and GITR which are important for Treg function have been found to be reduced in children with T1D (54). In a disease prevention study, NOD mice treated with low dose of IL-2 in the form of a IL-2/anti-IL-2 mAb complex led to a small increase in Treg cell percentage and a positive correlation with CD25 and Bcl-2 expression compared to control mice (14). No difference in expression of NK cells was reported.

Successful protection against islet β-cell destruction has also been observed with a combination therapy of rapamycin and LD IL-2 (13). Treatment with human recombinant IL-2 alone (4 ng/day) in NOD mice between the ages of 10–25 weeks did not prevent disease development while a dose-dependent decline in diabetes incidence in NOD mice treated with rapamycin alone (0.1 and 1.0 mg/kg/day) at the age of 10–33 weeks was seen. However, a synergistic effect was achieved using combination therapy with rapamycin plus human recombinant IL-2 that significantly decreased diabetes incidence in NOD mice compared to the vehicle-treated group. Disease prevention was maintained even after withdrawal of the combination therapy (13). Results like these encouraged the idea of using combinations to treat T1D, realizing the difficulty inherent in translating mouse studies to humans. We propose a LD IL-2 and antigen-specific therapy combination to induce immune tolerance occurring most likely through increase number and activity of antigen-specific Tregs. For example, a combination therapy of LD IL-2 with rapamycin has been shown to prevent allogeneic skin graft rejection in mice presumably through an increase in Treg production and decline of Teff cells detected in grafted mice (12). However, monotherapy with LD IL-2 (50,000 IU) or rapamycin did not prevent rejection (12). While rapamycin had adverse events in humans when tested in combination with LD IL-2, we propose the use of LD IL-2 in combination with an autoantigen like insulin or an insulin peptide (discussed below) be used as potential safe and efficacious therapy to prevent or reverse disease, in part by remedying the dysregulation of Treg and Teff cells, without impairing the immune response (53). The promising results in preclinical studies led to the use of LD IL-2 in the clinic. Since the therapeutic window of human recombinant IL-2 is narrow, further careful investigations are needed to determine a safe treatment strategy for LD IL-2. Evidence of the therapeutic potential of LD IL-2 in other immune diseases is compelling.

CLINICAL APPLICATION OF LD IL-2 IN PATIENTS WITH HCV

In a single-center, open-label, prospective phase 1/2 trial, Saadoun et al. investigated the efficacy and safety of low-dose Proleukin® in HCV-infected patients with mixed cryoglobulinemia who were refractory to previous antiviral therapies (17). Subcutaneous (s.c.) administration of LD IL-2 (1.5 million IU/day) was administered in four courses. First, patients received a 5-day course of 1.5 million IU of LD IL-2 followed by three 5-day courses of 3 million IU/day at weeks 3, 6, and 9. Clinical improvement of HCV was seen in eight out of 10 patients after receiving LD IL-2. They did detect an increase in the percentage of $CD4^+$, $FOXP3^+CD25$ high (17). In a recent audit of VASCU-IL-2 trial, errors lead to a correction and update of results that include loss of significance for both the decrease of cryoglobulinemia and the increase of C4 levels during administration of LD IL-2 in original report. In addition, a grade 2 serious adverse event was discovered and included in the correction (17).

In another study with patients coinfected with HIV/HCV administration of lower dose human recombinant IL-2 led to expansion and activation of Tregs, improvement of liver function, and reduction of inflammation (55, 56). These data indicate a promising new treatment option for patients with HCV but further testing in a larger number of patients is needed (17, 55, 56). Additionally, a dose must be identified that remains efficacious with minimal or no increase in eosinophils and NK cells. Future studies should also identify long-term efficacy and identify any additional adverse events for this indication (17).

EFFICACY OF LD IL-2 IN PATIENTS WITH GVHD

Administration of lower dose Proleukin® has been shown to improve the ratio between Tregs and Teff and to induce proliferation of peripheral Tregs while enhancing their resistance to apoptosis in patients with GVHD (19). In a phase 1 study, a dose-tolerance escalation trial was conducted for LD IL-2 in GVHD patients' refractory to glucocorticoids (20). For 8 weeks, a total of 29 patients received daily s.c. administration of LD IL-2. The patients were divided into three different dose levels (0.3×10^6, 1×10^6, or 3×10^6 IU/m^2 of body-surface area) (20). After a 4-week break in treatment, follow-up treatment was initiated only in responders. The dose of 1×10^6 IU/m^2 per day was the highest tolerated concentration. The higher dose of 3×10^6 IU/m^2 induced side effects that included fever, malaise, and arthralgia. In summary, there was no evidence of GVHD flare with LD IL-2 treatment, and 12 of 23 patients with GVHD showed partial response during the 8-week treatment period, with lower risk for erythema, higher joint mobility and gait, and improvement of liver function. One patient showed complete remission after 14 months even with discontinuation of both immunosuppressant and LD IL-2 (20). Additionally, two patients did not require glucocorticoid therapy after 30 and 36 months. After 4 weeks of LD IL-2 administration, the proportion of Tregs increased significantly to more than eight times the baseline level (20). However, the discontinuation of LD IL-2 led to a decline of Treg counts but remained higher than baseline. The median ratio of Treg:Teff was fivefold higher than the baseline level after 4 weeks LD IL-2 therapy. NK cells also increased during the treatment window but decreased after LD IL-2 was withdrawn. Similarly, LD IL-2 administration has been tested in patients receiving hematopoietic stem cell transplantation in order to prevent GVHD (57). No adverse events of grade 3 or 4 nor any induction of GVHD were reported. In addition to an expansion of Treg levels, viral infections were actually reduced in the LD IL-2 treated group compared to the control group (57). These data demonstrated that administration of LD IL2 was well tolerated and effective in preventing disease progression in patients with alloimmune disease. In the future, exciting clinical trials are expected for the clinical implication of LD IL-2 in GVHD (20, 57).

LD IL-2 THERAPY IN ALOPECIA AREATA

Alopecia areata is a T-cell-mediated disease involving the recognition of follicular autoantigens, resulting in inflammation-induced hair loss (58, 59). Patients with alopecia areata have a significantly higher number of Th17 cells but decreased Tregs in the peripheral blood compared to healthy controls (60). In a prospective, open pilot study, five patients with severe Alopecia areata received s.c. administration of LD IL-2 (1.5 million IU/day) for 5 days, and at weeks 3, 6, and 9 further 5-day courses of higher dose of 3 million IU/day of IL-2 (21). Using severity scoring scale for Alopecia areata, patients treated with LD IL-2 experienced a disease score improvement from 82 to 69. Furthermore, four out of five patients showed partial regrowth of scalp hair and an increased level of Tregs; however, this result was not statistically significant (60). Also, the number of recruited patients in this pilot study was very small, but the data offer promising results for a new treatment option in Alopecia areata.

Altogether, recent published clinical trials with LD IL-2 reported mild degrees of efficacy and safety and some evidence of

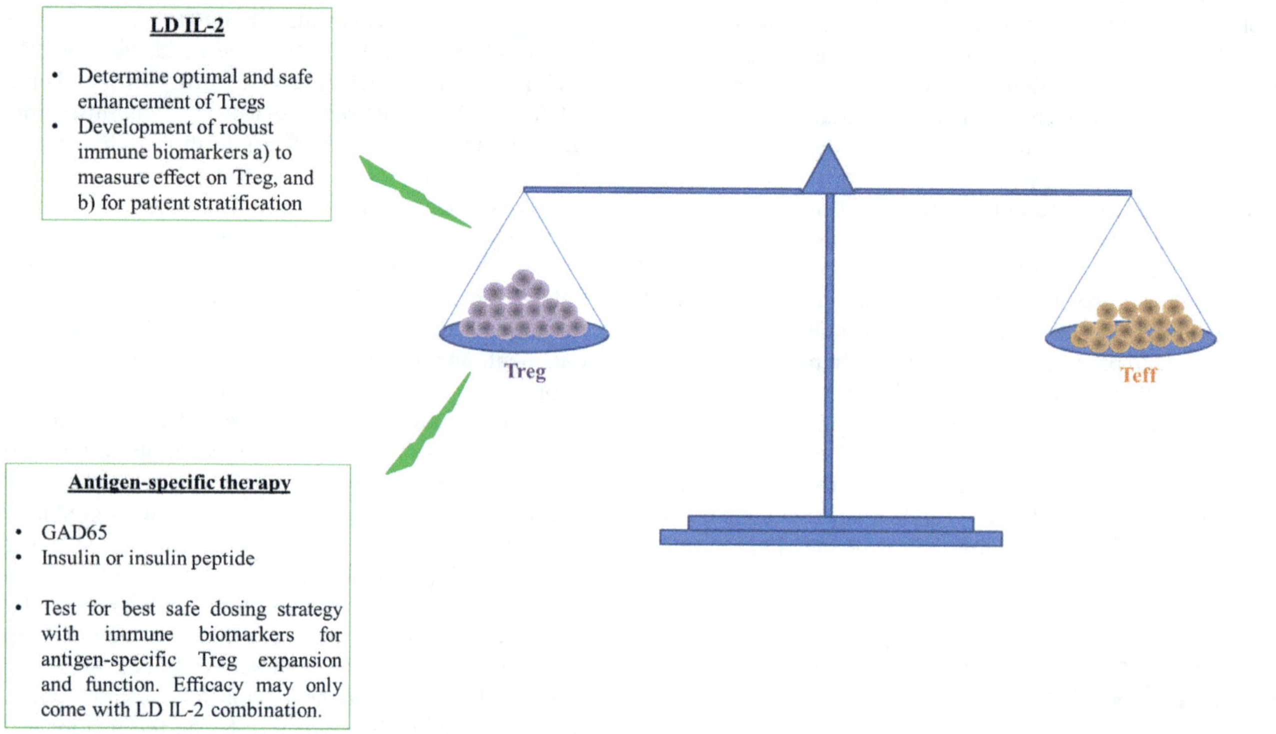

FIGURE 2 | Induction followed by maintenance of self-tolerance requires a balance between Treg and Teff to prevent or cure type 1 diabetes. The ability of LD IL-2 to improve the number and function of Tregs to restrain auto-reactive Teffs has shown promise in humans. However, human and T1D disease heterogeneity require better measures of Treg function and overall efficacy because this therapy may be more efficacious in a subset of individuals with T1D. The overall enhancement of Treg function will likely further benefit from targeted enhancement of Treg specific for islet antigens like insulin or insulin peptide. Antigen-specific therapy requires more early validation in humans with similar need of immune biomarkers that can access therapeutic effect or patient stratification. The measure of therapeutic effect is paramount for potential testing of both LD IL-2 and antigen-specific therapy in combination.

restoration of impaired Treg function (17, 19–21, 57). However, it is still not clear whether the promise of LD IL-2 for treatment of autoimmune diseases will be met. Nevertheless, we need to continue progress by focusing next on the identification of the therapeutic window of IL-2, which is no easy task given the heterogeneity inherent to human populations (61, 62). Development of good and reliable immune biomarkers and assays for prediction of the clinical efficacy and possible long-term adverse effects with LD IL-2 as well as a better understanding of the mechanism of action in heterogeneous responders are therefore urgently needed (see below and **Figure 2**).

LD IL-2 AS A NOVEL THERAPY FOR PATIENT WITH T1D

The efficacy of LD IL-2 was tested for the first time in a phase 1/2, double-blind, randomized, placebo-controlled trial with 24 T1D patients who were in an age range of 18–55 years and positive for at least one diabetes-associated autoantibody (15). The groups consisted of six patients each receiving either placebo, LD IL-2 at 0.33 MIU/day, LD-IL-2 at 1 MIU/day, or LD IL-2 at 3 MIU/day, for 5 days with a 60-day follow-up period. Overall, all patients appeared to tolerate the LD IL-2 well. The level of fasting C-peptide, incremental area under the curve (iAUC) plasma C-peptide, fasting plasma glucose, HbA1c, and insulin requirements were similar between treated groups. Significant incremental maximum effect and iAUC of Treg proportion were observed during the treatment period. A minimal but non-significant change in Teff and NK cells was also reported. Follow-up experiments tested increasing doses of LD IL-2 in an effort to determine a dose that would stimulate human Tregs without affecting other cells associated with the IL-2R (16, 62). Higher percentage of Tregs and enhanced levels of activation markers including CD25, GITR, CTLA-4, and basal pSTAT5 were detected and the data revealed that Tregs were 20-fold more sensitive to IL-2 than NK cells and memory T cells (16). In *in vitro* experiments, investigators found that increased expression of CD25 alone in activated $CD4^+$ T cells did not affect the high sensitivity of Tregs to IL-2 (62). Furthermore, this study reported that the EC50 level for IL-2 induction of STAT5 phosphorylation between T1D patients and healthy subjects was similar, and there is a response gap between Tregs and $CD4^+$ memory T cells in patients with T1D, which may be important in determining an effective therapeutic window for LD IL-2 for treatment of T1D (62). Additional, broader effects not directed at Tregs were also found and warrant further study and an improved understanding of Treg/Th17 balance (63) An important concern remains the potential unwanted activation of NK cells and eosinophils with LD IL-2. Overall, these studies pave the way for LD IL-2 therapy in T1D to enhance antigen-specific Tregs.

ANTIGEN-SPECIFIC THERAPY IN PATIENTS WITH T1D

Autoantigens have been of interest in T1D for treating the autoimmune component of the disease coinciding with the discovery of autoantibodies and T cells specific for GAD (GAD65), insulin, insulinoma-associated protein 2 (IA2), islet-specific glucose-6-phosphatase catalytic subunit related protein (IGRP), zinc transporter 8 (ZnT8), and others (64). Many of these autoantigens were identified as targets of the damaging immune response in the pancreas and then tested in preclinical models in a setting aimed at the induction of immunological tolerance to the autoantigens. Promising results seen in previous preclinical studies for preventing or reversal of T1D led to clinical trials (24, 65–69). Given the evidence in preclinical models, it is of great interest to test the efficacy of antigen-specific therapy in combination with LD IL-2. Unfortunately, most clinical trials testing autoantigens to prevent or cure T1D were disappointing. The trials focused primarily on three autoantigens insulin, GAD, and Hsp60, administered as intact protein or peptide derived from the autoantigen with very different routes of administration. In the case of insulin, the results have not indicated any significant effect despite attempts at the delivery of insulin orally, intranasally, and subcutaneously (24, 67, 68). A closer inspection of these disappointing results is important given the lack of information on optimal dosing strategy or route used in each trial. In the case of oral antigen administration, doses required in mice are larger than any used in clinical trial, and it is unclear how much insulin would remain undigested by the time it reached the small intestine without any encapsulation (70). The hsp60 peptide Diapep277 had marginal reduction in C-peptide and GAD65 in alum slowed beta cell loss, but the results were not repeated in Phase III (71–75). However, valuable information was obtained from these studies, including evidence of increased IL-10 and reduced T cell responses in patients treated with Hsp60, while patients treated with GAD alum had increased Tregs, T-cell proliferation, and inflammatory cytokines (76). It is imperative that we find appropriate immune biomarkers of response to antigenic therapy that measure immune responses to therapeutic self-antigens early during treatment (briefly mentioned below). The most promising antigen candidate for this therapy is insulin or an insulin-derived peptide. The basic idea would be to induce an infectious tolerance with the insulin-derived autoantigen that would provide protection from immune responses against other known T1D islet antigens. For example, it would be highly important if the number and function of Tregs specific for insulin could accurately and reliably be measured during and after treatment with the self-antigen. We believe that antigen therapy may not work alone but is better suited for use in combination with LD IL-2 or another induction agent and the antigen will likely have to be given continuously or as booster. Further studies are needed in both mice and human to validate the proposed combination in T1D. In addition, we must seriously consider the use of combination therapies that also work on metabolic dysregulation in the islets since there are likely components of T1D that are not immune related that could be of greater benefit if combined in the future (26). Biomarkers will have to be developed to better understand the natural history of T1D and that will inform clinical trials of the action or efficacy of a particular therapy.

TO MOVE THE FIELD FORWARD: RELIABLE AND ROBUST IMMUNE BIOMARKERS

The path toward a cure in T1D has been filled with many challenges (25, 64, 65). Many clinical trials have tested potential therapies for a cure or delay in the onset of T1D (24, 65–73, 77). However, the promising results seen in the NOD mouse model have, thus far, not translated to the clinic (24, 65–73). Unfortunately, reasons for failures are poorly understood in large part due to our lack of understanding about the cause or natural history of T1D and the difficulty of enrollment of younger age groups, where therapy may be more efficacious, but ethical and regulatory body restrictions limit or prevent participation.

In clinical trials, the C-peptide level has been relied on as a clinical endpoint together with blood glucose, HbA1c, and insulin requirement. C-peptide provides information about β-cell function and insulin production, but it is heterogeneous among patients depending on age, stage of diagnosis, disease progress, and sex with a slow decline in adults compared to children (26, 78, 79). For this reason, a more sensitive immune biomarker is required that could also allow for stratification of patients enrolling in clinical trials. From previous trials, it has been reported that higher C-peptide level is associated with lower HbA1c, reduced insulin requirement, reduced hypoglycemic events, and reduced retinopathy (80). Better stratification of patients would require immune biomarkers that could follow TID natural history (81, 82). Additional surrogate markers of β cells are needed to identify cell destruction, stress, or metabolic imbalance not limited to immune system parameters. Examples include miRNA, methods to measure pancreas size, or composition, and non-invasive imaging (26).

T1D is in part an immune-mediated and antigen-driven disease resulting in an imbalance between Tregs and Teff, we therefore need validated immune biomarkers and assays that can give us clear answers (1) about the functionality and quantity of islet antigen-specific T cells; (2) whether the intervention therapy will enhance Tregs; and (3) whether the restoration of antigen-specific or polyclonal Treg number and function will correlate positively with the pancreatic islet function.

Previous studies have reported that the disease development of T1D is associated with the presence of a specific signature of cytokines and adhesion molecules that can be captured by ELISA or Luminex assays (83). However, the organ that suffers most during the disease development of T1D is the pancreas; therefore, we need robust methods that can measure the activity and infiltration of immune cells in the pancreas and overall size and composition.

In the clinic, it is common to test for the existence of diabetes-associated autoantibodies, including GAD65, IAA, IA2, IGRP, and ZnT8 for diagnosis of patients with T1D (83, 84). It has been discussed that the titer and number of autoantibodies are a useful biomarker to predict disease progress in patients with T1D (84,

85). Currently, assays for measuring antigen-specific CD8 or CD4 T cells in both freshly isolated and cryopreserved peripheral blood mononuclear cells samples with flow cytometry-based HLA multimers are in progress and have been validated (84). Unfortunately, the percentage of autoantigen-specific T cells in the periphery is very low and often cannot be detected (84). Also, new barcoding with quantum dots has enhanced detection of autoreactive T cells but still require improvement (26, 84). In clinical trials, ELISpot is a common and widely used method to provide information about the functionality and quantity of immune cells (84–86). With ELISpot assays, we can measure cytokine responses to islet-specific antigens in T1D patients and healthy subjects (84). The number of cytokines that can be detected is increasing with improved fluorospot assays but still require development (84).

The failure for previous clinical trials may have not been only related to deficiencies in dosing and administration of tested therapies but also confounded by the late initiation of intervention therapy in patients. As T1D development is more prevalent in children and their disease progression more aggressive than in adults, we may also consider the effect of age in conducting a successful intervention trial. Some therapies may be more effective in children than in adult patients (26). However, we still do not know the exact window of opportunity for treatment in humans, and the therapy has to first be tested and proven safe in adults before given to children. To achieve a successful and effective intervention study, we need a better strategy that includes stratification for study participants for future clinical trials.

Given the promising data of LD IL-2 in patients with HCV, GVHD, and Alopecia areata, there is great interest in giving LD IL-2 to patients with T1D to specifically boost Treg numbers and activity (15, 16, 62). This treatment can then be enhanced with an antigen-based therapy to increase the number and activity of Tregs in patients with T1D. In order to make progress with the application of LD IL-2 with an antigen-mediated therapy in clinical trials, it is required to develop robust immune biomarker assays to determine the extent of expansion of Tregs in quantity and quality that can help stratify patients, tell us whether a given therapeutic hit the right pathway. Most importantly, we must develop biomarkers that teach us about the natural history of the disease. These reliable immune biomarkers will enable optimal clinical study plans and enrollment of the proper cohorts of patients, regardless of age, that would benefit most from LD IL-2 and antigen-based therapy. For more focus on biomarkers, please see Ryden et al. (77).

SUMMARY

In the present review, we discuss recent reports describing efficacy and side effects with LD IL-2 treatment in preclinical and clinical experiments of select autoimmune diseases. A common theme emerges: there is a mild increase and expansion of Tregs observed in murine models as wells as in patients. However, a slight increase of NK cells has been reported in some clinical trials even using lower dose of Proleukin®. Our need for a better and safer dosing strategy of low dose of Proleukin® is required for efficient and safe use in T1D and other autoimmune diseases (**Figure 2**). Importantly, biomarkers are needed to determine the safe expansion of Tregs in quantity and quality. The goal of developing robust immune biomarkers will help us to stratify and treat the patients in whom we know LD IL-2 therapy will be efficacious (**Figure 2**). At the moment, the lack of robust and reproducible immune biomarkers is a bottleneck. Further effort will be needed to make the treatment of LD IL-2 safer and more efficacious.

AUTHOR CONTRIBUTIONS

MP, JV, and MH contributed to concepts of the work, drafting, revising, and final approval of the review article.

ACKNOWLEDGMENTS

We thank Tamar Boursalian, Phil Pagni, and Nanette Schloot for reading and editing the manuscript.

REFERENCES

1. Morgan DA, Ruscetti FW, Gallo R. Selective in vitro growth of T lymphocytes from normal human bone marrows. *Science* (1976) **193**:1007–8. doi:10.1126/science.181845
2. Bayer AL, Pugliese A, Malek TR. The IL-2/IL-2R system: from basic science to therapeutic applications to enhance immune regulation. *Immunol Res* (2013) **57**:197–209. doi:10.1007/s12026-013-8452-5
3. Klatzmann D, Abbas AK. The promise of low-dose interleukin-2 therapy for autoimmune and inflammatory diseases. *Nat Rev Immunol* (2015) **15**:283–94. doi:10.1038/nri3823
4. Hanzly M, Aboumohamed A, Yarlagadda N, Creighton T, Digiorgio L, Fredrick A, et al. High-dose interleukin-2 therapy for metastatic renal cell carcinoma: a contemporary experience. *Urology* (2014) **83**:1129–34. doi:10.1016/j.urology.2014.02.005
5. Thomas JS, Kabbinavar F. Metastatic clear cell renal cell carcinoma: a review of current therapies and novel immunotherapies. *Crit Rev Oncol Hematol* (2015) **96**(3):527–33. doi:10.1016/j.critrevonc.2015.07.009
6. Bindon C, Czerniecki M, Ruell P, Edwards A, McCarthy WH, Harris R, et al. Clearance rates and systemic effects of intravenously administered interleukin 2 (IL-2) containing preparations in human subjects. *Br J Cancer* (1983) **47**:123–33. doi:10.1038/bjc.1983.15
7. Rosenberg SA, Yang JC, Topalian SL, Schwartzentruber DJ, Weber JS, Parkinson DR, et al. Treatment of 283 consecutive patients with metastatic melanoma or renal cell cancer using high-dose bolus interleukin 2. *JAMA* (1994) **271**:907–13. doi:10.1001/jama.1994.03510360033032
8. Yang JC, Sherry RM, Steinberg SM, Topalian SL, Schwartzentruber DJ, Hwu P, et al. Randomized study of high-dose and low-dose interleukin-2 in patients with metastatic renal cancer. *J Clin Oncol* (2003) **21**:3127–32. doi:10.1200/JCO.2003.02.122
9. Alric L, Thebault S, Peron JM, Balard P, Metivier S, Pipy B, et al. Pilot study of interferon-alpha-ribavirin-interleukin-2 for treatment of nonresponder patients with severe liver disease infected by hepatitis C virus genotype 1. *J Viral Hepat* (2006) **13**:139–44. doi:10.1111/j.1365-2893.2005.00694.x
10. Grinberg-Bleyer Y, Baeyens A, You S, Elhage R, Fourcade G, Gregoire S, et al. IL-2 reverses established type 1 diabetes in NOD mice by a local effect on pancreatic regulatory T cells. *J Exp Med* (2010) **207**:1871–8. doi:10.1084/jem.20100209
11. Ohl K, Wiener A, Schippers A, Wagner N, Tenbrock K. Interleukin-2 treatment reverses effects of cAMP-responsive element modulator alpha-over-expressing T cells in autoimmune-prone mice. *Clin Exp Immunol* (2015) **181**:76–86. doi:10.1111/cei.12629
12. Pilon CB, Petillon S, Naserian S, Martin GH, Badoual C, Lang P, et al. Administration of low doses of IL-2 combined to rapamycin promotes

allogeneic skin graft survival in mice. *Am J Transplant* (2014) **14**:2874–82. doi:10.1111/ajt.12944

13. Rabinovitch A, Suarez-Pinzon WL, Shapiro AM, Rajotte RV, Power R. Combination therapy with sirolimus and interleukin-2 prevents spontaneous and recurrent autoimmune diabetes in NOD mice. *Diabetes* (2002) **51**:638–45. doi:10.2337/diabetes.51.3.638
14. Tang Q, Adams JY, Penaranda C, Melli K, Piaggio E, Sgouroudis E, et al. Central role of defective interleukin-2 production in the triggering of islet autoimmune destruction. *Immunity* (2008) **28**:687–97. doi:10.1016/j.immuni.2008.03.016
15. Hartemann A, Bensimon G, Payan CA, Jacqueminet S, Bourron O, Nicolas N, et al. Low-dose interleukin 2 in patients with type 1 diabetes: a phase 1/2 randomised, double-blind, placebo-controlled trial. *Lancet Diabetes Endocrinol* (2013) **1**:295–305. doi:10.1016/S2213-8587(13)70113-X
16. Rosenzwajg M, Churlaud G, Mallone R, Six A, Derian N, Chaara W, et al. Low-dose interleukin-2 fosters a dose-dependent regulatory T cell tuned milieu in T1D patients. *J Autoimmun* (2015) **58**:48–58. doi:10.1016/j.jaut.2015.01.001
17. Saadoun D, Rosenzwajg M, Joly F, Six A, Carrat F, Thibault V, et al. Regulatory T-cell responses to low-dose interleukin-2 in HCV-induced vasculitis. *N Engl J Med* (2011) **365**:2067–77. doi:10.1056/NEJMoa1105143. Correction: *N Engl J Med* (2014) **370**:786.
18. Humrich JY, von Spee-Mayer C, Siegert E, Alexander T, Hiepe F, Radbruch A, et al. Rapid induction of clinical remission by low-dose interleukin-2 in a patient with refractory SLE. *Ann Rheum Dis* (2015) **74**:791–2. doi:10.1136/annrheumdis-2014-206506
19. Matsuoka K, Koreth J, Kim HT, Bascug G, McDonough S, Kawano Y, et al. Low-dose interleukin-2 therapy restores regulatory T cell homeostasis in patients with chronic graft-versus-host disease. *Sci Transl Med* (2013) **5**:179ra43. doi:10.1126/scitranslmed.3005265
20. Koreth J, Matsuoka K, Kim HT, McDonough SM, Bindra B, Alyea EP III, et al. Interleukin-2 and regulatory T cells in graft-versus-host disease. *N Engl J Med* (2011) **365**:2055–66. doi:10.1056/NEJMoa1108188
21. Castela E, Le DF, Butori C, Ticchioni M, Hofman P, Bahadoran P, et al. Effects of low-dose recombinant interleukin 2 to promote T-regulatory cells in alopecia areata. *JAMA Dermatol* (2014) **150**:748–51. doi:10.1001/jamadermatol.2014.504
22. Ludvigsson J, Cheramy M, Axelsson S, Pihl M, Akerman L, Casas R. GAD-treatment of children and adolescents with recent-onset type 1 diabetes preserves residual insulin secretion after 30 months. *Diabetes Metab Res Rev* (2014) **30**:405–14. doi:10.1002/dmrr.2503
23. Pozzilli P, Crino A, Schiaffini R, Manfrini S, Fioriti E, Coppolino G, et al. A 2-year pilot trial of continuous subcutaneous insulin infusion versus intensive insulin therapy in patients with newly diagnosed type 1 diabetes (IMDIAB 8). *Diabetes Technol Ther* (2003) **5**:965–74. doi:10.1089/152091503322641006
24. Skyler JS, Krischer JP, Wolfsdorf J, Cowie C, Palmer JP, Greenbaum C, et al. Effects of oral insulin in relatives of patients with type 1 diabetes: the diabetes prevention trial – type 1. *Diabetes Care* (2005) **28**:1068–76. doi:10.2337/diacare.28.5.1068
25. Walter M, Philotheou A, Bonnici F, Ziegler AG, Jimenez R. No effect of the altered peptide ligand NBI-6024 on beta-cell residual function and insulin needs in new-onset type 1 diabetes. *Diabetes Care* (2009) **32**:2036–40. doi:10.2337/dc09-0449
26. von Herrath MG, Korsgren O, Atkinson MA. Factors impeding the discovery of an intervention-based treatment for type 1 diabetes. *Clin Exp Immunol* (2015). doi:10.1111/cei.12656
27. Taniguchi T, Matsui H, Fujita T, Takaoka C, Kashima N, Yoshimoto R, et al. Structure and expression of a cloned cDNA for human interleukin-2. 1983. *Biotechnology* (1992) **24**:304–9.
28. Boyman O, Sprent J. The role of interleukin-2 during homeostasis and activation of the immune system. *Nat Rev Immunol* (2012) **12**:180–90. doi:10.1038/nri3156
29. Powell JD, Ragheb JA, Kitagawa-Sakakida S, Schwartz RH. Molecular regulation of interleukin-2 expression by CD28 co-stimulation and anergy. *Immunol Rev* (1998) **165**:287–300. doi:10.1111/j.1600-065X.1998.tb01246.x
30. Cheng LE, Ohlen C, Nelson BH, Greenberg PD. Enhanced signaling through the IL-2 receptor in CD8+ T cells regulated by antigen recognition results in preferential proliferation and expansion of responding CD8+ T cells rather than promotion of cell death. *Proc Natl Acad Sci U S A* (2002) **99**:3001–6. doi:10.1073/pnas.052676899
31. Malek TR, Castro I. Interleukin-2 receptor signaling: at the interface between tolerance and immunity. *Immunity* (2010) **33**:153–65. doi:10.1016/j.immuni.2010.08.004
32. Rickert M, Boulanger MJ, Goriatcheva N, Garcia KC. Compensatory energetic mechanisms mediating the assembly of signaling complexes between interleukin-2 and its alpha, beta, and gamma(c) receptors. *J Mol Biol* (2004) **339**:1115–28. doi:10.1016/j.jmb.2004.04.038
33. Stauber DJ, Debler EW, Horton PA, Smith KA, Wilson IA. Crystal structure of the IL-2 signaling complex: paradigm for a heterotrimeric cytokine receptor. *Proc Natl Acad Sci U S A* (2006) **103**:2788–93. doi:10.1073/pnas.0511161103
34. Wang X, Rickert M, Garcia KC. Structure of the quaternary complex of interleukin-2 with its alpha, beta, and gammac receptors. *Science* (2005) **310**:1159–63. doi:10.1126/science.1117893
35. Friedmann MC, Migone TS, Russell SM, Leonard WJ. Different interleukin 2 receptor beta-chain tyrosines couple to at least two signaling pathways and synergistically mediate interleukin 2-induced proliferation. *Proc Natl Acad Sci U S A* (1996) **93**:2077–82. doi:10.1073/pnas.93.5.2077
36. Wuest TY, Willette-Brown J, Durum SK, Hurwitz AA. The influence of IL-2 family cytokines on activation and function of naturally occurring regulatory T cells. *J Leukoc Biol* (2008) **84**:973–80. doi:10.1189/jlb.1107778
37. Sadlack B, Lohler J, Schorle H, Klebb G, Haber H, Sickel E, et al. Generalized autoimmune disease in interleukin-2-deficient mice is triggered by an uncontrolled activation and proliferation of CD4+ T cells. *Eur J Immunol* (1995) **25**:3053–9. doi:10.1002/eji.1830251111
38. Suzuki H, Kundig TM, Furlonger C, Wakeham A, Timms E, Matsuyama T, et al. Deregulated T cell activation and autoimmunity in mice lacking interleukin-2 receptor beta. *Science* (1995) **268**:1472–6. doi:10.1126/science.7770771
39. Thornton AM, Donovan EE, Piccirillo CA, Shevach EM. Cutting edge: IL-2 is critically required for the in vitro activation of CD4+CD25+ T cell suppressor function. *J Immunol* (2004) **172**:6519–23. doi:10.4049/jimmunol.172.11.6519
40. Todd JA. Etiology of type 1 diabetes. *Immunity* (2010) **32**:457–67. doi:10.1016/j.immuni.2010.04.001
41. Garg G, Tyler JR, Yang JH, Cutler AJ, Downes K, Pekalski M, et al. Type 1 diabetes-associated IL2RA variation lowers IL-2 signaling and contributes to diminished CD4+CD25+ regulatory T cell function. *J Immunol* (2012) **188**:4644–53. doi:10.4049/jimmunol.1100272
42. Hulme MA, Wasserfall CH, Atkinson MA, Brusko TM. Central role for interleukin-2 in type 1 diabetes. *Diabetes* (2012) **61**:14–22. doi:10.2337/db11-1213
43. Kitas GD, Salmon M, Farr M, Gaston JS, Bacon PA. Deficient interleukin 2 production in rheumatoid arthritis: association with active disease and systemic complications. *Clin Exp Immunol* (1988) **73**:242–9.
44. Lieberman LA, Tsokos GC. The IL-2 defect in systemic lupus erythematosus disease has an expansive effect on host immunity. *J Biomed Biotechnol* (2010) **2010**:740619. doi:10.1155/2010/740619
45. Linker-Israeli M, Bakke AC, Kitridou RC, Gendler S, Gillis S, Horwitz DA. Defective production of interleukin 1 and interleukin 2 in patients with systemic lupus erythematosus (SLE). *J Immunol* (1983) **130**:2651–5.
46. Plagnol V, Howson JM, Smyth DJ, Walker N, Hafler JP, Wallace C, et al. Genome-wide association analysis of autoantibody positivity in type 1 diabetes cases. *PLoS Genet* (2011) **7**:e1002216. doi:10.1371/journal.pgen.1002216
47. Chen Q, Kim YC, Laurence A, Punkosdy GA, Shevach EM. IL-2 controls the stability of Foxp3 expression in TGF-beta-induced Foxp3+ T cells in vivo. *J Immunol* (2011) **186**:6329–37. doi:10.4049/jimmunol.1100061
48. Rosenberg SA, Lotze MT, Muul LM, Leitman S, Chang AE, Ettinghausen SE, et al. Observations on the systemic administration of autologous lymphokine-activated killer cells and recombinant interleukin-2 to patients with metastatic cancer. *N Engl J Med* (1985) **313**:1485–92. doi:10.1056/NEJM198512053132327
49. Lentsch AB, Miller FN, Edwards MJ. Mechanisms of leukocyte-mediated tissue injury induced by interleukin-2. *Cancer Immunol Immunother* (1999) **47**:243–8. doi:10.1007/s002620050527
50. Mitra S, Ring AM, Amarnath S, Spangler JB, Li P, Ju W, et al. Interleukin-2 activity can be fine tuned with engineered receptor signaling clamps. *Immunity* (2015) **42**:826–38. doi:10.1016/j.immuni.2015.04.018
51. Spangler JB, Tomala J, Luca VC, Jude KM, Dong S, Ring AM, et al. Antibodies to interleukin-2 elicit selective T cell subset potentiation through distinct conformational mechanisms. *Immunity* (2015) **42**:815–25. doi:10.1016/j.immuni.2015.04.015

52. Churlaud G, Jimenez V, Ruberte J, Amadoudji ZM, Fourcade G, Gottrand G, et al. Sustained stimulation and expansion of Tregs by IL2 control autoimmunity without impairing immune responses to infection, vaccination and cancer. *Clin Immunol* (2014) **151**:114–26. doi:10.1016/j.clim.2014.02.003
53. Long SA, Rieck M, Sanda S, Bollyky JB, Samuels PL, Goland R, et al. Rapamycin/IL-2 combination therapy in patients with type 1 diabetes augments Tregs yet transiently impairs beta-cell function. *Diabetes* (2012) **61**:2340–8. doi:10.2337/db12-0049
54. Luczynski W, Wawrusiewicz-Kurylonek N, Stasiak-Barmuta A, Urban R, Ilendo E, Urban M, et al. Diminished expression of ICOS, GITR and CTLA-4 at the mRNA level in T regulatory cells of children with newly diagnosed type 1 diabetes. *Acta Biochim Pol* (2009) **56**(2):361–70.
55. Schlaak JF, Schramm C, Radecke K, zum Buschenfelde KH, Gerken G. Sustained suppression of HCV replication and inflammatory activity after interleukin-2 therapy in patients with HIV/hepatitis C virus coinfection. *J Acquir Immune Defic Syndr* (2002) **29**:145–8. doi:10.1097/00042560-200202010-00006
56. Velilla PA, Shata MT, Lages CS, Ying J, Fichtenbaum CJ, Chougnet C. Effect of low-dose IL-2 immunotherapy on frequency and phenotype of regulatory T cells and NK cells in HIV/HCV-coinfected patients. *AIDS Res Hum Retroviruses* (2008) **24**:52–61. doi:10.1089/aid.2007.0180
57. Kennedy-Nasser AA, Ku S, Castillo-Caro P, Hazrat Y, Wu MF, Liu H, et al. Ultra low-dose IL-2 for GVHD prophylaxis after allogeneic hematopoietic stem cell transplantation mediates expansion of regulatory T cells without diminishing antiviral and antileukemic activity. *Clin Cancer Res* (2014) **20**:2215–25. doi:10.1158/1078-0432.CCR-13-3205
58. Gilhar A, Etzioni A, Paus R. Alopecia areata. *N Engl J Med* (2012) **366**:1515–25. doi:10.1056/NEJMra1103442
59. Gilhar A, Shalaginov R, Assy B, Serafimovich S, Kalish RS. Alopecia areata is a T-lymphocyte mediated autoimmune disease: lesional human T-lymphocytes transfer alopecia areata to human skin grafts on SCID mice. *J Investig Dermatol Symp Proc* (1999) **4**:207–10. doi:10.1038/sj.jidsp.5640212
60. Han YM, Sheng YY, Xu F, Qi SS, Liu XJ, Hu RM, et al. Imbalance of T-helper 17 and regulatory T cells in patients with alopecia areata. *J Dermatol* (2015) **42**(10):981–8. doi:10.1111/1346-8138.12978
61. Tang Q. Therapeutic window of interleukin-2 for autoimmune diseases. *Diabetes* (2015) **64**:1912–3. doi:10.2337/db15-0188
62. Yu A, Snowhite I, Vendrame F, Rosenzwajg M, Klatzmann D, Pugliese A, et al. Selective IL-2 responsiveness of regulatory T cells through multiple intrinsic mechanisms supports the use of low-dose IL-2 therapy in type 1 diabetes. *Diabetes* (2015) **64**:2172–83. doi:10.2337/db14-1322
63. Kosmaczewska A. Low-dose interlekin-2 therapy: a driver of an imbalance between immune tolerance and autoimmunity. *Int J Mol Sci* (2014) **15**(10):18574–92. doi:10.3390/ijms151018574
64. Harrison LC, Wentworth JM, Zhang Y, Bandala-Sanchez E, Bohmer RM, Neale AM, et al. Antigen-based vaccination and prevention of type 1 diabetes. *Curr Diab Rep* (2013) **13**:616–23. doi:10.1007/s11892-013-0415-7
65. Peakman M, von HM. Antigen-specific immunotherapy for type 1 diabetes: maximizing the potential. *Diabetes* (2010) **59**:2087–93. doi:10.2337/db10-0630
66. Sarikonda G, Sachithanantham S, Manenkova Y, Kupfer T, Posgai A, Wasserfall C, et al. Transient B-cell depletion with anti-CD20 in combination with proinsulin DNA vaccine or oral insulin: immunologic effects and efficacy in NOD mice. *PLoS One* (2013) **8**:e54712. doi:10.1371/journal.pone.0054712
67. Diabetes Prevention Trial – Type 1 Diabetes Study Group. Effects of insulin in relatives of patients with type 1 diabetes mellitus. *N Engl J Med* (2002) **346**(22):1685–91. doi:10.1056/NEJMoa012350
68. Nanto-Salonen K, Kupila A, Simell S, Siljander H, Salonsaari T, Hekkala A, et al. Nasal insulin to prevent type 1 diabetes in children with HLA genotypes and autoantibodies conferring increased risk of disease: a double-blind, randomised controlled trial. *Lancet* (2008) **372**:1746–55. doi:10.1016/S0140-6736(08)61309-4
69. Thrower SL, James L, Hall W, Green KM, Arif S, Allen JS, et al. Proinsulin peptide immunotherapy in type 1 diabetes: report of a first-in-man phase I safety study. *Clin Exp Immunol* (2009) **155**:156–65. doi:10.1111/j.1365-2249.2008.03814.x
70. Bonifacio E, Ziegler AG, Klingensmith G, Schober E, Bingley PJ, Rottenkolber M, et al. Effects of high-dose oral insulin on immune responses in children at high risk for type 1 diabetes: the Pre-POINT randomized clinical trial. *JAMA* (2015) **313**:1541–9. doi:10.1001/jama.2015.2928
71. Huurman VA, Decochez K, Mathieu C, Cohen IR, Roep BO. Therapy with the hsp60 peptide DiaPep277 in C-peptide positive type 1 diabetes patients. *Diabetes Metab Res Rev* (2007) **23**(4):269–75. doi:10.1002/dmrr.691
72. Huurman VA, van der Meide PE, Duinkerken G, Willemen S, Cohen IR, Elias D, et al. Immunological efficacy of heat shock protein 60 peptide DiaPep277 therapy in clinical type I diabetes. *Clin Exp Immunol* (2008) **152**(3):488–97. doi:10.1111/j.1365-2249.2008.03656.x
73. Raz I, Elias D, Avron A, Tamir M, Metzger M, Cohen IR. Beta-cell function in new-onset type 1 diabetes and immunomodulation with a heat-shock protein peptide (DiaPep277): a randomised, double-blind, phase II trial. *Lancet* (2001) **358**(9295):1749–53. doi:10.1016/S0140-6736(01)06801-5
74. Axelsson S, Hjorth M, Akerman L, Ludvigsson J, Casas R. Early induction of GAD(65)-reactive Th2 response in type 1 diabetic children treated with alum-formulated GAD(65). *Diabetes Metab Res Rev* (2010) **26**(7):559–68. doi:10.1002/dmrr.1126
75. Ludvigsson J, Krisky D, Casas R, Battelino T, Castaño L, Greening J, et al. GAD65 antigen therapy in recently diagnosed type 1 diabetes mellitus. *N Engl J Med* (2012) **366**(5):433–42. doi:10.1056/NEJMoa1107096
76. Hjorth M, Axelsson S, Rydén A, Faresjö M, Ludvigsson J, Casas R. GAD-alum treatment induces GAD65-specific CD4+CD25highFOXP3+ cells in type 1 diabetic patients. *Clin Immunol* (2011) **138**(1):117–26. doi:10.1016/j.clim.2010.10.004
77. Ryden AK, Wesley JD, Coppieters KT, Von Herrath MG. Non-antigenic and antigenic interventions in type 1 diabetes. *Hum Vaccin Immunother* (2014) **10**:838–46. doi:10.4161/hv.26890
78. Bollyky JB, Xu P, Butte AJ, Wilson DM, Beam CA, Greenbaum CJ. Heterogeneity in recent-onset type 1 diabetes – a clinical trial perspective. *Diabetes Metab Res Rev* (2015) **31**:588–94. doi:10.1002/dmrr.2643
79. Greenbaum CJ, Beam CA, Boulware D, Gitelman SE, Gottlieb PA, Herold KC, et al. Fall in C-peptide during first 2 years from diagnosis: evidence of at least two distinct phases from composite Type 1 Diabetes TrialNet data. *Diabetes* (2012) **61**:2066–73. doi:10.2337/db11-1538
80. Lachin JM, McGee P, Palmer JP. Impact of C-peptide preservation on metabolic and clinical outcomes in the diabetes control and complications trial. *Diabetes* (2014) **63**:739–48. doi:10.2337/db13-0881
81. Eisenbarth GS. Type I diabetes mellitus. A chronic autoimmune disease. *N Engl J Med* (1986) **314**(21):1360–8. doi:10.1056/NEJM198605223142106
82. Campbell-Thompson ML, Kaddis JS, Wasserfall C, Haller MJ, Pugliese A, Schatz DA, et al. The influence of type 1 diabetes on pancreatic weight. *Diabetologia* (2016) **59**(1):217–21. doi:10.1007/s00125-015-3752-z
83. Purohit S, She JX. Biomarkers for type 1 diabetes. *Int J Clin Exp Med* (2008) **1**(2):98–116.
84. Rekers NV, von Herrath MG, Wesley JD. Immunotherapies and immune biomarkers in Type 1 diabetes: a partnership for success. *Clin Immunol* (2015) **161**(1):37–43. doi:10.1016/j.clim.2015.05.021
85. Tooley JE, Herold KC. Biomarkers in type 1 diabetes: application to the clinical trial setting. *Curr Opin Endocrinol Diabetes Obes* (2014) **21**:287–92. doi:10.1097/MED.0000000000000076
86. Odegard JM, Nepom GT, Wambre E. Biomarkers for antigen immunotherapy in allergy and type 1 diabetes. *Clin Immunol* (2015) **161**(1):44–50. doi:10.1016/j.clim.2015.05.023

20

Comorbidities in Recent-Onset Adult Type 1 Diabetes: A Comparison of German Cohorts

Oana P. Zaharia[1,2,3†], Stefanie Lanzinger[2,4†], Joachim Rosenbauer[2,5], Wolfram Karges[6], Karsten Müssig[1,7], Sebastian M. Meyhöfer[2,8], Volker Burkart[1,2], Michael Hummel[9], Dirk Raddatz[10], Michael Roden[1,2,3], Julia Szendroedi[1,2,11] and Reinhard W. Holl[2,4†] for the GDS Group and the DPV Initiative*

[1] Institute for Clinical Diabetology, German Diabetes Center, Leibniz Center for Diabetes Research at Heinrich Heine University, Düsseldorf, Germany, [2] German Center for Diabetes Research (DZD), München-Neuherberg, Germany, [3] Department of Endocrinology and Diabetology, Medical Faculty, Heinrich Heine University, Düsseldorf, Germany, [4] Institute of Epidemiology and Medical Biometry, Zentralinstitut für Biomedizinische Technik (ZIBMT), University of Ulm, Ulm, Germany, [5] Institute for Biometrics and Epidemiology, German Diabetes Center, Leibniz Center for Diabetes Research at Heinrich Heine University, Düsseldorf, Germany, [6] Division of Endocrinology and Diabetes, Rheinisch-Westfälische Technische Hochschule (RWTH) Aachen University, Aachen, Germany, [7] Department of Internal Medicine/Gastroenterology, Franziskus-Hospital Harderberg, Georgsmarienhütte, Germany, [8] Institute for Endocrinology and Diabetes, University of Lübeck, Rosenheim, Lübeck, Germany, [9] Diabetes Center Rosenheim, Rosenheim, Germany, [10] Division of Gastroenterology and Gastrointestinal Oncology and Endocrinology, University Medical Center Göttingen, Göttingen, Germany, [11] Department of Internal Medicine I and Clinical Chemistry, University Hospital Heidelberg, Heidelberg, Germany

***Correspondence:**
Julia Szendroedi
julia.szendroedi@ddz.de

† These authors have contributed equally to this work

Aims: Restrictive exclusion criteria from different study populations may limit the generalizability of the observations. By comparing two differently designed German cohorts, we assessed the prevalence of cardiovascular risk factors and diabetes-related complications in recent-onset adult type 1 diabetes.

Methods: This study evaluated 1511 persons with type 1 diabetes of the prospective diabetes follow-up registry (DPV) and 268 volunteers of the prospective observational German Diabetes Study (GDS) with a known diabetes duration <1 year. Participants had similar age (36 years), sex distribution (41% female) and BMI (26 kg/m^2) in both cohorts.

Results: The average HbA1c was 6.4 ± 0.8% in the GDS and 7.0 ± 1.1% in the DPV. Prevalence of hypertension (24%) was similar, while more DPV participants had dyslipidemia and lipid-lowering medication than GDS participants (77% vs. 41% and 7% vs. 2%, respectively; p<0.05). Prevalence of retinopathy and nephropathy was higher in DPV compared to GDS participants (10% vs. 3% and 18% vs. 7%, respectively; p<0.001).

Conclusions: Diabetic nephropathy and retinopathy are the most frequent complications in type 1 diabetes, affecting up to every 10th patient within the first year after diagnosis, underlining the need for more stringent risk factor management already at the time of diagnosis of type 1 diabetes.

Keywords: dyslipidaemia, hypertension, type 1 diabetes, complications, nephropathy, retinopathy

INTRODUCTION

The prevalence of comorbidities such as hypertension and dyslipidemia is often underestimated in patients with newly diagnosed type 1 diabetes (1, 2). However, a growing body of evidence emphasizes the frequent existence of cardiovascular risk factors also in newly manifested type 1 diabetes and underlines the need for effective cardioprotective measures from disease onset (2).

Seminal studies demonstrated that intensive glucose lowering therapy could reduce the incidence of microvascular complications (3). Consequently, preventive and therapeutic efforts have focused on optimizing glycemic control (4). Nevertheless, the discordance observed between glucose lowering treatment regimens and the prevalence of different complications suggests distinct risk factors associated with each of the diabetes-related complications (5). Hyperglycemia, hypertension, and dyslipidemia are well defined modifiable risk factors that promote the appearance of micro- and macrovascular complications in diabetes (6). Prompt and intensive treatment are critical for successful prevention or delay of micro- and macrovascular complications (7). However, treatment targets are frequently not met (8) and there is a paucity of data regarding sex specific differences in patterns of diabetes-related complications (9) in patients with type 1 diabetes.

Evidence from population-based studies addressing risk factors and predictors of severe complications can contribute to guidelines for clinical practice and large-scale management of diabetes (10, 11). Moreover, patient selection is crucial to the generalizability of the results of clinical studies on the distribution of risk factors and complications within the diseased population. Early detection and treatment of comorbid conditions is important as it has been indicated that health-related quality of life is preserved in persons with type 1 diabetes unless confronted with multiple comorbidities. Previous findings show the importance of tracking the presence of multiple comorbid conditions, by reviewing medical records, as well as screening for complications in routine diabetes care (12). Our study, therefore, assesses the risk profiles of voluntary study participants of a comprehensive longitudinal clinical study on one side and, on the other side, patients from a patient registry. This comparative evaluation of differently designed German cohorts gives the opportunity to focus on modifiable risk factors that can impact the development of complications in patients with type 1 diabetes in finer detail.

The aim was to compare the prevalence of comorbidities such as hypertension and dyslipidemia and the presence of diabetes-related complications in patients with recently diagnosed type 1 diabetes from the prospective cohort of the German Diabetes Study (GDS) and from the national diabetes prospective follow-up registry (DPV) and assess sex-specific differences in diabetes-related complications.

SUBJECTS, MATERIALS AND METHODS

Data Sources

We analyzed data from two cohorts, the GDS and the DPV. GDS is a prospective longitudinal observational multicenter cohort study investigating the phenotypes of diabetes and diabetes-related comorbidities and complications during the course of the disease (13). In addition to demographic and clinical data, baseline and follow-up assessments include deep metabolic phenotyping in order to identify prognostic factors and underlying mechanisms contributing to diabetes progression and the development of its comorbidities and complications. The GDS (Clinicaltrials.gov NCT01055093) was approved by the ethics boards of the Medical Faculty of the Heinrich Heine University Düsseldorf (reference number 4508) and is being performed according to the Declaration of Helsinki (13).

The DPV registry is an electronic health record-based documentation for both children and adults with any diabetes type. Relevant data pertaining to diabetes are documented by the physician/diabetes nurse specialist and are available for research purposes. Anonymized demographic and clinical data from patients are transmitted for central validation and analyses to Ulm University. The ethics committee of Ulm University as well as local review boards of the participating centers approved data collection and analysis for benchmarking and diabetes research. Data from 265 specialized centers in Germany, including 39 university hospitals or out-patient clinics and 226 private practices were studied (14). A rough estimate indicates that almost a quarter of German adults with diabetes are registered in the DPV.

Participants

Patients aged 18-69 years with newly diagnosed type 1 diabetes (disease duration <12 months) (13) from 2009 to 2017 were included. Diagnosis of diabetes was confirmed according to the criteria of the current guidelines: fasting plasma glucose ≥ 126 mg/dl or 2-hour plasma glucose during oral glucose tolerance test ≥ 200 mg/dl or HbA1c ≥ 6.5% (15, 16). Specific criteria for type 1 diabetes such as severe hyperglycemia and/or diabetic ketoacidosis as well as low or undetectable levels of plasma C-peptide were considered (15, 16). Exclusion criteria comprised specific types of diabetes due to other causes, including hereditary forms of diabetes (e.g. maturity onset diabetes of the young, MODY), pregnancy or poor glycemic control (HbA1c >9%) (13). For the GDS cohort, additional exclusion criteria were severe renal diseases (stage 3 and above; estimated glomerular filtration rate (eGFR) <60 ml*min^{-1}*1.73m^{-2}) and evidence for acute inflammatory syndromes (high-sensitivity C-reactive protein (hsCRP) >1 mg/dl) (17).

Risk Factors and Comorbidities

Patients' medical history, current medication as well as laboratory and clinical parameters were recorded. Blood pressure was measured in resting conditions. In patients of the GDS, serum levels of blood glucose, HbA1c, serum lipids (total cholesterol, LDL- and HDL-fractions and triglycerides) and creatinine were measured in fasted conditions as previously described (13). In the DPV cohort, analyses of blood parameters were performed in each center following standardized operating procedures (18).

Dyslipidemia was initially defined by serum levels of triglycerides were ≥150 mg/dl and/or total cholesterol ≥200 mg/dl and/or HDL-cholesterol ≤40 mg/dl and/or LDL-cholesterol ≥160 mg/dl. Thereafter, as newest guidelines (European Society of Cardiology, ESC) advocate for a stratified risk assessment with individualized targets for LDL cholesterol (19), the proportion of persons meeting these targets was also assessed. Hypertension was defined as systolic blood pressure ≥140 mmHg and/or diastolic blood pressure ≥90 mmHg.

Patient self-reported history of diabetes-associated complications such as myocardial infarction, stroke, diabetic foot syndrome and peripheral artery disease was recorded. In the DPV diagnosis of myocardial infarction, stroke, diabetic foot syndrome and peripheral artery disease is based on physician diagnosis (ICD based). Eye examinations were performed and evaluated by trained ophthalmologists differentiating between non-proliferative and proliferative retinopathy in accordance with ADA guidelines (20). Albuminuria was assessed as marker of diabetic nephropathy. Urine samples were analyzed and microalbuminuria was defined by urinary albumin levels between 30-300 mg/l and macroalbuminuria by albumin levels above 300 mg/l (21).

Statistical Analyses

Descriptive statistics are presented for both cohorts. Continuous variables are reported as mean ± SD and dichotomous variables as percentages. Kruskal-Wallis and chi-squared tests were performed to identify unadjusted differences between the GDS and DPV patient groups. Benjamini-Hochberg procedure was used to control the false discovery rate and to adjust for multiple testing. Event rates of acute complications per 100 patient years (PY) were calculated using Poisson regression models. Multivariable logistic regression models were used in order to evaluate differences in the presence of diabetes-related complications between the two cohorts. All models were adjusted for sex, age groups (<30, 30-<50, ≥50 years), BMI (categorized as <25, 25-<30, ≥30 kg/m^2) and migration background (at least one parent not born in Germany). A subsequent analysis additionally adjusting for hypertension and dyslipidemia was performed to study whether these parameters are associated with the presence of diabetes-related complications. Additionally, a pooled analysis of the GDS and DPV cohort was performed to identify sex-related differences in diabetes complications as well as age-stratified analyses for age groups (<30, 30-<50, ≥50 years). P-values for two-sided tests below 0.05 were considered to indicate statistical significance and analyses were conducted with SAS version 9.4 (SAS Institute Inc, Cary, NC, USA).

RESULTS

In total, 1779 patients (268 participants of the GDS and 1511 patients of the DPV registry) (**Figure 1**) were included and analyzed with regard to metabolic phenotypes, routine laboratory parameters, clinical data including disease duration, anthropometric variables, medication, the presence of diabetes-related comorbidities and complications and smoking status.

Anthropometry and Clinical Parameters

The baseline information on demographic variables, clinical parameters and behavioral risk factors is shown in **Table 1**.

Patients with type 1 diabetes did not differ between cohorts with regard to age, sex distribution or BMI. In DPV, 61% of participants had a BMI <25 kg/m^2, 26% were overweight (BMI 25-30 kg/m^2) and 13% were obese (BMI >30 kg/m^2). In GDS, 31% participants were overweight and 10% were obese.

While the GDS routinely screens for diabetes-associated autoantibodies, only 39% of the persons with type 1 diabetes in the DPV were investigated regarding diabetes-related autoimmunity. Diabetes-associated autoantibodies were detected in 92.5% of the participants with type 1 diabetes of the GDS and in 88.8% of the investigated patients of the DPV cohort.

Participants of the GDS were more frequently smokers, and consumed a higher number of cigarettes per day compared to patients of the DPV (**Table 1** all p<0.05). Of note, smoking habits were not systematically registered in both study cohorts (GDS 55%, DPV 73%).

Hyperglycemia and Glucose-Lowering Medication

Only patients with HbA1c <9% (75 mmol/mol) were included in this analysis in order to match for the inclusion criteria of the GDS (13). Of these individuals, 54% from DPV and 88% of GDS had good glycemic control (HbA1c <7%/53 mmol/mol). Current glucose-lowering medication is shown in **Figure 2**. As expected, newly diagnosed patients with type 1 diabetes were preferentially treated with insulin. In 14% of patients additional oral glucose-lowering medication was recorded. Metformin was the most frequently used oral therapy.

In the DPV registry event rates of acute complications were 13.8 events/100 patient years (PY) (95% confidence interval: 12.7-14.9) of severe hypoglycemia, 4.6 events/100 PY (4.0-5.3) of hypoglycemic coma and 0.6 events/100 PY (0.4-0.8) of ketoacidosis.

Dyslipidemia and Lipid-Lowering Treatment

Dyslipidemia, considering all cholesterol fractions and triglycerides, as defined above, afflicted 67% of the patients from both cohorts. There was a higher prevalence of dyslipidemia in the DPV cohort compared to the GDS cohort

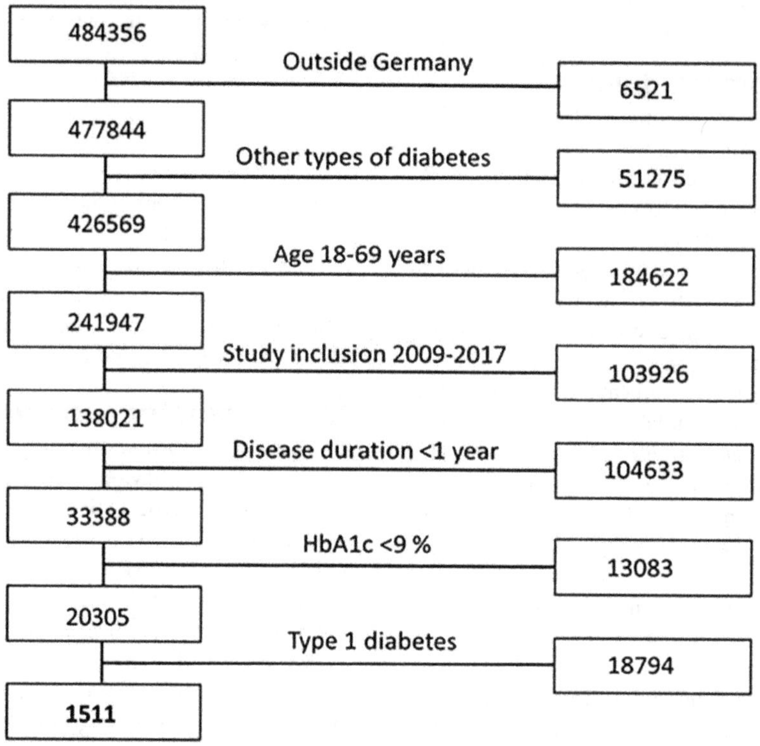

FIGURE 1 | Flow chart participants' selection criteria for the DPV registry. Flow chart showing the included and excluded participants of the DPV registry based on selection criteria matching the inclusion criteria of the GDS.

TABLE 1 | Anthropometric and clinical parameters of patients with newly diagnosed type 1 diabetes from the GDS and DPV cohorts.

	GDS		DPV		p-value
Variable	**n**		**n**		
Sex [% male]	268	59.3	1511	58.7	0.848
Age [years]	268	36.5 ± 11.6	1511	35.6 ± 14.6	0.050
Known diabetes duration [years]	268	0.52 ± 0.24	1511	0.38 ± 0.31	<0.001
Migration-background [%]	267	10.9	1511	6.3	0.020
Current smokers [%]	147	39.5	1109	28.2	0.007
Cigarettes/day [n]	44	12.9 ± 16.5	1109	3.7 ± 7.3	<0.001
BMI [kg/m^2]	268	25.0 ± 4.3	1443	24.9 ± 5.2	0.436
Systolic blood pressure [mmHg]	264	128.8 ± 16.3	1424	125.3 ± 14.8	0.003
Diastolic blood pressure [mmHg]	264	77.4 ± 9.7	1423	76.2 ± 10.4	0.239
Positivity for diabetes-related autoantibodies [%]	267	92.5	598	88.8	0.140
Fasted blood glucose [mg/dl]	264	129.1 ± 36.7	860	152.0 ± 88.8	<0.012
HbA1c [%]	267	6.4 ± 0.8	1511	7.0 ± 1.1	<0.001
HbA1c [mmol/mol]	267	46 ± 9	1511	53 ± 12	<0.001
Total cholesterol [mg/dl]	268	184.8 ± 38.4	926	190.0 ± 49.9	0.315
LDL-cholesterol [mg/dl]	267	110.4 ± 33.4	861	112.1 ± 36.5	0.606
HDL-cholesterol [mg/dl]	267	60.7 ± 17.1	874	55.4 ± 19.1	<0.001
Triglycerides [mg/dl]	268	89.7 ± 57.2	837	138.3 ± 114.1	<0.001
ALT [U/l]	268	21.9 ± 7.3	258	27.7 ± 31.7	0.108
AST [U/l]	268	24.0 ± 13.4	390	29.6 ± 27.2	0.018
GGT [U/l]	268	22.0 ± 21.2	376	53.3 ± 157.0	<0.001
Creatinin [mg/dl]	268	0.9 ± 0.2	1116	0.85 ± 0.53	<0.001
TSH [µIU/ml]	266	2.5 ± 2.6	984	0.9 ± 2.2	<0.001

n columns refer to the number of examined patients for each parameter. Data are shown as absolute numbers, percentages, mean ± standard deviation, as applicable. ALT, alanine aminotransferase; AST, aspartate aminotransferase; BMI, body mass index; DPV, Prospective Diabetes Registry; GDS, German Diabetes Study; GGT, gamma-glutamyl transferase; HbA1c, glycated hemoglobin A1c; HDL, high-density lipoprotein; LDL, low-density lipoprotein; TSH, thyroid stimulating hormone.

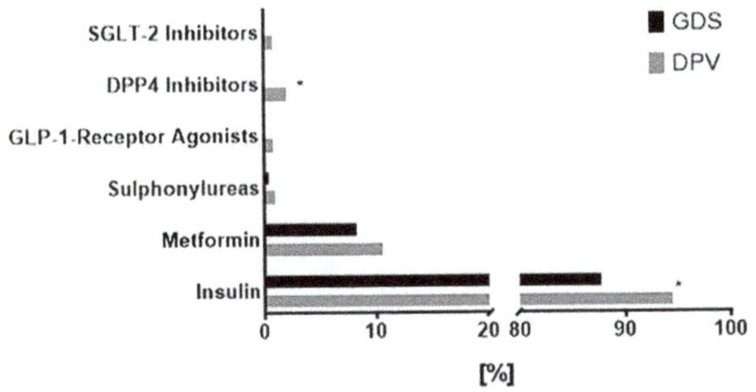

FIGURE 2 | Glucose-lowering medication in patients with newly diagnosed type 1 diabetes from the GDS and DPV cohorts. Choice of glucose-lowering medication in patients with newly diagnosed type 1 diabetes from the GDS (black) and DPV (grey) cohort. Data was collected on the frequency of use of sodium-glucose co-transporter-2 (SGLT-2) inhibitors, dipeptidyl peptidase-4 (DPP4) inhibitors, glucagon-like peptide-1 (GLP-1) receptor agonists, sulphonylureas, metformin and insulin. Data are expressed as percent from the total number of participants in each cohort. P values refer to comparison of unadjusted data. *p < 0.05.

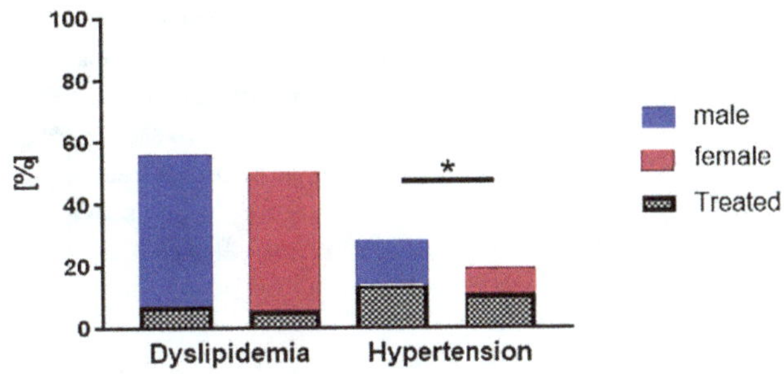

FIGURE 4 | Prevalence and management of hypertension and dyslipidemia in patients with newly diagnosed type 1 diabetes stratified by sex. Prevalence and management of modifiable cardiovascular risk factors (dyslipidemia and hypertension) in males (blue) and females (red) with newly diagnosed type 1 diabetes from the GDS and DPV cohort. 'Treated' refers to the frequency of lipid-lowering medication or antihypertensive, respectively. Data are expressed as percent from the total number of measured participants in each cohort. P values refer to comparison of unadjusted data. *p < 0.05 regarding the prevalence of comorbidities.

(77% vs 41%, p<0.001; **Figure 3**). When assessing the stratified ESC criteria for LDL cholesterol only (19), 40% of patients of the GDS and 47% of the DPV met the targeted levels. Of DPV patients, 7% had lipid-lowering medication compared to GDS where 2% had lipid-lowering medication (p<0.05). There was no difference in the prevalence of dyslipidemia between sexes (**Figure 4**).

Hypertension and Antihypertensive Treatment

Hypertension was present in 398 (24%) of the patients with type 1 diabetes from both cohorts with no difference between both cohorts (p=0.39, **Figure 3**). Of the patients in the DPV cohort, merely 13% had antihypertensive medication compared to the GDS participants of whom 9% had antihypertensive medication.

Men more frequently exhibited elevated blood pressure compared to women (p<0.001, **Figure 4**). In age-stratified analyses we observe an increase in prevalence of dyslipidemia and hypertension with age (**Figure 5**)

Diabetes-Related Complications

Figure 6 shows the prevalence of diabetes-related complications adjusted for age, sex, BMI, and migration background. There was a higher prevalence of both micro- and macrovascular complications in the DPV compared to the GDS cohort. Of note, largest differences were observed for nephropathy (18% vs.

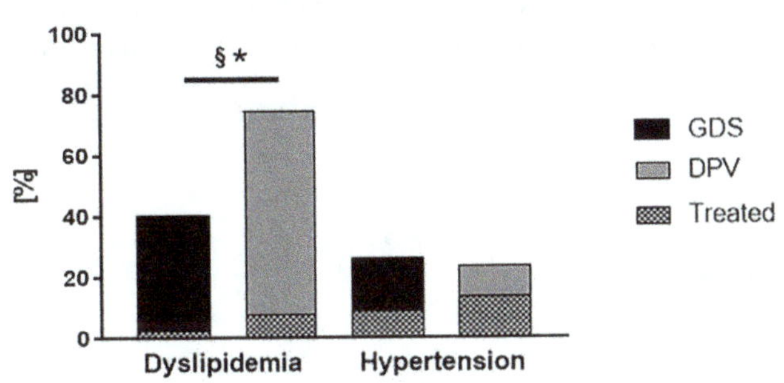

FIGURE 3 | Prevalence and management of hypertension and dyslipidemia in patients with newly diagnosed type 1 diabetes from the GDS and DPV cohorts. Prevalence and management of modifiable cardiovascular risk factors (dyslipidemia and hypertension) in patients with newly diagnosed type 1 diabetes from the GDS (black) and DPV (grey) cohort. 'Treated' refers to the frequency of lipid-lowering medication or antihypertensive, respectively. Data are expressed as percent from the total number of measured participants in each cohort. P values refer to comparison of unadjusted data. *p < 0.05 regarding the prevalence of comorbidities; §p < 0.05 regarding the percentage of treated patients.

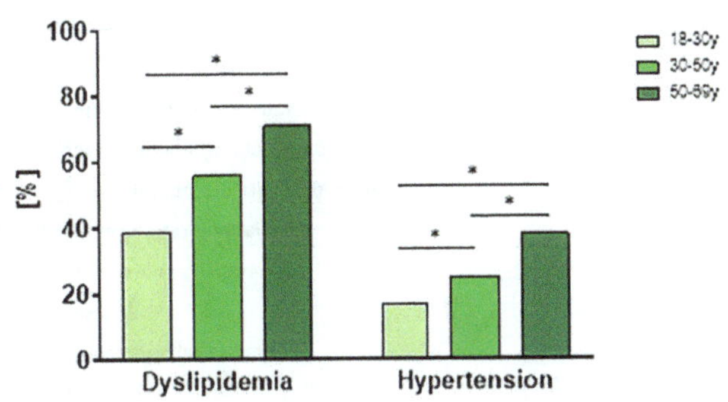

FIGURE 5 | Prevalence and management of hypertension and dyslipidemia in patients with newly diagnosed type 1 diabetes stratified by age. Prevalence and management of modifiable cardiovascular risk factors (dyslipidemia and hypertension) stratified by age tertiles in participants with newly diagnosed type 1 diabetes from the GDS and DPV cohort. P values refer to comparison of unadjusted data. *p < 0.05 regarding the prevalence of comorbidities.

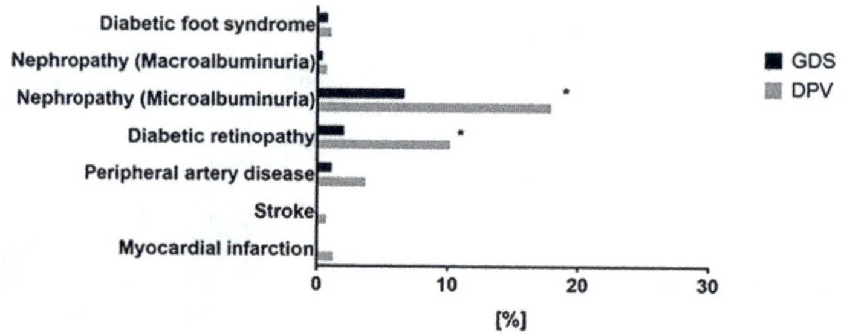

FIGURE 6 | Prevalence of diabetes related complications in patients with newly diagnosed type 1 diabetes from the GDS and DPV cohorts. Prevalence of diabetes-related complications in patients with newly diagnosed type 1 diabetes from the GDS (black) and DPV (grey) cohort. Data was collected on the prevalence of diabetic foot syndrome, diabetic nephropathy (micro- or macroalbuminuria), diabetic retinopathy, peripheral artery disease, myocardial infarction and stroke. Data are expressed as percent from the total number of measured participants in each cohort. P values refer to data adjusted for age, sex, BMI, migration background, hypertension and dyslipidemia for microalbuminuria, diabetic retinopathy, peripheral artery disease and myocardial infarction. P values for macroalbuminuria and diabetic foot syndrome are unadjusted because of the low case numbers. *p < 0.05.

7%) and diabetic retinopathy (10% vs 3%) (**Figure 6**). Additional adjustment for dyslipidemia and hypertension did not affect these results.

Regression analyses revealed that hypertension was positively associated with nephropathy (β=0.52, p=0.01) but neither hypertension nor dyslipidemia associated with the prevalence of retinopathy (p=0.17 and p=0.79, respectively).

Sex-specific analyses for diabetes related complications revealed no differences in the prevalence of retinopathy, nephropathy or peripheral artery disease after adjustments for age, BMI, migration background, dyslipidemia and hypertension (**Figure 7**). The low number of cases of other complications did not allow sex-specific evaluation.

Similarly, additional analyses were performed to address age-specific differences in the prevalence of retinopathy, nephropathy or peripheral artery disease. After adjustments for age, sex, BMI, migration background, hypertension and dyslipidemia the differences between groups with regard to nephropathy did not reach statistical significance, however the prevalence of retinopathy and peripheral artery disease increased with age (**Figure 8**).

DISCUSSION

The present study assessed the prevalence of diabetes-related complications in patients with newly diagnosed type 1 diabetes from two different types of cohorts – voluntary participants of a prospective longitudinal study and patients of a population-based patient registry. Both cohorts show on average very good glucometabolic control, but inadequate management of risk factors such as hypertension and dyslipidemia.

This comparative analysis of data from two different types of cohorts provides effective information on the distribution of risk factors and complications and identifies common factors, independent of study design. Subsequently, this analysis may improve the generalizability of data deriving from clinical trials to the general diseased population.

Glucose homeostasis was assessed by fasting blood glucose and HbA1c levels as parameters to determine the effectiveness of diabetes management. Even though the same inclusion criteria were applied for both cohorts, patients of the GDS had a slightly lower HbA1c and fasting glucose compared to patients of the

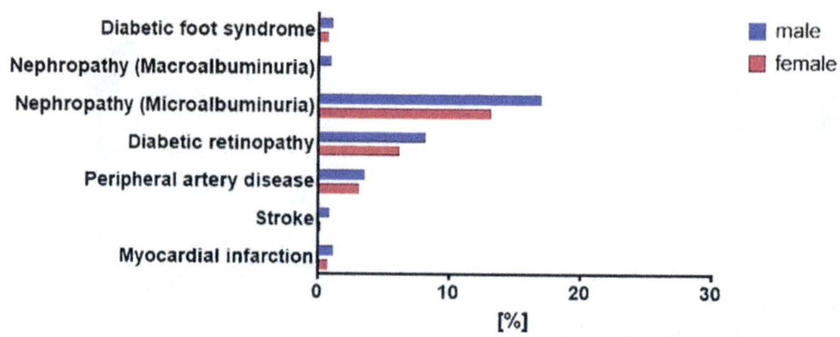

FIGURE 7 | Prevalence of diabetes related complications in patients with newly diagnosed type 1 diabetes stratified by sex. Prevalence of diabetes-related complications in males (blue) and females (red) with newly diagnosed type 1 diabetes from the GDS and DPV cohort. Data was collected on the prevalence of diabetic foot syndrome, diabetic nephropathy (micro- or macroalbuminuria), diabetic retinopathy, peripheral artery disease, myocardial infarction and stroke. Data are expressed as percent from the total number of measured participants in each cohort. P values refer to data adjusted for age, sex, BMI, migration background, hypertension and dyslipidemia.*p < 0.05.

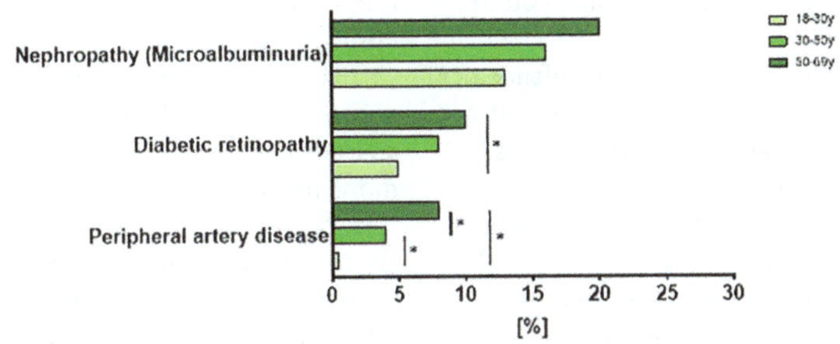

FIGURE 8 | Prevalence of diabetes related complications in patients with newly diagnosed type 1 diabetes stratified by age. Prevalence of diabetes-related complications stratified by age tertiles in participants with newly diagnosed type 1 diabetes from the GDS and DPV cohort. Data are expressed as percent from the total number of measured participants in each cohort. *$p < 0.05$ regarding the prevalence of complications adjusted for age, sex, BMI, migration background, hypertension and dyslipidemia.

DPV. Therefore, our data aligns with previous studies which suggested that patients voluntarily participating in clinical studies might be more inclined towards preserving a good glycemic control. This may be related to the opportunity to ask investigators for advice and recommendations, regular monitoring, as well as increased awareness and access to information compared to standard care (22). Other differences may reside in educational and social background. Some individuals with type 1 diabetes had no insulin treatment after diagnosis, possibly accounting for cases of preserved beta cell function in autoimmune diabetes (23) or may be related to partial remission (24) within the short time frame after diagnosis. Moreover, 14% of type 1 diabetes patients also received oral glucose lowering diabetes-medication. Metformin had been shown to reduce the insulin dose requirement in insulin resistant individuals, insulin-induced weight gain, and cholesterol levels (25). Therefore, recent studies focused on the assessment of the effects of metformin on the cardiovascular system in adults with type 1 diabetes. The results of these investigations suggest a possible role of metformin in the prevention of cardiovascular events in type 1 diabetes by reducing body weight and LDL-cholesterol levels (26). The addition of the glucagon-like peptide 1 (GLP-1) receptor agonists or of a sodium-glucose cotransporter 2 (SGLT2) inhibitor to insulin therapy was shown to trigger small reductions in HbA1c compared with insulin alone in people with type 1 diabetes and also reduced body weight (27–29). However, SGLT2 inhibitor use is also associated with adverse events including ketoacidosis (30), and was only prescribed off-label for patients with type 1 diabetes, as was also the case for GLP-1 receptor agonists, at the time of data acquisition in Germany, which could explain the low prescription frequency for newly diagnosed type 1 diabetes.

We further underline the need for multidisciplinary interventions focusing on groups at high risk for hyperglycemic crises in order to prevent ketoacidotic events. Diabetic ketoacidosis remains a serious endocrine emergency, associated with morbidity and mortality. Younger age, ethnicity, low income, and poor glycemic control were associated with an increased risk of hyperglycemic crises (31). Recent studies further these findings by analyzing the rate of readmission for diabetic ketoacidosis in type 1 diabetes. Multiple concomitant complications, hypertension, female sex, and incompliance towards medical advice were significant predictors of readmission (32).

In both cohorts, dyslipidemia was highly prevalent in type 1 diabetes and management of lipid abnormalities was suboptimal according to guidelines (33). The apparent inadequate treatment of these patients may have serious implications for the subsequent development of diabetes-related complications. The American Diabetes Association recommends lipid-lowering pharmacotherapy for patients with concomitant cardiovascular risk factors such as elevated LDL cholesterol, high blood pressure, smoking, obesity, and/or family history of premature cardiovascular events (33). In spite of a prevalence of dyslipidemia in 77% of the DPV patients and 41% of the GDS participants, only 7% and 2% were treated with lipid-lowering agents, respectively. Along these lines, only 40% of patients with diabetes of GDS and 47% of DPV met the stratified LDL cholesterol targets as defined by the ESC (19).

Hypertension, together with reduced insulin sensitivity and dyslipidemia, can contribute to an increased cardiovascular risk (34) in patients with diabetes. Nevertheless, only 8% of patients diagnosed with hypertension in the DPV cohort and 14% of those in the GDS cohort had antihypertensive medication, pointing to a considerable therapeutic inertia in the management of modifiable risk factors. Our study is in accordance to a previous comparison of the DPV registry with the American T1D Exchange Clinic Network showing that individuals with type 1 diabetes are inadequately treated for hypertension and dyslipidemia (35). Clinical inertia was discussed as one potential reason for the observed undertreatment while the authors emphasized the importance to strengthen physician and patient education on early treatment of cardiovascular risk factors. However, while we included individuals with recent-onset type 1 diabetes, Shah et al. only included individuals with type 1 diabetes aged ≥12 years and a diabetes duration of at least one year.

Socioeconomic factors and sex may have an impact on the adherence to lipid-lowering therapy as previous studies suggest that in individuals with type 1 diabetes lower adherence was associated with male sex, younger age, marital status and country of birth (36).

A previous study has also shown an increased prevalence of diabetes-related complications in the DPV cohort compared to an American registry (37), which was explained by a more frequent use of antihypertensive drugs and/or lower blood pressure of the 3297 participants aged > 60 years. This is also seen for the present comparison at a national level between the DPV and the GDS cohort with regard to both micro- and macrovascular complications. Nevertheless, it should be noted that the prevalence of dyslipidemia in individuals with type 1 diabetes varies markedly by country and age of the participants, with reported values between 3.8–72.5% (38). Initiating good glycemic control and strict monitoring of modifiable risk factors from onset of diabetes, irrespective of diabetes type, is essential to counteract pathogenetic processes causative for micro- and macrovascular complications (39). In this study, retinopathy and nephropathy, were more frequent compared to classical macrovascular complications such as myocardial infarction or stroke, irrespective of study cohort.

Diabetic retinopathy represents a frequent microvascular complication of diabetes and a leading cause of blindness among adults (40). In addition to hyperglycemia, dyslipidemia and hypertension may contribute to the onset and progression of diabetic retinopathy (41). Previous studies in type 1 diabetes showed that intensified glycemic control was highly effective in reducing the risk of developing microvascular complications (42). In the present analysis, in spite of predominantly good metabolic control and short diabetes duration, up to 10% of type 1 diabetes patients presented with diabetic retinopathy within the first year after diagnosis. As with peripheral artery disease, the prevalence of retinopathy increased with age, in line with previous observations showing that not only duration of diabetes but also advancing age independently predicts diabetes morbidity rates (43).

Nephropathy, another major microvascular complication, was linked to impaired glycemic control, increased body weight, and improper insulin dosage (44). Our study showed that microalbuminuria was present in 7% of the GDS population and was twice more frequent in DPV. As expected, microalbuminuria was positively associated with hypertension. Nevertheless, generally, it appears that renal dysfunction and hyperglycemia have improved considerably during recent years for people with type 1 diabetes. This finding has important implications for quality of life, health economics and prognosis regarding cardiovascular mortality (45).

Cardiovascular disorders are a major macrovascular complication which can increase the morbidity and mortality in patients with diabetes (46). However, evidence of cardiovascular risks and management of type 1 diabetes is often extrapolated from studies in type 2 diabetes patients (47). Overall, cardiovascular events are more common and occur earlier in patients with type 1 diabetes patients than in nondiabetic populations, with an even higher discrepancy in the female population (33). The prevalence of cardiovascular disease in patients with type 1 diabetes varies substantially based on disease duration, age of cohort, and sex, as well as possibly by ethnicity (9).

Factors related to sex seem to explain the consistently observed increased risk of incident type 1 diabetes for males of all age categories (48). However, females with type 1 diabetes are more likely to develop complications (9), possibly due to risk factors such as centrally distributed adipose tissue, which may contribute to their relatively higher risk for cardiovascular disease. The results of the present study did not reveal any differences in microvascular complication between male and female patients with type 1 diabetes. However, likely due to the short disease duration, patients with type 1 diabetes rarely presented with overt cardiovascular disease. Further mechanistic insights with regard to possible metabolic risk factors were limited due to the low number of cases.

The present comparative study may suffer from a certain degree of selection bias, since participants of the GDS are generally compliant, health-conscious patients with diabetes with an HbA1c below 9%. This could trigger a 'healthy user bias', whereas the DPV sample could be prone to the Berkson's fallacy, since a considerable fraction of the study population is selected from hospital care and therefore may be less healthy than the general population (49). This provides a sample population that may not be representative of the general population of persons with type 1 diabetes.

While for the GDS the baseline characteristics and blood chemistry have been done using standardized operating procedures in a centralized laboratory facility, this was not the case for patients of the DPV. Therefore, variations in sample collection and handling are to be expected between centers, and it cannot be guaranteed that DPV samples were collected in fasted conditions. Furthermore, for the GDS cohort the presented parameters are routinely screened in all study participants, while in the DPV some parameters are only measured if there is clinical suspicion (e.g. thyroid function, diabetes-related antibodies), increasing the likelihood of pathological levels. Recall bias cannot be excluded when addressing self-reported data. Also, other mediating factors that are not routinely quantified but may impact the results, such as physical activity behavior or smoking, could not be comprehensively assessed in the context of the present analysis.

Conclusion

The present analysis of data from different German diabetes cohorts allows for a better understanding of the distribution of risk factors and their association to diabetes-related complications and renders similar results irrespective of study design. The current mismanagement of known modifiable risk factors possibly contributes to the development of diabetes-related complications. We observed that diabetic nephropathy and retinopathy are the most frequent complications in type 1 diabetes affecting up to 10% of the patients within the first year after diagnosis. There were no differences in the prevalence of microvascular complication between male and female patients in our study. These observations warrant intensified and targeted treatment of modifiable risk factors from disease onset in order to prevent development and progression of diabetes-related complications.

AUTHOR CONTRIBUTIONS

OZ wrote the manuscript and researched data. SL, JR, RH performed the statistical analyses. WK, SM, MH, DR, SL, JR, JS, KM, VB, MR, RH researched data, contributed to the discussion and reviewed/edited the manuscript. All authors critically reviewed the manuscript. JS and RH are the guarantors of this work and, as such, had full access to all the data in the study and take responsibility for the integrity of the data and the accuracy of the data analysis. All authors read and approved the final manuscript.

ACKNOWLEDGMENTS

We would like to thank the staff of the German Diabetes Center for their excellent support. Also, we greatly appreciate the support of the centers involved in the German Diabetes Study as well as all centers participating in the DPV project.

REFERENCES

1. Wadwa RP, Kinney GL, Maahs DM, Snell-Bergeon J, Hokanson JE, Garg SK, et al. Awareness and Treatment of Dyslipidemia in Young Adults With Type 1 Diabetes. *Diabetes Care* (2005) 28(5):1051–6. doi: 10.2337/diacare.28.5.1051
2. Rawshani A, Sattar N, Franzen S, Rawshani A, Hattersley AT, Svensson AM, et al. Excess Mortality and Cardiovascular Disease in Young Adults With Type 1 Diabetes in Relation to Age at Onset: A Nationwide, Register-Based Cohort Study. *Lancet* (2018) 392(10146):477–86. doi: 10.1016/S0140-6736(18)31506-X
3. Reichard P, Nilsson BY, Rosenqvist U. The Effect of Long-Term Intensified Insulin Treatment on the Development of Microvascular Complications of Diabetes Mellitus. *N Engl J Med* (1993) 329(5):304–9. doi: 10.1056/NEJM199307293290502
4. Chillaron JJ, Flores Le-Roux JA, Benaiges D, Pedro-Botet J. Type 1 Diabetes, Metabolic Syndrome and Cardiovascular Risk. *Metabol: Clin Exp* (2014) 63(2):181–7. doi: 10.1016/j.metabol.2013.10.002
5. Nathan DM. Long-Term Complications of Diabetes Mellitus. *N Engl J Med* (1993) 328(23):1676–85. doi: 10.1056/NEJM199306103282306
6. Hammes HP, Welp R, Kempe HP, Wagner C, Siegel E, Holl RW. Risk Factors for Retinopathy and DME in Type 2 Diabetes-Results From the German/Austrian DPV Database. *PloS One* (2015) 10(7):e0132492. doi: 10.1371/journal.pone.0132492
7. Melendez-Ramirez LY, Richards RJ, Cefalu WT. Complications of Type 1 Diabetes. *Endocrinol Metab Clinics North America* (2010) 39(3):625–40. doi: 10.1016/j.ecl.2010.05.009
8. Schmittdiel JA, Uratsu CS, Karter AJ, Heisler M, Subramanian U, Mangione CM, et al. Why Don't Diabetes Patients Achieve Recommended Risk Factor Targets? Poor Adherence Versus Lack of Treatment Intensification. *J Gen Internal Med* (2008) 23(5):588–94. doi: 10.1007/s11606-008-0554-8
9. Huxley RR, Peters SA, Mishra GD, Woodward M. Risk of All-Cause Mortality and Vascular Events in Women Versus Men With Type 1 Diabetes: A Systematic Review and Meta-Analysis. *Lancet Diabetes Endocrinol* (2015) 3(3):198–206. doi: 10.1016/S2213-8587(14)70248-7
10. Karges B, Kapellen T, Neu A, Hofer SE, Rohrer T, Rosenbauer J, et al. Long-Acting Insulin Analogs and the Risk of Diabetic Ketoacidosis in Children and Adolescents With Type 1 Diabetes: A Prospective Study of 10,682 Patients From 271 Institutions. *Diabetes Care* (2010) 33(5):1031–3. doi: 10.2337/dc09-2249
11. Schwandt A, Best F, Biester T, Grunerbel A, Kopp F, Krakow D, et al. Both the Frequency of HbA1c Testing and the Frequency of SMBG Predict Metabolic Control: A Multicenter Analysis of 15,199 Adult Type 1 Diabetes Patients From Germany and Austria. *Diabetes Metab Res Rev* (2017) 33(7):e2098. doi: 10.1002/dmrr.2908
12. Shapira A, Harrington KR, Goethals ER, Volkening LK, Laffel LM. Health-Related Quality of Life in Youth With Type 1 Diabetes: Associations With Multiple Comorbidities and Mental Health Conditions. *Diabetic Med* (2021) 38(10):e14617. doi: 10.1111/dme.14617
13. Szendroedi J, Saxena A, Weber KS, Strassburger K, Herder C, Burkart V, et al. Cohort Profile: The German Diabetes Study (GDS). *Cardiovasc Diabetol* (2016) 15:59. doi: 10.1186/s12933-016-0374-9
14. Schwab KO, Doerfer J, Hecker W, Grulich-Henn J, Wiemann D, Kordonouri O, et al. Spectrum and Prevalence of Atherogenic Risk Factors in 27,358 Children, Adolescents, and Young Adults With Type 1 Diabetes: Cross-Sectional Data From the German Diabetes Documentation and Quality Management System (DPV). *Diabetes Care* (2006) 29(2):218–25. doi: 10.2337/diacare.29.02.06.dc05-0724
15. American Diabetes Association. Classification and Diagnosis of Diabetes: Standards of Medical Care in Diabetes—2020. *Diabetes Care* (2020) 43(Supplement 1):S14. doi: 10.2337/dc20-S002
16. Petersmann A, Müller-Wieland D, Müller UA, Landgraf R, Nauck M, Freckmann G, et al. Definition, Classification and Diagnosis of Diabetes Mellitus. *Exp Clin Endocrinol Diabetes* (2019) 127(S 01):S1–7. doi: 10.1055/a-1018-9078
17. Weber KS, Nowotny B, Strassburger K, Pacini G, Mussig K, Szendroedi J, et al. The Role of Markers of Low-Grade Inflammation for the Early Time Course of Glycemic Control, Glucose Disappearance Rate, and Beta-Cell Function in Recently Diagnosed Type 1 and Type 2 Diabetes. *Diabetes Care* (2015) 38(9):1758–67. doi: 10.2337/dc15-0169
18. Hermann JM, Hammes HP, Rami-Merhar B, Rosenbauer J, Schutt M, Siegel E, et al. HbA1c Variability as an Independent Risk Factor for Diabetic Retinopathy in Type 1 Diabetes: A German/Austrian Multicenter Analysis on 35,891 Patients. *PloS One* (2014) 9(3):e91137. doi: 10.1371/journal.pone.0091137
19. Cosentino F, Grant PJ, Aboyans V, Bailey CJ, Ceriello A, Delgado V, et al. 2019 ESC Guidelines on Diabetes, Pre-Diabetes, and Cardiovascular Diseases Developed in Collaboration With the EASD: The Task Force for Diabetes, Pre-Diabetes, and Cardiovascular Diseases of the European Society of Cardiology (ESC) and the European Association for the Study of Diabetes (EASD). *Eur Heart J* (2019) 41(2):255–323. doi: 10.1093/eurheartj/ehz486
20. Solomon SD, Chew E, Duh EJ, Sobrin L, Sun JK, VanderBeek BL, et al. Diabetic Retinopathy: A Position Statement by the American Diabetes Association. *Diabetes Care* (2017) 40(3):412. doi: 10.2337/dc16-2641
21. Cohen-Bucay A, Viswanathan G. Urinary Markers of Glomerular Injury in Diabetic Nephropathy. *Int J Nephrol* (2012) 2012:146987. doi: 10.1155/2012/146987
22. Zvonareva O, Kutishenko N, Kulikov E, Martsevich S. Risks and Benefits of Trial Participation: A Qualitative Study of Participants' Perspectives in Russia. *Clin Trials (Lond Engl)* (2015) 12(6):646–53. doi: 10.1177/1740774515589592
23. Zaharia OP, Bobrov P, Strassburger K, Bodis K, Karusheva Y, Scholz M, et al. Metabolic Characteristics of Recently Diagnosed Adult-Onset Autoimmune Diabetes Mellitus. *J Clin Endocrinol Metab* (2018) 103(2):429–37. doi: 10.1210/jc.2017-01706
24. Zhong T, Tang R, Gong S, Li J, Li X, Zhou Z. The Remission Phase in Type 1 Diabetes: Changing Epidemiology, Definitions, and Emerging Immuno-Metabolic Mechanisms. *Diabetes/Metabol Res Rev* (2020) 36(2):e3207. doi: 10.1002/dmrr.3207
25. Priya G, Kalra S. A Review of Insulin Resistance in Type 1 Diabetes: Is There a Place for Adjunctive Metformin? *Diabetes Ther Res Treat Educ Diabetes Relat Disord* (2018) 9(1):349–61. doi: 10.1007/s13300-017-0333-9

26. Petrie JR, Chaturvedi N, Ford I, Brouwers M, Greenlaw N, Tillin T, et al. Cardiovascular and Metabolic Effects of Metformin in Patients With Type 1 Diabetes (REMOVAL): A Double-Blind, Randomised, Placebo-Controlled Trial. *Lancet Diabetes Endocrinol* (2017) 5(8):597–609. doi: 10.1016/S2213-8587(17)30194-8
27. American Diabetes Association. Pharmacologic Approaches to Glycemic Treatment: Standards of Medical Care in Diabetes—2019. *Diabetes Care* (2019) 42(Supplement 1):S90. doi: 10.2337/dc19-S009
28. Dandona P, Mathieu C, Phillip M, Hansen L, Griffen SC, Tschöpe D, et al. Efficacy and Safety of Dapagliflozin in Patients With Inadequately Controlled Type 1 Diabetes (DEPICT-1): 24 Week Results From a Multicentre, Double-Blind, Phase 3, Randomised Controlled Trial. *Lancet Diabetes Endocrinol* (2017) 5(11):864–76. doi: 10.1016/S2213-8587(17)30308-X
29. Wang W, Liu H, Xiao S, Liu S, Li X, Yu P. Effects of Insulin Plus Glucagon-Like Peptide-1 Receptor Agonists (GLP-1ras) in Treating Type 1 Diabetes Mellitus: A Systematic Review and Meta-Analysis. *Diabetes Ther* (2017) 8 (4):727–38. doi: 10.1007/s13300-017-0282-3
30. Henry RR, Thakkar P, Tong C, Polidori D, Alba M. Efficacy and Safety of Canagliflozin, a Sodium–Glucose Cotransporter 2 Inhibitor, as Add-on to Insulin in Patients With Type 1 Diabetes. *Diabetes Care* (2015) 38(12):2258–65. doi: 10.2337/dc15-1730
31. McCoy RG, Galindo RJ, Swarna KS, Van Houten HK, O'Connor PJ, Umpierrez GE, et al. Sociodemographic, Clinical, and Treatment-Related Factors Associated With Hyperglycemic Crises Among Adults With Type 1 or Type 2 Diabetes in the US From 2014 to 2020. *JAMA Netw Open* (2021) 4(9): e2123471–e2123471. doi: 10.1001/jamanetworkopen.2021.23471
32. Shaka H, Aguilera M, Aucar M, El-Amir Z, Wani F, Muojieje CC, et al. Rate and Predictors of 30-Day Readmission Following Diabetic Ketoacidosis in Type 1 Diabetes Mellitus: A US Analysis. *J Clin Endocrinol Metab* (2021) 106 (9):2592–9. doi: 10.1210/clinem/dgab372
33. de Ferranti SD, de Boer IH, Fonseca V, Fox CS, Golden SH, Lavie CJ, et al. Type 1 Diabetes Mellitus and Cardiovascular Disease: A Scientific Statement From the American Heart Association and American Diabetes Association. *Diabetes Care* (2014) 37(10):2843. doi: 10.1161/CIR.0000000000000034
34. Marini MA, Fiorentino TV, Succurro E, Pedace E, Andreozzi F, Sciacqua A, et al. Association Between Hemoglobin Glycation Index With Insulin Resistance and Carotid Atherosclerosis in Non-Diabetic Individuals. *PloS One* (2017) 12(4):e0175547. doi: 10.1371/journal.pone.0175547
35. Shah VN, Grimsmann JM, Foster NC, Dost A, Miller KM, Pavel M, et al. Undertreatment of Cardiovascular Risk Factors in the Type 1 Diabetes Exchange Clinic Network (United States) and the Prospective Diabetes Follow-Up (Germany/Austria) Registries. *Diabetes Obes Metab* (2020) 22 (9):1577–85. doi: 10.1111/dom.14069
36. Hero C, Karlsson SA, Franzén S, Svensson AM, Miftaraj M, Gudbjörnsdottír S, et al. Impact of Socioeconomic Factors and Gender on Refill Adherence and Persistence to Lipid-Lowering Therapy in Type 1 Diabetes. *Diabetes Ther Res Treat Educ Diabetes Relat Disord* (2021) 12(9):2371–86. doi: 10.1007/s13300-021-01115-w
37. Weinstock RS, Schutz-Fuhrmann I, Connor CG, Hermann JM, Maahs DM, Schutt M, et al. Type 1 Diabetes in Older Adults: Comparing Treatments and Chronic Complications in the United States T1D Exchange and the German/Austrian DPV Registries. *Diabetes Res Clin Pract* (2016) 122:28–37. doi: 10.1016/j.diabres.2016.09.024
38. Vergès B. Dyslipidemia in Type 1 Diabetes: A Masked Danger. *Trends Endocrinol Metab* (2020) 31(6):422–34. doi: 10.1016/j.tem.2020.01.015
39. Inzucchi SE, Bergenstal RM, Buse JB, Diamant M, Ferrannini E, Nauck M, et al. Management of Hyperglycemia in Type 2 Diabetes, 2015: A Patient-Centered Approach: Update to a Position Statement of the American Diabetes Association and the European Association for the Study of Diabetes. *Diabetes Care* (2015) 38(1):140–9. doi: 10.2337/dc14-2441
40. Eshaq RS, Aldalati AMZ, Alexander JS, Harris NR. Diabetic Retinopathy: Breaking the Barrier. *Pathophysiol Off J Int Soc Pathophysiol* (2017) 24(4):229–41. doi: 10.1016/j.pathophys.2017.07.001
41. Duh EJ, Sun JK, Stitt AW. Diabetic Retinopathy: Current Understanding, Mechanisms, and Treatment Strategies. *JCI Insight* (2017) 2(14):e93751. doi: 10.1172/jci.insight.93751
42. Fullerton B, Jeitler K, Seitz M, Horvath K, Berghold A, Siebenhofer A. Intensive Glucose Control Versus Conventional Glucose Control for Type 1 Diabetes Mellitus. *Cochrane Database Syst Rev* (2014) 2:Cd009122. doi: 10.1002/14651858.CD009122.pub2
43. Huang ES, Laiteerapong N, Liu JY, John PM, Moffet HH, Karter AJ. Rates of Complications and Mortality in Older Patients With Diabetes Mellitus: The Diabetes and Aging Study. *JAMA Internal Med* (2014) 174(2):251–8. doi: 10.1001/jamainternmed.2013.12956
44. Dost A, Klinkert C, Kapellen T, Lemmer A, Naeke A, Grabert M, et al. Arterial Hypertension Determined by Ambulatory Blood Pressure Profiles: Contribution to Microalbuminuria Risk in a Multicenter Investigation in 2,105 Children and Adolescents With Type 1 Diabetes. *Diabetes Care* (2008) 31(4):720–5. doi: 10.2337/dc07-0824
45. Hallström S, Svensson AM, Pivodic A, Ólafsdóttir AF, Löndahl M, Wedel H, et al. Risk Factors and Incidence Over Time for Lower Extremity Amputations in People With Type 1 Diabetes: An Observational Cohort Study of 46,088 Patients From the Swedish National Diabetes Registry. *Diabetologia* (2021) 64 (12):2751–61. doi: 10.1007/s00125-021-05550-z
46. Tun NN, Arunagirinathan G, Munshi SK, Pappachan JM. Diabetes Mellitus and Stroke: A Clinical Update. *World J Diabetes* (2017) 8(6):235–48. doi: 10.4239/wjd.v8.i6.235
47. Lee SI, Patel M, Jones CM, Narendran P. Cardiovascular Disease and Type 1 Diabetes: Prevalence, Prediction and Management in an Ageing Population. *Ther Adv Chronic Dis* (2015) 6(6):347–74. doi: 10.1177/2040622315598502
48. Östman J, Lönnberg G, Arnqvist HJ, Blohmé G, Bolinder J, Schnell AE, et al. Gender Differences and Temporal Variation in the Incidence of Type 1 Diabetes: Results of 8012 Cases in the Nationwide Diabetes Incidence Study in Sweden 1983–2002. *J Internal Med* (2008) 263(4):386–94. doi: 10.1111/j.1365-2796.2007.01896.x
49. Hernan MA, Hernandez-Diaz S, Robins JM. A Structural Approach to Selection Bias. *Epidemiol (Cambridge Mass)* (2004) 15(5):615–25. doi: 10.1097/01.ede.0000135174.63482.43

Permissions

All chapters in this book were first published Frontiers; hereby published with permission under the Creative Commons Attribution License or equivalent. Every chapter published in this book has been scrutinized by our experts. Their significance has been extensively debated. The topics covered herein carry significant findings which will fuel the growth of the discipline. They may even be implemented as practical applications or may be referred to as a beginning point for another development.

The contributors of this book come from diverse backgrounds, making this book a truly international effort. This book will bring forth new frontiers with its revolutionizing research information and detailed analysis of the nascent developments around the world.

We would like to thank all the contributing authors for lending their expertise to make the book truly unique. They have played a crucial role in the development of this book. Without their invaluable contributions this book wouldn't have been possible. They have made vital efforts to compile up to date information on the varied aspects of this subject to make this book a valuable addition to the collection of many professionals and students.

This book was conceptualized with the vision of imparting up-to-date information and advanced data in this field. To ensure the same, a matchless editorial board was set up. Every individual on the board went through rigorous rounds of assessment to prove their worth. After which they invested a large part of their time researching and compiling the most relevant data for our readers.

The editorial board has been involved in producing this book since its inception. They have spent rigorous hours researching and exploring the diverse topics which have resulted in the successful publishing of this book. They have passed on their knowledge of decades through this book. To expedite this challenging task, the publisher supported the team at every step. A small team of assistant editors was also appointed to further simplify the editing procedure and attain best results for the readers.

Apart from the editorial board, the designing team has also invested a significant amount of their time in understanding the subject and creating the most relevant covers. They scrutinized every image to scout for the most suitable representation of the subject and create an appropriate cover for the book.

The publishing team has been an ardent support to the editorial, designing and production team. Their endless efforts to recruit the best for this project, has resulted in the accomplishment of this book. They are a veteran in the field of academics and their pool of knowledge is as vast as their experience in printing. Their expertise and guidance has proved useful at every step. Their uncompromising quality standards have made this book an exceptional effort. Their encouragement from time to time has been an inspiration for everyone.

The publisher and the editorial board hope that this book will prove to be a valuable piece of knowledge for researchers, students, practitioners and scholars across the globe.

List of Contributors

Juan Huang
National Clinical Research Center for Metabolic Diseases, Key Laboratory of Diabetes Immunology (Central South University), Ministry of Education, and Department of Metabolism and Endocrinology, The Second Xiangya Hospital, Central South University, Changsha, China
Section of Endocrinology, Department of Internal Medicine, School of Medicine, Yale University, New Haven, CT, United States

Zhiguang Zhou
National Clinical Research Center for Metabolic Diseases, Key Laboratory of Diabetes Immunology (Central South University), Ministry of Education, and Department of Metabolism and Endocrinology, The Second Xiangya Hospital, Central South University, Changsha, China
National Clinical Research Center for Metabolic Diseases, and Department of Metabolism and Endocrinology, The Second Xiangya Hospital of Central South University, Changsha, China
Key Laboratory of Diabetes Immunology, Ministry of Education, and Metabolic Syndrome Research Center, The Second Xiangya Hospital of Central South University, Changsha, China

Ningwen Tai, Lucy Zhang, Jian Peng, Youjia Hu and Li Wen
Section of Endocrinology, Department of Internal Medicine, School of Medicine, Yale University, New Haven, CT, United States

Chen Chao
National Clinical Research Center for Metabolic Diseases, Key Laboratory of Diabetes Immunology (Central South University), Ministry of Education, and Department of Metabolism and Endocrinology, The Second Xiangya Hospital, Central South University, Changsha, China

Qiyuan Tan
Section of Endocrinology, Department of Internal Medicine, School of Medicine, Yale University, New Haven, CT, United States
Department of Endocrinology and Metabolism, Shanghai Jiaotong University Affiliated Sixth People's Hospital, Shanghai, China

James Alexander Pearson
Section of Endocrinology, Department of Internal Medicine, School of Medicine, Yale University, New Haven, CT, United States
Division of Infection and Immunity, School of Medicine, Cardiff University, Cardiff, United Kingdom

F. Susan Wong
Division of Infection and Immunity, School of Medicine, Cardiff University, Cardiff, United Kingdom

Yangyang Li
Section of Endocrinology, Department of Internal Medicine, School of Medicine, Yale University, New Haven, CT, United States
Department of Endocrinology, The Second Hospital of Jilin University, Changchun, China

Yanpeng Xing and Luyao Zhang
Section of Endocrinology, Department of Internal Medicine, School of Medicine, Yale University, New Haven, CT, United States
Department of Gastrointestinal Surgery, The First Hospital of Jilin University, Changchun, China

Stephanie J. Hanna and Danijela Tatovic
Diabetes Research Group, Division of Infecti1on and Immunity, School of Medicine, Cardiff University, Cardiff, United Kingdom

Terri C. Thayer
Diabetes Research Group, Division of Infecti1on and Immunity, School of Medicine, Cardiff University, Cardiff, United Kingdom
Department of Biological and Chemical Science, School of Natural and Social Sciences, Roberts Wesleyan College, Rochester, NY, United States

Colin M. Dayan
Diabetes Research Group, Division of Infecti1on and Immunity, School of Medicine, Cardiff University, Cardiff, United Kingdom
Wellcome Centre for Human Genetics, University of Oxford, Oxford, United Kingdom

Ian Litchfield and Sheila Greenfield
Institute of Applied Health Research, University of Birmingham, Birmingham, United Kingdom

Rob C. Andrews
Medical School, University of Exeter, Exeter, United Kingdom
Taunton and Somerset NHS Foundation Trust, Musgrove Park Hospital, Taunton, United Kingdom

Parth Narendran
Institute of Immunology and Immunotherapy, University of Birmingham, Birmingham, United Kingdom
University Hospitals Birmingham NHS Foundation Trust, Queen Elizabeth Hospital, Birmingham, United Kingdom

Cathleen Petzold and Mangesh Jaykar
Molecular and Cellular Immunology/Immune Regulation, Center for Regenerative Therapies Dresden (CRTD), Center for Molecular and Cellular Bioengineering (CMCB), Technische Universität Dresden, Dresden, Germany

Deepika Watts, Marthe Janßen, Francesco Palmucci and Karsten Kretschmer
Molecular and Cellular Immunology/Immune Regulation, Center for Regenerative Therapies Dresden (CRTD), Center for Molecular and Cellular Bioengineering (CMCB), Technische Universität Dresden, Dresden, Germany
Paul Langerhans Institute Dresden (PLID) of the Helmholtz Zentrum München at the University Hospital and Medical Faculty Carl Gustav Carus of TU Dresden, Dresden, Germany
German Center for Diabetes Research (DZD e.V.), Neuherberg, Germany

Marc Weigelt and Angela Hommel
Regenerative Therapies for Diabetes, Center for Regenerative Therapies Dresden (CRTD), Center for Molecular and Cellular Bioengineering (CMCB), Technische Universität Dresden, Dresden, Germany

Ezio Bonifacio
Paul Langerhans Institute Dresden (PLID) of the Helmholtz Zentrum München at the University Hospital and Medical Faculty Carl Gustav Carus of TU Dresden, Dresden, Germany
German Center for Diabetes Research (DZD e.V.), Neuherberg, Germany
Regenerative Therapies for Diabetes, Center for Regenerative Therapies Dresden (CRTD), Center for Molecular and Cellular Bioengineering (CMCB), Technische Universität Dresden, Dresden, Germany

Tim Sparwasser
Institute of Infection Immunology, TWINCORE/ Centre for Experimental and Clinical Infection Research, Hanover, Germany

Pamela J. Lincez
Michael Smith Laboratories, The University of British Columbia, Vancouver, BC, Canada

Iryna Shanina and Marc S. Horwitz
Department of Microbiology & Immunology, Life Sciences Institute, The University of British Columbia, Vancouver, BC, Canada

Nicole K. Brockman
Augustana Faculty, University of Alberta, Camrose, AB, Canada

Jane E. Yardley
Augustana Faculty, University of Alberta, Camrose, AB, Canada
Physical Activity and Diabetes Laboratory, Alberta Diabetes Institute, Edmonton, AB, Canada
Faculty of Kinesiology, Sport and Recreation, University of Alberta, Edmonton, AB, Canada

Richard M. Bracken
Diabetes Research Unit and School of Sport and Exercise Science, Swansea University, Swansea, United Kingdom
Applied Sport, Technology, Exercise and Medicine Research Centre (A-STEM), College of Engineering, Swansea University, Swansea, United Kingdom
Diabetes Research Group, Medical School, Swansea University, Swansea, United Kingdom

Joanne Boldison
Institute of Biomedical & Clinical Science, University of Exeter, Exeter, United Kingdom

Richard B. Greaves, Dawei Chen and E. Allison Green
Centre for Experimental Medicine and Biomedicine, Hull York Medical School, University of York, York, United Kingdom

Jason Pitt
Applied Sport, Technology, Exercise and Medicine Research Centre (A-STEM), College of Engineering, Swansea University, Swansea, United Kingdom

Olivia McCarthy and Rachel Deere
Applied Sport, Technology, Exercise and Medicine Research Centre (A-STEM), College of Engineering, Swansea University, Swansea, United Kingdom
Diabetes Research Group, Medical School, Swansea University, Swansea, United Kingdom

Steve C. Bain
Diabetes Research Group, Medical School, Swansea University, Swansea, United Kingdom

Othmar Moser and Max L. Eckstein
Applied Sport, Technology, Exercise and Medicine Research Centre (A-STEM), College of Engineering, Swansea University, Swansea, United Kingdom
Cardiovascular Diabetology Research Group, Division of Endocrinology and Diabetology, Department of Internal Medicine, Medical University of Graz, Graz, Austria

Eliana Toren and Chad S. Hunter
Department of Medicine, Division of Endocrinology Diabetes and Metabolism, University of Alabama at Birmingham, Birmingham, AL, United States
Comprehensive Diabetes Center, University of Alabama at Birmingham, Birmingham, AL, United States

KaLia S. Burnette and Hubert M. Tse
Comprehensive Diabetes Center, University of Alabama at Birmingham, Birmingham, AL, United States
Department of Microbiology, University of Alabama at Birmingham, Birmingham, AL, United States

Ronadip R. Banerjee
Division of Endocrinology, Department of Medicine, Johns Hopkins University School of Medicine, Baltimore, MD, United States

Ivana Stojanović, Tamara Saksida, Đorđe Miljković and Nada Pejnovic
Department of Immunology, Institute for Biological Research “Sinisˇ a Stankovic´” – National Institute of the Republic of Serbia, University of Belgrade, Belgrade, Serbia

Adam Klocperk, Petra Vrabcova, Irena Zentsova, Anna Sediva and Zuzana Parackova
Department of Immunology, 2nd Faculty of Medicine Charles University, University Hospital in Motol, Prague, Czechia

Jana Vcelakova, Lenka Petruzelkova, Zdenek Sumnik and Stepanka Pruhova
Department of Pediatrics, 2nd Faculty of Medicine, Charles University and Motol University Hospital, Prague, Czechia

Sémah Tagougui
Institut de Recherches Cliniques de Montréal, Montreal, QC, Canada
Département de Nutrition, Faculté de Médicine, Université de Montréal, Montreal, QC, Canada

Nadine Taleb
Institut de Recherches Cliniques de Montréal, Montreal, QC, Canada
Département des Sciences Biomédicales, Faculté de Médicine, Université de Montréal, Montreal, QC, Canada

Rémi Rabasa-Lhoret
Institut de Recherches Cliniques de Montréal, Montreal, QC, Canada
Département de Nutrition, Faculté de Médicine, Université de Montréal, Montreal, QC, Canada
Département des Sciences Biomédicales, Faculté de Médicine, Université de Montréal, Montreal, QC, Canada
Division of Endocrinology, McGill University, Montreal, QC, Canada
Endocrinology Division, Montreal Diabetes Research Center, Montreal, QC, Canada

Maki Nakayama
Barbara Davis Center for Childhood Diabetes, University of Colorado School of Medicine, Aurora, CO, United States
Department of Pediatrics, University of Colorado School of Medicine, Aurora, CO, United States
Department of Immunology and Microbiology, University of Colorado School of Medicine, Aurora, CO, United States

Aaron W. Michels
Barbara Davis Center for Childhood Diabetes, University of Colorado School of Medicine, Aurora, CO, United States
Department of Pediatrics, University of Colorado School of Medicine, Aurora, CO, United States
Department of Immunology and Microbiology, University of Colorado School of Medicine, Aurora, CO, United States
Department of Medicine, University of Colorado School of Medicine, Aurora, CO, United States

Claudia Selck, Chun-Ting J. Kwong and Evan G. Pappas
St. Vincent's Institute, Fitzroy, VIC, Australia

Gaurang Jhala, Helen E. Thomas, Thomas W.H. Kay and Balasubramanian Krishnamurthy
St. Vincent's Institute, Fitzroy, VIC, Australia
Department of Medicine, The University of Melbourne, St Vincent's Hospital, Fitzroy, VIC, Australia

Jonathan Chee
National Centre for Asbestos Related Diseases, Institute of Respiratory Health, University of Western Australia, Perth, WA, Australia
School of Biomedical Sciences, University of Western Australia, Perth, WA, Australia

Qin Zeng, Jianfeng Song, Dandan Wang, Xiaoxiao Sun, Yalun Xiao, Haowei Zhang and Yang Xiao
National Clinical Research Center for Metabolic Diseases, and Department of Metabolism and Endocrinology, The Second Xiangya Hospital of Central South University, Changsha, China
Key Laboratory of Diabetes Immunology, Ministry of Education, and Metabolic Syndrome Research Center, The Second Xiangya Hospital of Central South University, Changsha, China

Tuo Deng
National Clinical Research Center for Metabolic Diseases, and Department of Metabolism and Endocrinology, The Second Xiangya Hospital of Central South University, Changsha, China
Key Laboratory of Diabetes Immunology, Ministry of Education, and Metabolic Syndrome Research Center, The Second Xiangya Hospital of Central South University, Changsha, China
Clinical Immunology Center, The Second Xiangya Hospital of Central South University, Changsha, China

Claudia Vetrani, Lutgarda Bozzetto, Giuseppe Della Pepa, Angela Albarosa Rivellese and Giovanni Annuzzi
Department of Clinical Medicine and Surgery, Federico II University, Naples, Italy

Arata Itoh, Lorenzo Ortiz, Kritika Kachapati, Yuehong Wu, David Adams, Kyle Bednar and William M. Ridgway
Division of Immunology, Allergy and Rheumatology, University of Cincinnati College of Medicine, Cincinnati, OH, United States

Shibabrata Mukherjee and Claire Chougnet
Division of Immunobiology, Cincinnati Children's Hospital Medical Center, Cincinnati, OH, United States

Robert S. Mittler
Department of Surgery, Emory University, Atlanta, GA, United States
Emory Vaccine Center, Atlanta, GA, United States

Yi-Guang Chen
Department of Pediatrics, Medical College of Wisconsin, Milwaukee, WI, United States

Laurence Dolan
Division of Endocrinology, Cincinnati Children's Hospital Medical Center, Cincinnati, OH, United States

Matthias G. von Herrath and Jose Luis Vela
Novo Nordisk Research Center, Seattle, WA, USA

Minh N. Pham
Novo Nordisk Research Center, Seattle, WA, USA
Pacific Northwest Diabetes Research Institute, Seattle, WA, USA

Volker Burkart
Institute for Clinical Diabetology, German Diabetes Center, Leibniz Center for Diabetes Research at Heinrich Heine University, Düsseldorf, Germany
German Center for Diabetes Research (DZD), München-Neuherberg, Germany

Oana P. Zaharia and Michael Roden
Institute for Clinical Diabetology, German Diabetes Center, Leibniz Center for Diabetes Research at Heinrich Heine University, Düsseldorf, Germany
German Center for Diabetes Research (DZD), München-Neuherberg, Germany
Department of Endocrinology and Diabetology, Medical Faculty, Heinrich Heine University, Düsseldorf, Germany

Stefanie Lanzinger and Reinhard W. Holl
German Center for Diabetes Research (DZD), München-Neuherberg, Germany
Institute of Epidemiology and Medical Biometry, Zentralinstitut für Biomedizinische Technik (ZIBMT), University of Ulm, Ulm, Germany

Joachim Rosenbauer
German Center for Diabetes Research (DZD), München-Neuherberg, Germany
Institute for Biometrics and Epidemiology, German Diabetes Center, Leibniz Center for Diabetes Research at Heinrich Heine University, Düsseldorf, Germany

Wolfram Karges
Division of Endocrinology and Diabetes, Rheinisch-Westfälische Technische Hochschule (RWTH) Aachen University, Aachen, Germany

Karsten Müssig
Institute for Clinical Diabetology, German Diabetes Center, Leibniz Center for Diabetes Research at Heinrich Heine University, Düsseldorf, Germany
Department of Internal Medicine/Gastroenterology, Franziskus-Hospital Harderberg, Georgsmarienhütte, Germany

Sebastian M. Meyhöfer
German Center for Diabetes Research (DZD), München-Neuherberg, Germany
Institute for Endocrinology and Diabetes, University of Lübeck, Rosenheim, Lübeck, Germany

Michael Hummel
Diabetes Center Rosenheim, Rosenheim, Germany

Dirk Raddatz
Division of Gastroenterology and Gastrointestinal Oncology and Endocrinology, University Medical Center Göttingen, Göttingen, Germany

Julia Szendroedi
Institute for Clinical Diabetology, German Diabetes Center, Leibniz Center for Diabetes Research at Heinrich Heine University, Düsseldorf, Germany
German Center for Diabetes Research (DZD), München-Neuherberg, Germany
Department of Internal Medicine I and Clinical Chemistry, University Hospital Heidelberg, Heidelberg, Ger-many

Index

www.ingramcontent.com/pod-product-compliance
Lightning Source LLC
LaVergne TN
LVHW082158200926
848484LV00008B/2178
9798887402512